N

Studies on Excitation and Inhibition in the Retina

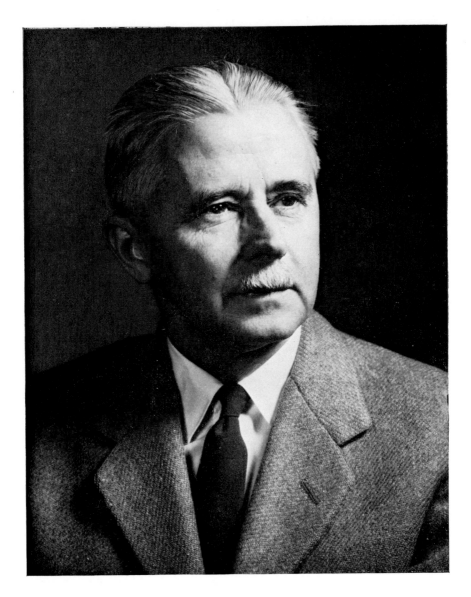

Studies on Excitation and Inhibition in the Retina

A collection of papers from the laboratories of

H. KEFFER HARTLINE

Edited by FLOYD RATLIFF
The Rockefeller University, New York

NEW YORK *The Rockefeller University Press*

First published in the U.S.A. 1974
by The Rockefeller University Press, New York

© *1974 Floyd Ratliff and H. K. Hartline*

Printed in Great Britain by
Fletcher & Son Ltd, Norwich

ISBN 0–87470–019–1
Library of Congress Catalog Card Number 73–89539

To
E. D. Adrian
and
D. W. Bronk

Contents

Preface

For nearly half a century, H. Keffer Hartline has conducted research on vision and the retina. His researches have extended into many and diverse branches of the field, and he has studied the retinas of various representatives of each of the three major phyla having well developed eyes – the arthropods, the vertebrates, and the mollusks. These comparative studies have elucidated numerous fundamental principles of retinal physiology which, over the years, have provided the foundation for many advances in the neurophysiology of vision. This collection of papers from his laboratory begins with one published early in his career when he and Clarence H. Graham first recorded the electrical activity of single optic nerve fibers and thereby initiated the quantitative unitary analysis of the roles played by excitation and inhibition in the integrative action of the retina. Ending with his recently published Nobel Lecture on the unitary analysis of retinal mechanisms of vision, the collection thus spans the entire history of this major branch of visual physiology.

Following an historical foreword by Professor Hartline, the papers are arranged, more or less in chronological order, in five parts. The first three parts are on the activity of single optic nerve fibers in: (i) the compound lateral eye of the horseshoe crab, *Limulus*, (ii) the retinas of various cold-blooded vertebrates, and (iii) the double retina of the eye of the scallop. The last two parts are on the inhibitory interaction in the lateral eye of *Limulus*: (iv) the steady state, and (v) the dynamics. Prefacing each part are a few introductory remarks on some significant aspects of the work in that area, with special reference to related contributions by other investigators.

These papers were assembled for publication as a collection to honor Professor Hartline on the occasion of his seventieth birthday, 22 December 1973. At his request, a few additional papers from his laboratory – but of which he is not a co-author – have been included in the collection in order to present a fuller account of some recent developments in the work.

ACKNOWLEDGEMENTS

Permission by the authors and publishers concerned to republish the several papers collected here is gratefully acknowledged. The date, place, and authorship of the original publication of each paper are given in full on its title-page.

I am most grateful to Mrs. Maria Lipski for her assistance in all phases of the editing of this collection. Special thanks are due to Miss Teresa Colaço, who prepared the name and subject indexes, and to Miss Marie Azzarello, who typed the Preface, Foreword, and Introductions.

FLOYD RATLIFF
The Rockfeller University
New York

Foreword

by HALDAN KEFFER HARTLINE

Surely every scientist feels that the time at which he began his career was an especially exciting era. To me, the late 1920s still seem to have been especially exciting for neurophysiology. This is perhaps more than personal bias; the vacuum tube amplifier was just being established as a research tool in the study of nervous systems, and it did revolutionize the field. In particular, in Adrian's laboratory it made possible the first studies of unitary neural action (Adrian and Zottermann, Adrian and Bronk) and today, unitary analysis occupies a central position in neurophysiology.

I was fortunate in entering my research career at just this time. I had had some experience, during my medical student years at Johns Hopkins, in retinal electrophysiology, monopolizing Professor C. D. Snyder's string galvanometer. I had been the first to record the form of the retinal action potential in human subjects, describing both its fast and slow components. Retinal action potentials of arthropods, especially insects, interested me: their fast transients had to be recorded faithfully in quantitative studies. I consequently appreciated the great advantages to be gained from a sensitive amplifier with high input impedance, driving a fast oscillograph. In the lively spirited Johnson Foundation, then but recently established under the inspiring directorship of Detlev W. Bronk, I built an amplifier which appalled the experts who looked inside it ('Jesus!' said John Hervey), but which worked. It was direct-coupled – following the lead of E. L. Chaffee, and for the same reasons – the need to record the relatively slow and long lasting components of the retinal action potential, as well as the fast transients at 'on' and 'off'.

Of the various arthropods I had studied, one, the arachnoid *Limulus polyphemus*, had held my interest since childhood. My father, a teacher of biology, called it 'King Crab', though, as he knew, it is not a true crab. Its domed carapace resembles a horse's hoof, hence the more common names 'horse foot' and 'horse-shoe "crab" '. Its sword-like tail (used by Indians for fishing spears, it is said) gives the name *Xiphosura* to the order. Through its lateral eyes, *Limulus* looks askance. These eyes are slight bulges on the carapace; they are compound, with facets large enough to be seen without a magnifier. The corneas are clear in young animals that molt frequently, and in adults caught in deep water. The optic nerves are long – they must cross almost half the breadth of the carapace to reach the optic lobes of the brain, and adult 'crabs' sometimes exceed half a meter in breadth. *Limulus* has a pair of small median ocelli which are closely set, but which are nothing to warrant the species' name 'polyphemus' – *Limulus* is no one-eyed giant.

My first work with *Limulus* was a repetition of Northrup and Loeb's amusing trick of tethering a 'baby' (4–6 cm broad) by its tail in the corner of an aquarium, and illuminating it by two lights shining at right angles through the aquarium corner walls. The angle which the tethered creature (selected for its negative phototaxis) took as it attempted to swim away from the lights varied, of course, with the intensities of the two lights. I was pleased to show, crudely, that the angle was independent of the absolute intensities, depending only on their ratios (Weber's 'law'). I also, soon afterwards, recorded the retinal action potential of the *Limulus* lateral eye, again from the small intact animals – a very simple monophasic transient at onset of light, with but a slight elevation during steady illumination. The direction of change made the cornea relatively more negative with respect to an indifferent electrode on the animal's body: this was in agreement with the findings in other invertebrates – insects, crayfish, cephalopods – all with 'direct' retinas in which the free ends of the retinal receptors point towards the cornea. To the early retinal electrophysiologists negativity of the sensory surface suggested a depolarization of the photoreceptors, with local currents in the right direction to excite the optic nerve fibers, a view that was ahead of its time, and not far from the mark for invertebrates, as we understand today. With this in mind, indeed, I tried to record electrical activity in the *Limulus* optic nerve, and succeeded to an extent limited by the slowness of the Einthoven galvanometer which had been made sensitive by a slack string. (For this work Professor Walter Garrey, with trepidation, allowed me to use his galvanometer at Woods Hole – I was a brash student, but expert at replacing broken strings, and he need not have worried.) The optic nerves of baby *Limulus* gave small but quite definite deflections on illumination of the eye, too small to be of much use, but significant nevertheless.

It was with this background that I built my amplifier, determined to do better with the optic nerve, and to investigate the relation between optic nerve activity and retinal action potential. Clarence Graham and I went to Woods Hole in the summer of 1931. With the amplifier driving a Matthews oscillograph there was now no trouble in recording the vigorous massed discharge of impulses in the optic nerve of small *Limulus*. We observed a strong transient outburst at the onset of light, steady activity during steady illumination, and no 'off' response – a simpler picture than the exciting records of massed activity that Adrian and Matthews had recently obtained from the eel's optic nerve. Fortunately, our interest in the retinal action potential waned, as we became intrigued by the idea of dissecting and recording from individual fibers – as Adrian and Bronk had done with the phrenic nerve of the rabbit. We could fray out the *Limulus* optic nerve readily enough, but the finest bundles from the young animals gave a jumble of spikes with only occasionally an exasperating promise of identifiable single-unit activity. On the next to the last day of our summer's stay at Woods Hole we had used all of the babies in our tank – only two adults remained – large, tough shelled, with dull, abraded eyes – miserable specimens compared to the fresh, beautiful, clear-eyed young ones, with their clean optic nerves. But the optic nerves of these adults could be dissected with ease, and promptly yielded records of beautifully regular trains of large impulses, rising from a smooth baseline. We had at last obtained the first records of the activity of a single optic nerve fiber. In *Limulus*, we had made a fortunate choice of material.

Exploration of the unitary photoreceptor activity was rewarding at every step. Many properties of the single receptor turned out to be old friends from classical visual physiology; many invited comparison with human psychophysics. One was the simple, approximately logarithmic relation between intensity of the light stimulus and response of the receptor as measured by the frequency of impulse discharge in its optic nerve fiber. Another was the marked sensory adaptation of the receptor following the strong initial transient in response to sudden onset of light – even if only a small increment. Reciprocity between intensity and duration of short flashes of light, familiar in the broad area of photobiology, could be investigated with precision in the *Limulus* single receptor. Graham and I exploited our technique to obtain 'action spectra' of single visual receptor units. Our data have stood the test of time well, for several decades later Hubbard and Wald could place our points with gratifying agreement on their curve of the absorption spectrum of the rhodopsin they extracted from the *Limulus* lateral eye. With Robb McDonald, I studied light and dark adaptation of the single units, and was astonished at how familiar our curves looked, and it was the same in preliminary studies on flicker, with Lorrin Riggs. More broadly, similarities and differences between the properties of the photoreceptor of *Limulus* and those of other receptors that were being enthusiastically explored by other workers in other laboratories at this same time lent great zest to these early studies.

For all the satisfaction to be had in exploring the properties of the

Limulus photoreceptor units, the lure of the vertebrate retina was not to be denied. But the vertebrate optic nerve presents a very different technical problem from that encountered in other nerves. Opening the sheath of the fresh optic nerve from a frog's eye reveals a pasty interior that defies any attempt to lift strands of fibers on to electrodes. But inside the eye, thinly spread over the vitreous surface of the retina, the layer of optic nerve fibers provides a natural dissection. Thin bundles of fibers can be coaxed up on to a cotton wick, and split with fine needles and scissors until only one fiber remains active. Successes were exasperatingly few, but they were welcome at that time, before Granit and his colleagues had developed their microelectrode for retinal recording. The rewards were exciting surprises. The fibers of this outlying brain tract that is the vertebrate optic 'nerve' exhibit a rich diversity of responses – a diversity that even today has not been completely explored. I catalogued the varieties of response patterns in three general classes – 'on', 'on-off', and 'off' – although I emphasized the existence of intermediate types. Now it is evident that there are many types that I did not see in these first exploratory studies. The quantitative studies of retinal ganglion cell physiology which were begun at that time are only now being taken up to the extent they merit. I worked principally with the frog retina. A cursory survey of other cold-blooded vertebrates suggested similar response patterns, but of course the varied mechanisms that a thorough comparative study can reveal remained untouched and even today are largely neglected, except for the rich returns yielded by numerous studies of the fish retina. The avian and mammalian retinas were beyond my dissection technique.

Retinal ganglion cells responding only to a decrease in illumination – the 'off' elements – intrigued me greatly (they still do!). I was reminded of an earlier interest in the 'shadow reactions' of many invertebrates. Indeed, I had made a minor study of the shadow response of the scallop, *Pecten*, in an effort to complement Hecht's studies of the light responses of the clam *Mya* – studies which had greatly influenced my interest in visual mechanisms. The well known double retina in the beautiful, gem-like blue eyes of *Pecten* turned out to be comprised of 'on' receptors in the proximal retina – responding to light much as do the visual receptors of *Limulus* – and 'off' receptors in the distal retina having properties almost indistinguishable from those of the 'off' elements of the frog or, for another example, the alligator retina.

To find a primary visual receptor responding to diminution of light was a surprise. It also posed a puzzle, for it was my opinion that the 'off' responses of the vertebrates are generated by neural mechanisms in the retina, rather than by primary receptors. Neural mechanisms do operate to generate 'off' responses in the optic ganglion of *Limulus*, as Wilska and I showed in a brief study, recently confirmed and extended by Snodderly, yet the input to that ganglion over the optic nerve is the conventional type of sensory 'on' activity. The recent findings from Tomita's laboratory, that cones and rods of the carp retina hyperpolarize in response to illumination adds renewed interest to the 'shadow receptors' of the *Pecten* eye – which in fact have also been shown, by Toyoda and Shapley, to hyperpolarize in response to light.

Two developments kept the *Limulus* eye in the foreground of interest. The first concerned the analysis of receptor mechanisms. A razor section of the eye, perpendicular to the cornea, exposes the sensory structures; individual ommatidia can be isolated by dissection. But more importantly, they are thus made accessible to penetration by fine glass micropipette electrodes. The development of these electrodes by Gerard and his colleagues was a major advance in neurophysiological technique. Henry Wagner, E. F. MacNichol and I, with others in our laboratory, were soon fully occupied by our intracellular recordings from the *Limulus* ommatidium. Others, too, have made use of this preparation, notably Tomita and his associates, and Fuortes and his.

The *Limulus* ommatidium is less simple than I first thought. It contains ten or more 'retinular cells' which bear the light-sensitive rhabdom and which are clustered about the dendritic process of what is presumably a second-order neuron, the 'eccentric cell'. It is the axon of this cell that carries the trains of nerve impulses that are generated by electrical depolarization of the sensory structure. In spite of the uncertainty that still exists concerning the exact functions of these two kinds of cells, intracellular recording contributes to the understanding of processes that intervene between the primary action of light and the initiation of trains of impulses in the optic nerve. Of special interest, in recent years, are the minute 'quantum bumps' (discovered by Steve Yeandle and studied later by Alan Adolph) which appear to superimpose to yield the generator potential.

The second development in our studies of the *Limulus* eye turned my attention away from receptor mechanisms. It began with the casual observation, in the late 1930s, that ambient illumination in the room often diminished the activity in an optic nerve fiber that was being prepared for study. I have no idea how often I had noticed this unthinkingly, without grasping its perversity. Once alert, I could easily show that shading the regions of the eye neighboring the receptor whose nerve fiber I had isolated restored its activity. Ommatidia in the lateral eye of *Limulus* inhibit one another. I should have paid attention to Grenacher's early description of the plexus of nerve fibers behind the layer of ommatidia, revealed by his methylene blue preparations. This retina of *Limulus* is derived from the branching of retinular and eccentric cell axons. It is very much simpler than the vertebrate retina or the optic ganglia in higher arthropods. It is devoid of ganglion cells, but has numerous clumps of neuropile, rich in synaptic regions, as W. H. Miller showed several years ago – a finding beautifully confirmed and extended in a recent study from Purple's laboratory.

A comparatively simple retina, exhibiting a purely inhibitory interaction provided an opportunity too good to be ignored, and the last two decades have been given over, increasingly, to exploiting this fortunate preparation. Floyd Ratliff, when he first came to work with me in 1950 with his interest fixed on the frog retina was immediately captivated by *Limulus*. Many others in our laboratory, and outside it, have been drawn to the study of the interactions in this primitive retina, which are just complicated enough to be interesting, yet seemingly simple enough to lead one to believe that they may eventually be understood.

Our attempts to analyze quantitatively the inhibitory interactions in the *Limulus* retina at first yielded puzzling and seemingly inconsistent results. These difficulties were resolved only after we realized that lateral inhibition acts mutually and in a 'recurrent' mode. That is, inhibition exerted by any ommatidium on its neighbors depends on its net activity, reduced as it may be by inhibition exerted on it by those very neighbors which it inhibits. To describe the responses of a set of interacting receptor units, a set of simultaneous equations must be written, each expressing the excitatory influence acting on the particular ommatidium to which that equation refers, diminished by terms expressing the combined inhibitory influences resulting from the responses of the neighboring ommatidia. Although strongly non-linear overall, these equations, mercifully, are piecewise linear to a good approximation. A number of years have been spent, in our laboratory, working out these quantitative relations, and exploring the role that inhibitory interaction plays in brightness contrast and, specifically, in the accentuation of edges, contours, and steep gradients of intensity in the retinal image.

Detailed analysis of the cellular mechanism provides an insight into the unitary events that are essential to the understanding of retinal interaction. Fuortes's experiments, and Rushton's analysis, followed by Richard Purple and Fred Dodge's work, established the relations between generator potential in the *Limulus* ommatidium and the membrane conductance change initiated by excitation of the receptor by light.

Purple and Dodge added the analysis of the lateral inhibitory synaptic potentials and their associated conductance changes. To this they made a further addition, demonstrating an inhibitory process associated with the discharge of each of the receptor's own nerve impulses. 'Self-inhibition' first appeared as a theoretical possibility in the formal analysis of steady-state interaction: completeness suggested the inclusion of non-zero diagonal terms in the matrix of inhibitory coefficients that is used to express the interaction of a set of receptor units. Charles Stevens, analyzing the transients in the train of impulses elicited by artificial injection of electric current into a *Limulus* eccentric cell, subsequently produced convincing evidence of the reality of a self-inhibitory process – quieting my own anguished protests that no neuron in its right mind would inhibit itself. Dodge and Purple's later experiments provided welcome direct evidence of the cellular basis for this process, which plays an essential role in the dynamics of receptor activity and retinal interaction.

These unitary cellular processes that underlie the interplay of excitation and inhibition in the *Limulus* retina are interesting in their own right, and fundamental to understanding, but they must also be considered in the context of their organized dynamic interrelationships. Direct studies of action of the system as a whole guide the development of this understanding. In recent years linear systems analysis, with the powerful Fourier methods that are used in it made practical by computer techniques, has been fruitful in our laboratory. The *Limulus* retina is especially favorable for this kind of analysis, for linearity applies in the *Limulus* eye over larger ranges of action than one would have dared to hope. Dodge and Bruce Knight, and with them for two years Jun-ichi Toyoda, have analyzed the excitatory and inhibitory processes by using light sinusoidally modulated about a mean ambient value; by electric current sinusoidally modulated, injected into the eccentric cell, and by trains of antidromic volleys – Tomita's technique – with similarly modulated repetition rates to activate the lateral inhibitory mechanisms. From the understanding thus gained, synthesis then provides substantial insights into the dynamics of the receptors and their interactions. To this is to be added the very latest studies of spatial transfer functions by Ratliff, Knight, and Norma Graham, based on Robert Barlow's painstaking, unit by unit, mapping of the field of inhibitory influences about a small group of receptors. Thus both the temporal and the spatial aspects of retinal integration in the eye of *Limulus* are being brought under study.

We are encouraged to believe that we have made good progress towards our goal of understanding the *Limulus* retina as an integrative system which processes the raw data of the retinal image preparatory to transmitting it, as useful visual information, to the higher centers in the animal's brain. We are also encouraged to believe that our recent work, for all of its being a single-minded study of the eye of an archaic animal, has yielded certain broad principles of visual physiology and indeed of neural integrative function in general.

If there is any merit in republishing a collection of papers extending back over forty years, it lies in exhibiting a short segment of a thread of work that is now woven almost unrecognizably into the fabric of visual science. This thread is spun of many strands, whose origins are easily traced to the beginnings of modern science – the optics of Kepler, the 'animal electricity' of Galvani. The influence of Helmholtz, of course, and of Mach is clear. Adrian's influence is fundamental to this entire study, and Adrian and Bronk's technique and their inspiration and example invited its development. Sherringtonian concepts pervade its later phases basically, spurred by Granit's interpretations. The early retinal electrophysiologists contributed much, but it would be hard to sort out specific influences. And it is almost as hard to recognize the ideas contributed by one's contemporaries, interacting with one's own. Origins of ideas soon become obscured, just as the ideas developed in these papers will inevitably share the anonymity that soon graces most of the contributions of individual workers as patterns in the fabric of understanding emerge.

Part One

Neural Activity Generated by Single Photoreceptor Units in the Eye of *Limulus*

INTRODUCTION by F. Ratliff

> '*By the methods of comparative physiology, or of experimental biology, by the choice of a suitable organ, tissue or process, in some animal far removed in evolution, we may often throw light upon some function or process in the higher animals, or in man.*'
>
> A. V. Hill, *The Lancet*, 1929.

The prophetic remark above by the noted biophysicist A. V. Hill is an almost perfect characterization of research that was to follow, within a few years, on the compound lateral eye of the horseshoe 'crab', *Limulus*. This ancient marine arthropod (which is not a crab at all, but rather is a not too distant relative of the desert scorpion) has changed little over the past 200 million years or so, according to fossil evidence. It is undoubtedly 'far removed in evolution' from man – even according to the views of Patten (1912), who claimed that *Limulus* was the ancestor of the vertebrates. However distant the kinship and whatever may be the lines of descent, many fundamental processes in the retina of the compound lateral eye of *Limulus* do none the less resemble certain aspects of vision in higher animals, including man. Indeed, for many years the results of electrophysiological experiments on the *Limulus* eye seemed to parallel human vision more closely than did some of the early experiments on the vertebrate retina itself (cf. Ratliff, 1962). But this was only because the *Limulus* eye was such a favorable preparation for the study of certain basic processes that all photoreceptors and nervous systems share in common – processes which, at that time, could not be observed directly in the vertebrate retina and had to be inferred from psychophysical experiments. The resemblance to human vision of some of these basic processes in the visual system of our distant relative, *Limulus*, is the main subject of these introductory remarks.

The Weber-Fechner Law. The first of the several parallels between retinal physiology and visual experience to be demonstrated in Hartline's work was that of the near linear relation between the logarithm of the intensity of illumination and the steady-state frequency of discharge of impulses in the *Limulus* photoreceptor and the similar logarithmic relation between intensity and brightness in human vision known as the Weber-Fechner Law. Thus, as in our own eyes, constant relations in a pattern of light and shade – whatever the absolute levels – produce more or less constant visual effects; we do not enter a new and vastly different visual world every time a cloud passes in front of the sun.

Another important consequence of this logarithmic compression from light intensity to impulses is that it enables the single photoreceptor to respond over enormous ranges from 1 to 10^6 or more – even without the aid of the changes in sensitivity that result from prolonged adaptation to light or to darkness. Complete dark adaptation of the eye, in the intact animal, extends the range to about 10^{10} (Barlow and Kaplan, 1971). The range over which the human eye operates is very similar; from noonday sun to faintest visible star is about 10^{14}. It is clear that in *Limulus* this compression occurs in the early stages of the transduction from photochemical to neuro-electric events, and recent intracellular records of the electrical activity of vertebrate rods and cones reveal in them a similar compression, partly linear, partly logarithmic (see Tomita, 1968 and 1970). Exactly how this receptor activity is transmitted across the whole of the more complex vertebrate retina and eventually is converted to nerve impulses in the axons of the retinal ganglion cells, however, is only beginning to be understood (see, for example, Werblin and Dowling, 1969, and Kaneko, 1971).

Spectral Sensitivity. The 'visibility curve' for the single photoreceptor unit of the *Limulus* eye and the luminosity curve for rod vision in the human eye (in each case, the reciprocal of the intensity to elicit a specified response at various wavelengths) are strikingly similar. There is good reason for this – both are basically measures of the absorption spectrum of the photopigments involved. And what matters, in such experiments, is how much light the pigment absorbs. In so far as the pigments are the same, so will the results be the same – even though the dependent variable in the one case is impulses discharged in the optic nerve, and in the other the threshold of visibility of a small spot of light.

The similarity of the photopigments in the eyes of such distant relatives as man and *Limulus* has proven to be most remarkable. The human rod pigment, of course, is a rhodopsin, and – as was demonstrated not long ago by Hubbard and Wald (1960) – so is the pigment of the *Limulus* photoreceptor. Furthermore, the absorption spectrum of this pigment that they extracted from the *Limulus* eye, and which they identified as a retinene$_1$ rhodopsin, parallels almost exactly the electrophysiological measurements made some thirty years earlier by Graham and Hartline. It is evident that many aspects of optic nerve activity are direct manifestations of the physico-chemical properties of the individual receptor cells.

The Bunsen-Roscoe Law. In photography (and in photochemistry in general) the total effect produced by light depends very little upon when it is absorbed. Indeed, duration of exposure and aperture of lens opening can simply be interchanged – one for the other – over very wide ranges, and still produce a constant photographic effect. This interchangeability of shutter speed and aperture stop is a specific example of the more general reciprocity law of Bunsen and Roscoe which states that the photochemical effect of a flash of light depends only upon its energy (intensity × duration).

Similar effects, below certain critical times, have long been known to occur in human vision and were demonstrated also in some very early studies of the electroretinograms of lower animals (cf. de Haas, 1903 and Hartline, 1928). It was not until 1934, however, that Hartline finally succeeded in demonstrating the reciprocal relation between intensity and duration in the stimulation of the single photoreceptor unit in the compound eye of *Limulus*. The parallels between these latter results and the results of similar experiments on human vision subsequently carried out by Graham and Margaria (1935) and by Long (1951) are striking. As in the studies on spectral sensitivity mentioned above, all the experiments were so designed that primary photochemical reactions were the principal controlling factors. In so far as these basic reactions are similar in the human eye and in the *Limulus* eye; the results of the experiments must be similar, too.

Light and Dark Adaptation. The loss of sensitivity by a single photoreceptor unit of the *Limulus* eye, following exposure to light, the time in the dark required to regain full sensitivity, and the effects of the intensity and duration of the previous exposure on the time course of these changes, resemble in considerable detail the familiar phenomena of light and dark adaptation in our own eyes (cf. Hecht, Haig, and Chase, 1937). The demonstration of these phenomena in isolated receptor units, by Hartline and McDonald, was taken as strong presumptive evidence that the underlying mechanisms reside in the receptors themselves. Indeed, their studies were based upon and seemed, in turn, to support strongly the quantitative photochemical interpretation of light and dark adaptation formulated by Hecht (1937).

Although Hecht's formulation was then widely accepted, an alternative suggestion that there might be a 'neural' component in the processes of light and dark adaptation had already been made by Granit, Holmberg, and Zewi (1938). Hartline and McDonald's finding that different features of the neural response (e.g. number and temporal pattern of impulses) are affected differently by adaptation offered potential methods for isolating the photochemical and neural mechanisms. But these effects, and the effects of adaptation on minute variations in the generator potential discussed below, have not been exploited fully, and the mechanisms of light and dark adaptation in the lateral eye of *Limulus* (and in the vertebrate retina, also) are by no means fully understood as yet.

Uncertainty of Response at Threshold. In 1942, Hecht, Shlaer, and Pirenne carried out a study on the fluctuations in sensitivity, at threshold, in the human eye. This uncertainty of response they attributed to statistical fluctuations in the number of quanta absorbed from the supposedly constant test flash. As their experiments (and many others) have shown, the minimum amount of light energy necessary for vision is extremely small. At the absolute threshold, the quantal nature of light itself seems to set the lower limit; only one quantum per receptor being required. Although more than one receptor must be stimulated at the same time to reach the threshold of vision, the total number of quanta required on the average is still so small that fluctuations about this mean may therefore be expected to have a profound influence on the visual response. The uncertainty of response at threshold in the *Limulus* photoreceptor unit is remarkably similar to that observed by Hecht, Schlaer, and Pirenne in the human eye and has been interpreted in much the same way.

As an eye becomes light-adapted more and more quanta are required, on the average, to reach threshold. In the end, several hundred times as many quanta may be needed. There is also a concomitant narrowing of the range of uncertainty of the response. This decrease in uncertainty with light adaptation, first observed in the *Limulus* photoreceptor unit, is similar to the analogous effects subsequently reported for the human eye by Mueller and Wilcox (1954). Unfortunately, these latter investigations were originally reported only in brief abstracts. Some of the work on *Limulus* has since been published in more detail, however, in the revised edition of Pirenne's book on *Vision and the Eye* (1967).

The Generator Potential and Flicker Fusion Phenomena. The changes in electrical potential across the whole retina (the retinal action potential) that result from changes in the light incident on the retina have always been regarded as a manifestation – in part at least – of primary photochemical processes. The equally natural assumption that this potential, or some component of it, somehow generates the impulses in the optic nerve which ultimately give rise to vision stimulated

Hartline's early interest in the retinal action potential. Indeed, one of the aims of his researches on the human electroretinogram in 1925 was to devise a method for the simultaneous observation, in one and the same subject, of the objective retinal action potential and the corresponding subjective visual experience. But it was not until ten years later that he managed to isolate, by dissection, a single photoreceptor unit of the *Limulus* eye and thus to record the 'action current' of a single sensory unit in response to light and to observe its relation to the discharge of nerve impulses. This was the realization, at last, of the unitary 'generator potential' which other investigators (notably Granit) had long assumed to be manifested externally, in composite form, as the retinal action potential.

The later development by Graham and Gerard (1946) and Ling and Gerard (1949) of micropipette electrodes with tips small enough to penetrate cells without seriously damaging them provided methods for more direct and more meaningful observations of many of the electrical signs of the mechanisms underlying all of the various processes described above. For example, Hartline, Wagner, and MacNichol were thus enabled to record the actual depolarization of photoreceptor cells and to find the direct relation of this depolarization to the discharge of nerve impulses. In brief, it now appears that the magnitude of the potential across the cell membrane at or near the site of impulse generation determines the frequency of impulses. For a review, see Dodge (1969).

The minute irregular fluctuations that Yeandle (1957) first observed in the generator potential may represent still more basic electrochemical processes that sum to yield it. Whatever affects these fluctuations can therefore be expected to affect the generator potential and, ultimately, the discharge of impulses. As Fuortes and Yeandle (1964) and Adolph (1964) showed, the amplitudes of these minute variations vary markedly with the state of light and dark adaptation. The intervals between impulses discharged were later shown by Ratliff, Hartline and Lange to vary similarly, suggesting a close correlation between the two, which has since been demonstrated more directly (Shapley, 1969, 1971a, and 1971b). Using techniques of linear system analysis, Dodge, Knight, and Toyoda have shown that the durations and amplitudes of the minute fluctuations, and conditions which affect them, appear to determine the frequency characteristics of the generator potential (tested with sinusoidally modulated stimuli). These transfer functions show a very close qualitative correspondence with the analogous flicker responses of other visual systems, including that of the human (see de Lange,

1958). The similar results of these similar experiments on the *Limulus* retina and on the human eye indicate once again that similar basic mechanisms may be involved in both.

The Central Ganglion and Behavior. How the central nervous system of *Limulus* further processes the visual information transmitted to it by the optic nerve and how this information eventually influences the animal's behavior has only begun to be explored. The inaccessibility of the *Limulus* central ganglion (it surrounds the oesophagus almost exactly in the center of the body) has forestalled much work on the projections of the retina to the central nervous system. Wilska and Hartline (1941) and Oomura and Kuriyama (1953) have recorded from ganglion cells in the brain of *Limulus*, however, and shown that responses there have considerable similarity to the responses of ganglion cells of the vertebrate retina – that is, the cells in the optic ganglion respond principally to changes in the stimuli incident on the eye. A further and more extensive investigation along these lines, and also a mapping of the receptive fields of central neurons, has been carried out recently by Snodderly (1969).

Although *Limulus* is an excellent subject for electrophysiological studies on vision, it appears not to be so well suited for comparable behavioral studies. The numerous attempts that have been made over the past fifty years or so to measure its visual capacities have met with but limited success. For brief reviews of some of this work see von Campenhausen (1967) and Makous (1968). The fault may not be in the ability of *Limulus* to see, however; in its natural state it leads a long, active, and complicated life in which vision probably plays an important role. Perhaps new experimental techniques based on the natural behavior of *Limulus* itself, rather than adaptations of old techniques based upon and designed for the study of the behavior of other animals, will be required to reveal this role.

REFERENCES

Adolph, A. R. (1964), 'Spontaneous Slow Potential Fluctuations in the *Limulus* Photoreceptor', *J. Gen. Physiol.*, **48**, 297–322.

Barlow, R. B., and Kaplan, E. (1971), 'Properties of Receptor Units in the unexcised Eye', *Science*, **174**, 1027–1029.

Campenhausen, C. von (1967), 'The Ability of *Limulus* to See Visual Patterns', *J. Exp. Biol.*, **46**, 557–570.

De Haas, H. K. (1903), *Lichtprikkel en retinastroomen in hun quantitatief verband*, Inaug. Diss. Leiden.

De Lange, H. (1958), 'Research into the Dynamic Nature of the Human Fovea→Cortex Systems with Intermittent and Modulated Light. I. Attenuation Characteristics with White and Colored Light', *J. Opt. Soc. Amer.*, **48**, 777–784.

Dodge, F. A. (1969), 'Excitation and Inhibition in the Eye of *Limulus*', Conference on Processing of Optical Data by Organisms and by Machines, *Proceedings of the International School of Physics 'Enrico Fermi'*, XLIII, pp. 341–365, W. Reichardt, editor, Academic Press, New York and London.

Fuortes, M. G. F., and Yeandle, S. (1964), 'Probability of Occurrence of Discrete Potential Waves in the Eye of *Limulus*', *J. Gen. Physiol.*, **47**, 433–463.

Graham, C. H., and Margaria, R. (1935), 'Area and the Intensity Relation in the Peripheral Retina', *Amer. J. Physiol.*, **113**, 299–305.

Graham, J., and Gerard, R. W. (1946), 'Membrane Potential and Excitation of Impaled Single Muscle Fibers', *J. Cell Comp. Physiol.*, **28**, 99–117.

Granit, R., Holmberg, T. and Zewi, M. (1938), 'On the Mode of Action of Visual Purple on the Rod Cell', *J. Physiol.*, **94**, 430–440.

Hartline, H. K. (1925), 'The Electrical Response to Illumination of the Eye in Intact Animals, Including the Human Subject, and in Decerebrate Preparations', *Amer. J. Physiol.*, **73**, 600–612.

Hartline, H. K. (1928), 'A Quantitative and Descriptive Study of the Electrical Response to Illumination of the Arthropod Eye', *Amer. J. Physiol.*, **83**, 466–483.

Hartline, H. K. (1935), 'The Discharge of Nerve Impulses from the Single Visual Sense Cell', *Cold Spring Harbor Symposia on Quantitative Biology*, III, 245–250.

Hecht, S., Haig, C. and Chase, A. M. (1937), 'The Influence of Light

Adaptation on Subsequent Dark Adaptation of the Eye', *J. Gen. Physiol.*, **20**, 831–850.

Hecht, S. (1937), 'Rods, Cones, and the Chemical Basis of Vision', *Physiol. Rev.*, **17**, 239–290.

Hecht, S., Shlaer, S., and Pirenne, M. H. (1942), 'Energy, Quanta, and Vision', *J. Gen. Physiol.*, **25**, 819–840.

Hubbard, R., and Wald, G. (1960), 'Visual Pigment of the Horseshoe Crab, *Limulus polyphemus*', *Nature*, **186**, 212–215.

Kaneko, A. (1971), 'Physiological Studies of Single Retinal Cells and their Morphological Identification', *Vision Research Supplement No. 3*, 17–26.

Ling, G., and Gerard, R. W. (1949), 'The Membrane Potential and Metabolism of Muscle Fibers', *J. Cell. Comp. Physiol.*, **34**, 413.

Long, G. E. (1951), 'The Effect of Duration of Onset and Cessation of Light Flash on the Intensity-Time Relation in the Peripheral Retina', *J. Opt. Soc. Amer.*, **41**, 743–747.

Makous, W. L. (1969), 'Conditioning in the Horseshoe Crab', *Psychon. Sci.*, **14**, pp. 4 and 6.

Mueller, C. G., and Wilcox, L. R. (1954), 'Probability of Seeing Functions for Near-Instantaneous Thresholds', *Science*, **120**, 786.

Oomura, Y., and Kuriyama, H. A. (1952/1953), 'On the Action of the Optic Lobe of *Limulus longspina*', *Japanese J. Physiol.*, **3**, 165–169.

Patten, W. (1912), *The Evolution of the Vertebrates and their Kin*. P. Blakiston's Son & Co., Philadelphia.

Pirenne, M. H. (1967), *Vision and the Eye*. Science Paperbacks, Chapman & Hall, London.

Ratliff, F. (1962), 'Some Interrelations among Physics, Physiology, and Psychology in the Study of Vision', in *Psychology: A Study of a Science*, S. Koch, ed., McGraw-Hill, New York, Vol. 4, 417–482.

Shapley, R. M. (1969), 'Fluctuations in the Response to Light of Visual Neurones in *Limulus*', *Nature*, **221**, 437–440.

Shapley, R. M. (1971a), 'Fluctuations of the Impulse Rate in *Limulus* Eccentric Cells', *Journal of General Physiology*, **57**, 539–556.

Shapley, R. M. (1971b) 'Effects of Lateral Inhibition on Fluctuations of the Impulse Rate', *Journal of General Physiology*, **57**, 557–575.

Snodderley, D. M. (1969), Processing of Visual Inputs by the Ancient Brain of *Limulus*, Thesis, The Rockefeller University.

Tomita, T. (1968), 'Electrical Response of Single Photoreceptor', *Proc. of the IEEE*, **56**, 1015–1023.

Tomita, T. (1970), 'Electrical Activity of Vertebrate Photoreceptors', *Quarterly Reviews of Biophysics*, **3**, 179–222.

Werblin, F. S., and Dowling, J. E. (1969), 'Organization of the Retina of the Mudpuppy, *Necturus maculosus*. II. Intracellular Recording', *J. Neurophysiol.*, **32**, 339–355.

Wilska, A., and Hartline, H. K. (1941), 'The Origin of "Off-Responses" in the Optic Pathway', *Amer. J. Physiol.*, **133**, 491P.

Yeandle, S. (1957), *Studies on the Slow Potential and the Effects of Cations on the Electrical Responses of the* Limulus *Ommatidium (with an Appendix on the Quantal Nature of the Slow Potential)*. Ph.D. Thesis, The Johns Hopkins University.

Nerve impulses from single receptors in the eye

H. KEFFER HARTLINE AND C. H. GRAHAM [1]

Eldridge Reeves Johnson Foundation for Medical Physics, University of Pennsylvania, Philadelphia, and Marine Biological Laboratory, Woods Hole, Massachusetts

Reprinted from the JOURNAL OF CELLULAR AND
COMPARATIVE PHYSIOLOGY, Vol. 1, no. 2, pp. 227–295, April 1932

Recent studies in sensory physiology have provided a new approach to the problem of the mechanism of sense organs. The discharge of nerve impulses in the afferent fibers from various receptors has been studied in preparations in which the activity can be limited to a single end organ and its attached nerve fiber. The more complete analysis characteristic of this approach is best exemplified in the work done on tension, touch, and pressure receptors (Adrian, '26; Adrian and Zotterman, '26; Bronk, '29; Matthews, '31; Adrian, Cattell, and Hoagland, '31; Adrian and Umrath, '29; Bronk and Stella, '32). In the case of these relatively simple end organs it has been possible to study the effect of various intensities of stimulation upon the nervous discharge and to investigate the processes of adaptation and fatigue. It is highly desirable to extend this method to the photoreceptor.

Within the last few years Adrian and Matthews ('27 a, '27 b, '28) have succeeded in demonstrating the passage of impulses in the optic nerve of the eel, Conger vulgaris, upon stimulation of the retina by light. These investigations on the discharge in the entire optic nerve have yielded such valuable information regarding the mechanism of the visual process and especially regarding the synaptic factors that the possibility of

[1] National Research Fellow in the Biological Sciences.

studying the response of a single photoreceptor unit becomes a most attractive one. For this purpose two conditions must be met which are not fulfilled by the eye of the eel. It is necessary to have a preparation in which the nerve can be readily separated into its constituent fibers and there should be no intervening neurones between the receptor cell and the nerve fiber in which the impulses are recorded.

The present paper[2] is concerned with a study of the nerve message in a more primitive eye, that of Limulus polyphemus, which admirably meets these requirements. In this eye the fibers in the optic nerve come directly from the receptor cells with no intervening neurones. Moreover, we have been able to develop a technique whereby the discharge from a single receptor unit is recorded.

THE PREPARATION

The lateral eye of the horseshoe crab[3] (Limulus polyphemus) is a facetted eye containing about 300 large, coarsely spaced ommatidia. The histological structure of this organ has been studied in detail by Grenacher ('79) and Exner ('91). In each ommatidium there are fourteen to sixteen sense cells ('retinula cells') grouped about a central rhabdom. From each sense cell a nerve fiber runs uninterruptedly in the optic nerve to the central ganglion. Grenacher was unable to find any evidence of the presence of ganglion cells in the eye itself. On this basis we believe that in the optic nerve of Limulus we are dealing with a true sensory nerve, the activity of which is uncomplicated by synapses or ganglion cells. The nerve is unusually long, and in the adult animal may reach a length of 10 cm.

The carapace of the animal is opened from the dorsal side and the optic nerve is readily found at the point where it leaves the eye. It is dissected free of surrounding tissue and

[2] A preliminary report of this study has been published in Proc. Soc. Exp. Biol. and Med., Hartline and Graham ('32). We wish to thank Mr. M. G. Larrabee for his assistance in the experiments during the summer of 1931.

[3] Prof. C. E. McClung, of the Department of Zoölogy, has kindly provided us with facilities for keeping the animals during the experiments in Philadelphia.

severed at a convenient length (1 to 3 cm.). The eye, with a margin of carapace surrounding it, is then loosened from the animal and removed with its attached length of nerve. It is mounted on the front wall of a moist chamber by means of melted paraffin and the nerve, extending through a slot, is slung on silk thread electrodes. This preparation will survive for ten to twelve hours.

METHOD AND APPARATUS

The method used in these experiments is to obtain in the usual manner oscillograms of the potential changes between the cut end and an uninjured portion of the nerve upon stimulation of the eye by light. The scheme of the experimental layout is given in figure 1. The eye-nerve preparation in its moist chamber (MC) is placed in an electrically shielded and thermally insulated box (B) with the front surface of the eye (E) at the focus of a 16-mm. microscope objective (M). Illumination is provided by a 500-watt projection lamp. An image of the filament is focused on a metal diaphragm (D), the rays first passing through a heat filter consisting of 7 cm. of distilled water. The aperture in the diaphragm may be either a slit (about 10 mm. $\times$ 1 mm.) or a pinhole (about 0.5-mm. diameter), and it is the image of this aperture which is focused by means of the objective onto the cornea of the eye. Provision is made for the control of intensity by means of Wratten neutral-tint filters (F) placed immediately behind the diaphragm, and the exposure is regulated by a hand-operated shutter (S) situated in front of it. The moist chamber containing the eye-nerve preparation is mounted on a platform (P) carried by a vernier micrometer manipulator.[4] This manipulator is placed with its controls (X, Y, Z) outside the dark box and permits accurately controlled motion in three perpendicular directions. With this arrangement it is possible to adjust accurately the position of the image on the eye and to reproduce a given setting to within 0.01 mm. The nerve (N) is slung over two silk threads soaked in sea-

[4] Designed and built by Mr. A. J. Rawson.

water which serve as electrodes. These threads run in glass tubes through the wall of the moist chamber and at *C* make contact with the non-polarizable Ag-AgCl electrodes connected to the input of a vacuum-tube amplifier (leads *I* in fig. 1).

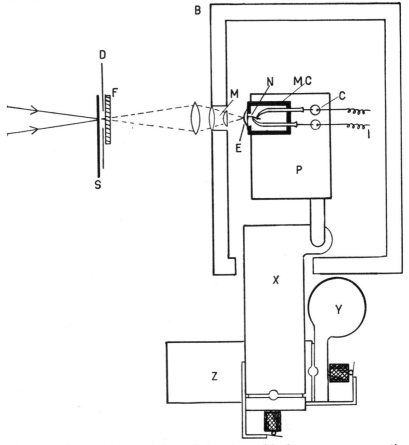

Fig. 1 Diagram of part of the optical system, with the eye-nerve preparation and micrometer manipulator. Explanation in text.

The amplifier consists of three stages of direct-coupled amplification and one power stage. The design is similar in principle to that used by Chaffee, Bovie, and Hampson ('23), and recently Adrian ('31) has described a circuit which is almost identical with the one which we have been using. In the first stage is a high-mu tube (UX-240) de-based and carefully mounted in such a manner as to minimize microphonic disturbances. This tube operates at a grid bias of —1.5 volts. The next two stages are screen-grid tubes (UY-224). These three stages in cascade yield a maximal voltage amplification of 80,000. This maximum, however, is seldom used, the amplification being reduced by means of volume controls in the screen-grid stages. Adjustable grid bias in the first and last stages provides for balancing the amplifier, the output of which feeds into a power stage consisting of four power pentodes (RCA-247) in parallel. The recording instrument, a Matthews' moving-reed oscillograph, is placed in the output of the power stage (compare Matthews, '29). At maximum sensitivity 3 microvolts applied to the input of the first stage produces a deflection of 1 mm. of the oscillograph beam at the camera (distance of 5 meters). In most experiments, however, it was necessary to reduce the sensitivity to about one-tenth of this. Within the range used the deflections are proportional to the applied E.M.F. and a rectangular wave is reproduced with inappreciable distortion (fig. 2, C).

RESPONSES OF THE WHOLE NERVE

The electrical changes taking place in the whole nerve are best studied in the young animal (3 to 8 cm. across carapace). A typical record of the changes when the whole eye is illuminated is shown in figure 2, A. After a short latent period there is an irregular variation of potential, followed immediately by an increase in negativity of the lead nearer the eye. This secondary rise reaches a maximum in about a fifth of a second and then sinks slightly to a steady value which is maintained throughout the duration of the illumination. Superimposed on these slow changes of potential is seen the fine structure associated with the passage of nerve impulses. When the light is turned off the impulses cease after a short latent period and the potential returns to its original level.

Except for the slow changes this record is quite similar to those obtained by Adrian and Matthews from the optic nerve of the conger eel ('27 a). Control experiments show that when the nerve is crushed between the eye and the lead nearer it neither slow change nor impulses can be detected.

It is interesting to compare the response from the nerve with the retinal potentials obtained by placing one lead on the cornea and one on the tissue at the back of the eye. These retinal potentials in Limulus have already been described by one of us (Hartline, '28) and a typical record obtained with the present apparatus is reproduced in figure 2, B. It is to be noted that this retinal action potential is a simple wave entirely devoid of fine structure. Its maximum is reached before that of the slow change in the nerve and is indeed approximately synchronous with the first burst of nerve activity.

The size of the slow change in the nerve may be materially modified by changes in the position of the electrode nearer the eye. When this electrode is close to the point where the nerve leaves the back of the eye, the slow changes are large; if it is more than 5 mm. from this point, the slow change may be almost absent, although the impulses are still recorded unchanged. If the retina and nerve are included in the electrical circuit, i.e., if leads are taken from the cornea and nerve, both the nerve impulses and slow change may be quite large.

The interpretation of the relationship between the slow potential changes in the nerve, the discharge of nerve impulses, and the retinal potentials must be left for further experimentation.

RESPONSES OF SINGLE PHOTORECEPTOR UNITS

Isolation of single units

The lateral eye and optic nerve of the adult Limulus are exceptionally good material for the recording of single fiber responses. The nerve is practically free of connective tissue and when floated on the surface of a drop of sea-water may

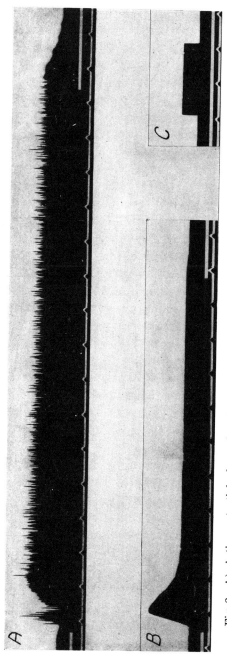

Fig. 2 A) Action potentials from the whole optic nerve. Deflection upward indicates increasing negativity of lead next the eye. (Height of maximum rise, 0.4 millivolt.) Lower white line indicates time in fifths of seconds. Line above time record signals the onset and cessation of illumination. B) Retinal action potential. Deflection upward indicates increasing negativity of the cornea with respect to the back of the eye. (Height of maximal rise, 1.35 millivolts.) Time record and signal as in A. C) Record of a calibrating potential of 0.16 millivolt applied to the amplifier input (sensitivity as in A). Time in fifths of seconds.

readily be dissected apart with glass needles under a binocular microscope. In this manner it is possible to obtain very small bundles of nerve fibers. In the young animal such bundles show evidence of a fair number of active fibers, but in the adult it appears that considerable areas of the eye have undergone degeneration of both ommatidia and nerve fibers. Consequently, many of the bundles obtained by dissection show no electrical response. A few trials, however, usually yield a bundle in which the response shows the striking regularity characteristic of the impulse discharge in a single nerve fiber (fig. 3).

A typical experiment makes clear the procedure used. An eye-nerve preparation was mounted in the manner described. The moist chamber was then flooded with sea-water, and by means of fine-pointed glass needles the nerve was split into several large bundles. The sea-water in the chamber was then drawn off and one of the bundles slung over the electrodes. This preparation was placed in the dark box and a trial record taken. Several bundles were tried in succession and the one giving the most favorable discharge was chosen. The moist chamber was again flooded with sea-water and a fine strand dissected off this bundle. When the sea-water was withdrawn and the eye stimulated, it was found that there were still several active fibers. One more dissection, however, gave a very delicate strand in which there was but one active fiber.

A record from this fiber is given in figure 3 (A, B, C, D). The impulses are unusually large (0.3 millivolt), due in part, at least, to the fact that there was in this fine strand very little material short-circuiting the active fiber. In other preparations we have obtained impulses as large as 0.6 milli-

Fig. 3 Action potentials of a single nerve fiber. Recording as in figure 2. Complete dark adaptation of eye. A to D) Intensity of stimulation, respectively, 0.1, 0.01, 0.001, and 0.0001 in arbitrary units (1 unit = 630,000 meter candles on the surface of the eye). The gap in each of the records represents an interval of 2.8 seconds, 1.4 seconds, 4.5 seconds, and 3.3 seconds, respectively. E) From another preparation, showing effect of high frequency of response on height of individual action potentials (compare text).

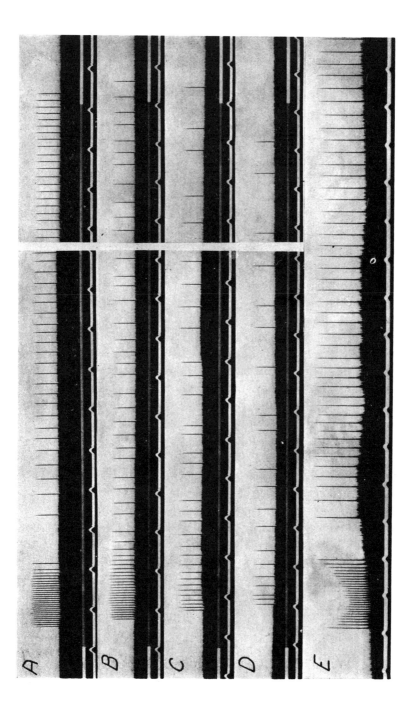

volt. That we are dealing with impulses in one fiber only is evidenced by the following considerations: 1) The discharge exhibits a regularity typical of that in a single fiber. Moreover, there is never any type of response intermediate between that figured here and no response at all. Further subdivision of the nerve strand invariably yields one portion which gives no response, the other showing the same regular succession of impulses as before. Adrian and Zotterman ('26) have discussed this point fully, and it has become generally recognized that the discharge of a train of regularly spaced nerve impulses of uniform size is typical of the functioning of a single nervous unit. This is true not only for various end organs and their nerve fibers, but also for the efferent impulses in motor units (Adrian and Bronk, '28). 2) Matthews ('31) has found in the case of the tension receptors in muscle that such a regularity of response occurs when stimulation is restricted to a portion of the muscle found histologically to contain a single muscle spindle. We have performed an experiment which has certain features similar to his. When the pinhole diaphragm was placed at D (fig. 1) and the preparation adjusted so that the image of the pinhole fell on the surface of the eye, it was found that no response to illumination occurred unless the image fell upon a definitely restricted region. The response obtained in this position consisted of the same regular series of impulses as had been obtained with illumination of the entire eye. By means of the micrometer manipulator it was possible to determine the extension of this region from which a response could be obtained. This was done by taking micrometer readings at the points where impulses first appeared as the region was approached from either side. This area was found to have a vertical diameter of 0.12 mm. and a horizontal diameter of 0.17 mm. The surface of the eye in this region was then examined by means of the following device. A half-silvered mirror was introduced into the light beam between the diaphragm (D) and the microscope objective (M, fig. 1) at an angle of 45° to the optical axis. With the help of a suitably placed eyepiece a region of the front surface of the eye 1.5 mm. in diameter could be observed at a magnification of about 40 ×. In the center of this field the small illuminated region could be seen where the image of the pinhole fell upon the eye. In the present experiment this examination was made with the eye so situated that a maximum frequency of response was elicited from the nerve fiber. It was found that the image of the pinhole lay directly over one ommatidium. This image was a circular patch of light 0.12 mm. in diameter and the ommatidium was slightly smaller. There were no other ommatidia illuminated by this patch of light, the average separation of adjacent ommatidia being about 0.3 mm. That we are dealing with the synchronous discharge of all the fibers from one ommatidium is rendered unlikely by the fact, already mentioned, that when a strand showing a uniform series of impulses is further subdivided the one part gives the same discharge and the other none at all. Further, it has been impossible to obtain a simple regular series of impulses by confining the stimulus to a single ommatidium without previous dissection of the nerve. We must rely upon the good fortune of the dissection to include only one active fiber from a given ommatidium.

If several active elements are present in the nerve bundle, it is frequently possible, if their number is not too great, to recognize their respective impulses in the responses obtained when the region of illumination is large, and to effect a separation physiologically by means of confining the stimulus to the respective end organs supplied. An example of this is given in the experiment of figure 4. In this experiment a region of the eye known to contain active elements was first mapped by means of the microscope and micrometer manipulator. The method was to adjust the manipulator until the center of the small patch of light coincided with the center of an ommatidium. Readings of the micrometer heads, X and Y, were then taken. Ommatidia were found in the following positions:

Ommatidium no.	X mm.	Y mm.
1	15.72	13.91
2	15.86	14.97
3	16.00	14.61
4	16.07	14.28
5	16.30	14.20

The diagonal mirror was then removed and the response tested at each of these settings of the micrometers. No

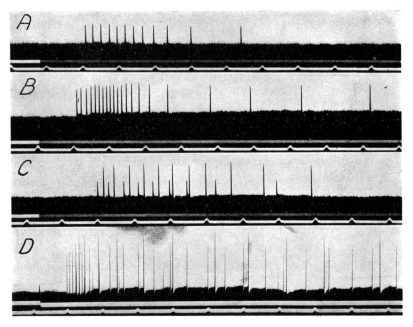

Fig. 4 Action potentials from nerve strands containing several active fibers. A to C) From bundle containing two active fibers. A and B) Stimulation of respective end organs separately. Intensity, 0.1. C) Stimulation of both end organs simultaneously. Intensity, 0.03. D) Record showing discharge in three active fibers. Recording as in figure 2.

responses were obtained when the preparation was adjusted for the illumination of the first two and the last of the ommatidia listed. Stimulation of the other two ommatidia (3 and 4) resulted in responses in both cases. From no. 3 the greatest frequency of response was obtained with a micrometer setting of X = 16.00, Y = 14.60. A record of the response of this ommatidium is given in figure 4, A. From no. 4 the maximum response was obtained with a setting X = 16.00, Y = 14.30. A record of this response is given in figure 4, B. It is seen that the impulses in the two cases differ in magnitude, a result which is in keeping with the fact that two different nerve fibers are involved. The micrometer was next set at X = 16.00, Y = 14.45 (halfway between the two ommatidia), and by means of the Z control (motion parallel to optical axis) the eye was moved back 4.2 mm. and was illuminated by an out-of-focus patch of light, which in this case had a diameter of 2.1 mm. and a correspondingly reduced intensity. The response obtained when both ommatidia were thus equally illuminated is given in figure 4, C. There is no difficulty in recognizing the small impulses from no. 3 and the large ones from no. 4. Another example of responses in several fibers is given in figure 4, D. This is from another preparation (whole eye illuminated), and the record shows the presence of three active fibers in the nerve bundle, the respective impulses being of different magnitudes and discharged at different frequencies.

Nature of the response

As examples of typical single fiber responses we may take the records reproduced in figure 3, B, and figure 4, B. The discharge begins after a latent period at a relatively high frequency which may rise to a maximum and then sinks, rapidly at first, and then more slowly, tending to reach a constant level. The discharge continues as long as the light is shining on the eye, and at the higher intensities is quite regular. When the light is turned off, the discharge persists for a very short period and then stops abruptly.

The effect of intensity upon the discharge is marked. It is shown in four records of figure 3. At the higher intensities the initial maximum frequency and the final steady value are both increased, as has been found to be the case for all other end organs studied by other investigators. At lower intensities the frequency is less, the discharge tends to become irregular, and the latent period increases. At still lower intensities the discharge becomes very short in spite of continued illumination and just above the threshold consists of only a single impulse. Figure 5 gives the graphs of the frequency-time relation for three intensities. The curves are taken from the records A, C, and D of figure 3. In figure

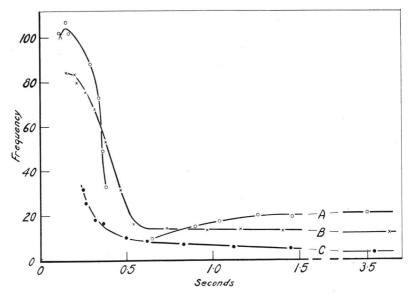

Fig. 5 Frequency of impulses (number per second) versus time after the onset of illumination. Curve A, from figure 3, A; intensity, 0.1. Curve B, from figure 3, C; intensity, 0.001. Curve C, from figure 3, D; intensity, 0.0001. Intensity in arbitrary units (1 unit = 630,000 meter candles on the surface of the eye). The points give the average frequency of four successive impulses; the time value is assigned to the second impulse.

6 is plotted the frequency of discharge against the logarithm of the stimulating intensity; curve A gives the initial maximum frequencies; curve B, the frequencies after three and one-half seconds. The linear relation over a moderate range of intensities parallels that found by Matthews ('31) for the muscle spindle.

A striking feature of the response of the completely dark-adapted eye to high intensities (fig. 3, A and E) is the brief pause in the discharge after the initial maximum. Following this 'silent period' the discharge is resumed at a much lower frequency, rises slightly to a secondary maximum, and then declines slowly toward a steady level. (In figure 3, A, this second maximum is reached in about three seconds; in figure 3, E, in about one second.) When the eye is not completely

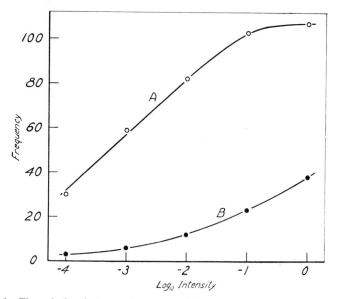

Fig. 6 The relation between frequency of impulses (number per second) and logarithm of the intensity of stimulating light. Intensity in arbitrary units (1 unit = 630,000 meter candles). Curve A, frequency of the initial maximal discharge. Curve B, frequency of discharge 3.5 seconds after onset of illumination. The data for this graph were obtained from the experiments of figure 3, A to D (the record supplying the data for the highest intensity is not given in fig. 3).

dark-adapted, the initial maximum is of lower frequency and the discharge is an unbroken sequence of impulses. The presence of the silent period in the response of the completely dark-adapted eye to lights of high intensity appears to be a true property of the receptor. Matthews ('31) has reported a similar pause in the discharge of a single muscle spindle, less marked than in these records but quite definite.

In the present case there can be no possibility of irregularity in the application of the stimulus to the sense cell. It is to be noted that the silent period also appears in records from the whole nerve (fig. 2, A), so that it cannot be due to injury of the fiber during dissection. That it is not alone due to the high frequency of the initial discharge is shown by an experiment in which the eye, having had sixteen minutes of dark adaptation, gave a response reaching a maximum of 80 per second and showed no trace of silent period or discontinuity in the rate of fall of discharge frequency. Previous to this, with complete dark adaptation (over one hour), this same preparation was stimulated with a light one-tenth as bright and responded with a maximum initial frequency of 78 per second, following which there was a marked silent period lasting for more than 0.2 second.

An interesting phenomenon which has manifested itself was shown by the preparation represented in figure 3, E. From this nerve the impulses recorded in the initial burst show a decrease and subsequent increase in height paralleling closely the rise and fall of the frequency of the discharge. In the succeeding discharge (after the silent period) the impulses are of uniform height. These decreased action potentials are clearly to be interpreted as being due to the impulses following each other so closely that each falls within the relative refractory period left by the preceding one. This finding is by no means the rule. We have observed it in several preparations, but have failed to find it in others where the frequency actually reaches a higher value (fig. 3, A), but where presumably the time constants of the fiber were different. By rapid repeated stimulation of the tactile end organs of the frog skin, Cattell and Hoagland ('31) have demonstrated the same effect. It is evident that only during the first burst does the nerve respond with a frequency which is close to its physiological limit.

DISCUSSION

The discharge of impulses recorded in a single nerve fiber when its attached photoreceptor is stimulated by light closely resembles that found in similar preparations from other sense organs. Initially discharging at a high frequency, this photoreceptor unit adapts fairly rapidly, but maintains a steady discharge as long as the stimulus is applied. In this respect it may be classed with the tension and pressure receptors as opposed to the tactile. Moreover, as in other sense organs, the frequency of discharge is greater with higher intensities of stimulation. At the highest intensity employed the maximum frequency we have observed is about 130 per second. At low intensities the discharge becomes irregular and may even stop. These experiments on the isolated photoreceptor unit, uncomplicated by synapses or ganglion cells, agree in revealing a typical nervous unit discharging a regular sequence of nerve impulses. The photoreceptor is thus seen to fit into the general picture of sense-organ activity developed from the study of other receptors.

The relation of these findings to visual physiology has not been touched upon in this paper. It is of interest to notice that the familiar linear relation between the response and the logarithm of the stimulating intensity is present in the behavior of the single photoreceptor unit. Of particular significance is the fact that a single receptor unit is capable of responding at different frequencies over such a wide range of intensities. In figure 6, where the intensity range is 1 to 10,000, it is evident that the lower limit has not been reached. Other experiments have shown us that the range may be as great as 1 to 1,000,000.

SUMMARY

1. The lateral eye of Limulus polyphemus when excised with a portion of its optic nerve attached provides a preparation well suited for the study of the nerve discharge associated with the process of photoreception. In this primitive eye there are neither ganglion cells nor synapses.

2. The method used in this study has been to stimulate the eye by light and record the action potentials in the optic nerve by means of an oscillograph.

3. In the whole nerve the response to light consists of slow potential changes, superimposed upon which are rapid, irregular fluctuations associated with the passage of nerve impulses.

4. The optic nerve may be subdivided into strands, which, if sufficiently small, may show a regular sequence of uniform nerve impulses, which from analogy with other sense organs are interpreted as being due to the discharge from a single fiber.

5. This regular discharge is associated with stimulation of a single ommatidium.

6. When several active fibers are present in a strand from the optic nerve, their respective discharges may be recognized by differences in the corresponding size of impulses. In one case each discharge was shown to be associated with the stimulation of separate ommatidia.

7. The discharge in a single fiber begins after a short latent period at a high frequency, which has been found to be as high as 130 per second. The frequency falls rapidly at first, and finally approaches a steady value, which is maintained for the duration of illumination.

8. Frequency of discharge is greater at high intensities of illumination and the latent period is shorter.

9. The response of the completely dark-adapted eye to high intensities is characterized by a short pause in the discharge after the first initial burst. Following this 'silent period' the discharge is renewed at a lower frequency.

10. The behavior of this photoreceptor is analogous to that of other receptor organs, particularly those of tension and pressure.

11. The range of intensities to which a single photoreceptor unit responds with varying frequency may be as great as 1 to 1,000,000.

LITERATURE CITED

ADRIAN, E. D. 1926 The impulses produced by sensory nerve endings. Part I. J. Physiol., vol. 61.

———— 1931 Potential changes in the isolated nervous system of Dytiscus marginalis. J. Physiol., vol. 72.

ADRIAN, E. D., AND BRONK, D. W. 1928 The discharge of impulses in motor nerve fibres. Part I. J. Physiol., vol. 66.

ADRIAN, E. D., CATTELL, McK., AND HOAGLAND, H. 1931 Sensory discharges in single cutaneous nerve fibres. J. Physiol., vol. 72.

ADRIAN, E. D., AND MATTHEWS, R. 1927 a The action of light on the eye. Part I. J. Physiol., vol. 63.

———— 1927 b The action of light on the eye. Part II. J. Physiol., vol. 64.

———— 1928 The action of light on the eye. Part III. J. Physiol., vol. 65.

ADRIAN, E. D., AND UMRATH, K. 1929 The impulse discharge from the pacinian corpuscle. J. Physiol., vol. 68.

ADRIAN, E. D., AND ZOTTERMAN, Y. 1926 The impulses produced by sensory nerve-endings. Part II. J. Physiol., vol. 61.

BRONK, D. W. 1929 Fatigue of the sense organs in muscle. J. Physiol., vol. 67.

BRONK, D. W., AND STELLA, G. 1932 Afferent impulses in the carotid sinus nerve. Part I. J. Cell. and Comp. Physiol., vol. 1.

CATTELL, McK., AND HOAGLAND, H. 1931 Responses of tactile receptors to intermittent stimulation. J. Physiol., vol. 62.

CHAFFEE, E. L., BOVIE, W. T., AND HAMPSON, A. 1923 The electrical response of the retina under stimulation by light. J. Opt. Soc. Amer., vol. 7.

EXNER, S. 1891 Die Physiologie der facettirten Augen. Franz Deuticke, Leipzig und Wien.

GRENACHER, H. 1879 Untersuchungen über das Sehorgan der Arthropoden. Vandenhoeck und Ruprecht, Göttingen.

HARTLINE, H. K. 1928 A quantitative and descriptive study of the electric response to illumination of the arthropod eye. Am. J. Physiol., vol. 83.

HARTLINE, H. K., AND GRAHAM, C. H. 1932 Nerve impulses from single receptors in the eye of Limulus. Proc. Soc. Exp. Biol. Med., vol. 20.

MATTHEWS, B. H. C. 1929 A new electrical recording system. J. Sci. Inst., vol. 6.

———— 1931 The response of a single end organ. J. Physiol., vol. 71.

The response of single visual sense cells to lights of different wave lengths

C. H. GRAHAM* AND H. KEFFER HARTLINE†

*Eldridge Reeves Johnson Foundation for Medical Physics,
University of Pennsylvania, Philadelphia*

Reprinted from the JOURNAL OF GENERAL PHYSIOLOGY,
20 July 1935, Vol. 18, no. 6, pp. 917–931

Any adequate theoretical explanation of color vision and its related effects involves a consideration of how the single visual sense cell responds to different wave lengths of light. Up to the present time this has been a matter of inference and hypothesis, and no direct information has been available concerning the response of the single sense cell to light from different parts of the spectrum. In an earlier paper (Hartline and Graham, 1932) we have described a method for observing nerve impulses in single fibers of the optic nerve of *Limulus polyphemus* in response to stimulation of the attached sense cells by light. The present paper is concerned with a discussion of the effect of wave length of the stimulating light upon this response.

Method and Apparatus

The method for obtaining records of action potentials in the single optic nerve fibers is as follows: The lateral eye of an adult *Limulus* is excised with a centimeter or so of optic nerve and mounted in a moist chamber. With the aid of glass needles the nerve is frayed out into small bundles and the amplified action potentials in such bundles are recorded by means of an oscillograph. In several trials, splitting the bundles into still finer strands if necessary, one can obtain the response typical of a single active fiber, and locate in the eye the ommatidium which contains the corresponding receptor unit. Records from such a preparation provide the data for this report. Details of the method, the arrangement for the stimulating light,[1] and the devices for controlling its constancy and the duration of its

---

* Department of Psychology, Clark University.

† A part of the expenses of this investigation was met by a Grant-in-Aid from the National Research Council to one of us.

[1] The pointolite lamp used in the previous studies has been replaced in these experiments by a tungsten filament lamp (photocell exciter lamp used in talking pictures) working at a 20 per cent overvoltage.

exposure have been described in a recent paper by one of us (Hartline, 1934). In the present experiments a condition of complete dark adaptation is maintained and the temperature is controlled to within ±0.2°C.

To obtain spectral lights of different wave lengths and known energy content we have employed Wratten monochromatic filters (Nos. 70 to 76) in conjunction with Wratten neutral tint filters and a liquid filter of 1 per cent $CuCl_2$ (31 mm. in thickness) to remove the near infrared (*cf.* Hecht, 1928). While the Wratten filters do not yield strictly monochromatic light their transmission bands are narrow enough for the present purpose, and they have been used by other workers for a similar purpose (Hecht, 1928; Grundfest, 1932 *b*; Crozier, 1924). The transmission spectrum of each filter was corrected for the transmission of the $CuCl_2$ solution and the central wave length of this band was determined for each filter by the method described by Hecht (1928).[2] A direct calibration of the relative

TABLE I

Relative energies of spectral lights supplied by seven Wratten monochromatic filters. The light source is a tungsten filament. A filter consisting of 31 mm. of a 1 per cent aqueous solution of $CuCl_2$ is used to remove the near infrared.

Filter No.	Central wave length	Relative energy
	$m\mu$	
70	690	1.72
71*A*	640	1.36
72	610	0.96
73	575	1.01
74	530	1.00
75	490	0.74
76	440	0.67

energy of the light provided by each filter was obtained by means of a thermopile and a galvanometer, the thermopile being in the position of the eye. Table I gives the results of these calibrations. In it are entered the central wave length and the relative energy of the light supplied to the eye when the various filters are used. The energy with filter 74 has been arbitrarily assigned a value of unity.

Wratten neutral tint filters were employed to vary the intensity of the stimulating lights. Photometric determinations of these filters have been made several times during the course of the work and their values found to be constant within 3 per cent. Moreover, they have been checked directly by means of the thermopile. Under these conditions their densities with each of the monochromatic

---

[2] We have neglected the correction due to the emission spectrum of the tungsten filament of the light source. This will slightly affect the value of the central wave length.

filters were found to be the same and within 5 per cent of the rating given by the manufacturers. Both the monochromatic filters and the neutral tint filters transmit a large amount of the near infrared. This does not affect the *Limulus* eye, but, of course, it is measured by the thermopile and galvanometer. It is for this reason that the CuCl₂ filter has been used in all the experiments reported in this study.

RESULTS

The response of the single receptor cell in the eye of *Limulus*, in terms of impulses discharged in its attached nerve fiber, has been described in two previous publications (Hartline and Graham, 1932; Hartline, 1934). When stimulating lights of different wave lengths but of approximately equal energy content are used it is found that the response to green light is stronger than the response to either red or violet; *i.e.*, the latent period is shorter, the initial and maximum frequency is higher and, for short flashes, the total number of impulses is larger; with prolonged exposure the final level of frequency is higher. These are all characteristic of higher intensity of stimulation, and hence it should be possible to make up for the lower level of response in the red and violet by supplying more energy at these wave lengths. This has been done as shown in Fig. 1. In this figure the intensities for the different wave lengths have been so adjusted that the responses are approximately equal. The first column gives the central wave length of the stimulating light, the second column gives the relative energy content of the light (referred to filter 74 as unity), and the right hand column contains records of the responses to a short flash (0.04 second) of each of these lights. The response consists of a burst of seven impulses (plus or minus one) and it is seen that the latent periods and frequencies are approximately the same. It is clear that when the intensities are properly adjusted there is no effect of wave length *per se*.

To test this point more carefully we have chosen three spectral lights in the red, green, and violet portions of the spectrum and we have taken pains to adjust their intensities to yield responses as nearly identical as possible. The close adjustment of intensity was obtained by varying the current through the tungsten filament of the light source and the energy values were obtained by direct calibration with

$\lambda_{m\mu}$ I *Response*

690   690

640   55

610   9.6

575   2.0

530   1.0

490   1.5

440   6.7

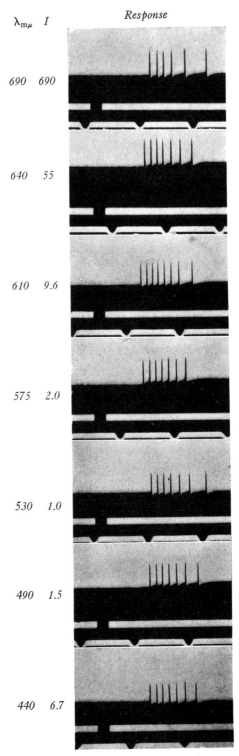

Fig. 1

the thermopile. The responses for the three different colors agree with each other impulse for impulse as closely as the reproducibility of the results will allow. The experimental findings are summarized in Table II. In this table the duration of the exposure, the central wave length, and the relative energy are given in the three left hand columns. In the upper part of this table are given results obtained with a flash of 0.04 second duration. The features of response measured are latent period, initial frequency (impulses 1 to 3), maximum frequency, and total number of impulses in the initial burst. The lower part of the table summarizes results obtained with prolonged illumination. In it are entered measurements of latent period, initial frequency, maximum frequency, the level of frequency reached after 3 seconds, and the time of the fiftieth impulse. The experiments with the short flash were performed at two different levels of intensity, one level having one hundred times the energy value of the other.

It may be seen that the responses to the three wave lengths whose energies have been properly adjusted are in close agreement, and that this agreement is maintained regardless of the energy level or duration of the illumination. The agreement between the responses to the three wave lengths is as close as could be obtained at any one wave length with a repetition of the same stimulus. To show the marked effect of intensity upon these features of the response we have added in Table II *a* a summary of results obtained in the same experiment with one wave length (filter 74) at different intensities. Reference to Table II *a* shows within what small limits of intensity we have succeeded in matching the responses in Table II.

Table II shows that the responses to different wave lengths may be equated at two different levels of the response and that the relative energies of the different wave lengths are in the same ratios regardless of the level of the response. Thus, in Table II the energies of the

---

FIG. 1. Oscillographic records of the impulse discharge in a single optic nerve fiber in response to stimulation of the eye by lights of different wave lengths. The wave lengths are given in the first column. The intensities have been adjusted to give approximately equal responses and their values are given in the second column. In each record the lower line marks time in fifths of seconds. In the line above this appears the signal indicating the time during which the eye is illuminated (exposure = 0.04 second).

TABLE II

Comparison of matched responses to lights of different wave lengths, together with the relative energies necessary to produce them. The comparison with short flashes (0.04 sec.) at two levels of intensity (2.0 log units apart) and with prolonged illumination. The energy of the green light (filter no. 74) of highest intensity is assigned a value of unity.

Exposure	Central wave length	Logarithm relative energy Log$_{10}$ I	Latent period	Initial frequency	Maximum frequency	Number of impulses (first burst)	Frequency at 3 sec.	Time of fiftieth impulse
sec.	*mμ*		*sec.*	*per sec.*	*per sec.*		*per sec.*	*sec.*
	640	$\bar{1}$.64	0.329	39	39	7		
	530	$\bar{2}$.00	0.325	39	39	7		
	440	$\bar{2}$.64	0.356	38	38	7		
0.04								
	640	1.64	0.121	78	98	29		
	530	0.00	0.112	78	97	30		
	440	0.64	0.123	79	96	29		
	640	$\bar{1}$.64	0.246	44	65		14.7	2.08
∞	530	$\bar{2}$.00	0.238	47	64		14.7	2.42
	440	$\bar{2}$.64	0.251	43	63		14.6	2.52

TABLE IIa

Data from the same experiment as Table II, showing the effect of intensity of light of a given wave length (filter no. 74) on the various features of the response.

Exposure	Central wave length	Logarithm relative energy Log$_{10}$ I	Latent period	Initial frequency	Maximum frequency	Number of impulses (first burst)	Frequency at 3 sec.	Time of fiftieth impulse
sec.	*mμ*		*sec.*	*per sec.*	*per sec.*		*per sec.*	*sec.*
		$\bar{3}$.60	0.409	27	27	6		
		$\bar{2}$.00	0.323	42	42	7		
		$\bar{2}$.30	0.267	56	56	9		
0.04	530							
		$\bar{1}$.60	0.134	73	88	24		
		0.00	0.109	78	100	31		
		0.30	0.094	87	106	38		
		$\bar{3}$.60	0.262	35	58		11.4	3.40
∞	530	$\bar{2}$.00	0.238	47	64		14.7	2.42
		$\bar{2}$.30	0.198	57	74		17.3	1.46

brighter flashes are all 100 times (2 log units) greater than the energies of the less bright flashes at the corresponding wave lengths; but it is to be noted that the responses which are matched at one level are still matched at the other level. Obviously, no Purkinje effect is exhibited by the single visual sense cell of *Limulus*. This is in agreement with all our findings in thirteen other experiments over even greater ranges of intensity; the curves relating magnitude of response to log intensity of stimulus are parallel for all wave lengths. These experiments show that within the limits of the reproducibility of results there is no specific effect of wave length other than one of brightness.

The relative energies of lights of different wave lengths required to produce the same response yield the visibility curve for the single visual sense cell. In accordance with established usage the reciprocal of the energy at a given wave length necessary to produce a constant response is defined as the visibility at that wave length (Hecht and Williams, 1922). Thus in Fig. 1 the reciprocals of the values of intensity in the second column are the visibility values of the light whose central wave length is given in the first column (approximate only, since the responses are not perfectly matched).

We have obtained visibility curves for sixteen single sense cells in six animals. In Fig. 2 is plotted the logarithm of the visibility against the different wave lengths from these different experiments. The three sets of points are the values for each of three single sense cells; the curve is drawn through the average values of all sixteen experiments. The detailed method for obtaining visibility values of the different wave lengths was as follows: For each spectral light the combination of Wratten neutral filters was selected which would give an approximate equality of response. These lights were presented in random order and records of the responses obtained. Short flashes were used (0.04 second). The green filter (No. 74) was chosen as a control stimulus and repeated more frequently than any of the others. The effect of intensity at a given wave length, *i.e.* green, was also obtained over a range which would embrace the range of response inequality. (Ordinarily an intensity series covering a range of 1 log unit is sufficient for this purpose.) Some convenient feature of the response was chosen (*e.g.*, latent period, frequency of first 5 impulses, *etc.*) and this feature was measured for all the responses. That portion of the experiment showing least variation in the control response was chosen and the responses to each wave length were averaged. These values are only approximately matched. To obtain the visibility it is necessary to

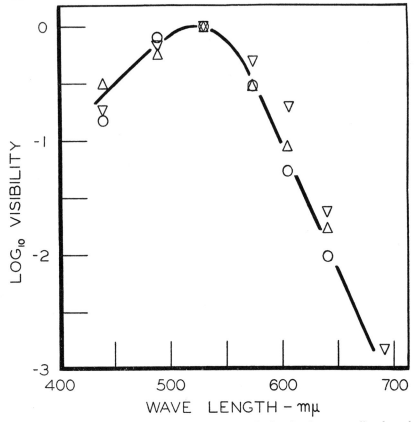

FIG. 2. The logarithms of the visibility for single visual sense cells plotted against wave length. The curve is drawn through the average values from sixteen experiments. The points are values of the visibilities for single sense cells. The circles and base-down triangles are the values for two cells from the same eye. The base-up triangles are values for a sense cell from another eye. The visibility of green light ($\lambda 530 \; m\mu$) is assigned a value of unity.

know what energy of stimulus should have been used to give a response which would be exactly matched for all wave lengths. From the curve relating magnitude of response to intensity we determined the amount of energy by which the actual stimulus should have been increased or decreased to equal exactly the average control response. This is valid because the curves relating response and logarithm of energy for all wave lengths are parallel as has been shown. We thus obtain the exact energy at each wave length necessary to produce a given constant response. The value for the green is arbitrarily assigned a value of unity, and the reciprocals of the relative energies in the other wave lengths yield the visibilities at these wave lengths in terms of a visibility of unity for green. In the light of the previous discussion it is clear that it makes no difference to the final result what feature of the response or what level of intensity is chosen for the calculation. Indeed, in some experiments a whole intensity curve was obtained for each wave length. As has been stated above, these curves, on a logarithmic scale, are parallel for all wave lengths, and the amount that each is displaced from the green gives the logarithm of the visibility (Hecht, 1928; Chaffee and Hampson, 1924).

In Fig. 2 it is seen that the visibility curves for different experiments do not agree at their extremes. This is not surprising when different animals are used, but in Fig. 2 two of the sets of points are from different cells in the same animal, and their lack of agreement is greater than the limits of error. This indicates that light of a given wave length does not have exactly the same visibility in all of the sense cells in the eye of *Limulus*. We have performed nine experiments which agree in indicating a true differential sensitivity for wave length among receptor cells in the same eye.

There are two methods for testing this differential sensitivity. Instead of dissecting the nerve bundle until it contains a single active fiber we choose a strand in which there are several active fibers. In the first method an analysis of the relative effects of wave lengths in different receptor cells depends upon the fact that the impulses in the different nerve fibers can be identified by their characteristics of form and magnitude. The whole region supplied by the active fibers is illuminated by lights of different wave lengths whose energies have been adjusted to give approximately matched responses. In effect this amounts to performing several experiments simultaneously upon sense cells located close together under conditions which are presumably identical. Records from such an experiment are reproduced in Fig. 3.

Response

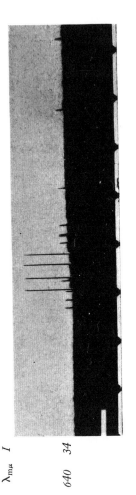
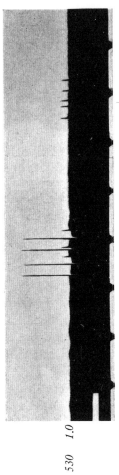
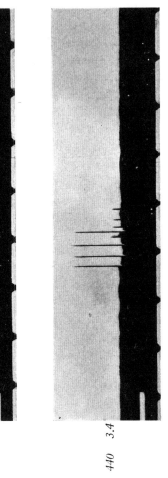

$\lambda_{m\mu}$ I

640 34

530 1.0

440 3.4

FIG. 3. Oscillographic records of responses from two sense cells in the same eye to three different wave lengths. The relative intensities have been adjusted so that the responses of one sense cell (large impulses) are approximately matched. Recording as in Fig. 1.

In this experiment there are two active fibers whose impulses are readily identifiable by their size and form. The intensities have been so adjusted that the response in the fiber giving the large impulses is constant for all wave lengths. It is seen that these intensities do not constitute a match for the fiber giving the small impulses, but that this fiber gives a stronger response with the red light. In passing to the green and violet it is seen that the latent period progressively increases and the number of impulses decreases. The visibility for this sense cell, then, must be lower in the violet and higher in the red than the visibility for the cell giving the larger impulses.

With this method high intensity responses are unobtainable since the illumination must be spread over a considerable area. Threshold

TABLE III

Negative logarithms of relative visibilities in the red and violet (basis of visibility of λ 530 mμ equal to unity) for four different sense cells in the same eye.

Sense cell No.	λ 640 mμ	λ 440 mμ
I*	$\begin{cases} 1.70 \\ 1.75 \end{cases}$	$\begin{cases} 0.55 \\ 0.48 \end{cases}$
II	1.67	0.43
III	1.89	0.37
IV	1.98	0.81

* The two values for this sense cell are repetitions at the beginning and end of the experiment.

responses are apt to be quite variable and the impulse discharge (as shown in Fig. 3) is irregular. Moreover, the records are analyzable only provided they contain few active fibers. For these reasons we have employed a second method. This method depends upon the fact that the active fibers in a small bundle from the optic nerve frequently come from sense cells located in different ommatidia. It is possible to locate these ommatidia and illuminate them separately with a small intense spot of light (Hartline and Graham, 1932). By means of an improved micrometer manipulator (constructed by Mr. A. J. Rawson of this Foundation) similar to the one described in an earlier paper (Hartline and Graham, 1932) it has been possible for us to examine as many as six separate sense cells in the same eye in rapid succession. In one experiment done by this method we obtained the entire visibility curve for each of four fibers. The visibilities for two of these fibers (Nos. I and IV) are plotted in Fig. 2 (triangles with base down and circles). The logarithms of the visibilities for all of the fibers of the red and violet are given in Table III. It is seen that the sense cells were not equally sensitive to the different wave lengths. The visibility values in this experiment were reproducible within 0.1 log unit and the level of stimulation was high (initial frequency of impulses, 50 to 60 per second) so that there can be no question as to threshold variability. We have performed four experiments by this method (eighteen fibers) and five by the first method (twelve fibers). These experiments all agree in showing that, while many fibers have visibilities which agree closely with each other in both the red and the violet, there is a large percentage of cases (*ca.* 50 per cent) in which the visibilities for different fibers differ from each other by significant amounts. The differences are frequently 0.3 or 0.4 log unit, and go as high as 0.6 log unit. The reproducibility of results is usually within 0.15 log unit; it is always closer than 0.2 log unit.

DISCUSSION

The present finding, that the wave length of the stimulating light has no specific effect in the stimulation of the single visual sense cell other than one of brightness is in keeping with the current conceptions of visual physiology. Phenomena such as the Purkinje effect and specific effects of wave length *per se, e.g.,* perception of color, are commonly ascribed to the activity of populations of sense cells. Nevertheless we believe that it is of value to be able to present direct evidence for the correctness of these views, even though the findings are for a comparatively primitive eye. In spite of the fact that the spectral lights used are not strictly monochromatic, we believe that the present experiments do give at least an approximate idea of the shape of the visibility curves for single receptor cells. It is to be noted that there are no striking differences between the curves of the individual sense cells such as might be lost when the visibility curve of a large group is determined. These findings indicate that each visual sense cell is sensitive to practically the entire range of wave lengths to which the whole eye can respond.

It is of interest to compare the visibility curve for the *Limulus* eye with that of the human eye. This is done in Fig. 4 where the data of Hecht and Williams (1922) for the dim vision of the human subject can be compared with the averaged data of the present experiments. As shown by this figure the visibility curve of the *Limulus* eye is a simple curve with a maximum at about λ520mμ, falling symmetrically

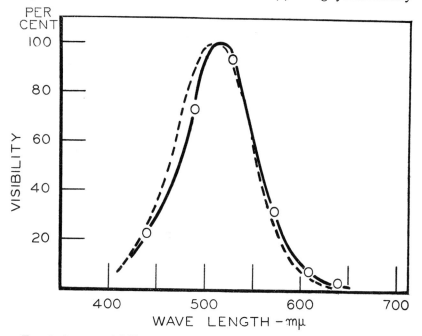

Fig. 4. Average visibility curve for the *Limulus* eye (points and solid curve) compared with the human dim vision visibility curve (dashed line) after Hecht and Williams (1922). The visibilities are expressed on the basis of maximum visibility equals unity.

on either side to low values in the red and violet. The similarity between the human curve and that for *Limulus* is striking. Following the interpretation of visibility curves given by Hecht and Williams (1922) (*cf.* also Grundfest, 1932 *a*) we may say that the stimulation of the single visual sense cell by light depends upon the absorption spectrum of the primary photosensitive substance.

It has been seen that while the visibility curves for single sense cells in the same eye are approximately similar they do differ by significant amounts. It is true that many of the visibility values fall close to the average, but a good number deviate appreciably. In view of the evidence we do not believe that this can be ascribed to experimental error and feel that it represents a true differential sensitivity to wave length among the sense cells of the eye. In view of the primitive nature of the *Limulus* eye this finding is somewhat surprising, for it is, of course, precisely such a mechanism as is postulated to explain color vision in the higher animals (*cf.* Hecht, 1930). While any single sense cell cannot distinguish wave length differences it is clear that, for example, the two sense cells whose responses are given in Fig. 2 can together distinguish violet from red, and the presence of differential sensitivity to wave length in the *Limulus* eye may be considered a possible peripheral mechanism for color discrimination. Whether the animal possesses the adequate central and motor equipment to make use of this mechanism is not known.

The present data do not allow us to discuss in detail the types of variation in the visibility curves. Apparently, however, the variations are not confined to any particular portion of the range of wave lengths but are to be observed over the entire curve. Moreover, the different curves cannot be obtained from a single curve by a shift in the position of the maximum. We have been unable to distinguish any tendency on the part of the curves to fall into groups within which the visibility curves are identical or even nearly so. As to the causes which might underlie the differences in the visibility curves of the various sense cells: whether, for example, they are due to overlying pigment or to slight differences in the photosensitive substance itself, we are not in a position to speculate.

SUMMARY

The effect of various wave lengths of visible light in the stimulation of single visual sense cells has been studied by means of the single fiber preparation from the eye of *Limulus*. Oscillographic records were made of the impulse discharge in a single optic nerve fiber in response to stimulation of the attached sense cell by lights of different wave lengths. Wratten monochromatic filters supplied the means for obtaining the different spectral lights; the total intensity supplied to the eye being determined by a thermopile and galvanometer.

With lights of approximately equal energy content the strongest response occurs to the green region of the spectrum. The response, however, does not vary qualitatively with wave length. By the proper adjustment of intensity, responses can be obtained which are identical, impulse for impulse, for all the spectral lights used. Moreover the ratios of the intensities for the various wave lengths necessary to produce a constant response do not vary with the intensity level of the stimulating lights; there is no Purkinje effect. The single visual sense cell can gauge brightness but cannot distinguish wave length.

The reciprocals of the intensities necessary to produce a constant response when plotted against wave length give the visibility curve for the single sense cell. This curve is symmetrical about a maximum at $\lambda 520m\mu$, falling off to low values in the red and violet. It closely resembles the visibility curve for human rod vision.

Bundles from the optic nerve containing several active fibers whose impulses can be distinguished by differences in form and magnitude or whose attached sense cells can be located and illuminated independently were used to determine whether there is any differential sensitivity among sense cells in the same eye for different regions of the spectrum. Such a differential sensitivity has been found to exist in the eye of *Limulus* and may be considered a peripheral mechanism of color vision.

REFERENCES

Chaffee, E. L., and Hampson, A., *J. Opt. Soc. America*, 1924, **9,** 1.
Crozier, W. J., *J. Gen. Physiol.*, 1924, **6,** 647.
Grundfest, H., *J. Gen. Physiol.*, 1932 a, **15,** 307.
Grundfest, H., *J. Gen. Physiol.*, 1932 b, **15,** 507.
Hartline, H. K., *J. Cell. and Comp. Physiol.*, 1934, **5,** 229.
Hartline, H. K., and Graham, C. H., *J. Cell. and Comp. Physiol.*, 1932, **1,** 277.
Hecht, S., *J. Gen. Physiol.*, 1928, **11,** 657.
Hecht, S., *J. Opt. Soc. America*, 1930, **20,** 231.
Hecht, S., and Williams, R. E., *J. Gen. Physiol.*, 1922, **5,** 1.

Intensity and duration in the excitation of single photoreceptor units

H. KEFFER HARTLINE

*Eldridge Reeves Johnson Foundation for Medical Physics,
University of Pennsylvania, Philadelphia*

Reprinted from the JOURNAL OF CELLULAR AND
COMPARATIVE PHYSIOLOGY, Vol. 5, no. 2, pp. 229–247, October 1934

The effect upon the eye of a short flash of light depends not only upon its intensity, but also upon its duration. Many investigators have studied the relative roles of intensity and duration of a stimulating flash in the excitation of photosensory end-organs and particular attention has been paid to the applicability to the visual process of the reciprocity law of Bunsen and Roscoe. This law of photochemistry— which can only be expected to hold for uncomplicated systems —states that the photochemical effect of a flash of light depends only upon its energy (product of intensity into duration). Bloch (1885) was the first to show that to produce a given constant visual effect, it is necessary that the product of intensity of the stimulating flash into its duration be approximately constant, at least within a certain range of durations. Subsequent work, notably by Blondel and Rey ('11) and by Piéron ('20) has indicated a significant failure of the reciprocity law for longer durations, and the question arises as to whether or not this is due to a failure of the Bunsen-Roscoe law for the photochemical system concerned with vision. Such failure is by no means unknown in photochemistry and Hecht ('29, '31) has shown that deviations from the reciprocity law may be expected in the visual system. However, Adrian and Matthews ('27), recording nerve action potentials from the eel's eye, and Hartline ('28), measuring the retinal potential of the insect eye, find no significant

47

failure of the law, provided the durations used are less than those needed to produce the maximum effect possible at the corresponding intensities. These latter methods have obvious advantages over subjective measurements, but they both deal with the activity of many sense cells, and it is desirable to have information concerning the single receptor unit. The application of the single fibre technique to the eye and optic nerve of Limulus polyphemus, described in a previous paper (Hartline and Graham, '32), makes it possible to obtain such information. In that paper a method was described for obtaining oscillographic records of impulses in the optic nerve from a single receptor unit in the eye, and evidence was presented to show that these impulses are from single nerve fibres, and that the units in the eye are the single retinula cells making up the sensory structures of the ommatidia. In the eye of Limulus there are no neurones intervening between the sense cells and the fibres in the optic nerve. It is thus possible to record the response of the single visual sense cell, in terms of the impulses it discharges in its attached nerve fibre. It is the purpose of the present paper[1] to investigate this response when the receptor cell is stimulated by flashes of light of various intensities and durations.

MATERIAL AND METHOD

The method for obtaining oscillographic records of action potentials of single optic nerve fibres, in response to stimulation of the eye by light has been described in the paper referred to above (Hartline and Graham, '32). Briefly, it is as follows: the lateral eye of adult Limulus polyphemus[2] is excised, with a centimeter or two of optic nerve, and mounted in a moist chamber. The nerve sheath is removed, and with the aid of glass needles the nerve is frayed out into small bundles. The action potentials in such bundles are amplified and observed by means of a Matthews oscillograph. In

[1] A preliminary report of this work was presented before the American Physiological Society (Hartline, '33).

[2] I wish to express my appreciation to Dr. Van Dusen, of the Philadelphia City Aquarium, for facilities for keeping the animals.

several trials, splitting the bundles into still finer strands if necessary, it is possible to obtain the typical records of a single active fibre, and to locate in the eye the ommatidium which contains the corresponding receptor unit. Records from such a preparation constitute the material on which this paper is based.

Certain precautions of method have been adopted in the present investigation. The chitinous growth which nearly covers the back of the eye of adult crabs is carefully removed to permit freer diffusion of gases, and the moist chamber is partly filled with defibrinated blood so as to bathe the lower half of the eye. Temperature control is effected by circulating water at constant temperature ($\pm 0.2°$C.) through the hollow metal walls of the light-tight box surrounding the preparation.

A condition of complete dark adaptation is maintained for all of the present experiments. One to 2 hours are allowed to elapse between setting up the preparation and the beginning of the experiments—a sufficient time for complete dark adaptation to become established, as well as temperature equilibrium. Preliminary experiments have shown that short flashes of moderate intensity do not disturb the condition of dark-adaptation if repeated at intervals of not less than about 10 minutes. Flashes which yield very vigorous responses require an interval of 20 minutes before the control response can be shown to have returned to the completely dark-adapted value.

Under these conditions, the control response to a constant stimulus will usually settle down to a steady value which will be maintained to within a few per cent for 4 or 5 hours, or at worst will show a slow but steady drift over a period of 10 to 12 hours.

APPARATUS

a. Stimulus. The arrangement for the stimulating light is essentially the same as that described in the previous paper (Hartline and Graham, '32). An image of the light source is focused upon an elliptical pin-hole, 1.2 mm. long by 0.8 mm. wide, in a metal diaphragm, the rays first passing through 10 cm. of water. At the diaphragm is located the shutter for regulating the duration of the exposure, and a box for the filters which regulate the intensity. An image for the illuminated pin-hole is focused upon the surface of the eye by means of a Zeiss achromatic objective, 5 mm. focus, N. A. 0.8, forming a small spot of light ca. 0.14 mm. in diameter, just large enough to cover one ommatidium. The system is carefully shielded to exclude stray light, and all experiments are done with the room in semidarkness. The source of light in the present experiments is the incandescent electrode of a tungsten arc ('Pointolite') lamp.[3]

To control the constancy of the illumination upon the eye a prism has been arranged to slide into position so that the light from the pin-hole, instead of falling upon the eye, is reflected onto the surface of a photoelectric element (Weston photronic cell) and the current consumed by the lamp adjusted to give a constant photoelectric current. In this way the intensity of the light is kept constant to within about 2 per cent.

To vary the intensity of the stimulating light in a known manner Wratten 'neutral tint' filters are used. The densities of these filters were checked photometrically several times in the course of the work and found to be within 3 per cent of the rating given them by the manufacturers. The spectrophotometric calibrations by the manufacturers of these filters claim neutrality to within 5 per cent over the visible range. These calibrations were not checked in the present experiments. However, the photometric checks of the filters are sufficient, since the visibility curve of the Limulus eye (Hartline and Graham, '34) is closely similar to that of the human eye.

---

[3] As these lamps age, they tend to become unstable and it is difficult to maintain constant illumination of the pin-hole. They have been replaced in later experiments by a small tungsten filament lamp (photocell exciter lamp, used in talking pictures) operating at an overvoltage.

Since only relative intensities are of interest, a value of 1 is arbitrarily assigned to the highest intensity in a given experiment—i.e., the value of the intensity with no filters in the beam. The absolute value of the intensity is computed from measurements of the average intensity over the circle of illumination cast by the microscope objective at a given distance from the tiny image of the pin-hole. This intensity, and the diameter of the circle of illumination, gives the total amount of luminous flux, all of which has passed through the area of the small image. The average illumination over the area of the image computed in this manner is 3×10^6 meter candles.

The control of the duration of the exposures over a wide range is accomplished by means of a motor-driven rotating-disc shutter, similar in principle to one used in an earlier study (Hartline, '30). The present shutter was designed and built by Mr. A. J. Rawson, of this Foundation. It consists of a high speed rotating disc from which is cut a sector of known angular aperture. As this disc rotates in front of the pin-hole, it exposes the eye to light for a duration of time which depends upon the angular aperture in the disc and its speed of rotation. Interchangeable discs provide a choice of several different angular apertures, and the speed of rotation can be varied by an adjustable resistance in series with the armature of the driving motor. The speed can be adjusted to any desired value, to within about 4 per cent by the aid of a stroboscopic device; its exact value is determined by means of a mirror on the high-speed shaft which shines a light-signal onto the photographic record at each revolution of the shaft. Geared to the high-speed shaft is a low-speed disc with apertures large enough to permit passage of a single flash with the high speed disc of largest aperture. This serves to reduce the frequency of flashes to the point where a cam-operated shutter, which can be engaged at will by the operator, can single out one of them and close automatically before the next. The interval during which the eye is illuminated is recorded by a light signal from a second pin-hole exposed simultaneously with the pin-hole illuminating the eye.

With this exposure device it is possible to obtain flashes ranging in duration continuously from 0.0001 second to 1.0 second, accurate to about 1 per cent. The dimensions of the sector apertures and pin-hole are such that over most of this range the fraction of the flash during which the light is increasing and decreasing in intensity is small. Only for the very shortest flashes, from 0.0001 to 0.0005 second, is it large enough to be of possible significance—it is then 32 per cent of the total duration. From 0.0005 to 0.002 second it is 8 per cent of the total duration, from 0.002 to 0.04 second it is 2 per cent and from 0.04 second up it is 0.25 per cent. For exposures of 1.0 second the flash begins to lose its 'suddenness' of onset, since it then takes 0.00125 second for the edge of the sector to cross the pin-hole; hence longer durations are generally obtained by a manually operated shutter.

There is little possibility for error in the apparatus. Shutter and diaphragm are bolted securely to concrete bases to minimize mutual vibration. The cam-operated shutter is very light and has a positive action; even at the highest shutter speeds the parts which actuate it move slowly, and it is so arranged that if it operates at all it will be fully open before the beginning of the flash, and cannot close until after the end. The signal on the high speed shaft has shown that two consecutive revolutions take place in times constant to within 2 per cent for all speeds, to within less than 0.5 per cent for the higher speeds. It is believed that in this study both intensity and duration have been controlled with an accuracy of approximately 3 per cent.

b. Recording. The recording instruments have been described in the previous paper. The action potentials are passed through three stages of direct-coupled amplification to a power stage which actuates a Matthews oscillograph. The deflections are photographed on moving bromide paper along with the signal marking the period of illumination, and the one marking the revolutions of the high-speed shutter disc. The camera is driven by a synchronous motor geared directly to its shaft, giving a film speed which is uniform to within less than 0.5 per cent.

RESULTS

The response of a photoreceptor unit to illumination has been described in the previous paper (Hartline and Graham, '32). The discharge of nerve impulses from these sense cells is in all respects similar to the responses of other sense organs excited by their adequate stimuli. Beginning after a short latent period, the impulses come initially at a high frequency, which may rise slightly to a maximum, but then sinks in a regular manner, at first rapidly, then more slowly, approaching a final steady value which is maintained as long as the illumination lasts. The higher the intensity of the stimulating light, the higher is both the initial and final steady value of the discharge frequency, and the shorter is the initial latent period. When the stimulus is a short flash of light, the sense cell may still respond with a burst of impulses, the response being determined by the intensity and duration of the exposure. In figure 1 is reproduced an array of records obtained from a single photoreceptor unit. They show the effect of the two elements of the exposure—intensity and duration—upon the response. The horizontal rows of this figure show the effect of varying duration of the stimulating flash at a given constant intensity, the values of the durations being in geometric progression so that the flash in any given record has a duration ten times as long as the one immediately to the left of it. The vertical columns of the figure show the effect of varying intensity of the stimulating flash at a given constant duration, the values of the intensities being likewise in geometric progression, so that the flash in any given record has an intensity ten times as great as the one immediately below it. This choice of the intensities and durations results in the diagonals of the figure—from upper left to lower right —containing flashes for which the energy (product of intensity into duration) is constant. The energy of the flashes in a given one of these diagonals is ten times that in the diagonal immediately below and to the left of it.

Figure 1 shows that the effect of intensity described above for prolonged illumination is also to be seen in the responses to short flashes. The higher the intensity of a short flash of given duration, the shorter is the latent period of the response, the higher the frequency of the discharge and the greater the total number of impulses produced. It is furthermore seen that for short flashes the effect of duration is the same as the effect of intensity—the greater the duration of a short flash of given intensity, the stronger is the response of the sense cell. Figure 1 also shows that responses standing in a given diagonal, for which energy of flash is constant, are practically identical in all respects, provided one considers only short flashes—excluding the column on the extreme right (duration = 1 second). Moreover, this is true for each diagonal, from an energy just slightly above the threshold to one a hundred times as great, where the response is quite vigorous. There is thus a reciprocal relation existing between intensity and duration, in the stimulation of the single photoreceptor unit by short flashes which may be stated as follows: to produce a given constant response of a single photoreceptor cell, as measured by the impulses discharged over its attached nerve fibre, it is necessary that:

(1) $$I \cdot \tau = K_E$$

where I is the intensity of the light illuminating the sense cell, τ the duration of the flash, and K_E a constant whose value depends upon the magnitude of the response.

Fig. 1 Oscillograph records of action potentials from single optic nerve fibres of Limulus, in response to illumination of the eye by flashes of light of various intensities and durations. Horizontal rows contain responses to flashes of constant intensity and varying duration. Vertical columns contain responses to flashes of constant duration and varying intensity. Values of intensity of flash (in arbitrary units: 1 arbitrary unit = 3.0×10^6 meter candles on the surface of the eye) given at the right, opposite the respective rows. Values of duration of flash (in seconds) given at the top, above the respective columns.

In any given record the lower white line marks fifths of seconds; above this is a white line containing the light signal recording the interval during which the eye is illuminated. For very short flashes this signal does not reproduce clearly; its position is shown by the arrows. The black edge records electric potential between two points on the nerve fibre. At the top of each record is a row of black dots giving the speed of rotation of the shutter disk.

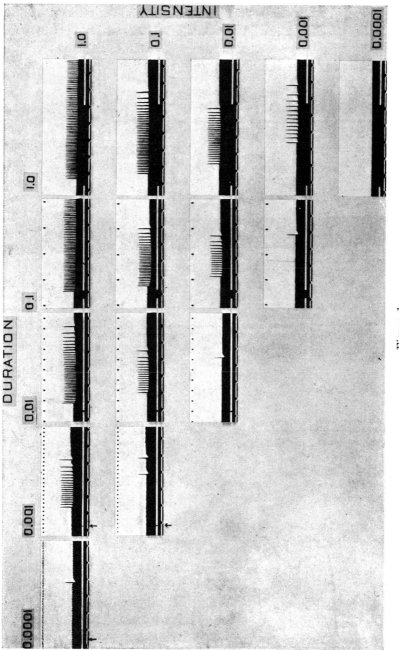

Figure 1

The validity of this statement as an approximation of the truth is evident from an inspection of figure 1. To provide a quantitative test for equation (1) certain features of the responses may be singled out and entered in a table, arranged

TABLE 1

Duration

0.0001	0.001	0.01	0.1	1.0		Intensity
a) 0.676 d) 1	a) 0.223 b) 31 c) 41 d) 18	a) 0.100 b) 50 c) 60 d) 39	a) 0.088 b) 53 c) 66 d) 101	a) 0.077 b) 54 c) 67 d) ca. 200	1.0	
	a) 0.610 b) 5 d) 2	a) 0.224 b) 31 c) 40 d) 16	a) 0.143 b) 46 c) 57 d) 31	a) 0.136 b) 44 c) 59 d) 43	0.1	
		a) 0.632 d) 1	a) 0.259 b) 32 c) 39 d) 16	a) 0.249 b) 32 c) 48 d) 27	0.01	
			a) 0.750 d) 1	a) 0.505 b) 18 c) 23 d) 13	0.001	
					0.0001	
				d) 0		

Measurements of the records of figure 1. Four features of the responses have been measured: a) latent period (time in seconds from the beginning of the stimulus flash to the first impulse); b) initial frequency for the first three impulses (reciprocal of one-half the interval of time between the first and the third impulses; c) maximum frequency (3 adjacent impulses); d) total number of impulses.

The measurements are arranged in the table so that each group of numbers occupies the same relative position as its corresponding record in figure 1.

as in figure 1. The features chosen are, a) latent period, b) initial frequency (first three impulses), c) maximum frequency (three impulses), d) total number of impulses. These four measurements, properly labeled, are entered in table 1, each group occupying the space corresponding to the position in figure 1 of its respective record. It is seen that corresponding numbers in a given diagonal of equal energy are in quite close agreement, provided again that the column on the extreme right is excluded.

The validity of the intensity-duration relationship of equation (1) can be more rigorously tested using a series of flashes of various intensities and durations, all having the same energy content ($I \cdot \tau =$ constant). The flashes are presented in a random order, and records obtained for several repetitions of each flash. That part of the experiment is then chosen over which time the control response to some one given flash shows as little and as uniform a drift in its various features as possible, and the measurements of all responses over this period are averaged. Several such experiments have been performed, using energies ranging from those only slightly above threshold to those for which the responses were quite vigorous. In all cases the reciprocity relation between intensity and duration (equation (1)) was substantiated, for short flashes within the limits of reproducibility of the results. An example is given in table 2.

Both tables 1 and 2 show a clear deviation from constancy of response for the flashes of longer duration. A little consideration shows that this is to be expected from the nature of the response with which we are dealing. In the first place, the latent period of the response shows a distinct lengthening with increased duration, an effect which is readily understood, for the deviations from constancy are first apparent in those cases where the duration of the flash is an appreciable fraction of the latent period itself. When the energy of the flash is spread out so that it is still accumulating at a time well into the latent period, it is to be expected that the appearance of the first impulse will be delayed.

A further restriction of equation (1) is rendered necessary by the consideration that an event in the response, such as appearance of the first impulse (determining the latent period), occurs at a given time with a given intensity of prolonged illumination. It is obviously meaningless to discuss the effect upon such an event of durations of flashes which are not yet over when this event takes place. The same logical restriction applies to such features of the response as the initial frequency, the maximum frequency, or any measurement involving the interval between any two impulses in the response. Consequently, a consideration of the reciprocity

TABLE 2

INTENSITY	DURATION (SECONDS)	LATENT PERIOD (SECONDS)	INITIAL FREQUENCY (IMPULSES PER SECOND)	MAXIMUM FREQUENCY (IMPULSES PER SECOND)	NUMBER OF IMPULSES
1.0	0.0010	0.242	42	56	13
0.50	0.0020	0.269	37	58	17
0.25	0.0040	0.244	42	57	14
0.10	0.010	0.257	40	56	14
0.050	0.020	0.267	38	55	15
0.025	0.040	0.268	40	56	14
0.010	0.10	0.299	37	56	14
0.0050	0.20	0.344	33	56	17
0.0025	0.40	0.373	26	46	15
0.0010	1.0	0.500	16	26	15

Responses of a single receptor to flashes of constant energy.

In the first and second left-hand columns are given respectively the intensities (in arbitrary units: 1 unit = 3×10^6 meter candles on the surface of the eye) and the durations (in seconds) of the flashes used to stimulate the eye. The energy (product of intensity into duration) of each of these flashes is the same (3×10^3 meter candles seconds). Four features of the responses were measured and are entered in the appropriately labeled column. Each figure is the average of 3 to 5 separate determinations, excepting those in the fourth row, which served as a control and was repeated thirteen times. The individual determinations for the control flash show an average deviation from the mean of about 5 per cent for latent period, 8 per cent for initial frequency, 6 per cent for maximum frequency and 20 per cent for total number of impulses. The deviation is in the form of a drift, all the numbers showing an increase with time. This is also apparent in the repetitions of flashes other than the control. Since all the individual determinations were taken in random order, it is legitimate to take the average for each flash. The experiment lasted about 7 hours.

relationship for any feature of the response which is of the nature of an 'event' taking place at a given time after the onset of illumination must be limited to those durations of exposure which are shorter than this time. This limitation clearly cannot be considered a failure of the reciprocity relationship in the photosensory process.

If, for any reason, this logical restriction is unrecognized, equation (1) will appear to fail for all durations greater than a certain critical value, which is the time at which the response of the sense cell takes place. Above this critical value of the duration only intensity can affect the response, and the condition for a constant response is simply that the intensity be constant. Equation (1) will then appear to be abruptly superseded at a duration τ_c, and the expression of the requirements for a constant response will be:

(1) $$I \cdot \tau = K_E \ ; \ \tau \leqslant \tau_c$$

(2) $$I = \text{Const.} = \frac{K_E}{\tau_c} \ ; \ \tau_c < \tau$$

It is not difficult to see how this logical restriction might be unrecognized in experiments such as those involving a subjective or reflex method in which the direct response of the sense cell is not recorded in its true time relations. Indeed the presence in the data of a transition from equation (1) to (2) might be the best evidence as to when the actual response of the sense cell takes place.

There is possibility for such a deviation even in the present experiments, for an impulse is determined within the sense cell at an instant which may be an appreciable time before its appearance under the electrodes. For flashes ending within this time the reciprocity relationship (1) will be superseded by equation (2). Evidence of this is to be seen in table 1. Choosing the second row ($I = 0.1$), it is seen that the initial frequency of the response increases with increasing duration of the stimulation flash, up to 0.1 second. Beyond this an increase of duration has no further effect, so the maximal initial frequency at this intensity is obtained in 0.1 second or less, even though the first of the two impulses determining this event does not appear until 0.143 second. Likewise in the row below this ($I = 0.01$) the highest value the initial frequency can have at this intensity, no matter how long the duration, is 32. This frequency can be obtained with a flash of this intensity lasting only 0.1 second, even though the impulses do not begin to appear until 0.259 second. Moreover, the initial frequency in the responses standing in the same diagonal as ($I = 0.01$, $\tau = 0.1$, but at higher intensities, are both 31. Equation (1) is thus seen to hold up to 0.1 second, equation (2) above that.

In studies similar to this it is customary to determine the energy of the flash ($I \cdot \tau$) necessary to produce a constant effect, and plot it against the duration (τ). With the help of additional information from the experiment, giving the effect of intensity on the response for various durations, it is possible to put the data of table 2 in this form. The result is plotted in figure 2, for initial and maximum frequency. In such a graph, equation (1) is a horizontal line, equation (2) an inclined line with a slope of unity, since logarithmic plotting has been employed. The critical duration is marked by the break in the line, and it is seen that it occurs at a distinctly shorter duration than the instant of appearance of the impulses concerned, marked in each case by arrows. It is also to be noted that the critical duration for the initial frequency is shorter than that for the maximum frequency.

The above remarks have been concerned with latent period, initial frequency, and maximum frequency—features which are of the nature of an event within the response. They may be applied to any feature which is of this nature. The total number of impulses, however, is clearly in a different category. It is not reckoned until everything is over. Both tables 1 and 2 indicate that for it, too, the reciprocity relation holds, and for even longer durations than any of the other features considered. It is clear that it cannot continue to hold for all durations, first, because of the linear relation between frequency and logarithm of intensity (Hartline and Graham, '32) for the steady level of discharge; second, because very long exposures would necessitate an intensity which is below threshold, for which no impulses are produced at all. This threshold intensity constitutes an additional limitation of the reciprocity relation, and is well illustrated in table 1. The very lowest intensity ($I = 0.0001$) produced no impulses at all when shining for 1 second, al-

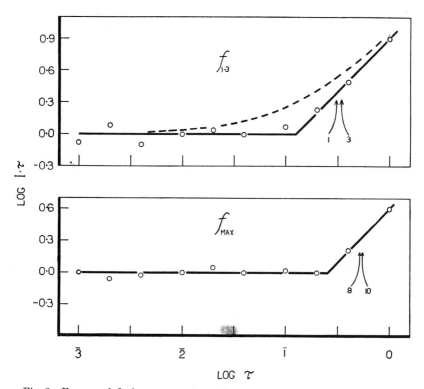

Fig. 2 Energy of flash necessary to produce a constant response as a function of duration of flash from the data of table 2. The ordinates give the logarithms (base 10) of energy of flash necessary to produce a constant response (1 unit of energy $= 3 \times 10^3$ meter candle seconds). Abscissae give the logarithms (base 10) of the duration of flash (seconds). The upper curve gives the energy necessary to produce an initial frequency (first three impulses) of 40 per second. The lower curve gives the energy necessary to produce a maximum frequency (three impulses) of 56 per second. In order to present the data of table 2 in this way it is necessary to measure the effect of varying intensity of a flash of given duration upon the initial and maximum frequencies. This was done for $\tau = 0.01$ second, and serves for all flashes of 0.1 second and less; separate determinations of the effect of intensity were made for each duration greater than 0.1 second.

The time of appearance of each of the impulses concerned in the measurement is indicated by an arrow with the number of the respective impulse.

The solid lines are graphs of equation (1) and (2). The dotted curve is the graph of equation (3) (see text). The circles are experimental points.

though flashes of equal energy, but higher intensity, were able to produce at least one impulse. Indeed, this same intensity (0.0001) when allowed to shine for 10 seconds was still unable to produce any impulses, and experience has shown that if none are produced within 2 or at most 3 seconds, then no matter how long the light continues to shine, no impulses will appear. This intensity limits, not only the diagonal of lowest energy, but all the others as well.

DISCUSSION

The present experiments on excitation of single visual sense cells show that a reciprocal relation exists between the intensity of a stimulating flash and its duration, provided the duration is small with respect to the time of appearance of the response. In this they are in agreement with the other experiments (compare Hecht, '29; '31). The present experiments have shown that when certain features of the response, such as initial or maximum frequency, are considered this reciprocity relationship is limited by a critical duration. The critical duration for a given feature of the response is, moreover, shorter than the time of appearance of the impulses concerned. The suggestion is made that the response of the sense cell actually occurs at an appreciably earlier time than the appearance of impulses under the electrodes, and that this time marks the critical duration. Preliminary experiments indicate that only a small fraction of the interval between critical duration and time of appearance of the response is delay due to conduction time from sense cell to electrodes. This interval presumably is occupied by processes intervening between the photochemical activity and the elaboration of impulses.

The existence of a 'critical duration,' and its importance in limiting the reciprocity law, has been discussed by Adrian and Matthews ('27), who related it to McDougall's ('04) 'action time,' and by the present author ('28). In both of these papers the delimiting action of the critical duration appears to be fairly sharp, as though the action of the light is abruptly interrupted by the reaction of the sense cells. Subjective measurements on the human eye, however (Blondel and Rey, '11, and Piéron, '20), show instead of a distinct critical duration a gradual deviation from the reciprocity law at longer durations. Blondel and Rey fit their data quite successfully by the equation:

(3) $$I \cdot \tau = A + B \cdot \tau ,$$

which has as asymptotes equations (1) and (2).

It is not unreasonable to suppose that the absence of a clearly marked critical duration in these subjective experiments may be due to the activity of many sense cells, and to the long nervous paths involved. On the other hand, Hecht ('29) has shown that the 'back' reaction of the photosensory process, whereby products of photolysis combine independently of light to re-form the photosensitive substance, will produce a deviation from the reciprocity law which can be described by equation (3). This interpretation might also be applied to the present experiments, to account for the deviation from the reciprocity law in the short range of durations immediately preceding the appearance of the impulses. However, this would not account for the longer critical durations of features which appear later in the response, nor for the fact that for total number of impulses, for which there is no critical duration, the reciprocity relationship holds for even longer durations than have been investigated here. Moreover, the 'back' reaction was postulated to account for dark adaptation—a process which is very slow (compare Hartline, '30), and it seems doubtful if it could be appreciable in the very short flashes under consideration, especially since the amount of light adaptation induced by the total flash is very small.

These considerations support the position that for the intensities and durations used in the present experiments the photochemical basis of the sensory process may be considered a simple system, to which the reciprocity law of Bunsen and Roscoe may be applied, and that the apparent deviations from this law for the latter part of the range of durations which may logically be considered is due to the active response of the sense cell occurring at an appreciable time before its impulses are observed.

SUMMARY

Action potentials in single fibres of the optic nerve of Limulus polyphemus have been recorded by means of amplifier and oscillograph. The response of the single visual sense cell, in terms of the impulses it discharges in its attached nerve fibre, has been investigated when the sense cell is stimulated by flashes of light of various intensities and durations.

Increasing the intensity of a flash of given duration shortens the latent period of the response, raises the frequency and increases the total number of impulses discharged. Increasing the duration of a flash of given intensity has a similar effect, provided only short flashes are considered (less than the latent period). There is a reciprocal relation between intensity and duration in the stimulation of the single receptor cell: to produce a given constant effect, it is necessary that the energy of the stimulating flash (product of intensity into duration) be constant. This holds strictly for all features of the response, provided the duration is short compared to the latent period. This is taken as indicating that the photosensory mechanism has a simple photochemical basis to which the Bunsen-Roscoe law may be applied.

It is pointed out that for features which are of the nature of an event in the response (such as initial or maximum frequency), only those durations which are shorter than the time of appearance of the event may be considered logically. If this restriction should be unrecognized, the reciprocity relationship will appear to fail, and the condition for constant response will be that the intensity must be constant. The experiments show that, for both initial and maximum frequency, the reciprocity relationship fails, and is superseded by the condition $I =$ constant, at a critical duration which is appreciably shorter than the time of appearance of the impulses determining the particular feature of the response. This is interpreted as indicating that the impulses are determined within the sense cell at a time which is appreciably earlier than their appearance under the electrodes.

Part of the expenses of this study were met by a grant-in-aid from the National Research Council.

LITERATURE CITED

ADRIAN, E. D., AND R. MATTHEWS 1927 a The action of light on the eye. J. Physiol., vol. 64, p. 279.

BLOCH, A. M. 1885 Expériences sur la vision. C. r. Soc. Biol., T. 2, p. 493.

BLONDEL, A., AND J. REY 1911 Sur la perception des lumières brèves à la limite de leur portée. J. d. Physique, series 5, T. 1, p. 530.

HARTLINE, H. K. 1928 A quantitative and descriptive study of the electric response to illumination of the arthropod eye. Am. J. Physiol., vol. 83, p. 466.

———— 1930 The dark adaptation of the eye of Limulus, as manifested by its electric response to illumination. J. Gen. Physiol., vol. 13, p. 379.

———— 1933 The discharge of impulses in the optic nerve in response to flashes of light of short duration. Am. J. Physiol., vol. 105, p. 45.

HARTLINE, H. K., AND C. H. GRAHAM 1932 Nerve impulses from single receptors in the eye. J. Cell. and Comp. Physiol., vol. 1, p. 277.

———— 1934 The spectral sensitivity of single visual sense cells. Am. J. Physiol., vol. 109, p. 49.

HECHT, S. 1929 The nature of the photoreceptor process. Found. Exp. Psychol., p. 216. Clark Univ. Press, Worcester, Mass.

———— 1931 Die Physikalische Chemie und die Physiologie des Sehaktes. Ergebnisse d. Physiol., Bd. 32, S. 243.

McDOUGALL, W. 1904 The variation of the intensity of visual sensation with the duration of the stimulus. Brit. J. Psychol., vol. 1, p. 151.

PIÉRON, H. 1920 De la variation de l'énergie luminaire en fonction de la durée d'excitation pour la vision fovéale. C. r. Acad. Sci., T. 170, p. 525.

———— 1920 De la variation de l'énergie luminaire en fonction de la durée d'excitation pour la vision périphérique. C. r. Acad. Sci., T. 170, p. 1203.

Light and dark adaptation of single photoreceptor elements in the eye of *Limulus*

H. KEFFER HARTLINE[1] AND P. ROBB MCDONALD[2]

Johnson Research Foundation and Department of Ophthalmology,
University of Pennsylvania, Philadelphia

Reprinted from the JOURNAL OF CELLULAR AND
COMPARATIVE PHYSIOLOGY, Vol. 30, no. 3, pp. 225–253, December 1947

It is generally believed that the salient features of light and dark adaptation are determined by basic changes in the individual receptor cells of the visual mechanism. Biochemical studies of the visual pigments of the receptors of the vertebrate retina support this view and provide a possible explanation of these changes. As yet, however, there have been no systematic studies of the effects of light and dark adaptation on the action of individual visual receptor elements, in terms that are of known neurological significance. Such studies might be expected to yield direct information concerning the extent to which the receptor elements contribute to light and dark adaptation of the visual system and to provide a link between the biochemistry of visual pigments and the action of the higher visual centers. It is the purpose of this paper to report the extent to which the sensitivity changes generally ascribed to the photoreceptor endings may actually be demonstrated in them; how the discharge of nerve impulses by a single receptor cell is modified by light and dark adaptation, and the effects of various intensities and durations of light

[1] Preparation of this paper was made under Contract N6-onr-249 Task Order II, between the University of Pennsylvania and the Office of Naval Research, U. S. Navy.

[2] Research Fellow in Ophthalmology, 1938–1940.

adaptation upon the subsequent recovery of sensitivity of a single receptor element during dark adaptation.[3]

The discharge of nerve impulses by single photoreceptor elements may be investigated by using the excised lateral eye of *Limulus,* from which single optic nerve fibers are isolated. In *Limulus,* the fibers of the optic nerve are axones of the visual receptor cells in the eye; there are no neural elements intervening (Hartline and Graham, '32).

METHOD

The methods used in this study have been described in previous papers (Hartline and Graham, '32; Hartline, '34). In each experiment, the excised lateral eye and optic nerve of an adult *Limulus* was mounted in a moist chamber; a small bundle of fibers was dissected from the optic nerve and placed on recording electrodes to permit the oscillographic recording of its amplified action potentials. This bundle was dissected until the action potential spikes showed the regularity of discharge and uniformity of size and shape that may be taken as evidence that only a single nerve fiber remained active in the bundle. The eye was stimulated by a small spot of light imaged on it by a low power microscope objective, confined to the facet containing the visual sense cell which gave rise to activity in the particular nerve fiber under observation.

In all experiments reported here, temperature was controlled at 18°C. ± 0.1°.

APPARATUS

In the early experiments reported in this paper the arrangements for illuminating the eye were identical with those described in previous papers. An image of an incandescent tungsten filament was formed upon a pinhole which in turn was imaged on the eye by a microscope objective. Intensity was varied by the insertion of calibrated Wratten neutral tint

---

[3] An abstract of a brief report of the present investigations has been published (Hartline and McDonald, '41).

filters in the beam (Hartline and Graham, '32). Duration of exposure for short test flashes was controlled by the rotating-disk shutter described in a previous paper (Hartline, '34). In later experiments, greater flexibility was achieved by a re-design of this equipment.[4] Two independently controlled channels of illumination were provided, one for the light-adapting exposures, the second for providing test exposures. For each channel, an image of the incandescent filament of the common source was formed on an aperture 1 mm $\times$ 4 mm controlled by a pulse-operated electro-magnetic shutter. The intensity[5] of the source was monitored by a vacuum photocell, to a constancy of 1%. Calibrated Wratten neutral-tint filters for the control of intensity were placed in the beam 2 cm beyond the aperture. Light passed through the aperture to illuminate a condensing lens, 10 cm in diameter at a distance of 40 cm, which formed an image of the aperture on half of an objective lens system located 100 cm beyond, each channel utilizing its respective half. The objective system formed superposed images of each illuminated condensing lens on the eye at a demagnification of 40 to 1. The resulting circular area of illumination, 25 mm in diameter, could be further restricted by the insertion of diaphragms close to the condensing lenses. Thus small spots of light could be caused to fall anywhere within an area 25 mm in diameter on the eye. The spots formed by the different channels of illumination could be adjusted independently in size and location within the 25-mm circle, but in the present experiments they were kept equal in size (0.2 mm diameter) and were both adjusted to illuminate the same facet of the eye. The intensities and times of exposure of the

[4] Constructed by Mr. A. J. Rawson. Funds for the construction of this equipment were furnished by the John and Mary Markle Foundation, through the Department of Ophthalmology, University of Pennsylvania Hospital.

[5] Since only relative values of intensity are of interest, it is convenient throughout this paper to express intensities in terms of an arbitrary unit of illumination (approximately 25 lumens per cm^2, measured on the surface of the eye). This was the highest intensity available with the 2-channel optical system; the earlier system provided approximately 10 times as much illumination.

2 superimposed spots were, however, varied independently in accordance with the requirements of the experiments.

Each of the electro-magnetic shutters [6] controlling the exposure consisted of a soft iron armature (20 mm × 5 mm × ¼ mm) mounted on a stiff steel wire shaft between 2 iron pole-pieces attached to a small "horse-shoe" permanent magnet. The pole pieces were U-shaped, mounted with their open ends toward each other and the ends of their limbs separated by a gap of about 1¼ mm. The armature was so mounted that it could take up 1 of 2 positions of equilibrium diagonally across the gap between the U's. A fixed coil of wire encircling the armature and filling the space inside the U's permitted the armature to be driven from 1 position of equilibrium to the other by suitably directed short pulses of current (½ millisecond duration, 150 milliamperes). Attached to 1 end of the iron armature was a light, strong vane (20 mm × 5 mm) made of black paper impregnated with celluloid which served as the shutter to occlude the aperture through which the light passed. The distance travelled by the vane in moving from 1 position of equilibrium to the other was 3 mm; the width of the aperture was 2 mm, allowing a small extra margin of movement to take care of possible "bounce" and vibration of the armature and vane. Observation with a cathode-ray oscilloscope and photocell showed that the shutters opened (or closed) in ½ millisecond and once properly adjusted were free from any evidence of bounce. Operation of the shutter was perfectly reliable for all exposures down to 2 milliseconds. A "signal" beam was diverted from the main beam of illumination through each aperture and reflected into the recording camera.

Duration of exposure was controlled by electronic timers [7] consisting of mono-stable multivibrators triggering the pulses to the shutters. With these timers the interval between the "on" pulse and the "off" pulse could be varied from 2 milliseconds (limit set by the speed of action of the shutters) to 10

[6] Designed and constructed by A. J. Rawson.

[7] Designed by John P. Hervey.

seconds, and the operation of the shutter in 1 channel could be delayed with respect to the other by any desired interval within these time limits. Time calibrations were constant to within $\frac{1}{2}\%$. For exposures and delays longer than 10 seconds, manual switches were used to control the shutters.

RESULTS

Prolonged illumination of a visual receptor in the eye of *Limulus* elicits a discharge of nerve impuses at a frequency that is high initially. Within a few seconds the frequency of discharge decreases markedly, then more slowly, and although it never ceases as long as light of moderate intensity continues to shine steadily, the effectiveness of the stimulus after several seconds is less than at first. When the light is turned off, this process of light adaptation is reversed; a test flash of constant magnitude applied to the eye elicits bursts of impulses discharged in greater number and at higher frequency the longer the eye remains in the dark, until the maximum sensitivity of the receptor has been recovered. The present experiments deal mainly with this recovery of sensitivity of the visual sense cell following periods of light adaptation of various intensities and durations.

An illustrative experiment is recorded in figure 1. An eye that had been kept in the dark for more than an hour was illuminated by light of moderately high intensity for a period of 2 minutes; at various times after turning off this light, test flashes of constant intensity and duration were applied. Records of the brief bursts of impulses discharged in response to the test flashes are reproduced in the figure, showing the progressive increase in the number of nerve impulses elicited by the test flash as the preparation was allowed to remain in darkness. The increase was rapid for the first few minutes, then more gradual; the receptor required approximately an hour to reach a final level of maximum sensitivity. At the end of this time, the response was equal to that elicited by an equal test flash prior to the light adapting exposure.

Not only did the total number of impulses in the response increase as dark adaptation progressed, but the duration of the activity lengthened and the frequency of the discharge also increased, although in a less striking manner (cf. Hartline, '32). The latency of the response, on the other hand, showed very little change. Thus exposure to light decreased the ability of the receptor to discharge nerve impulses in response to a test flash of fixed magnitude; following the return to darkness, the receptor gradually recovered its ability to respond to the test flash. Light adaptation and dark adapta-

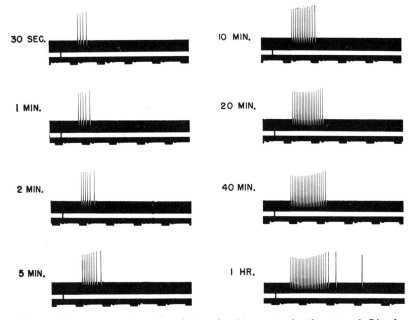

Fig. 1 Dark adaptation of a single visual receptor in the eye of *Limulus*. Oscillograms of the amplified action potentials of a single optic nerve fiber, showing the discharge of impulses in response to a test flash of light of fixed intensity applied to the eye at various times in the dark (given at the left of each record) following a period of light adaptation. In each record, deflections of the upper black edge are the amplified action potential spikes of a single active fiber in a small bundle dissected from the rest of the optic nerve and slung across electrodes connected to the input of a vacuum tube amplifier. On the lower black edge are time marks (1/5 second); the white band just above contains the signal of the test flash (narrow black stripe near the left hand edge; flash duration: 0.008 second).

tion are thus shown to be properties of the single visual sense cell, in the eye of *Limulus*.

This experiment parallels the familiar experience, that a light of fixed intensity seen faintly by the light-adapted observer appears brighter and brighter as dark adaptation progresses. Measurement of this subjective experience has been made by Wright ('34, '37), Johannsen ('34) and Schouten and Ornstein ('39) by the method of binocular matching.

It is evident from the preceeding description that the visual receptor undergoes large changes in sensitivity during light and dark adaptation. The strict usage of the term "sensitivity," however, requires the determination of the intensity of stimulus necessary to elicit a response of fixed magnitude in some particular attribute, rather than measurement of the magnitude of that attribute of the response elicited by a stimulus of fixed intensity. In this paper, sensitivity will be defined as the reciprocal of the energy of test flash necessary to elicit just 1 nerve impulse. Figure 2 presents the results of an experiment in which the increase of sensitivity during dark adaptation was measured directly and recorded by plotting the fall of threshold as a function of time in the dark. In this experiment the test flashes applied after a period of light adaptation were varied in intensity and duration, and the energy value required to elicit a response of just 1 nerve impulse was determined by trial. This determination of threshold was repeated a number of times during the course of the recovery from the exposure to light. In figure 2 the logarithms of the threshold energies are plotted as ordinates against the time after cessation of the light adaptation as abscissae. After 40–60 minutes in darkness, another exposure to light was made, and the course of recovery was followed again. Several such repetitions are plotted in figure 2. The initial fall in threshold was rapid, becoming more and more gradual, the threshold approaching asymptotically a level close to its value prior to light adaptation. The total change in threshold between the value a few seconds after the adapting light was turned off, and the level finally attained

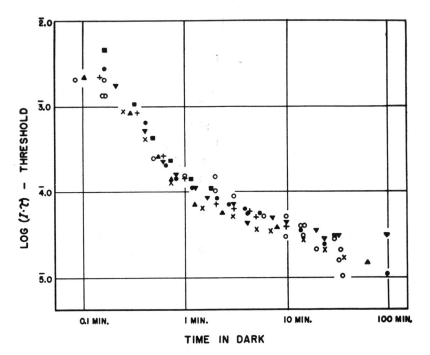

Fig. 2 Dark adaptation of a single receptor in the eye of *Limulus*. Fall in threshold following a period of light adaptation. Ordinates: logarithm of the energy $(1 \cdot \tau)$ of test flash just necessary to elicit the discharge of 1 impulse in a single optic nerve fiber. Intensity (I) of test flash in arbitrary units (1 arb. unit = 25 lumens cm^2). Duration (τ) of test flash in seconds. Flash intensity was varied by filters in steps of 0.3 or 0.4 logarithmic units; smaller energy steps were obtained by varying the duration in 1 millisecond steps between 5 and 10 milliseconds. Abscissae: time in the dark (in minutes, plotted on a logarithmic scale) after the cessation of the light adapting exposure. Light adapting exposure: 1 arb. unit for 1 second.

Five consecutive ''runs'' were made; in each, the threshold change was followed for an hour or more, after which the light adapting exposure was repeated and the threshold change followed again. The various solid symbols show the results for the separate runs. Interspersed with the threshold determinations, records were obtained of the discharge of impulses elicited by a test flash of fixed energy (1 arb. unit, 0.010 second); from the number of impulses in the responses and from a curve relating number of impulses and energy of test flash (obtained after complete dark adaptation), the threshold was calculated as explained in the text. The values of threshold so calculated are plotted as open circles in this figure.

after an hour in darkness, was over 2 logarithmic units; even greater changes have been observed in other experiments. The agreement among the various repetitions in this experiment is noteworthy since the eye was excised and devoid of its normal circulation of blood. In most of our experiments the results were quantitatively reproducible over the period of 6 or 8 hours.

The fall in threshold recorded in figure 2 is typical of the course of dark adaptation as measured in a wide variety of animals by numerous investigators; the way in which this experiment has been done makes it exactly analogous to the determination of the course of dark adaptation in human observers. As is well known, human dark adaptation curves usually show 2 distinct segments, as first the cones and subsequently the rods adapt, whereas the *Limulus* receptor yields only a single smooth recovery curve. In its approximate form, however, and in the range covered by the sensitivity changes, the recovery curve of figure 2 resembles the curve of human dark adaptation. It is generally believed, for good reasons, that the sensitivity changes in the visual system which take place during light and dark adaptation are mainly to be ascribed to the receptor elements of the eye. The present results provide direct evidence that, for the eye of *Limulus*, the receptor cells do indeed manifest typical adaptation effects in their discharge of nerve impulses. They show, moreover, that the sensitivity changes of an individual receptor element cover a range comparable to that undergone by the entire visual system of most animals. They do not, of course, entirely exclude the possibility of additional factors in the light and dark adaptation of visual systems in general, associated with the functional organization of the receptors and higher neurones (Schouten and Ornstein, '39; Lythgoe, '40).

The experiments of figure 1 and figure 2 present 2 ways of describing the fundamental change in sensitivity of the *Limulus* visual sense cell during dark adaptation. These 2 presentations are related, as is demonstrated in the experiment of figure 3. This figure shows the relation between the number of impulses discharged by a visual sense cell and the intensity (log I) of the stimulating flash of light, for the condition of complete dark adaptation and for 3 levels of light adaptation. The responses in the light adapted conditions were obtained by exposing the eye to the desired intensity for 10 minutes; the illumination was then interrupted at 2-minute intervals for a period of 2 seconds; in the middle of each interruption a test flash was applied. The figure shows that the brighter the adapting light the fewer were the

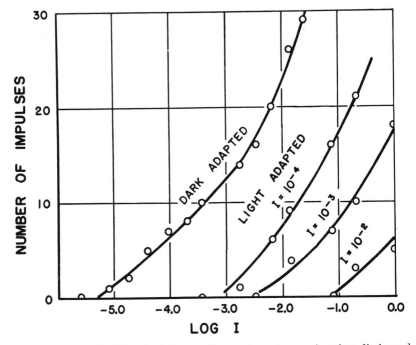

Fig. 3 Effect of light adaptation on the number of nerve impulses discharged by a single receptor in response to flashes of light of various intensities. Ordinates: number of impulses elicited by a test flash (duration: 0.010 second). Abscissae: logarithm of test flash intensity (in arb. units). Points on the left hand curve were obtained with the eye completely dark adapted (2 hours or more after previous light adaptation). Right hand curves were obtained with the eye light adapted to various intensities (values given on each curve, in arb. units). For each curve, eye was exposed for 10 minutes or more to adapting light, which was then interrupted at intervals of 2 minutes for a period of 2 seconds; in the middle of each interruption a test flash was applied.

number of impulses discharged in response to a test flash
of given intensity; alternatively, the more intense was it necessary to make the test flash to produce a given constant number
of impulses. Within the limits of reproducibility of the results, the points on the 3 right hand curves of figure 3 may all
be considered to be fitted by the left-hand curve shifted to the
right by various amounts. Since a logarithmic intensity scale
has been used in figure 3, it follows that the variation of
number of impulses in the response with the ratio of the
intensity of the test flash to its threshold value was not affected by light adaptation; the receptor was merely adjusted
to lower levels of sensitivity. The amount that the "dark-
adapted" curve of figure 3 must be displaced horizontally to
fit the points for a given condition of light adaptation may be
taken as a measure (in terms of log I) of the decrease in sensitivity induced by the light adaptation. It is clear, of course,
that the measurement of a threshold by trial constitutes a
direct determination of this displacement for a response of
just 1 impulse, but figure 3 shows in addition that any other
arbitrary number of impulses could be chosen as a criterion
of response without greatly affecting the value of the measured sensitivity change. Other experiments similar to that
of figure 3 gave analogous results.[8]

Since the number of impulses in a response to a test flash
is determined by the ratio of the flash intensity to the threshold, for any condition of adaptation, it is possible to compute
the value of the threshold from the number of impulses in a
supra-threshold response to a flash of known intensity. For

[8] In a previous paper one of us (Hartline, '30) has shown that the course of
dark adaptation in intact *Limulus* could be followed by recording "retinal"
action potentials from the eye. The same kind of analysis as that just presented
was made in this earlier study. It was shown that dark adaptation could be followed either by recording the responses to a test flash of constant intensity, or by
calculating the sensitivity on the basis of intensity required to produce a response
of constant magnitude (amplitude of the initial "wave" of potential change).
The similiarity between the rise and fall of retinal action potential, recorded
from an isolated ommatidium, and the frequency of discharge of nerve impulses
in the axones of the retinula cells (Hartline, '35) suggests that these 2 signs
of sense-cell activity are intimately related.

this purpose, it is only necessary to obtain 1 curve relating intensity of test flash and number of impulses at some fixed level of adaptation. In the experiment of figure 2, the direct determinations of thresholds during dark adaptation were interspersed with records of responses to a test flash of fixed intensity, and when the eye was dark adapted a curve was obtained relating test flash intensity with number of impulses in the response. The corresponding "computed thresholds" are plotted (open circles) in figure 2. These points show that the values of threshold thus computed agree satisfactorily with those observed by direct trial (solid symbols).

It is often more convenient to map the course of dark adaptation by recording the responses to a test flash of fixed intensity than by the more laborious method of determining threshold by direct trial. Consequently, the demonstration that the 2 methods are equivalent is of practical utility; in most of the experiments to be reported in the remainder of this paper a test flash of constant intensity was employed.

The loss of sensitivity following exposure to light, and the time required for the receptor to regain its dark adaptation were strongly affected by the duration of the light adapting exposure. This is shown in figure 4 where the number of impulses elicited by a test flash of fixed magnitude was determined at various times during the recovery from various durations of exposure to illumination of a fixed intensity. Each one of these curves shows the same general time-course of dark adaptation as that indicated by figure 1, i.e., a rapid recovery of sensitivity at the beginning, proceeding with steadily diminishing rate to approach the final dark adapted level asymptotically. The greater the light adapting exposure, the greater was the initial loss of sensitivity and the longer was the time required for complete recovery. The light adapting effect increased rapidly with increasing short exposures, then more gradually; this is shown in figure 4 by the necessity of choosing durations that increase by factors of 10 in order to yield approximately equal spacing of the first points (time in dark = 10 seconds) of the respective recovery

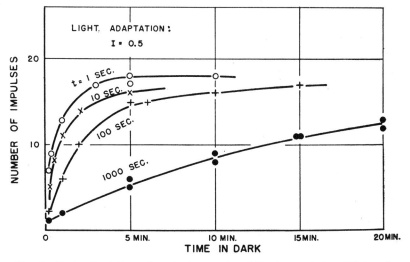

Fig. 4   Dark adaptation of a single receptor following periods of light adaptation of various durations. Ordinates: number of impulses elicited by a test flash of constant intensity (5 arb. units) and duration (0.010 seconds). Abscissae: time in the dark (in minutes, linear scale) following the end of the period of light adaptation. Intensity (I) of light adapting exposures; 0.5 arb. units. Durations (t) of light adapting exposures on respective curves.

curves. These results demonstrate that light adaptation of single receptor elements increases progressively during prolonged exposure to light.[9] We have found light adaptation at moderate intensities to be approximately complete only after many (10–20) minutes of illumination. This is comparable to the course of light adaptation when measured by comparable

[9] Riggs and Graham ('40) investigated light adaptation of single receptor elements in *Limulus* by measuring the increment in frequency in the extra burst of impulses elicited by adding a short test flash to the steady adapting illumination. The "sensitivity," defined by them as the reciprocal of the intensity required to elicit a constant increment in frequency, was found to rise during the first 30 seconds of illumination, and then to fall steadily thereafter. Perhaps their choice of criterion was responsible for this phenomenon. In our experiments, determination of the threshold after the adapting light was turned off has shown only a decreased sensitivity, compared with the dark-adapted condition. This loss in sensitivity resulting from the pre-exposure has been found to increase steadily with increasing duration of light adaptation, as described above.

methods in visual systems of human observers (Wald and Clark, '37).

Not only the duration, but also the intensity of the light-adapting exposure affected the subsequent recovery of sensitivity by the visual receptor units. In figure 5, recovery curves are shown that were obtained following exposures of 10 seconds duration to light of various intensities. The

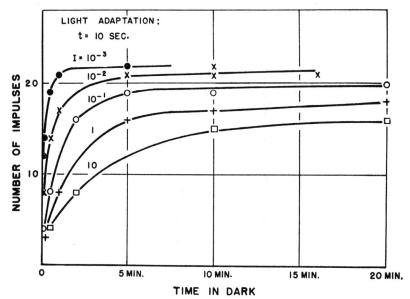

Fig. 5 Dark adaptation of a single receptor following periods of adaptation to light of various intensities. Ordinates: number of impulses elicited by a test flash of constant intensity (1 arb. unit) and duration (0.010 second). Abscissae: time in the dark (in minutes, linear scale). Duration (t) of light adapting exposures; 10 seconds. Intensities (I) of light adapting exposures given on respective curves, in arbitrary units.

greater the intensity of the adapting exposures, the greater was the initial loss of sensitivity and the longer was the time required for recovery. It is noteworthy that the light-adapting effect of intensity covered a considerable range; eventual recovery (in 1½ hours) took place even after the highest intensity available, and yet an exposure to 1/10,000 of this intensity produced significant loss of sensitivity that required at least 1 minute for its restoration. Measurable losses have been shown following intensities as low as $I = 10^{-6}$, which were themselves just too weak to elicit any impulses from the receptor. Uusually, light adapting effects failed to appear only when the intensity was less than approximately 1/10 of the threshold value.

These effects of intensity and duration of the light adapting exposure on the subsequent dark adaptation of the visual receptor elements of the *Limulus* eye resemble very closely those that have been described extensively for most of the visual systems that have been studied, especially with human observers. This similarity includes many significant details, as will now be described.

In the curves of figures 4 and 5 it may be noted that the long recovery time following strong light adaptation was partly the result of the large initial loss of sensitivity which had to be recovered, but also because of an over-all slowing of the dark-adaptation process. If the slopes of the curves of figures 4 or 5 are measured at a fixed level of sensitivity, it may be seen that the rate of dark adaptation was greatest following the smallest amount of light adaptation and decreased progressively with increasing intensity or duration of pre-exposure. Thus, in figure 5 the slopes of the recovery curves measured at an ordinate level of 15 impulses (7 impulses less than the number in the response after complete recovery) are 14 impulses in the response per minute of recovery ($I = 10^{-3}$ curve), 6 impulses per minute (10^{-2}), 3 impulses per minute (10^{-1}), 1.2 impulses per minute (1) and 0.3 impulses per minute (10). Translated into terms of sensitivity by means of a curve relating intensity of test flash to number of impulses in the response, this means that at a level 0.5 logarithmic units below the final dark-adapted sensitivity, recovery proceeded at a rate of 0.95, 0.4, 0.2, 0.08 and 0.02 logarithmic units per minute for the respective curves. Similar results may be obtained for the curves of figure 4.

If the recovery process of dark adaptation were a simple one, governed for example by a simple chemical reaction of regeneration of photosensitive material in the sense cell, the rate of recovery would be expected to depend only on how far the system was displaced from its final level of equilibrium. Such a property has been demonstrated by Clark ('38) for the dark adaptation of *Dineutes;* recovery curves following various amounts of light adaptation were shown to be fragments of a single curve and could all be superimposed by shifting horizontally by various amounts. It is evident from figures 4 and 5 that this simple property does not apply to the dark adaptation of the *Limulus* visual sense cell. Instead, *Limulus* recovery curves resemble the rod portions of the family of curves obtained with human observers (Müller, '31; Winsor and Clark, '36; Hecht, Haig and Chase, '37; Wald and Clark, '37; Haig, '41; Crawford, '47). Indeed, if the data are translated into terms of logarithm of threshold change (as may be visualized roughly by imagining figures 4 and 5 reflected in a horizontal axis); the resemblance to the data of human dark adaptation is striking. For the human eye, Winsor and Clark ('36) and Wald and Clark ('37) have suggested that the slow recovery characteristically following long or intense light adaptation is the result of the conversion of a large fraction of retinene into vitamin A. From vitamin A the regeneration of visual purple is much slower than from retinene directly. An analogous visual cycle could be invoked to explain the present data.

The similarity between the curves of figures 4 and those of figure 5 suggests that they are all members of 1 family, and that within limits recovery can be caused to follow one or another of the members of this family by changing either the intensity or the duration of the light adapting exposure. Comparison of the figures suggests, moreover, that changing the intensity by a given factor had much the same effect as changing its duration by the same factor, that is, the light adapting effect of an exposure appears to depend only upon its total quantity of light (product of intensity by duration). Direct experimental evidence in support of these observations is presented in figures 6 and 7.

In figure 6 are plotted points representing the course of dark adaptation following 4 different light adapting exposures for which the intensities and durations were adjusted to yield equal "initial" losses in sensitivity (measured 10 seconds after turning off the adapting light). In the subsequent recoveries, it is to be noted that the points all fall along

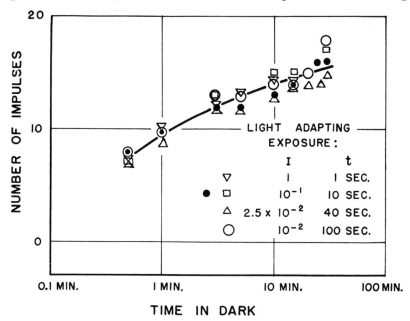

Fig. 6   Dark adaptation of a single receptor following periods of adaptation to light of different intensities (I) and durations (t) such that the total energy (I·t) of the adapting exposure was constant. Ordinates: number of impulses elicited by a test flash of constant intensity (0.1 arb. unit) and duration (0.008 seconds). Abscissae: time in the dark (minutes, logarithmic scale). Intensities (arb. units) and durations of light adapting exposure as given for respective symbols.

a single curve, even though the exposure components were varied by a factor of 100. Figure 7 is similar, and is from another experiment in which the range covered was even greater. It is to be noted, furthermore, that the necessary adjustment of intensity and duration was that which gave their product the same value. With notable exception (to be described below), the dark adaptation of the *Limulus* visual sense cell can be made to follow any one of the family of recovery curves represented in figures 4 and 5 by adjusting either the intensity or the duration of the light adapting exposure. To achieve this, it is necessary only that the total quantity of light in the exposure be given the proper value. This reciprocity relation holds over a surprisingly large range of values of intensity and duration.

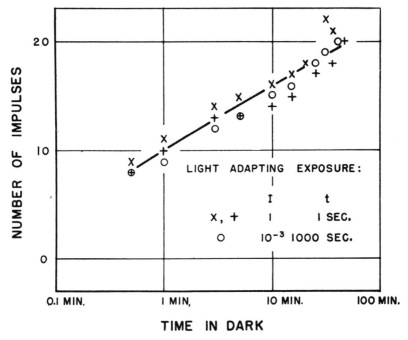

Fig. 7 Dark adaptation of single receptor, as in figure 6.

Analogous properties have been reported for light and dark adaptation of human observers by Haig ('41) for scotopic vision, and by Crawford ('46) for both photopic and scotopic visual mechanisms. Not only were similar dark adaptation curves obtained by suitable adjustment of either intensity or duration of the previous light adaptation, within wide limits, but the reciprocity relation was found to govern the necessary adjustment over a considerable range. Here is further resemblance between the properties of the *Limulus* visual sense cell and measurements of visual function in human subjects.

The excitation of the receptor units in the eye of *Limulus* by flashes of light has been shown by one of us (Hartline, '34) to be governed by intensity and duration reciprocally. It was pointed out that this was to be expected from a simple photo-sensory system if the exposures were of short enough duration (less than 0.2 second) to be uninfluenced by the relatively slow recovery processes. In the present case, however, the durations of exposure were often long, and quite comparable to the time during which considerable recovery could take place, after the eye was returned to darkness. Nevertheless, the light adapting effect was found to be governed only by the total amount of light that was applied to the sense cell, within wide limits. Haig (loc. cit.) suggested that the slowing of the recovery process of dark adaptation by light adaptation may be the explanation for the wide range over which a reciprocity relation holds for human light adaptation (cf. also Crawford, '46). This same consideration, if it can be shown to be an adequate explanation, could be applied to the present experiments.

The reciprocity relation in light adaptation does have a limit to its range of application. That this must be true for the *Limulus* visual sense cell follows from the observation that very weak intensities of light, well below the limen at which nerve impulses are discharged, have no measurable effect upon the sensitivity of the receptor no matter how long they may continue to shine. Even intensities that do produce demonstrable light adaptation may do so inefficiently as compared with the same amount of luminous energy applied in a short flash. This is shown by the 2 curves on the left in figure 8. In this experiment, exposure to a weak light ($I = 10^{-4}$) for 10 seconds resulted in a sensitivity loss from which recovery was 80% complete in approximately 30 seconds. On the other hand, recovery from an exposure to the same quantity of light condensed within a 0.01 second flash ($I = 10^{-1}$) required nearly 2 minutes. Short intense flashes are exceptionally efficient in light adapting the visual sense cell, and the reciprocity relation fails most notably when their effects are compared with those of long, weak exposures.

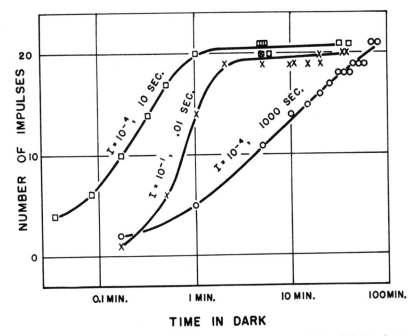

Fig. 8 Dark adaptation of a single receptor following periods of light adaptation of different intensities and durations, as given on respective curves. Logarithmic time scale.

In the experiment of figure 8, an attempt was made to determine how great an increase in adapting exposure time would be necessary to obtain, with the weak light, the same depression in sensitivity that had been effected by the short flash of strong light. The result revealed an additional property of the visual sense cell. In figure 8, the right hand curve (circles) shows the recovery from an exposure to the weak light for 1000 seconds. This was sufficient exposure to reduce the sensitivity of the receptor measured 10 seconds after the end of the exposure to nearly the same value that had been effected by the short flash (2 impulses in response to the test flash as compared with 1 impulse). The subsequent recovery, however, was very much slower following the long exposure to the weak light, requiring 30 minutes to reach 80% of complete recovery. In another experiment (fig. 9) the reduction in sensitivity following a long exposure to a weak light

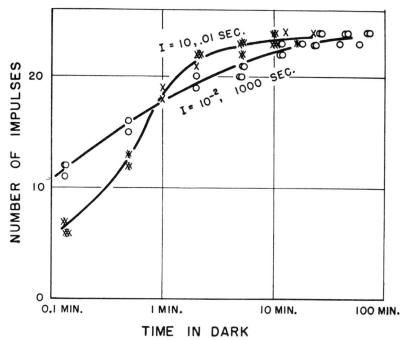

Fig. 9 Dark adaptation of a single receptor following periods of light adaptation of different intensities and durations, as given on respective curves. Logarithmic time scale.

was considerably less than after a short flash of higher intensity; nevertheless, dark adaptation following the long exposure was so much slower that the recovery curves actually crossed.

In still another experiment (fig. 10) thresholds were determined by direct trial during the course of recovery from light adapting exposures of high intensity ($I = 1$) for 1 second and of weak intensity ($I = 10^{-2}$) for 1000 seconds. These exposures were such that the thresholds measured 10 seconds after the end of the light adaptation were the same in both cases, to within the limits of the method (approx. 0.05 log unit). Although starting from the same point, dark adaptation following the long exposure to weak light was considerably slower than that following the short exposure to strong

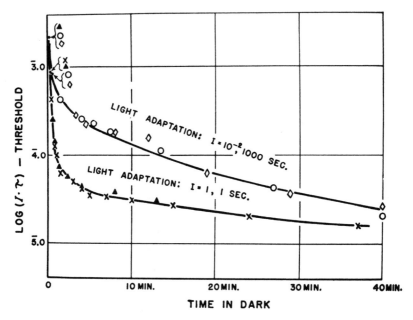

Fig. 10 Dark adaptation of a single receptor, as shown by the fall in threshold, following periods of light adaptation of different intensities and durations, as given on respective curves. Ordinates: logarithm of threshold energy, as in figure 2. Abscissae: time in dark (in minutes, linear scale). Same experiment as figure 2.

light. Not only did the reciprocity law fail, but it was no longer possible to duplicate the recovery curve following the short intense exposure by adjusting the duration of the weak one. Thus a simple family of recovery curves similar to those of figures 4 or 5 does not describe all of the possible courses of dark adaptation in extreme cases. The course of dark adaptation does not depend solely on how great an initial loss

of sensitivity has been induced by the foregoing light adaptation, but also upon the particular values of intensity and
duration of the light adapting exposure.

Here again analogous effects have already been described
for vertebrate vision. Johannsen ('34) has reported that intensity and duration of light adaptation are not interchangeable in their effect on the subsequent dark adaptation of cone
vision of human subjects. Especially important is Wald and
Clark's ('37) demonstration that the dark adaptation of the
rod mechanism of subjects exposed to a brief flash of very
high intensity proceeds so rapidly, that the recovery curve
sometimes crosses curves obtained after a long exposure to a
weak adapting intensity[10]— an observation similar to that
we have just described for the single visual receptor of
Limulus. Recently Crawford ('46) has demonstrated this
crossing of dark adaptation curves for both photopic and
scotopic vision in human subjects. For the eye of the frog
Riggs ('37) reported a similar crossing of the curves of cone
dark adaptation derived from retinal action potential measurements.

Wald and Clark explain this effect in terms of Wald's visual
cycle, according to which prolonged exposure to a weak light
results in the conversion of retinene into a certain amount of
vitamin A, from which regeneration of visual purple is slow.
The similarities of the present experiments suggest that an
analogous explanation could be applied to the adaptation of
the *Limulus* visual sense cell.

---

[10] Haig ('41) explains his failure to verify Wald and Clark's finding by the
fact that he used an artificial pupil in his experiment, while Wald and Clark
did not. Wald ('44), however, reports that a repetition of the experiment, using
an artificial pupil, yielded results identical with those reported originally. An
artificial pupil was used in Johannsen's ('34, I) experiments, and some of the
recovery curves she obtained also cross. The point is settled conclusively in favor
of Wald and Clark's observation by Crawford's recent experiments, in which
a Maxwellian view of both conditioning and test fields was used, providing an
effective pupil fixed at 0.5 mm diameter.

DISCUSSION

Light and dark adaptation, which are manifested so universally by photosensory systems, have long been considered to have their origin in the light receptors. In higher animals, it is generally believed that the eye, rather than the brain, is the seat of the principal sensitivity changes which characterize these processes. To cite only 2 lines of evidence, the extensive studies that have been made of the retinal action potential both in excised eyes and in intact animals lead to this conclusion, and in vertebrates the discharge of nerve impulses by single retinal ganglion cells has been shown to be greatly affected by light and dark adaptation of the retina (Hartline, '38; Granit, '44). The vertebrate retina, however, is highly organized, and has neural components in addition to the receptor cells. Indeed, it has been suggested that these other components participate in the retinal changes that take place during light and dark adaptation. Thus Schouten and Ornstein thought it necessary to postulate the spread of electric influences over the retina during "indirect adaptation," which they believe has its seat in the retinal synapses. Furthermore, Lythgoe ('40) has postulated changes in the functional connections of the receptor elements, to explain the progressive deterioration of the finer visual judgments during dark adaptation.

By avoiding the complexity of the vertebrate retina, we have been able to show that fundamental aspects of light and dark adaptation are manifested in an eye containing, as far as is known, no neural elements other than receptor cells and their axons. Moreover, we have shown this for individual receptor units, and have used for our measurements a response of known neurological significance. Our experiments do not, of course, exclude the possibility of additional effects in the vertebrate retina, nor can the comparison between the *Limulus* receptor unit and the vertebrate rod or cone be made without reservation. However, the faithful resemblance between the present experiments and the results of studies of visual function in the vertebrate eye suggests that the properties of receptor cells are quite sufficient to account for most of the sensitivity changes which take place in higher animals during light and dark adaptation.

The present studies do more than provide information concerning the sensitivity changes of the visual receptor cell, as measured (either directly or indirectly) by changes in threshold. In addition, the responses to flashes of light considerably above threshold have been recorded during the course of dark adaptation. One result of this study has been to demonstrate that the individual receptor preserves its ability to respond in a graded manner to stimuli of different intensities, although adjusted to different levels of sensitivity by the state of its adaptation. Quantitatively, moreover, the variation of response with the intensity *relative to threshold* is unaltered by the level of adaptation, if the number of impulses in the response be taken as a criterion. The total number of impulses elicited by a test flash, however, is but one of the attributes of a receptor's response which may be considered in studying the effects of light and dark adaptation. Other features, such as duration of the activity and frequency of impulse discharge are also affected by adaptation, as was noted in the discussion of figure 1. If the only effect of adaptation were to adjust the sensitivity of the receptor to a new level, the burst of impulses elicited by a flash of light from a dark adapted preparation might be expected to be matched in all respects by the burst elicited by a more intense flash from the same receptor after light adaptation. It would then make no difference which of the attributes of the response were chosen for measurement. However, this is not the case. We will show in a subsequent paper that such a match between responses obtained in light and dark adapted conditions cannot be made by any adjustment of stimulus intensity; different features of the response are differently affected by adaptation, and it is evident that the "sensitivity" of the receptor is not the only one of its properties that changes during adaptation.

SUMMARY

Light and dark adaptation of single visual receptor units of the excised lateral eye of *Limulus* have been studied by recording the discharge of impulse in single fibers of the optic nerve, by means of their amplified action potentials.

Exposure to light decreased the ability of the receptor to respond to a short test flash of light; during the subsequent stay in darkness the discharge of impulses that could be elicited by a test flash of constant intensity and duration increased, both in the number of impulses in the burst and the frequency at which they were discharged. The recovery of sensitivity of single receptors during dark adaptation was also followed by determining the energy of test flash just sufficient to elicit 1 nerve impulse in an isolated optic nerve fiber. The threshold thus determined fell comparatively rapidly immediately after an exposure to light, then more slowly in a smooth curve, approaching its dark adapted value asymptotically. Recovery following moderate exposures to light was practically complete in 1 hour (18°C.).

Light adapted receptor units were able to respond in a graded manner to test flashes of various intensities, although at levels of sensitivity that were lower the higher the intensity of the adapting light. The relation between the number of impulses elicited by a test flash and the ratio of its intensity to threshold at any given level of sensitivity was unchanged by light adaptation. Knowledge of this relation for a given receptor therefore permitted the calculation of threshold from the number of impulses elicited by a test flash of known intensity, at any level of adaptation.

The loss of sensitivity following exposure to light, and the time required to regain dark adaptation, were strongly affected by the duration of the light adapting exposure, and by its intensity. The effects of light adaptation increased rapidly with increasing short exposures, more gradually with longer ones, and were complete (at moderate intensities) after 10–20 minutes of exposure. With an exposure of constant duration, the effects of light adaptation were greater the higher its intensity: a slight but measurable effect could be demonstrated at intensities just too weak to elicit a discharge of impulses; following exposure to very high intensities the intial loss of sensitivity was great and eventual recovery in darkness took an hour or more.

Strong light adaptation caused an overall slowing of the subsequent dark adaptation; the recovery rate, measured at a fixed level of sensitivity, was less the longer the duration or the higher the intensity of the previous light adapting exposure. Within limits, intensity and duration of the exposure were interchangeable in determining the course of the subsequent recovery, and over a wide range only the constancy of their product (total energy of the exposure) was required to produce a given constant recovery curve. However, recovery was faster following extremely short intense exposures than after very long weak ones, even though the initial loss of sensitivity was the same or greater; for these extreme conditions of light adaptation the reciprocity relation failed, and moreover intensity and duration were no longer interchangeable in their effects on the subsequent dark adaptation.

The course of the recovery of sensitivity during dark adaptation of the single visual receptor of *Limulus,* and the effects upon it of intensity and duration of the previous light adapting exposure, resemble in detail the phenomena exhibited by visual mechanisms of higher animals, including the human subject. The demonstration of this for isolated receptor units is strong presumptive evidence that the mechanism responsible for light and dark adaptation of many visual systems does indeed reside in the receptor elements of the eye, as is commonly assumed. Chemical mechanisms analogous to those revealed by biochemical investigations of the vertebrate retina may be postulated to explain the present results.

Recording the nervous activity of receptor axones provides the means for investigating visual responses at supra-threshold levels during light and dark adaptation. There is evidence, requiring further investigation, that the "sensitivity" of the receptor is not the only one of its properties that changes during adaptation.

LITERATURE CITED

CLARK, L. B. 1938 Dark adaptation in *Dineutes*. J. Gen. Physiol., *21:* 375–382.

CRAWFORD, B. H. 1946 Photochemical laws and visual phenomena. Proc. Roy. Soc. London, ser. B, *133:* 63–75.

———— 1947 Visual adaptation in relation to brief conditioning stimuli. Proc. Roy. Soc. London, Ser. B, *134:* 283–302.

GRANIT, R. 1944 The dark adaptation of mammalian visual receptors. Acta Physiol. Scand., *7:* 216–220.

HAIG, C. 1941 The course of dark adaptation as influenced by the intensity and duration of pre-adaptation to light. J. Gen. Physiol., *24:* 735–751.

HARTLINE, H. K. 1930 The dark adaptation of the eye of *Limulus*, as manifested by its electric response to illumination. J. Gen. Physiol., *13:* 379–389.

———— 1932 The effect of dark adaptation on the discharge of impulses in single optic nerve fibers (abstr.). Am. J. Physiol., *101:* 50.

———— 1934 Intensity and duration in the excitation of single photo-receptor units. J. Cell. and Comp. Physiol., *5:* 229–247.

———— 1935 The discharge of nerve impulses from the single visual sense cell. Cold Spring Harbor Symposia on Quantitative Biology., *3:* 245–249.

———— 1938 The response of single optic nerve fibers of the vertebrate eye to illumination of the retina. Am. J. Physiol., *121:* 400–415.

HARTLINE, H. K., AND C. H. GRAHAM 1932 Nerve impulses from single receptors in the eye. J. Cell. and Comp. Physiol., *1:* 277–295.

HARTLINE, H. K., AND R. MCDONALD 1941 Dark adaptation of single visual sense cells (abstr.). Am. J. Physiol., *133:* P321.

HECHT, S., C. HAIG AND A. M. CHASE 1937 The influence of light adaptation on subsequent dark adaptation of the eye. J. Gen. Physiol., *20:* 831–850.

JOHANNSEN, D. E. 1934 Duration and intensity of the exposure light as factors determining the course of the subsequent dark adaptation. J. Gen. Psychol., *10:* (I) pp. 4–19, (II) pp. 20–41.

LYTHGOE, R. J. 1940 The mechanism of dark adaptation. Brit. J. of Ophthol., *24:* 21–43.

MÜLLER, H. K. 1931 Ueber den Einfluss verschieden langer vorbelichtung auf die Dunkeladaptation und auf die Fehlergrösse der Schwellenezbestimmung während der Dunkelanpassung. Graefe's Arch. f. Ophthal., *125:* 624–642.

RIGGS, L. A. 1937 Dark adaptation in the frog eye as determined by the electrical response of the retina. J. Cell. and Comp. Physiol., *9:* 491–509.

RIGGS, L. A., AND C. H. GRAHAM 1940 Some aspects of light adaptation in a single photoreceptor unit. J. Cell. and Comp. Physiol., *16:* 15–23.

SCHOUTEN, J. F., AND L. S. ORNSTEIN 1939 Measurements on direct and indirect adaptation by means of a binocular method. J. Opt. Soc. Am., *29*: 168–182.

WALD, G. 1944 Vision: Photochemistry. Medical Physics, Otto Glasser, editor. Year Book Publishers, Chicago, pp. 1658–1667.

WALD, G., AND A. B. CLARK 1937 Visual adaptation and chemistry of rods. J. Gen. Physiol., *21*: 93–105.

WINSOR, C. P., AND A. B. CLARK 1936 Dark adaptation after varying degrees of light adaptation. Proc. Nat. Sci., *22*: 400–404.

WRIGHT, W. D. 1934 The measurement and analysis of color adaptation phenomena. Proc. Roy. Soc. London, ser. B, *115*: 49–87.

——————— 1937 The foveal light adaptation process. Proc. Roy. Soc., London, ser. B, *122*: 220–245.

Fluctuations of response of single visual sense cells

H. K. HARTLINE, LORUS J. MILNE (by invitation), AND
I. H. WAGMAN

*Johnson Research Foundation, University of Pennsylvania and
Department of Physiology, Jefferson Medical College*

Reprinted from FEDERATION PROCEEDINGS, Vol. 6, no. 1, March 1947

The uncertainty of response of single visual sense cells to repeated flashes of light of 'constant' intensity has been studied by recording the action potentials of single fibers dissected from the optic nerve of *Limulus*. A series of short flashes delivered to the eye at a given intensity near threshold elicits occasional responses of one or more nerve impulses, interspersed among failures to respond. Occurrence of responses in any given series is random, according to statistical tests. The frequency of occurrence of responses increases with increasing intensity of the flashes. In most dark-adapted preparations, the intensity range within which frequency of responses is greater than zero and less than 100 per cent covers approximately one logarithmic unit. This range is not measurably affected by a temperature change of 10°C. A similar uncertainty has been found for eliciting responses equal to or exceeding some fixed number of impulses greater than one; the greater this number, the narrower is the range of uncertainty.

Light adaptation raises the threshold of the sense cell; at the same time the range of uncertainty is narrowed, on a logarithmic scale of intensity. This effect is reversed by dark adaptation.

The uncertainty of response might be explained by statistical fluctuations in the number of quanta absorbed from the 'constant' flash,

[1] Work done under Contract N5–ORI–122, proj. 4, between the University of Pennsylvania and the Office of Naval Research.

following the explanation that has been suggested for the uncertainty of seeing by human observers. Possibility of fluctuations in sensitivity of the receptor cell and its axone, analogous to those reported for axones stimulated electrically, must also be considered.

The peripheral origin of nervous activity in the visual system

H. K. HARTLINE, HENRY G. WAGNER,[1] AND
E. F. MACNICHOL, JR.

Thomas C. Jenkins Laboratories of Biophysics, Johns Hopkins University, Baltimore, Maryland

Reprinted from COLD SPRING HARBOR SYMPOSIA ON
QUANTITATIVE BIOLOGY, Vol. XVII, 125–141, 1952

It is the function of the sense organs to reflect, in the nervous activity they generate, the state of the organism's environment, initiating chains of neural events that regulate behavior. The mechanisms whereby environmental influences excite activity in afferent nerve fibers have been discussed by many authors. Nevertheless, it is not yet possible to trace, step by step, the physical and chemical events that intervene between the action of a stimulus on a receptor and the response of the associated afferent fiber. This paper will consider some of the ideas that have been developed, and add new observations that bear on the problem of the origin of nervous activity, with particular reference to the visual system.[2]

The activity that is generated in afferent nerve fibers, when their sense organs are stimulated, consists of trains of nerve impulses such as are observed elsewhere in the nervous system. In any one fiber, the frequency of the discharge of impulses depends upon the intensity of the stimulus and upon the state of the receptor, as determined by the various factors affecting its responsiveness. These are now familiar facts of neurophysiology (Adrian, 1935). An example of such neural activity is given in Fig. 1, which shows oscillograms of the action potentials recorded from a single optic nerve fiber from the eye of *Limulus*. In this case, a visual receptor element, stimulated by light, initiated the activity. As a result of the work of many investigators, beginning with Adrian and his associates, the discharge of impulses in afferent fibers has been recorded for almost all the major types of sense organs. The fact has emerged that, except for differences in the amount of sensory adaptation shown by different types of end-organs under continuous stimulation, the patterns of response are essentially alike. Evidently, the

---

[1] Naval Medical Research Institute, Bethesda.

[2] Work done under contract Nonr–248(11), between the Johns Hopkins University and the Office of Naval Research.

various kinds of sensory end-organs with their associated afferent fibers possess certain fundamental properties in common.

However, specificity of sensory pathway is essential to the discrimination of different kinds of stimuli. Each sense organ is especially sensitive to a particular stimulating agent. Although an important part of this specificity arises from the secondary structures of the various sense organs, much of it depends on specialized mechanisms in the receptors

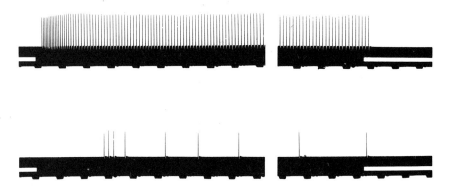

Fig. 1. Oscillograms of action potentials of a single optic nerve fiber of *Limulus*, in response to prolonged illumination of the eye. For the top record, the intensity of stimulating light was 10,000 times that used for the bottom record. Eye partially light adapted. Signal of exposure to light blackens out the white line above time marks. Each record interrupted for approximately 7 sec. Time marked in ¼ sec.

themselves. Thus one may expect to find two aspects to the study of the receptor mechanisms. On the one hand, general principles governing the excitation of all irritable tissue should be discernible, determining properties that are common to all sense organs and, indeed, to all nervous tissue. On the other hand, specific mechanisms concerned with the translation of particular external influences into sensory excitation may be expected to possess properties that differ widely from the one type of receptor to another.

In the case of the visual system, the component that gives to the receptor its specific sensitivity to light is a photosensitive chemical compound contained in the structure of the visual end-organ. In the rods of the vertebrate retina the specific photosensitive substance has been known for almost 100 years as visual purple, or rhodopsin. The biochemistry of extracted rhodopsin and other compounds related to it is being actively explored and much is understood about it. It is a conjugated protein in which the prosthetic group responsible for photo-sensitivity is a carotenoid closely related to vitamin A. When acted upon by light, rhodopsin undergoes a succession of chemical changes, ending in the liberation of the carotenoid fraction (retinene). Only the first step in this process is photochemical in nature, the rest are thermal. In the eye, visual purple is constantly being replenished by other chemical mechanisms. In part at least, these can be duplicated in the test tube, and considerable knowledge has been gained concerning the enzyme mechanisms involved. Not only has the photosensitive substance of the vertebrate retinal rods been investigated, but that of the cones as well, and biochemical studies of visual pigments have been extended to a few invertebrates. Some of the recent developments in this field have been reviewed by Wald (1949, 1951), in whose laboratory many of the important advances have taken place.

The initial step in the action of light on the visual receptor is the absorption of energy from the incident radiation by the photosensitive substance. Not all of the radiation in the electro-magnetic spectrum is 'visible', and in the visible spectrum not all wavelengths are equally effective. This simply reflects the fact that the photosensitive substance of the visual receptor has an absorption spectrum that is not uniform. The more efficiently light of a given wavelength is absorbed by the visual receptors, the greater is the sensitivity at that wavelength. The absorption spectrum of rhodopsin has been measured, and, after suit-able correction, has been found to explain satisfactorily the spectral distribution of sensitivity of the vertebrate rods (see Wald, 1949).

Several other familiar properties of the visual system have been related directly to the chemistry of the photosensitive substance. In the excitation of the receptor, the familiar reciprocal relation between the intensity of the stimulating light and duration of the exposure has been attributed to this photochemical system (Hecht, 1919a; Hartline, 1934). This relation is looked upon simply as the expression of the Bunsen–Roscoe law of photochemistry. Furthermore, the very large changes in sensitivity during light and dark adaptation have been attributed to a decrease in the concentration of the photosensitive substance by photolysis, and to its regeneration by chemical mechanisms that are independent of light (Hecht, 1919b; Wald and Clark, 1937; Hartline and McDonald, 1947). Here it may be well to exercise caution in inter-pretation, for sensory adaptation is a universal property of receptors of all kinds. It scarcely seems reasonable to ignore this and ascribe all of the sensitivity changes in the visual receptor to alterations in its highly specialized photochemical component.

The processes that intervene between the initial photochemical re-action in the receptor and the initiation of nervous activity are almost completely unknown. However, we have made some experimental observations relating to the time required for these processes. One of them concerns the persistence of excitatory effects in a photoreceptor after a brief exposure to light. As recorded in a single optic nerve fiber of *Limulus*, the entire discharge of impulses in response to a very short flash of light acting upon the receptor takes place after the flash is over,

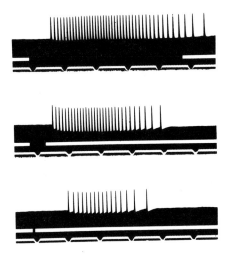

Fig. 2. Discharge of impulses in a single optic nerve fiber of *Limulus*, in response to exposures of the eye to light of the same intensity for durations of 0.97 sec., 0.096 sec., and 0.010 sec. (top to bottom). Signal marking period of exposure blackens out white line above time marks. Time in $\frac{1}{5}$ sec. The times from the onset of illumination to the successive occurrences of corresponding impulses in the upper and middle records were the same for the first 10 impulses. From the 11th impulse on, the occurrences were significantly earlier in the upper record than in the middle. Therefore, 0.096 sec. was the 'critical duration' for the 10th impulse, for which the time of occurrence = 0.32 sec. For the 1st impulse (time of occurrence = 0.14 sec.) the critical duration at this intensity was 0.04 sec.

and often lasts for several tenths of a second (Fig. 2). A very intense flash can elicit a discharge lasting for a minute or more. Even after a flash of light too weak to elicit a response, excitatory effects can be shown to persist for one or two seconds (Wagman, Hartline, and Milne, 1949). In the experiment illustrated in Fig. 3 this was demonstrated by using a second flash to test the sensitivity of the receptor at various times after the exposure to the subliminal flash. (Following the period of enhanced excitability in this experiment there was a transitory period of diminished sensitivity. Except for the much longer time constants, these changes in excitability are reminiscent of those well known in peripheral nerve subjected to subliminal electrical shocks.) The persistence of the exciting effects of light can be ascribed either to the properties of the photochemical system of the receptor or, equally well, to later events in the process leading to the discharge of nerve impulses.

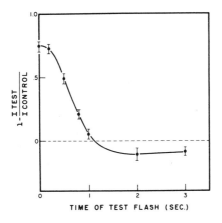

TIME OF TEST FLASH (SEC.)

Fig. 3. Persistence of excitatory effects in a photoreceptor element in the eye of *Limulus* at various times following a short flash (0.02 sec. duration) of light of sublimal intensity (70 per cent of normal threshold). At various times after the subliminal flash (abscissae), the receptor was illuminated by test flashes (0.02 sec. duration) the intensity of which was adjusted until the receptor would respond to 50 per cent of the flashes. The amount by which the test flash had to be diminished from its normal threshold value was taken as the measure of the excitation remainder (ordinates). Normal threshold = 1 unit of intensity. After approximately 1 sec. the remainder became negative (post-excitatory depression), after which the receptor recovered slowly, until at 15 sec. its threshold had returned to normal. Each point is the weighted mean of several determinations; the limits of ± 1 standard error are indicated by the lengths of the vertical lines through the points. (From Hartline, Wagman, Wagner, and Milne, in preparation.)

However, these observations do show that the excitatory effects in the photoreceptor are not limited to the period during which light energy is being absorbed and active photolysis is taking place.

It has long been known that there is an interval of time between the absorption of light and the first sign of response by the organism. Many years ago Hecht (1919b) attributed most of this delay to a latent period in the photoreceptor itself, subsequent to photolysis. The analysis of the electrical response of isolated photoreceptors has shown his interpretation to be correct. When the discharge of impulses is recorded in nerve fibers coming directly from the receptor elements, as in the eye of *Limulus*, there is an interval of time between the onset of illumination and the beginning of the discharge (Fig. 1). At 18°C the latent period may range in value from several hundredths of a second at high intensities to one or two seconds, or even more, when the receptor is dark adapted and the intensity near threshold. Lowering the temperature slows the latent period very markedly. The response to a short flash (Fig. 2) also shows a latent period, so that, as we mentioned above, the entire response may take place when the receptor is in darkness. Evidently the products of photolysis that are generated during illumination take some time to exert their effects.

The latent period of the *Limulus* photoreceptor may be analyzed further. In the response to a short flash of fixed intensity the latent period decreases with increasing duration of the flash up to a certain critical value. Beyond this 'critical duration' continuation of the exposure has no further effect on the time of appearance of the first impulse. It is as though the processes determining the beginning of the response are completed at the end of the critical duration, even though the impulses themselves do not appear until sometime later. This is very similar to the 'sensitization period' described by Hecht for the response of *Mya*, although his theory fails to describe the *Limulus* data quantitatively.

This experimental analysis may be extended to the timing of the impulses that occur after the first one. Continuation of the exposure beyond the duration that is 'critical' for the first affects later impulses, but for these, too, 'critical durations' are observed that are longer in proportion to the times of appearance of the respective impulses (see Fig. 2). (This analysis has not been extended to the timing of impulses that occur later than those determining the maximum frequency of the discharge, usually 10–20 impulses). The significance of the 'critical duration' for the present problem has been discussed at an earlier symposium (Hartline, 1935). Since then, we have found (in collaboration with Dr. J. H. Stover) that, for any one preparation, the 'critical duration' for a given impulse is a nearly constant fraction (usually between one-third to one-half) of the time at which that impulse appears in response to prolonged illumination, irrespective of conditions of temperature, adaptation, and intensity of stimulation. The interval between the end of the 'critical duration' for a given impulse, and the time of its appearance in the nerve discharge, being a constant fraction of that time, is shorter the higher the intensity of illumination. Whatever the process may be that occupies this final interval, it proceeds more rapidly the stronger the stimulus to the receptor, although it is independent of whether or not the light is shining on the receptor while it is taking place.

Another demonstration of the time-lag between the stimulating light and the response it elicits is seen when the receptor, illuminated steadily and discharging a steady train of impulses, is subjected to a sudden increase (or sudden decrease) in light intensity. In response there is an increase (or decrease) in the frequency of the discharge (MacNichol and Hartline, 1948). This change begins after an appreciable latency (0.1 to 0.2 sec.), during which time the original discharge rate is entirely unaltered.

These observations show that excitatory effects in the photoreceptor take time to develop to the point where they result in the discharge of nerve impulses. They suggest the concept of a photochemical stimulus distinct from subsequent reactions that finally excite the axon. These intervening processes limit the speed with which a photoreceptor can respond to a change in the stimulus. However, except to show that the processes involved consume time, such studies have contributed little to the understanding of the physical nature of the mechanisms whereby the products of photochemical action generate nerve activity. A more direct experimental approach is needed.

Nearly 100 years ago Holmgren discovered the retinal action potential. Since then, many investigators have studied the electrical responses to illumination that can be obtained from the eyes of a variety of animals merely by placing electrodes on either side of the layer of sensory elements and recording fluctuations in electric potential by a suitable instrument. Of the many treatises on this extensive subject, those of Kohlrausch (1931) and Granit (1947) may be recommended. An eye need not be especially highly developed to yield a simple retinal action potential (Fig. 4). It is only necessary that it be sufficiently well organized so that the sensory elements are similarly oriented and closely packed, presenting favorable electrical conditions for recording. It is now believed that a large component of the retinal action potential in all eyes arises from the sensory elements themselves, and that its behavior parallels closely the activity of these cells. For these reasons, and because of the importance of electrical phenomena in the initiation and propagation of nervous activity, it seems reasonable to hope that a study of the retinal action potential may provide a direct method of investigating the origin of nervous activity in the visual receptor.

This idea is made particularly inviting by a consideration of the polarity of the electrical response from a layer of visual receptor elements. In all eyes so far studied, a large component of the electrical response to light is usually in a direction indicating increased negativity of the free distal ends of the receptor cells with respect to the ends from which their nerve fibers arise. In peripheral nerve, the propagated impulse is associated with local negativity of the excited region. The direction of the local currents that are set up are then such as to cause spread of the excitation. It is tempting to postulate that as an ultimate

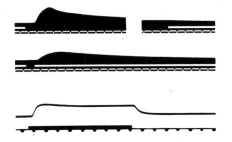

Fig. 4. Upper and middle records: Retinal action potentials recorded from an eyespot of a star-fish (*Asterias* sp.). (Direct-coupled amplifier was used for this and for all other retinal action potentials recorded in this paper.) Leads: corneal surface to back of eye. Deflection upward indicates corneal lead becoming more negative with respect to lead on back of eye. Duration of exposure indicated by signal, which blackens the white line just above the time marks (interruption of upper record was for approx. 3 sec.). Time in ½ sec. Lower record: Retinal action potential from an eye of a spider (species undetermined). Leads: surface of cornea to optic nerve. Deflection upward indicates increasing negativity of corneal lead relative to lead on nerve. Amplitude of initial maximum = 0.9 mv. Period of illumination signalled by heavy black band above time marks. Time in ½ sec.

consequence of the initial photochemical reaction a potential gradient is set up in the photoreceptor, causing local currents in the direction favorable to the spread of excitation in the receptor's nerve fiber. By this hypothesis a large component of the retinal action potential would be the external sign of an electrical event in the receptors that is one of the essential links in the chain of processes relating the action of light with a discharge of nerve impulses. This would be in line with ideas that are currently held relating the discharge of impulses to slow-action potentials in other sense organs and in nerve cells.

Many authors have expressed or implied this interpretation of the significance of the retinal action potential, but there are difficulties to be met before this hypothesis can be accepted. In many highly developed eyes, as in the insects and vertebrates, the receptor elements have associated with them extensive ganglionic structures, the activity of which may contribute notably to the retinal action potential (Fig. 5; see Granit, loc. cit.). Moreover, the afferent nerve activity to which the retinal potential is related, according to this hypothesis, should be recorded from fibers arising from the receptors rather than from more proximal neurones in which the activity may be affected by very complex interactions within the optic ganglia, as in the vertebrate retina. By using a simpler eye, or one in which the ganglionic structures can be removed or inactivated (Bernhard, 1942), some of these complications can be avoided. The visual receptors in an eye are often of diverse types, as for example the rods and cones in the vertebrates, or they may

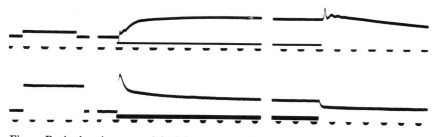

Fig. 5. Retinal action potential of the compound eye of the house fly. Upper record taken from the intact insect, leads: cornea to indifferent lead on head. Lower record taken after removal of the optic ganglion, leads: cornea to inner surface of sensory layer. Calibration: upper record 2.0 mv; lower record 0.5 mv. Deflection upward indicates increasing negativity of corneal lead. Time in $\frac{1}{5}$ sec. Illumination signal indicated by black line just above the time marks.

have a statistical distribution of their properties that would cloud an attempt to relate their nerve fiber activity to the retinal action potential. Ideally, it would be desirable to record simultaneously, from a single receptor, both its action potentials and the activity in its nerve fiber. As yet this has not been possible. However, in the compound eye of *Limulus* we have been able to isolate intact single ommatidia, and in experiments on such preparations to record both the discharge of impulses in the nerve leading from the ommatidium and the slow-action potential of the group of cells comprising its sensory structure (Hartline, 1948).

The structure of the eye of *Limulus* is not yet satisfactorily understood. Current studies by Waterman (1951) and some in our own laboratory (Miller, 1952) are making progress, and may help to clarify the uncertainties. Because the *Limulus* eye has been so favorable for physiological study, we will describe briefly what we know of its histology.

The compound, lateral eye of *Limulus* contains, on the average, some

600 ommatidia. The lenticular portion of each ommatidium is a thickening of the transparent chitinous cornea, forming a small conical projection into the interior of the eye. At the end of each cone, embedded in heavily pigmented tissue, is a cell-complex, the sensory portion of the ommatidium (see Fig. 6). There are several types of cells in this complex, of which two seem to be neuroepitheleal and concerned with the light receptive process. One of these, generally termed the retinula cell, is a fairly large cell, some 150 μ in length. From ten to twenty of these cells are grouped about a central axis much like the segments in an orange (Grenacher, 1879; see Fig. 7). Each appears to have a nerve fiber emerging from the base; this fiber runs proximally, converging with nerve fibers from neighbouring retinula cells of the same and other ommatidia to form the optic nerve. The retinula cell is pigmented, except at the axial border. Here specialization into a laminated hyaline structure, the rhabdomere, is evident. The other neuropithelial cell, of which there is usually only one in each ommatidium, is frequently termed the eccentric cell, from the observation that its cell body is situated on one side of the axis, near the proximal end of the sensory ommatidium (Watase, 1887; Demoll, 1917; see Fig. 8). It is distinguished in a number of other ways. There is a distal process that penetrates to the axis of the ommatidium and runs axially almost to the chitinous cone. It, too, has a nerve fiber that runs proximally with the nerve fibers of the surrounding retinula cells. Because this cell is not pigmented like the surrounding retinula cells and has a bipolar appearance, Watasé was tempted to refer to it as a ganglion cell. However, both he and Demoll regarded the eccentric cell as a sense cell and

Figs. 6–8. Sections taken from lateral eye of *Limulus*. (From Wagner and Miller, in preparation; photomicrographs by W. H. Miller.)

Fig. 6. Horizontal section, showing seven entire ommatidia. Contrast between different corneal layers (C, C') and crystalline cones (CO) is exaggerated. Sections moderately bleached to show retinula (R). Only a portion of the plexus is shown (P). Lee Brown modification of Mallory's aniline blue stain.

Fig. 7. Cross-section through sensory portion of an ommatidium, showing rosette configuration of retinula cells (RC). Light region in center is occupied by the rhabdomeres of the retinula cells, surrounding the central process of the eccentric cell. Portion of eccentric cell body shown on right (EC). Thionine stain; sections unbleached.

Fig. 8. Axial section through sensory portion of an ommatidium (corneal end at top). Shows eccentric cell body (EC), two retinula cells (RC) flanking the axial canal (light streak) in which is the central process of the eccentric cell. The rhabdomeres of the retinula cells appear as dark-staining bands bordering the axial canal. (Similar details may be seen in Fig. 6.) Lee Brown modification of Mallory's aniline blue stain; sections unbleached.

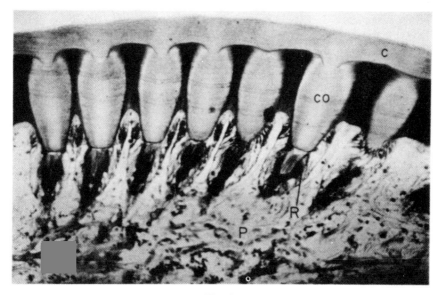

Fig. 6

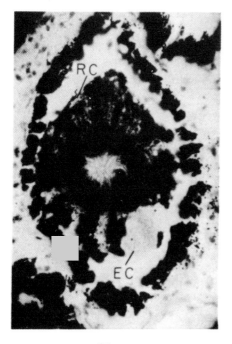

Fig. 7

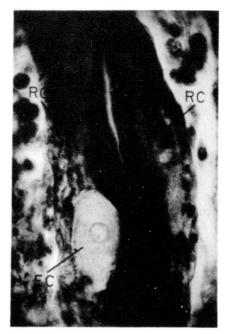

Fig. 8

photoreceptor. Patten (1912) reported 'a loose layer of ganglion cells lying just beneath the inner surface of the lateral eye'. Grenacher (loc. cit.) could find no separate layer of ganglion cells.

The course of the nerve fibers after leaving the sensory ommatidia is not entirely clear. Behind the ommatidia there is a network of nerve fibers and connective tissue, that was termed by Watasé a 'plexus'. Indeed, Watasé felt that the bundles of nerve fibers from the ommatidia broke up in this plexus, made 'peculiar' connections with other fibers, then recombined to form the optic nerve.

In our own preparations, the bundles of fibers emerging from the bases of the ommatidia can often be identified for a fair distance as they penetrate into the substance behind the eye. They can frequently be followed until they join together into larger bundles that can be seen ultimately to converge to form the optic nerve. Study of the optic nerve sections suggests that all of the sense cell fibers reach to and become part of the optic nerve (see also Waterman, loc. cit.). Still, the exact course of any individual nerve fiber is usually obscure in the network of fibers and cells that the bundles enter as soon as they leave the ommatidia. The histological detail of this region is difficult to determine. That some sort of functional connection exists between ommatidia we are confident, from physiological evidence that we shall present later in this paper. Although the anatomy of the *Limulus* eye is not as simple as early descriptions would leave one to believe, it is far less complex than the eyes of higher animals.

In our experiments on the isolated ommatidia of the *Limulus* eye we have begun by making a cut with a sharp razor-blade through a freshly excised eye perpendicular to the corneal surface. From a little below the surface exposed by the cut a small nerve strand from one of the ommatidia can be snipped out with sharp, finely pointed scissors. If it has not been damaged by the dissection, such a bundle shows action potentials typical of the activity of a single nerve fiber, even though (as we have shown above) the nerve strand from each ommatidium contains ten or more fibers. We doubt that this simple response arises because all of the fibers discharge synchronously. From the rather uncertain evidence now at hand, we are inclined to believe that it is the activity of the axon from the eccentric cell that is recorded.

If the dissection has been successful up to this point, it is then possible to isolate the ommatidium from which this nerve strand arises by snipping away adjacent ommatidia, and finally stripping off all the rest of the tissue of the eye, leaving only this one ommatidium attached to the cornea. The situation is shown schematically in Fig. 9. Fine cotton wicks leading to Ag-AgCl electrodes are then applied in the positions indi-cated. Leads 1 and 2 are taken to the input of a direct-coupled amplifier (which is always used for recording slow-action potentials). Leads 3 and 4 are connected to a capacitance-coupled amplifier for the simultaneous recording of the action potential spikes in the nerve.

The slow, 'retinal' action potential recorded from the body of an isolated ommatidium (Figs. 10, 13, and 14) is a simple fluctuation in the potential difference between its ends, the distal (corneal) end be-coming more negative with respect to the proximal end. We will term this the 'ommatidial action potential'. It begins suddenly after a latent period, rises steeply to a maximum and then subsides. At the same time that the ommatidial action potential starts to rise (or a little later) the discharge of impulses in the nerve fiber begins. The frequency of the discharge also rises to a maximum and then subsides.

The precise placement of the leads has an appreciable effect on the size of the ommatidial action potential that is recorded. To obtain the maximum response, the distal lead (1) should be on the cornea, or close to it on the body of the ommatidium, and the proximal lead (2) should be near the proximal tip of the ommatidium. If part of the nerve strand is included between leads (1) and (2), spike potentials are recorded superimposed on the slow ommatidial potential (Fig. 11). Traces of these spikes are sometimes seen even when the proximal lead is on the ommatidium itself (see Figs. 13 and 14). When some of the nerve is included with the ommatidium between leads 1 and 2, the action potential spikes are usually (but not always) in the downward direction on the records, indicating increased positivity of the distal lead with respect to the proximal lead; when only the nerve strand is between the electrodes (leads 3–4), the spike action potentials are in the usual direction, the distal lead becoming relatively more negative in the initial deflection.

Slight mechanical stretch of the ommatidium, or puncture with a fine glass needle, often results in a preparation that no longer discharges nerve impulses but still produces an ommatidial action potential in response to light (Fig. 12). More extensive mechanical disturbance will abolish all response; the preparation is very delicate.

The higher the intensity of the stimulating light, and, for short flashes, the longer its duration, the greater is the amplitude of the initial maximum of the slow-action potential from an isolated ommatidium, and the higher the frequency of the discharge of impulses in its nerve strand in the initial outburst of activity (Figs. 10 and 13). In response to test flashes of constant intensity, both the ommatidial action potential

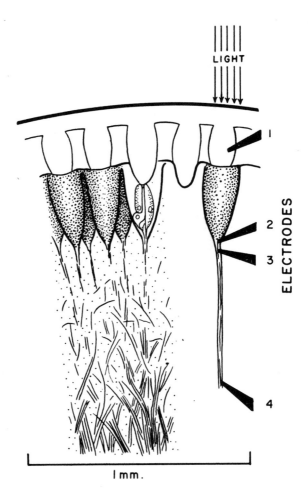

Fig. 9. Schematic drawing, representing a section of lateral eye of *Limulus* in a plane perpendicular to surface of cornea, as seen in fresh preparations. Transparent cornea at top, showing crystalline cones of the ommatidia; the heavily melanin-pigmented conical bodies of these form a layer on the inner surface of the cornea. On the left, a group of ommatidia is represented, with indications of bundles of nerve fibers traversing the plexus behind the ommatidia, collecting in larger bundles that become the optic nerve still farther back. One of these ommatidia has been represented as if the section had passed through it, revealing the sensory component, also as if sectioned. On the right an ommatidium with its nerve fiber bundle is represented as it appears after having been isolated by dissection and suspended, in air, on electrodes (moist cotton wicks, from chlorided silver tubes filled with seawater) represented by solid black triangles.

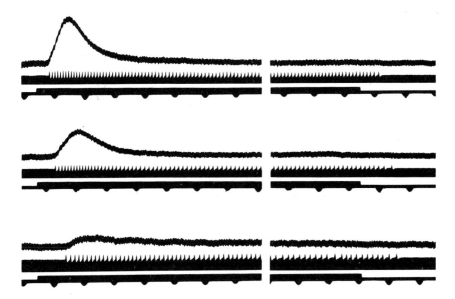

Fig. 10. Simultaneously recorded nerve and 'retinal' action potentials of an isolated ommatidium from the eye of *Limulus*, in response to illumination at three intensities of relative value (top to bottom) 1.0, 0.1, 0.01. Upper trace in each record: action potential of the body of the ommatidium (leads 1–2, cf. Fig. 9), D.C. amplification. Lower trace (black edge) in each record: spike action potentials of the nerve strand from the ommatidium (amplifier time constant = 0.1 sec.). For both traces, deflection upward indicates increasing negativity of distal leads (1, 3) with respect to proximal leads (2, 4). Peak deflection of upper trace in top record = 0.4 mv. In each record, signal marking period of illumination blackens lower half of white band above time marks. Time marked in ⅕ sec.

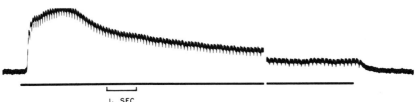

Fig. 11. Action potential of isolated ommatidium (*Limulus* eye) and its nerve strand (leads 1–4, Fig. 9) in response to prolonged steady illumination. Deflection upward indicates increasing negativity of cornea (lead 1) with respect to cut end of nerve strand (lead 4). D.C. amplification. Black line above time-scale signals period of illumination (record interrupted for approx. 8 sec.).

and the frequency of the discharge in the nerve fiber are decreased by light-adapting the receptor unit, and recover in a parallel manner during subsequent dark adaptation (Fig. 14). Thus, the maximum amplitude of the ommatidial action potential and the maximum frequency reached in the corresponding discharge of impulses are closely correlated under various conditions of stimulation and adaptation. The slow-action potentials recorded from the body of the ommatidium and the discharge of impulses in the nerve strand appear to be comparable manifestations of the initial phase of the activity of the sensory element.

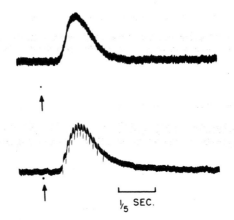

$\frac{1}{5}$ SEC.

Fig. 12. Action potentials recorded from an isolated ommatidium and its nerve strand (leads 1–4; same preparation as in Fig. 11) in response to a flash of light 0.01 sec. long (signals marked by arrows). Lower record: from intact ommatidium. Upper record: after piercing body of ommatidium with glass needle (somewhat higher amplification).

However, comparison of these two signs of activity during the course of any single response reveals discrepancies that cannot be neglected. If the frequency of discharge is measured at various times during the course of a response, and compared with the corresponding values of the ommatidial action potential at these same times, it is seen (Fig. 15) that the two measures are not related in a simple manner. Indeed, a single value of potential is not uniquely associated with a single value of frequency. This is perhaps not too surprising, for the properties of the irritable mechanism may be expected to change during activity. However, in the later phases of the responses to continued illumination the relation between the discharge of impulses and the level of potential appears to break down almost completely. After one or two seconds of illumination the potential difference between the ends of the

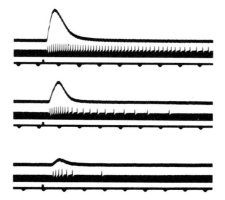

Fig. 13. Action potentials of an isolated ommatidium and its nerve strand recorded simultaneously, in response to short flashes of light (0.02 sec.) at three intensities (relative value, top to bottom, 1.0, 0.1, 0.01). Signal of light flash appears as black square near beginning of each record in lower half of white band just above time marks. Same preparation as in Fig. 10; see legend for details.

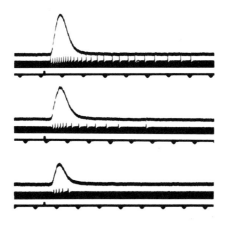

Fig. 14. Ommatidial and nerve fiber action potentials, recorded simultaneously from an isolated ommatidium (*Limulus*) in response to test flashes of fixed intensity at various times during dark adaptation (2 min., 4 min., 10 min., bottom to top) after a one-minute exposure to a bright light. Same preparation as in Figs. 10 and 13; see legends for details.

ommatidium subsides almost to its original resting value, while the discharge of nerve impulses is maintained at a steady level as long as the light continues to shine. This is true even for high intensities that elicit a brisk discharge of impulses.

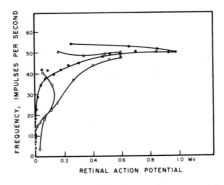

Fig. 15. Relation between the value of the slow action potential of an isolated ommatidium and the frequency of impulses in the nerve fiber attached to it, during the course of prolonged exposures to light. These curves were plotted from the records shown in Fig. 10 (● = top record, △ = middle record; ○ = bottom record. See legend of Fig. 10 for details). For each point the ordinate is the reciprocal of the time interval between successive impulses. The abscissa is the difference between the resting value of the retinal potential and its value at the time midway between these impulses. The upper left-hand point on each curve indicates the reciprocal of the interval between the first and second impulse in the discharge, and successive points indicate the frequencies determined by selected pairs of impulses during the course of the record.

Limulus happens to be rather exceptional in showing only very slight elevations in retinal action potentials during steady illumination. The eyes of most other animals show distinct plateaus of potential, even when no ganglionic elements are present (Figs. 4 and 5). The retinal action potential of the cephalopod eye, in which the retina is a simple mosaic of receptor elements, is a particularly good example (Fröhlich, 1913; Therman, 1940). Perhaps in *Limulus*, steady potential gradients associated with steady nerve discharge develop in regions of the cellular elements not favorably oriented for recording by the arrangement of external leads that we have employed. Indeed, we have evidence of slow electrical processes that are associated with activity of the sensory element, but not recorded by leads confined to the body of the ommatidium. In records obtained with both the nerve strand and the body of the ommatidium included between the leads to the amplifier (Fig. 11) the level of the slow-action potential can often be somewhat more satisfactorily correlated with frequency of impulse discharge than when the electrical response of the body of the ommatidium alone is considered (see Hartline, 1935). The nerve strand itself appears to contribute significantly to the potential gradients thus recorded. This contribution can be seen directly in some preparations, especially in those that have been slightly damaged so that the repetitive discharge of nerve impulses no longer takes place. When these slow potential changes in the nerve strand can be observed, their time course is very similar to the rise and fall of frequency of impulses discharged from undamaged preparations (Fig. 16), although no exact quantitative comparisons have yet been made.

The slow potential changes in the nerve strand, elicited by illumination of the receptor element, appear to be the result of electrotonic spread of electrical changes originating in the ommatidium. They resemble the electrotonic potentials recorded by Katz (1950) from the terminal nerve twigs of the muscle stretch receptor. Electrotonic spread of potential changes along nerve pathways from the receptor layer of the eye has been observed by other investigators (Bernhard, 1942; Parry, 1947); it may well contribute an important component of the total retinal action potential.

The isolated ommatidium of the *Limulus* eye affords an opportunity to study in detail the electrical responses of a structural element that appears to function as a single receptor unit. Still, our preparation does not consist of a single photoreceptor cell alone, and the electrical responses of the cell actually responsible for the discharge of nerve impulses may be partially masked by the activity of other cellular components of the retinula whose functions we do not understand (see Wulff, 1950). If, in addition, the geometrical arrangement of the cellular elements interferes with the faithful recording of the significant potential gradients, the interpretation of the action potentials recorded by external leads may be difficult, indeed. At best, in any preparation, the retinal action potential, as it is usually recorded, should be regarded only as an external manifestation of summated electrical events in the cellular components responsible for the generation of propagated impulses.

The recent development of micropipette electrodes small enough to penetrate single cells without killing them (Graham and Gerard, 1946; Ling and Gerard, 1949; Nastuk and Hodgkin, 1950; Brock, Coombs, and Eccles, 1951) offers great promise of resolving some of the difficulties that we have encountered in identifying electrical processes leading to the generation of nerve impulses. Our own investigations along these lines are as yet preliminary. Examples of the electrical response

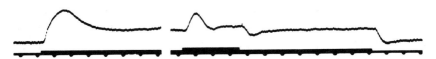

Fig. 16. Slow-action potentials recorded from the nerve bundle attached to a single ommatidium that had been injured deliberately in such a way that nerve impulses were no longer discharged. The potential difference was obtained from a pair of wick electrodes, one of which was placed close to the point at which the nerve bundle emerged from the ommatidium; the other supported the cut end (electrode separation approx. 0.5 mm). The amplitude of the initial maximum of potential was 0.18 mv. (Deflection upward indicates electrode nearest ommatidium became more negative with respect to cut end.) The period of illumination is indicated by the black band above the time line (interval between time marks = ½ sec.). After interruption of the record (approx. 5 sec.), the light intensity was increased by 50 per cent. (Signalled by upper black band.)

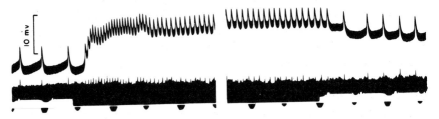

Fig. 17. Simultaneous records of the potentials arising within an ommatidium (upper trace) and from the nerve-bundle attached to the ommatidium (lower trace) in response to prolonged illumination. The black band under the lower trace indicates the duration of illumination. The activity of the ommatidium was recorded between a micropipette (tip diameter < 1 μ) inserted into it, and an indifferent electrode in the solution covering the eye. D.C. amplification was used; the resting potential having been cancelled by means of a potentiometer. Wick electrodes and a capacitance-coupled amplifier were used for recording the potentials from the nerve. Interval between time marks = ½ sec.

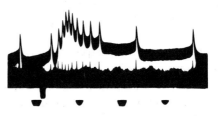

Fig. 18. Simultaneous records of potentials arising within a single ommatidium (micropipette recording) and from the attached nerve-bundle in response to a short flash of light (0.02 sec.). Other conditions as in Fig. 17.

recorded by a micropipette inserted into an isolated ommatidium are shown in Figs. 17 and 18. Many probings by the pipette were necessary before the responses illustrated were obtained, even though the group of retinula cells always comprises a sizable fraction of the volume of the ommatidium. This would seem to support our belief that it is the eccentric cell that is responsible for the discharge of nerve impulses. In the experiment from which Figs. 17 and 18 were taken, the final successful probing resulted in a sudden change in the potential of the micropipette, the electrode becoming more negative with respect to an indifferent lead by at least 50 mv. At the same time, the nerve bundle from the ommatidium suddenly began to discharge impulses spontaneously, and, synchronously with each nerve impulse, spike-like positive deflections were recorded by the micropipette.

Upon illumination of the ommatidium (Fig. 17) the potential of the micropipette became less negative and remained at a nearly constant value, elevated above the resting level, as long as the light continued to shine. At the same time there was an increase in the frequency of the spikes recorded by means of the microelectrode and their concomitant impulses in the nerve. Upon cessation of illumination the frequency of discharge decreased and the potential of the microelectrode returned slowly to its resting value. The higher the intensity of the stimulating light, the greater was the elevation of potential of the microelectrode, and the greater was the increase in the frequency of the discharge of impulses. In response to a short flash (Fig. 18) there was a transitory increase in the potential of the microelectrode, and a simultaneous transitory increase in the frequency of the impulses. Both of these effects began after a latent period of 0.07 sec. It may be noted at this point that in Fig. 17 the frequency of the impulses discharged by this element in response to light reached a high value initially, and then declined to a lower level that was maintained for the rest of the period of illumination, but that no corresponding maximum occurred in the initial development of the slow potential change. Our experience with this type of preparation is too limited to permit us to discuss the relation between the potential level and the frequency of nerve discharge, or to relate the potential changes recorded by means of the micropipette to the slow-action potentials recorded with external electrodes on the ommatidium or its nerve bundle. However, we are encouraged to believe that the use of the micropipette enables us to observe directly a depolarization of the sensory element under the action of light, a depolarization that is intimately related to the initiation of nerve impulses and that is manifested externally as the retinal action potential.

Since electrical processes initiated by the action of light appear to be of importance in the generation of nervous activity, it is profitable to examine the effects of electrical current passed through the eye. An excised eye of *Limulus* was arranged so that current from a battery could be passed through it, while activity was recorded in a single optic nerve fiber (Hartline, Coulter, and Wagner, 1952). Records from a typical experiment are shown in Fig. 19. When the corneal surface of the eye

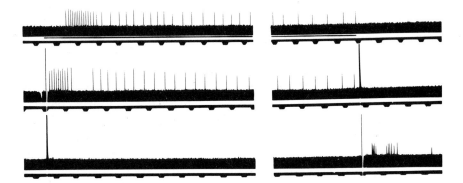

Fig. 19. Discharge of impulses in a single optic nerve fiber (*Limulus*, whole-eye preparation) in response to illumination and to electric current. Upper record: eye illuminated during the interval indicated by the black line in the white band above the timing line. Middle record: constant current (5 ma.) passed through the eye; cornea cathodal. Bottom record: constant current (5 ma.) passed through the eye; cornea anodal. Area of eye approximately 1 cm². The beginning and end of the constant currents were signalled in the middle and bottom records by the large artifacts near the start and finish of each record. A time-constant of 0·001 sec. was used in the amplifier to avoid displacement of the base-line during the passage of current through the eye. (Time in ⅕ sec.). (From Hartline, Wagner, and Coulter, in preparation.)

was made cathodal, trains of impulses were discharged in the fiber during the passage of the current. When the cornea was made anodal, no impulses appeared in the nerve fiber during the time the current was flowing, but after it was stopped a burst of impulses was discharged. With the surface of the cornea cathodal, the discharges resembled those obtained in response to illumination of the eye, beginning at a high frequency and subsiding to a lower steady level. The stronger the exciting current, the shorter was the latency and the higher the frequency of the discharge, just as in the responses to stimulation by light. Only the latent period differed significantly: for responses of comparable frequency, the discharge always began in a much shorter time after the onset of the stimulating current than when light was the stimulus. When a current was passed through the eye in such a direction that the cornea was anodal, the burst of impulses that occurred after cessation of the current had a longer duration, a higher frequency and a shorter latency, the greater the intensity or duration (up to one or two seconds) of the stimulus.[1] Very similar responses to the passage of electric current have been observed in peripheral nerve by Fessard (1936), Arvanitaki (1938), and by Hodgkin (1948).

The effects of electric current passed through the eye of *Limulus* combine with the excitatory effects of light. In the experiments cited above, the frequency of discharge in a nerve fiber responding to steady illumination of the eye was increased when the cornea was made cathodal. Current passed in the opposite direction slowed the discharge, and if strong enough would stop it. During current flow in the inhibiting direction (cornea anodal) the threshold to a short flash of light was raised. Subliminal current, flowing in the exciting direction (cornea cathodal) lowered the threshold to a flash of light, showing that the excitatory effects of subliminal current and subliminal light can summate to yield a response. So, evidently, light and electric current exert some of their effects at a common locus in the receptor or its nerve fiber.

Thus it appears that the visual receptors and their associated nerve fibers resemble other components of the nervous system, both in the action potentials they manifest when excited by their natural stimulus and in their reactions to applied electrical currents. Although many details remain to be clarified, it seems reasonable at the present time to predict that electrical aspects of the excitatory process in the photoreceptor will prove to play the same essential role as in the axons and cell bodies of neurones.

Even if we accept the hypothesis that the agent that generates activity in the afferent nerve fiber is an electrical process in the receptor, there still remains the question of how the initial photochemical reaction is linked to this electrical process. We may recall the well established fact that the retinal action potential, like the discharge of optic nerve impulses, does not begin immediately with the onset of illumination, but

---

[1] These responses following cessation of a current passed in a direction opposite to that causing excitation are of special interest, for they resemble 'off' responses to sudden darkening of the eye that are often observed in visual systems, such as the distal retina of *Pecten* (Hartline, 1938a) and certain of the ganglion cells of the vertebrate retina (Hartline, 1938b; Granit, 1947). While elements responding to a decrease in illumination have never been observed in the lateral eye of *Limulus*, such responses have been found in the optic lobe of the central ganglion in this animal (Wilska and Hartline, 1941).

has an appreciable latency. Following a short flash of light it, too, may take place entirely in darkness (see Figs. 4, 12, 13, and 14). This is universally true of retinal action potentials, whatever may be the animal form from which they are recorded. Simple eyes, in which there can be no question of ganglionic delays, show appreciable latencies in the appearance of the retinal potentials (see Fig. 4). In the isolated ommatidium of the *Limulus* eye, the retinal action potential recorded by external leads does not begin to rise until just slightly before the first nerve impulse of the response is discharged (see especially Figs. 11 and 12). The same is true of the electrical responses recorded by a micropipette in the ommatidium (Figs. 17 and 18). Analysis of the latent period of the retinal potential of the isolated ommatidium shows that it, like the latent period of the optic nerve discharge, has a 'critical duration'. Thus there must be an appreciable time-lag between photolysis and the beginning of the electrical response. The short latency of the nerve response to an applied electrical current, as contrasted with that of a comparable response to light, suggests that much of the delay in the generation of nerve impulses must be attributed to the elaboration of products of photolysis, and to their action in initiating the basic electrical process that in turn is assumed to generate nerve activity. Recently Wald and Brown (1952) have made the specific suggestion that the liberation of sulf-hydryl groups in the bleaching of rhodopsin may generate electrical potential gradients in the receptor, but it is still too early to judge whether this will account for the observed facts of receptor excitation. The links between the special photochemical mechanism of the visual receptor and the more general neural excitation processes remain obscure.

A comprehensive discussion of the properties of a sensory system would not be complete without reference to the complex neural interactions that take place between component cells. In a paper restricted to the consideration of the peripheral origin of nervous activity such a topic might properly be excluded, were it not for the fact that in some sensory systems, the very origin of nervous activity in the most peripheral receptor unit is affected by such interactions. This is true in the eye of *Limulus*, as the next section shows, and has also been reported for the sensory structure of the cochlea of the vertebrate ear (Galambos, 1944). The principle involved may well be of general importance.

In the compound lateral eye of *Limulus*, activity in a single optic nerve fiber can be elicited by illumination of one, and only one, ommatidium. Nevertheless, if a given ommatidium is illuminated steadily, giving rise to a steady train of impulses in its nerve fiber, illumination of other regions of the eye not too far distant from it produces a pronounced slowing of the discharge (Fig. 20; Hartline, 1949). The brighter the light on these regions, and the larger the area illuminated, the greater is this inhibiting effect upon the discharge. The effect becomes weaker for regions farther removed from the specific ommatidium, but often extends for a radius of several millimeters, over a third or more of the total area of the eye. If the activity is recorded from nerve fibers from two ommatidia not too widely separated, it can be shown that the inhibitory effect is reciprocal, each one affecting the other. Thus the activity of each ommatidium inhibits, and in turn is inhibited by, activity of many other ommatidia in surrounding regions of the eye.

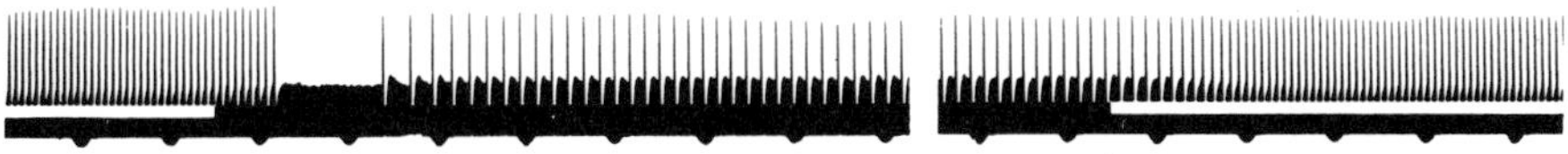

Fig. 20. Inhibition of the activity of a receptor element by illumination of a nearby retinal area. A single optic nerve fiber (*Limulus* whole-eye preparation) was caused to discharge impulses by shining a small spot of light on the cornea, focussed upon the ommatidium of the fiber. The illumination had commenced 5 sec. before the start of the record and continued throughout its duration. During the period indicated by the blackening of the white line above the time record a region of the cornea several millimeters distant from the excited ommatidium was illuminated. (Time in ⅕ sec.).

We do not yet understand how this inhibitory action is exerted, except that it appears to be dependent on the integrity of the nervous pathways in the network of fibers back of the ommatidia. In a few experiments, we have been able to show that if the bundle of nerve fibers from an ommatidium is snipped out, as in the first step of isolating an ommatidium (described above), the inhibitory effects are thereby abolished. Moreover, a microelectrode inserted into the ommatidium itself, thus recording the discharge of impulses at their point of origin, shows the same slowing of the rate of discharge when inhibiting areas of the eye are illuminated, provided the connections back of the ommatidia are intact.

Although we cannot explain the mechanism of this inhibitory influence in the *Limulus* eye, it is easy to understand its role in visual function. Since the inhibition of any receptor element is greater the higher the intensity of light shining on the surrounding regions, it is evident that brightly illuminated areas of the eye inhibit the activity of dimly lighted regions more than the latter inhibit the activity of the former. Thus contrast is enhanced. By a relatively simple type of interaction among elements of the eye an important visual effect is achieved.

For this paper the significance of the interaction observed in the eye of *Limulus* is that the degree of nervous activity initiated by any single photoreceptor unit is determined not only by the conditions of stimulation and adaptation of that unit, but also by the degree of activity of adjacent receptors. Each individual sensory element does not function as an isolated detecting device for luminous energy, totally independent of the action of all its fellows. The process of integration of nervous activity may extend peripherally to the very elements in which that activity is generated.

REFERENCES

Adrian, E. D. (1935), *The Mechanism of Nervous Action*. The University of Pennsylvania Press, Philadelphia.

Arvanitaki, A. (1938), *Les Variations Graduées de la Polarization des Systèmes Excitables*. Hermann et Cie. Paris.

Bernhard, C. G. (1942), 'Isolation of retinal and optic ganglion response in the eye of *Dytiscus*', *J. Neurophysiol.* **5,** 32–48.

Brock, L. G., Coombs, J. S., and Eccles, J. C. (1951), 'Action potentials of motoneurones with intracellular electrodes', *Proc. Univ. of Otago Med. School*, **29,** 14–15.

Demoll, R. (1917), *Die Sinnesorgane der Arthropoden ihr Bau und ihre Functionen*. Friedrich Vieweg & Sohn, Braunschweig.

Fessard, A. (1936), *Recherches sur L'Activité Rythmique des Nerfs Isolés*. Hermann et Cie, Paris.

Fröhlich, F. W. (1913), 'Beiträge zur allegemeinen Physiologie der Sinnesorgane', *Zeitschr. Sinnesphysiol.*, **48,** 28–165.

Galambos, R. (1944), 'Inhibition of activity in single auditory nerve fibers by acoustic stimulation', *J. Neurophysiol.*, **7,** 287–303.

Graham, J., and Gerard, R. W. (1946), 'Membrane potential and excitation of impaled single muscle fibers', *J. Cell. Comp. Physiol.*, **28,** 99–117.

Grenacher, H. (1879), *Untersuchungen über das Sehorgan der Arthropoden*. Göttingen.

Granit, R. (1947), *Sensory Mechanisms of the Retina*. Oxford University Press.

Hartline, H. K. (1934), 'Intensity and duration in the excitation of single photoreceptors', *J. Cell. Comp. Physiol.*, **5,** 229–247.

(1935), 'The discharge of nerve impulses from the single visual sense cell', *Cold Spr. Harbor Symposia Quant. Biol.*, **3,** 245–249.

(1938a), 'The discharge of impulses in the optic nerve of *Pecten* in response to illumination of the eye', *J. Cell. Comp. Physiol.* **11,** 465–478.

(1938b), 'The response of single optic nerve fibers of the vertebrate eye to illumination of the retina', *Amer. J. Physiol.*, **121,** 400–415.

(1948), 'Retinal action potentials of photoreceptor cells and the discharge of nerve impulses in their axons', *Federation Proceedings*, **7,** 51–52. (Abstr.)

(1949), 'Inhibition of activity of visual receptors by illuminating nearby retinal areas in *Limulus*', *Federation Proceedings*, **8,** 69. (Abstr.)

Hartline, H. K., and McDonald, P. R. (1947), 'Light and dark adaptation of single photoreceptor elements in the eye of *Limulus*', *J. Cell. Comp. Physiol.*, **30**, 225–254.

Hartline, H. K., Coulter, N. A., Jr., and Wagner, H. G. (1952), 'Effects of electric current on responses of single photoreceptor units in the eye of *Limulus*', *Federation Proceedings*, **11**, 65–66. (Abstr.)

Hecht, S. (1919a), 'The photochemical nature of the photosensory process', *J. Gen. Physiol.*, **2**, 229.

—— (1919b), 'Sensory equilibrium and dark adaptation in *Mya arenaria*', *J. Gen. Physiol.*, **1**, 545.

Hodgkin, A. L. (1948), 'The local electric changes associated with repetitive action in non-medulated axons', *J. Physiol.*, **107**, 165–181.

Katz, B. (1950), 'Depolarization of sensory terminals and the initiation of impulses in the muscle spindle', *J. Physiol.*, **111**, 261–282.

Kohlrausch, A. (1931), 'Elektrische Erscheinungen am Auge', *Handb. Norm. Path. Physiol.*, **12**, 1393–1496.

Ling, G., and Gerard, R. W. (1949), 'The membrane potential and metabolism of muscle fibers', *J. Cell. Comp. Physiol.*, **34**, 413.

MacNichol, E. F., Jr., and Hartline, H. K. (1948), 'Response to small changes in light intensity by the light-adapted photoreceptor', *Federation Proceedings*, **7**, 76. (Abstr.)

Miller, W. H. (1952), 'The neural structure and function of an invertebrate eye', *Bull. Johns Hopkins Hospital*, **91**, 72. (Abstr.)

Nastuk, W. L., and Hodgkin, A. L. (1950), 'The electrical activity of single muscle fibers', *J. Cell. Comp. Physiol.*, **35**, 39–73.

Parry, D. A. (1947), 'The function of the insect ocellus', *J. Exp. Biol.*, **24**, 211–219.

Patten, W. (1912), *The Evolution of the Vertebrates and their Kin* (see p. 153). Blakiston, Philadelphia.

Therman, P. O. (1940), 'Electrical response of eyes', *Amer. J. Physiol.*, **130**, 239–248.

Wagman, I. H., Hartline, H. K., and Milne, L. J. (1949) 'Excitability changes of single visual receptor cells following flashes of light of intensity near threshold', *Federation Proceedings*, **8**, 159–160. (Abstr.)

Wald, G. (1949), 'The photochemistry of vision', *Documenta Ophthalmologica*, **3**, 94–137.

—— (1951), 'The photochemical basis of rod vision', *J. Opt. Soc. Amer.*, **41**, 949–956.

Wald, G., and Brown, P. K. (1952), 'The role of sulfhydryl groups in the bleaching and synthesis of rhodopsin', *J. Gen. Physiol.*, **35**, 797–821.

Wald, G., and Clark, A. B. (1937), 'Visual adaptation and chemistry of the rods', *J. Gen. Physiol.*, **21**, 93–105.

Watasé, S. (1887), 'On the morphology of the compound eyes of arthropods', *Studies Biol. Lab.*, Johns Hopkins Univ., **4**, 287–334.

Waterman, T. H. (1951), 'Polarized light navigation by arthropods', *Trans. N.Y. Acad. Sci.*, **14**, 11–14.

Wilska, A., and Hartline, H. K. (1941), 'The origin of "off-responses" in the optic pathway', *Amer. J. Physiol.*, **133**, 491–492. (Abstr.)

Wulff, V. J. (1950), 'Duality in the electrical response of the lateral eye of *Limulus polyphemus*', *Biol. Bull.*, **98**, 258–265.

DISCUSSION

MONNIER: Among the remarkable results obtained by Dr. Hartline one appeared to me particularly striking. It is the parallelism between the subliminal photo-excitation of a receptor and the subliminal electrical excitation of a nerve. This observation indicates that both modes of excitation bear upon the same processes. It is therefore possible that photoexcitation may disclose oscillatory phenomena just as those shown in certain cases, by electrical stimulation. This situation seems to appear in human vision. The apparent brilliancy of a source of light presents a marked overshoot above its normal value, at the beginning of the illumination. This overshoot is more and more apparent as the true brilliancy increases, and is finally followed by several oscillations. This oscillatory behavior has been accurately accounted for by the late Dr. Lassalle according to the kinetics of the photo-chemical cycle of reactions which appear to be actually involved.

HARTLINE: The excitability of the *Limulus* photoreceptor unit shows a marked 'overshoot' at the beginning of a period of prolonged subliminal illumination, but after this initial maximum the excitability subsides to a steady level, greater than its value in darkness, without any oscillations that we have been able to detect. However, the responses to supraliminal excitation of the dark-adapted, isolated ommatidium usually show a minimum in the frequency of the discharge of nerve impulses following the initial maximum. This is more pronounced the higher the intensity of the stimulating light. Sometimes a small second maximum is present before the discharge settles down to a steady frequency. Thus, as Dr. Monnier suggests, these photoreceptors do show oscillatory phenomena, but the oscillations are heavily damped.

Voltage noise in *Limulus* visual cells

F. A. DODGE, JR.,[1] B. W. KNIGHT,[2] AND J. TOYODA[3]

IBM Research and *Rockefeller University, New York, 10021*[1]
Cornell University Graduate School of Medical Sciences and
Rockefeller University[2]
Rockefeller University[3]

Reprinted from SCIENCE, 5 April 1968, Vol. 160, pp. 88-90

Abstract. *Intracellular recordings from* Limulus *eccentric cells suggest that the generator potential arises from the superposition of numerous discrete fluctuations in membrane conductance. If this is so, a relation between frequency response to flickering light and noise characteristics under steady light may be predicted. This prediction is verified experimentally. If a discrete fluctuation model is assumed, the data indicate that increased light has two major effects: (i) the discrete events are strongly light adapted to smaller size, and (ii) the time course of each event becomes briefer.*

The eccentric cell in the compound eye of *Limulus polyphemus*, the horseshoe crab, is particularly well suited for investigation of the generator potential which apparently underlies visual sense perception. Here we present evidence from our observations on this cell in support of three suggestions concerning the nature of the generator potential.

(1) The generator potential arises from a superposition of discrete voltage 'shot' events or 'bumps', which are triggered by the absorption of light.

(2) The average size of the bumps decreases markedly as the ambient light intensity is increased, and this is the major mechanism for light adaptation.

(3) The improved time-resolution of visual response that occurs with increasing level of ambient light can be attributed to two factors – a more rapid rate at which the average bump size adjusts to light intensity and a small decrease in the duration of an individual bump.

Rushton (1) has discussed the possibility that the generator potential is the summation of bumps and has outlined the essential ideas embodied in the suggestions cited above. Yeandle (2), Fuortes and Yeandle (3), and Adolph (4) have extensively investigated several properties of the bumps which are resolved as discrete events in the dark-adapted

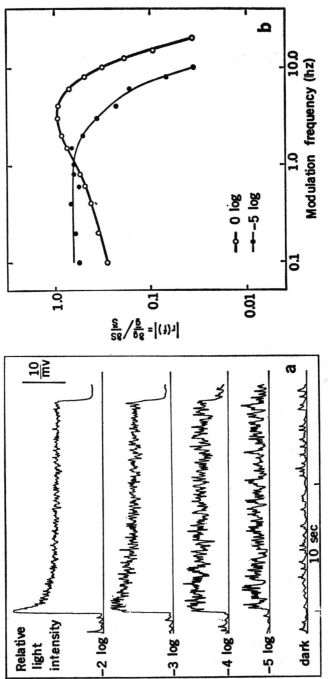

Fig. 1. (a) Representative records of generator potentials at different light intensities measured from an eccentric cell in which the nerve spikes were blocked by tetrodotoxin. (b) Transfer functions for the modulation of the generator potential in response to sinusoidal modulation of the light intensity, normalization described in text. The mean amplitude of generator petontial was 25 mv for o log and 4.0 mv for −5 log.

ommatidium. Some important results of these studies are that the rate at which bumps occur increases proportionally to light intensity (2–4), that the times of occurrence appear to be random and independent (3, compare with 4), and that the statistics of the bumps elicited by brief flashes is consistent with the idea that a bump is triggered by absorption of a single photon (3).

Physically, the bumps are discrete transitory increases in the membrane conductance of the visual cell (4). These bumps differ from the analogous quantal conductance changes underlying the miniature end-plate potentials of the neuromuscular junction (5) in that the duration of a bump is long compared to the membrane time constant and that the average amplitude of the bumps varies markedly as a consequence of normal function. In a study of the electrical equivalent circuit of the eccentric cell, Purple (6) has shown that the equilibrium potential associated with the excitatory conductance change is about 50 mv above the resting potential. Because the amplitude of the generator potential can be an appreciable fraction of this equilibrium potential, we have taken into account the non-linear relation between membrane potential and conductance in the analysis of our data, in the way routinely used in the analysis of end-plate potentials (7).

Figure 1(a) shows a sequence of generator potentials measured at several different light intensities from an eccentric cell (action potentials of the nerve were suppressed by a minimal amount of tetrodotoxin in the bathing solution). In examining these records we note: (i) in darkness, the spontaneous bumps are recorded as discrete events; (ii) in response to dim light, the very noisy generator potential appears to be the superposition of more frequent 'dark' bumps; (iii) the mean amplitude of the generator potential does not increase proportionally with the light intensity, but increases more nearly as its logarithm; (iv) the amplitude of the noise in the generator potential decreases with increasing light intensity; and (v) no large bumps are seen immediately following a bright light. All these remarks are qualitatively consistent with suggestions 1 and 2.

A quantitative relation between the noise observed under steady light and the response to a sinusoidally flickering light will be utilized below. We have measured the flicker response by a method similar to that of Pinter (8) except that our measurements were made on eccentric cells, rather than retinular cells, and that our frequency responses were refined by a narrow-pass digital filter (9). In these experiments the peak-to-peak modulation of the light intensity was about 40 per cent of the mean, and the linearity of response was excellent, as checked by the

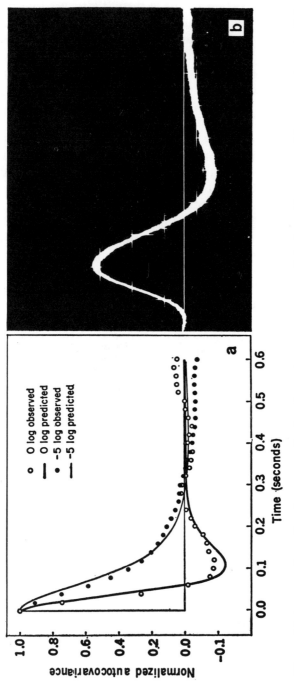

Fig. 2. (a) Autocovariance functions, normalized to the variance, at two mean light intensities measured from generator potentials (points) and predicted from the transfer functions (curves); same cell as Fig. 1 (b). The variance $(mv)^2$/mean amplitude (mv) was 0.0032/25 for 0 log; 0.17/4.0 for −5 log. (b) Direct measurement of the response to a brief (40 msec) flash superimposed on a steady bright background. Sweep duration, 0.5 second; response amplitude, about 5 mv; and generator potential amplitude, 16 mv.

absence of harmonics. Typical results are illustrated in Fig. 1(b) by plots of the amplitude of the frequency response measured at two greatly different mean light intensities. For this plot, the measured voltage changes (modulated component and mean value) were normalized so that the ordinate is the ratio of the fractional variation $\delta g/\bar{g}$ in excitatory conductance to the fractional variation $\delta S/\bar{S}$ in light intensity. For the very low mean light intensity, the frequency response shows simply the steep high frequency cut-off, which we ascribe to the shape of the bumps. For the high mean light intensity, the frequency response also shows a prominent low frequency cut-off, which we ascribe to the readjustment of the average bump size in response to the variation in light intensity.

Important temporal features of a (stationary) shot-noise process are conveniently given by its autocovariance function, that is, the time average of the lagged products of the instantaneous departure of the signal from its mean value:

$$C(\tau) = \overline{[g(t) - \bar{g}]\,[g(t + \tau) - \bar{g}]} \tag{1}$$

where the average is taken over the time t. Thus $C(0)$ is the variance of the signal, and roughly speaking $C(\tau)$ gives a picture of how the signal remembers its past. For the same cell that yielded Fig. 1(b), we have computed the autocovariance functions according to Eq. (1) from records of the response to constant light at the same two intensities (50 seconds of data were used for the dim light and 130 seconds for the bright). The results, normalized to $C(0)$, are plotted as the points in Fig. 2(a).

For a wide variety of shot-noise phenomena, a relation can be deduced between the autocovariance of the steady-state response and the expected response to small sinusoidal variations in a parameter of the system. The relation may be expressed as

$$C(\tau) = A \int_0^\infty |\,r(f)\,|^2 \cos\,(2\pi f \tau)\,df \tag{2}$$

where A is a constant of proportionality and $|\,r(f)\,|$ is the frequency response amplitude, as shown in Fig. 1(b). Equation (2) is easily demonstrated for an inhomogeneous Poisson (uncorrelated) shot noise (10, 11) where the parameter is the expected rate. More general models, in which the occurrence of a bump may influence the sizes of subsequent bumps (as suggestion 2 would imply), also lead to Eq. (2) (12). We have evaluated the integral in Eq. (2) by the Cooley–Tukey fast Fourier algorithm (13), using the data of Fig. 1(b), and the results are plotted as the solid lines in Fig. 2(a). We emphasize that the points and lines in Fig. 2(a) have been generated directly by the two kinds of data; there has been no fitting of parameters.

The degree of agreement in Fig. 2(a) encourages us to accept suggestion 1 provisionally and to examine suggestions 2 and 3 by deducing how the parameters of the shot noise depend on light intensity.

The mean and variance of a shot-noise signal are related by a pair of expressions of the form:

$$\bar{g} = \lambda \, T \, a \tag{3}$$

$$\overline{(g - \bar{g})^2} = \lambda \, T \, a^2 \tag{4}$$

where λ is the shot rate; T, the effective shot duration; and a, the effective shot amplitude. Equations (3) and (4), together with rigorous expressions for T and a, are known as Campbell's theorem (10). (If the shots, of which a shot noise is composed, are of constant amplitude for a finite duration, Eqs. (3) and (4) are satisfied if the amplitude is a and the duration is T.) If the effective duration T is known, then Eqs. (3) and (4) may be solved together for the rate λ and the amplitude a from measured values of the mean and variance. [This has previously been done by Hagins (14) for voltages recorded in the squid retina and by Adolph (4) for the *Limulus* generator potentials under very dim illumination.] Even for correlated shot processes, following from suggestion 2, the effective duration T may be evaluated rigorously from the frequency response of Fig. 1(b) (12). We have evaluated these parameters over a broad span of light intensities, with results shown in Fig. 3. Several features of these results deserve comment. (i) Over the span of a factor of 10^5 in light intensity the effective duration decreases by a factor of 4, of which about a factor of 2 results from the correlation of bump size (as indicated by attenuation of low frequencies in Fig. 1(b)), and the remainder may be attributed to a shortening in the time scale of the underlying bump as implied by the shift of the high frequency cut-off by about a factor of 2 in Fig. 1(b). (ii) With increasing light intensity the rate departs from strict proportionality to light intensity, which is indicative of a reduced quantum efficiency. (iii) The steady-state bump size decreases continuously, approximately as the inverse square root of the light intensity.

Suggestion 2 implies that even a momentary flash of light should cause a slight readjustment of bump sizes towards smaller values. A flash has been superimposed on steady bright light and the result is shown in Fig. 2(b). It is seen that, after an initial voltage surge in response to the flash, the voltage drops briefly below its steady-state value, as predicted. Similar experiments, in which the cell resistance was measured simultaneously, have shown that there is a definite minimum of the conductance at the minimum of the potential change. This observation speaks against the alternative interpretation that the underlying bumps might be diphasic at high light intensities, as high conductance at the minimum of Fig. 2(b) would be implied.

The undershoot of the response to a flash superimposed on a bright background (Fig. 2(b)) is reflected in the prominent negative phase of the corresponding autocovariance function (Fig. 2(a)). This implies that

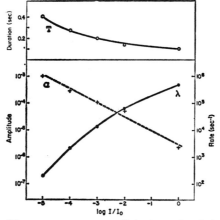

Fig. 3. Dependence of bump parameters on light intensity deduced from the noise on the generator potential. The effective bump amplitude (a) is given as the fraction of the conductance of the cell in the resting state. Same cell as in Figs. 1(b) and (2a). At intermediate light intensities the variance (mv)²/mean amplitude (mv) was 0.016/16 for −3 log; 0.032/12 for −3 log; and 0.077/6.9 for −4 log.

a positive fluctuation predisposes the generator potential to undergo a subsequent negative fluctuation. If the individual bumps are monophasic, this lends additional support to suggestion 2, with the further implication that it is the rate of bump occurrence that regulates the sizes of subsequent bumps.

Fuortes and Hodgkin (15) have investigated the quantitative relation between the changes in sensitivity and time scale that occur when the eye of *Limulus* is light- or dark-adapted. A major conclusion from their study is that a 200-fold reduction in the sensitivity is associated with a halving of the time constant of the response. If these responses were the summation of many quantum bumps triggered nearly synchronously by the test flash, their conclusion might be readily interpreted in terms of the results summarized by Fig. 3, in which the adaptation of the bump size by a factor of 200 was also associated with a shortening of the time scale of the bump by about a factor of 2.

A difficulty, which precludes the quantitative comparison of the two types of experiments, is our ignorance of how the dispersion in the time of bump occurrence, observed by Fuortes and Yeandle (3), depends on the past history of light intensity. Pinter (8) has pointed out that the formal model developed by Fuortes and Hodgkin (15) to describe the time course of the response to a flash is quantitatively consistent with the high frequency cut-off seen in the frequency response of the generator potential.

We close with two additional comments. First, not every eccentric cell shows the precision of agreement seen in Fig. 2(a). The time scale of the autocovariance predicted from flicker is often a bit slower than that directly observed, especially at low levels of light. This suggests an additional response feature that is relevant only when the input is time-dependent, and a good presumptive candidate is the time dispersal of bumps triggered by light (3). Second, the close qualitative correspondence between our Fig. 1(b), the wolf-spider retinograms of De Voe (16), and the frequency responses measured psychophysically by de Lange (17) for human subjects raises the possibility that the mechanisms discussed here may have applicability to other visual systems.

REFERENCES

1. W. A. H. Rushton, in *Light and Life*, W. D. McElroy and H. B. Glass, Eds. (Johns Hopkins Press, Baltimore, 1961), p. 706.
2. S. Yeandle, thesis, Johns Hopkins University (1957).
3. M. G. F. Fuortes and S. Yeandle, *J. Gen. Physiol.* **47,** 443 (1964).
4. A. R. Adolph, *ibid.*, **48,** 297 (1964).
5. J. del Castillo and B. Katz, *J. Physiol.* **124,** 560 (1954).
6. R. L. Purple, thesis, Rockefeller University (1964); summarized by R. L. Purple and F. A. Dodge, Jr., *Cold Spring Harbor Symp. Quant. Biol.* **30,** 529 (1965).
7. A. R. Martin, *J. Physiol.* **130,** 114 (1955).
8. R. B. Pinter, *J. Gen. Physiol.* **49,** 565 (1966).
9. Described briefly by J. Toyoda, F. A. Dodge, Jr., B. W. Knight, in *Abstr. Biophys. Soc.*, (1967), abstr. FA9, p. 94, or R. L. Purple and F. A. Dodge, Jr., in *The Functional Organization of the Compound Eye*, C. G. Bernhard, Ed. (Pergamon, Oxford, 1966), p. 462.

10. S. O. Rice, in *Selected Papers on Noise and Stochastic Processes*, N. Wax, Ed. (Dover, New York, 1954).

11. E. Parzen, *Stochastic Processes* (Holden-Day, San Francisco, 1962), chap. 4; also, A. Papoulis, *Probability, Random Variables, and Stochastic Processes* (McGraw-Hill, New York, 1965), p. 358.

12. B. W. Knight, J. Toyoda, F. A. Dodge, Jr., *J. Gen. Physiol.*, **56**, 421–437 (1970).

13. J. W. Cooley and J. W. Tukey, *Math. Comput.* **19**, 297 (1965).

14. W. A. Hagins, *Cold Spring Harbor Symp. Quant. Biol.* **30**, 403 (1965).

15. M. G. F. Fuortes and A. L. Hodgkin, *J. Physiol.* **172**, 239 (1964).

16. R. D. DeVoe, *J. Gen. Physiol.* **50**, 1993 (1967) (see also p. 2008).

17. H. DeLange, *J. Opt. Soc. Amer.* **48**, 777 (1958).

18. Partially supported by research grant B864 from the National Institute of Neurological Diseases and Blindness and grant GB-654OX from the National Science Foundation. We thank H. K. Hartline and D. Lange for major help with this project.

Variability of interspike intervals in optic nerve fibers of *Limulus*: effect of light and dark adaptation

FLOYD RATLIFF, H. KEFFER HARTLINE, AND
DAVID LANGE†

The Rockefeller University, New York, N.Y.

Reprinted from the PROCEEDINGS OF THE NATIONAL ACADEMY
OF SCIENCES, Vol. 60, no. 2, pp. 464-469, June 1968

The intervals between the impulses discharged by afferent neurons under steady conditions usually vary considerably. This variability is of interest for several reasons: (1) It must depend in some way on the underlying receptor and neural mechanisms that generate and propagate the impulses. An analysis of the factors that influence variability can therefore be expected to yield some indication of the nature of those mechanisms. (2) The information transmitted to the central nervous system by afferent neurons is coded in terms of the intervals between impulses, that is, in terms of the temporal pattern of the discharge rather than in terms of the shapes or amplitudes of the individual impulses. Any intrinsic variability in the intervals between impulses discharged by the neuron must therefore limit its capacity to carry information about extrinsic events. (3) Although the intrinsic variability may be "noise" as far as external events are concerned, there is nevertheless the possibility that it may actually carry useful information to the central nervous system about the state of the receptor or neuron and the influences that contribute to the variability of the discharge.

The variation of the intervals between impulses has been investigated and described for many different types of neurons,[1-3] but the causes of the variability are largely unknown. One supposed cause is "biological noise"—minute haphazard fluctuations in membrane potential such as those first observed by Fatt and Katz[4] at motor nerve endings in muscle. Recently, for example, it was shown that such random fluctuations, observed in spinal motoneurons of the cat, are adequate to account for the variability of the intervals between impulses discharged by these neurons.[5]

It is usually difficult to control the random fluctuations or "noise" in the membrane potential of a discharging neuron. But such fluctuations are unlikely to be altogether haphazard, and with adequate knowledge of factors that influence their frequency, amplitude, and other characteristics, they may sometimes be brought under control. This is the case with the irregular fluctuations in membrane potential observed by Yeandle[6] in eccentric cell bodies of ommatidia in the compound lateral eye of *Limulus*. At low intensities of illumination, the fluctuations are maximal and occur infrequently. The higher the intensity of illumination, the greater the frequency of occurrence of the fluctuations and, in the steady state, the smaller their amplitudes. Furthermore, the amplitudes of the fluctuations vary markedly with the state of light and dark adaptation of the ommatidium.[7, 8] After some time in the dark, the fluctuations elicited by low-level illumination of an ommatidium are large and distinct, but following a long exposure of the ommatidium to strong light, the amplitudes of the fluctuations become so small that they are barely discernible (Fig. 1).

FIG. 1.—Intracellular records of generator potential in an eccentric cell in response to a steady low level of illumination, below the threshold of impulse generation. The record on the left was obtained after the ommatidium had been in the dark for about half an hour. The record on the right was obtained after the ommatidium had been exposed to strong illumination for about 60 sec.

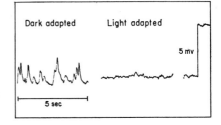

It was suggested by Rushton[9] that these fluctuations in membrane potential may sum to yield, or at least contribute to, the larger so-called generator potential upon which excitation of the eccentric cell and generation of impulses in its axon depends. A recent experimental analysis and theoretical treatment of the relation between the fluctuations and the generator potential by Dodge, Knight, and Toyoda[10] supports this view. Since the amplitudes of these fluctuations in membrane potential and the resulting irregularities in the generator potential vary with intensity and with the state of light and dark adaptation, the variations in interspike interval should be similarly affected. The following experiments were undertaken to make some preliminary tests of this idea.

A lateral eye of *Limulus* was excised and mounted in a moist chamber. Impulses generated by the eccentric cell of an ommatidium were recorded either (first set of experiments) by dissecting the optic nerve and placing a bundle containing a single active fiber on cotton wick silver/silver chloride electrodes or (second set of experiments) by inserting a micropipette electrode directly into the eccentric cell body. In the first set of experiments (Figs. 2 and 3), the ommatidium was stimulated by a small spot of steady light confined to its facet. In the second set of experiments (Fig. 4), the ommatidium was stimulated either by steady light on its facet or by steady electric current passed through the micropipette electrode.

For the "light-adapted" condition in the various experiments, the ommatidium was exposed repeatedly to 20-second periods of fixed high-intensity "adapting" illumination spaced four minutes apart. The intensity of this illumination was such that after a few repetitions a steady state was reached in which a discharge

FIG. 2.—Instantaneous frequency (reciprocals of intervals) of impulses discharged by an eccentric cell in response to steady illumination when the ommatidium was dark-adapted (*left*) and light-adapted (*right*). The sample records extend from the 15th to the 20th sec of 20-sec periods of illumination. The numerical data (*above*) are based on a set of records that included these samples but extended from the 10th to the 20th sec of illumination. Intensities of illumination were chosen (low on the dark-adapted ommatidium, high on the light-adapted) that yielded nearly equal frequencies of discharge.

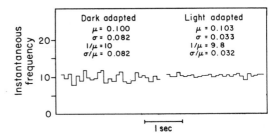

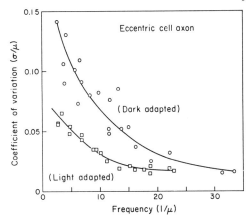

FIG. 3.—Variability of intervals between impulses recorded from the axon of an eccentric cell of an ommatidium when dark-adapted (*upper curve*) and when light-adapted (*lower curve*). The two curves were fitted to the points by eye. (The sample records and numerical data illustrated in Fig. 2 are from this set of observations.)

of about 35 impulses per second was elicited. Midway between these repeated "adapting" exposures the ommatidium was tested by exposure for 20 seconds to steady illumination at various intensities or, in parts of the second set of experiments, by stimulation with steady current. For the "dark-adapted" condition, the procedure was the same as above, except that the repeated exposures to the fixed high-intensity "adapting" illumination were omitted. The differences in these two schedules of illumination were sufficient to produce large differences in the state of adaptation of the eye. Complete dark adaptation was not achieved, however, since the testing exposures themselves, particularly at the higher intensities, inevitably produced some light adaptation.

The times of occurrence of the impulses were recorded on-line by a small digital computer,[11] and the mean length (μ) of the interspike intervals, the mean rate or frequency ($1/\mu$), the standard deviation (σ), and the coefficient of variation (σ/μ) were computed for the final ten seconds of each period. (The first ten seconds were omitted from the computation to avoid the transient changes in frequency that accompany the onset of illumination. Since a slight downward "drift" in the frequency of the discharge always remained, even in these last ten seconds of the 20-second exposure, a smoothed ramp was fitted to the data, and the deviations about it were used to compute σ.) Samples of typical data are illustrated in Figure 2.

In the steady state, the frequency of discharge of impulses increases with increasing intensity of illumination; that is, the mean interval (μ) decreases. But the standard deviation (σ) of the distribution of the intervals about the mean interval decreases more rapidly with increasing frequency than does the mean interval itself. Therefore, the coefficient of variation (σ/μ) decreases with increasing frequency of discharge of impulses. The exact form of the function is markedly affected, however, by the state of light and dark adaptation: the coefficient of variation is greater, for any given frequency, when the ommatidium is dark-adapted (Fig. 3).

These effects cannot be attributed to any long-term changes in the state of the excised eye as a whole. Alternating between light- and dark-adapted conditions

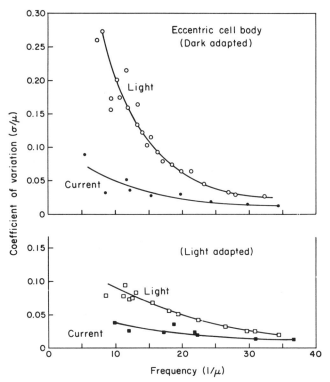

FIG. 4.—Variability of intervals between impulses recorded with a micropipette electrode from the eccentric cell body of an ommatidium when dark-adapted (*upper graph*) and when light-adapted (*lower graph*). The upper curve in each graph represents the normal discharge of impulses in response to steady lights of various intensities. The lower curve in each graph represents the discharge of impulses in response to depolarizing current of various strengths passed through the recording electrode. The curves were fitted to the points by eye.

during the experiment ruled this out. Furthermore, we have observed the same differences in variability while recording simultaneously from two ommatidia in the same eye—one light-adapted and the other dark-adapted. The dependence of the variability of interspike intervals on light and dark adaptation is the principal finding of the research reported here. This result is to be expected if the fluctuations in membrane potential, which are associated with the photo-excitatory process and which are markedly affected by light and dark adaptation, are indeed the underlying cause of the variability.

Further evidence that these fluctuations in membrane potential underlie the variability of interspike intervals was obtained in the second set of experiments. In these experiments, a micropipette electrode was inserted directly into the eccentric cell body and used both to stimulate the cell and to record its activity. This technique is based on the finding of some years ago that the ultimate action of light on an ommatidium is to produce a depolarization of the eccentric cell (the so-called generator potential), which in turn results in the discharge of impulses in the eccentric cell axon.[12] The depolarization results from a flow of current released by a photically induced increase in the conductance of the cell membrane.[13] The discharge may therefore be generated artificially by the passage of a steady current from an external source through the micropipette electrode in the proper direction to depolarize the eccentric cell.[14] Since the impulses originate in the axon near the cell body, they may be recorded by this same electrode.

The results obtained when the ommatidium was stimulated in the dark by a current passed through the recording electrode were very striking. In all cases and under all conditions, the variation of the interspike intervals was much reduced (lower curve in each of the two graphs in Fig. 4). Indeed, only very slight changes in the coefficient accompanied very large changes in the frequency of discharge. The results obtained lend strong support to the view that the fluctuations in membrane potential resulting from the photoexcitatory process are the principal cause of the variability of the interspike intervals since the variability is much reduced, as expected, when the photoexcitatory mechanism is bypassed in this way. Furthermore, as one would also expect, there is very little difference between the variability in the light-adapted and in the dark-adapted conditions. What little difference there is may be attributed to either the "spontaneous" appearance of some of the minute fluctuations or to their elicitation by very low-intensity light leakage into the box containing the preparation. In either event, whatever fluctuations may occur would be expected to be larger in the dark-adapted than in the light-adapted eye.

The reduced variability is not a consequence of the penetration of the eccentric cell by the micropipette. Indeed, when the ommatidium is stimulated normally by light, rather than by a current passed through the electrode, the results (upper curve in each of the two graphs shown in Fig. 4) are essentially the same as those obtained when the discharge is recorded from a point on the axon several millimeters distant from the cell body (Fig. 3). That is, for any given frequency, the coefficient of variation is greater when the ommatidium is dark-adapted than when it is light-adapted. If there is any difference at all between the variability observed with the recording electrode inserted into the eccentric cell body and that observed with extracellular electrodes in an axon some distance from the cell body, it is usually an increase rather than a decrease, presumably because of injuries caused by the penetration of the ommatidium.

The results obtained when the ommatidium is stimulated with current rather than light must be interpreted with a degree of caution, however. The paths followed by the flow of current passed through the recording electrode and cell membrane were undoubtedly quite different from the paths followed when the eye was stimulated normally by light.

The marked influence of light and dark adaptation on the variability of interspike intervals, which we have demonstrated in the experiments above, is perhaps related to similar changes, with light and dark adaptation, in the "sharpness" of visual thresholds. For example, Hartline, Milne, and Wagman[15] observed that the range of intensities required to elicit a fixed number of impulses, at threshold, in an optic nerve fiber of *Limulus* is quite large in the dark-adapted eye, but is greatly reduced by light adaptation. Similar effects in human vision were subsequently reported by Mueller and Wilcox.[16]

In summary, the results of these preliminary investigations are in accord with the view that the generator potential in the *Limulus* receptor is the sum of discrete photically induced fluctuations in membrane potential and that these fluctuations are the principal source of the variations in interspike interval. Whether these variations are mere "noise" or are actually carriers of useful information to the central nervous system remains to be determined.

We gratefully acknowledge the assistance of Dr. Jun-ichi Toyoda in carrying out the experiment on which Figure 4 is based.

* This research was supported by grant B864 from the National Institute of Neurological Diseases and Blindness, the National Institutes of Health, U.S. Public Health Service, and by grant GB-6540X from the National Science Foundation. A preliminary report of this work was presented at the Symposium on Processing of Data by the Visual System, The Max-Planck-Institute, Tübingen, Germany, August 29–31, 1966.

† Present address: Department of Neurosciences, School of Medicine, University of California at San Diego, La Jolla, California.

[1] Moore, G. P., D. H. Perkel, and J. P. Segundo, "Statistical analysis and functional interpretation of neuronal spike data," *Ann. Rev. Physiol.*, **28**, 493–522 (1966).

[2] Stein, R. B., "Some models of neuronal variability," *Biophys. J.*, **7**, 37–68 (1967).

[3] Perkel, D. H., G. L. Gerstein, and G. P. Moore, "Neuronal spike trains and stochastic point processes," *Biophys. J.*, **7**, 391–418 (1967).

[4] Fatt, P., and B. Katz, "Some observations on biological noise," *Nature*, **166**, 597–598 (1950).

[5] Calvin, W. H., and C. F. Stevens, "Synaptic noise as a source of variability in the interval between action potentials," *Science*, **155**, 842–844 (1967).

[6] Yeandle, S., "Evidence of quantized slow potentials in the eye of *Limulus*," *Am. J. Ophthalmol.*, **46** (3), 82–87 (1958).

[7] Fuortes, M. G. F., "Discontinuous potentials evoked by sustained illumination in the eye of *Limulus*," *Ext. Arch. Ital. Biol.*, **97** (3), 243–250 (1959).

[8] Adolph, A. R., "Spontaneous slow potential fluctuations in the *Limulus* photoreceptor," *J. Gen. Physiol.*, **48**, 297–322 (1964).

[9] Rushton, W. A. H., "The intensity factor in vision," in *Light and Life*, ed. W. D. McElroy and Bentley Glass (Baltimore, Md.: Johns Hopkins Press, 1961), pp. 706–722.

[10] Dodge, F. A., Jr., B. W. Knight, and J. Toyoda, "Voltage noise in *Limulus* visual cells," *Science*, **160**, 88–90 (1968).

[11] Lange, D., H. K. Hartline, and F. Ratliff, "Inhibitory interaction in the retina: techniques of experimental and theoretical analysis," *Ann. N. Y. Acad. Sci.*, **128**, 955–971 (1966).

[12] Hartline, H. K., H. G. Wagner, and E. F. MacNichol, Jr., "The peripheral origin of nervous activity in the visual system," in *Cold Spring Harbor Symposia on Quantitative Biology*, vol. 17 (1952), pp. 125–141.

[13] Fuortes, M. G. F., "Initiation of impulses in visual cells of *Limulus*," *J. Physiol.*, **148**, 14–28 (1959).

[14] MacNichol, E. F., Jr., "Visual receptors as biological transducers," in *Molecular Structure and Functional Activity of Nerve Cells* (Washington, D.C.: American Institute of Biological Sciences, 1956), publ. 1, pp. 34–53.

[15] Hartline, H. K., L. J. Milne, and I. H. Wagman, "Fluctuations of response of single visual sense cells," *Federation Proc.*, **6**, 124 (1947). For details see: Pirenne, M. H., *Vision and the Eye* (London: Associated Book Publishers, Ltd., 1967), chap. 9.

[16] Mueller, C. G., and L. R. Wilcox, "Probability of seeing functions for near-instantaneous thresholds," *Science*, **120**, 786 (1954).

Part Two

The Activity of Single Optic Nerve Fibers of the Vertebrate Retina

INTRODUCTION by F. Ratliff

> '*The retinal region occupied by visual sense cells whose connections converge upon a given retinal ganglion cell shall be termed the receptive field of that ganglion cell. . . . Not only do excitatory influences converge upon each ganglion cell from different parts of its receptive field, but . . . inhibitory influences converge as well.*
> '*The study of these retinal neurons has emphasized the necessity for considering patterns of activity in the nervous system. Individual nerve cells never act independently; it is the integrated action of all the units of the visual system that gives rise to vision.*'
> H. K. Hartline, The Harvey Lecture, 1942.

How individual cells and unitary processes are organized into the complex structural and functional systems that make up organs and organisms is one of the most fundamental, and yet one of the most neglected, of the many problems facing modern biological science. It is fundamental because this elaborate organization alone, perhaps, distinguishes living beings from non-living things. It has been somewhat neglected, however, largely because of the productivity of, and resulting recent emphasis on, the analytic approach to biology – the study of the structure and behavior of single cells and of the molecular and sub-molecular events within them. But to understand the neurophysiological basis of even the simplest and most ordinary aspects of visual perception, which is so rich and so varied in its content, requires far more than a knowledge of the specific properties of the individual cellular components of the visual system. The very first stage in the visual system, the retina, is a network. The functional units in it are interdependent and interact with one another; consequently many visual phenomena may depend as much upon the properties of this network, acting as a whole, as they do upon the properties of its individual components, acting alone. The Sherringtonian concept of the receptive field, first applied by Hartline to the study of retinal ganglion cells, is basic to an understanding of this integrative action of the retina and of how the responses that result from it are projected to, and further integrated in, the central nervous system.

Types of Responses. The most prominent features of the responses of vertebrate retinal ganglion cells are the bursts of impulses that occur when the conditions of illumination on their receptive fields are changed abruptly. Only a very small proportion of retinal ganglion cells typically yield a steady discharge of impulses to steady illumination – and even this steady discharge, when it does occur, is likely to be of relatively low frequency. The majority respond vigorously only when the illumination is changed: some yield impulses when the light is turned on, and another burst when the light is turned off – others remain completely inactive during maintained illumination and then respond with a burst of activity when the light is turned off. Hartline named these basic types of ganglion cells 'on', 'on-off', and 'off', respectively. He noted the existence of intermediate types, however, and it has since become evident that there are many others that are highly specialized in other respects. But no matter how complex and highly specialized, all types subsequently discovered appear to be variations of, and elaborations on, the three basic types that Hartline first saw.

The receptive fields in the retinas of cold-blooded vertebrates described by Hartline were more sensitive in the center than in the periphery, but yielded more or less the same type of response throughout their whole extent. He did notice, however, that in the eye of the frog an 'off' response could be inhibited by illuminating another area in the same receptive field, and Barlow (1953) later observed a similar inhibitory influence surrounding the excitatory region of the receptive field. Kuffler (1953) found an even more complex spatial organization in the eye of the cat: all three of the response types first described by Hartline may occur in one and the same receptive field, but with a clear-cut concentric arrangement – the typical form being an 'on' center and 'off' periphery, with an intermediate 'on-off' zone (or the converse). Similar more or less concentric fields, with antagonistic centers and surrounds, have since been found in the retinas of many other animals – both warm-blooded and cold-blooded.

Recent developments in the techniques of intra-retinal and intra-cellular recording and marking (see Dowling and Werblin, 1971, and Kaneko, 1971 for reviews) have now made feasible the direct investigation of the integrative mechanisms underlying these and other response patterns of retinal ganglion cells. Most of our knowledge of these mechanisms is still indirect, however, having been deduced from analyses of the responses of ganglion cells to various spatial, temporal, and spectral patterns of illumination. The dependence of the responses of certain ganglion cells on color provided an especially fruitful method of analysis which has contributed much to our present understanding of the nature and organization of the receptive field.

Color Coding. Wagner, MacNichol, and Wolbarsht (1960), in a study of the goldfish retina, found that the 'on' and 'off' character of the responses of some ganglion cells depended on the wavelength of illumination. (This 'coding' of color had previously been observed by De Valois, Smith, Kitai, and Karoly (1958), in the lateral geniculate of the rhesus monkey.) Similar effects were observed later by Hubel and Wiesel (1960) in the retina of the spider monkey and by Michael (1968) in the ground squirrel. A further investigation of color-coded ganglion cells in the goldfish retina, carried out by Daw (1968), showed the receptive fields to be more extensive than first supposed, but confirmed the basic observations made earlier, that some wavelengths of illumination are excitatory and others are inhibitory. Spekreijse, Wagner, and Wolbarsht (1972) have since shown that there are at least a dozen different types of ganglion cells in the goldfish retina classified according to the spatial and spectral characteristics of the 'on' and 'off' responses. Since the goldfish eye has only three different kinds of cones with three spectral sensitivities, this great variety of a dozen or more response types must result from the integrative action of the retina. Thus, it appears that although the photoreceptors in the retina operate in accord with the Young-Helmholtz three-color receptor theory of color vision, the neural network in the retina operates in accord with the Hering opponent-colors theory. As is so often the case in controversial issues, there is an element of truth on both sides. For a brief review of this issue, see MacNichol (1966).

The Spatial and Temporal Organization of Receptive Fields. The finding of the dependence of the excitatory and inhibitory influences upon wavelength has not only been of great significance for color vision, it has also provided a means for understanding the organization of the receptive field in general. Consider, for example, cells that have an 'on' center and an 'off' surround, with an intermediate 'on-off' zone in response to white light. With monochromatic light these same cells might be maximally excited by short wavelengths and maximally inhibited by long wavelengths (or the converse). Although it might appear that the center of these fields are purely excitatory, the surrounds purely inhibitory, and the intermediate zones a mixture of the two – this turns out not to be the case. Excitatory and inhibitory influences both extend over the whole receptive field, and the response at any point is governed by the relative amounts of the two influences. Wagner, MacNichol, and Wolbarsht (1963) demonstrated this by mapping a receptive field first with excitatory wavelengths and then with inhibitory wavelengths. This spatial and spectral organization has since turned out to be more complicated than it first seemed (Spekreijse, Wagner, and Wolbarsht, 1972), but it still appears that some combination of excitation and inhibition at a particular point in the field, rather than one influence on the other alone, usually determines the character of the response at that point. Although this view was based mainly on the experiments on color coding cited above, strong support has since been provided by several theoretical formulations derived from quantitative experiments on the exact timing and balance of opposed excitatory and inhibitory influences within the receptive field. See Bicking (1965), Bishop and Rodieck (1965), and Rodieck (1965). Supporting evidence comes also from a number of studies on responses to steps and edges of illumination in the receptive field; see, for example, Baumgartner (1961), Rodieck and Stone (1965), Enroth-Cugell and Robson (1966), Levick (1967), and Gordon (1969). The latter study, especially, shows how the relative contributions of excitatory and inhibitory influences may be deduced from responses to a step.

Motion. Retinal ganglion cells that respond to the onset and cessation of a stationary spot of illumination, Hartline observed, may respond equally well to a movement of the same spot. (See also Maturana, Lettvin, McCulloch, and Pitts, 1960.) That is, the cell responds to change and it matters little how the change is brought about.

Grüsser-Cornehls, Grüsser, and Bullock (1963), however, have since observed ganglion cells in the frog that respond little or not at all to changes in illumination without movement, but which respond vigorously to changes in the location of the pattern of illumination. Certain retinal ganglion cells are even more highly specialized and show a selective sensitivity to direction of motion; impulses are discharged in response to movement in one direction, but not to movement in the opposite direction. Such directionally sensitive ganglion cells have been observed in the pigeon retina (Maturana and Frenk, 1963), in the rabbit retina (Barlow, Hill, and Levick, 1964), in the grey squirrel (Cooper and Robson, 1966), and in the ground squirrel (Michael, 1968).

Experiments by Barlow and Levick (1965) indicate that asymmetrical lateral inhibition may account for the directionally selective responses. When the stimulus moves in the preferred direction the inhibition trails behind the excitation within the retina and has little or no effect on the ultimate response of the ganglion cell. With movement in the opposite (null) direction, the inhibition 'collides' with the excitation in the retina and thus suppresses the response. Again, the specialization appears to depend on the balance and timing of opposed excitatory and inhibitory influences. However, a possible role of the lateral spread of adaptation in motion sensitivity has been proposed by Burkhardt and Berntson (1972).

Configuration. The size and shape of a pattern of illumination, as well as its intensity and color, significantly affect the response of a retinal ganglion cell. In his studies of spatial summation Hartline found that, in general, increasing the area of illumination on a receptive field of a frog retinal ganglion cell increases the response. Subsequently, however, Barlow (1953) noted that some frog retinal ganglion cells may respond preferentially to small stimuli. These he called 'fly detectors'. Maturana, Lettvin, McCulloch and Pitts (1960) later observed similar effects and also noted that a relatively large pattern with a straight edge might yield no response at all when moved into the receptive field of a particular type of frog retinal ganglion cell, while a small circular stimulus might yield a vigorous response when moved into the same field. This type of cell they called a 'convexity detector'. According to Gaze and Jacobson (1963), however, such cells do not respond to convexity *per se*; rather, it is a particular balance of excitation and inhibition that determines the response, and different conditions – including both straight and convex edges – can be equally effective. For an experimental critique of some of the early studies on various classes of detectors, see Varju (1969).

It is clear from the work of Taylor (1956), Reichardt and Mac-Ginitie (1962), and others that the output of an inhibitory network depends very much upon the configuration of the stimulus. For review, see Ratliff (1965). In particular, since inhibitory influences generally diminish with distance, the amount of interaction will depend upon whether the stimulus is compact or spread out. Such mechanisms may well play a role in shaping preferential responses to small stimuli. Similarly, the amount of inhibition produced by the corner of a rectangular stimulus is less than that produced by the center, since points excited by the corner are only partially surrounded by other excited points, while those at the center are completely surrounded. Such effects may account, in part, for preferential responses of some ganglion cells to marked curvature of edges or sharp corners of stimuli. In any event, it appears almost certain that it is the distribution of excitation and inhibition within the receptive field of a ganglion cell that determines the character of its response to various configurations of illumination. And this distribution, of course, must depend in some way upon the arrangement of the retinal structures over which the excitation and inhibition are mediated (see Dowling, 1970, for a review of the structure of the retina).

Variations in Receptive Fields. The character of a receptive field is by no means fixed. Most noticeable is that the antagonistic surround tends to drop out in the dark adapted condition leaving the center with its characteristic response. See Kuffler (1952) and Barlow, Fitzhugh, and Kuffler (1957). Recent studies by Maffei, Fiorentini, and Cervetto (1971) show a further complication, however: 'on' center and 'off' center ganglion cells do not change in exactly the same way as they adapt. Thus not only size, but the overall character of the field, too, changes with adaptation. The reduction in effective size of the receptive field may be the basis for the increase in transmission of low spatial frequencies in the dark adapted state, observed both in psychophysical studies on the human eye (Patel, 1966) and in electrophysiological studies on the cat retina (Enroth-Cugell and Robson, 1966).

It has been suggested that changes in the relative contributions of rods and cones to particular ganglion cells during adaptation may account for these changes in receptive field organization. In support of this view are experiments by Barlow, Fitzhugh, and Kuffler (1957) on the cat, and Donner and Rushton (1959) on the frog. See Dowling (1967) for a review of work on the site of adaptation, and Dowling and Ripps (1970, 1971, and 1972) and Werblin (1971) for examples of more recent studies on adaptation.

The different parts of a receptive field not only share in common the final common pathway through the axon of the ganglion cell, they probably also share a great many intermediate structures as well. Any long-lasting changes in those common structures produced by stimulating any one local region of the receptive field might alter the response produced by stimulating another part, even at some later time. Lipetz (1961) and (1962) has reported two effects of this kind in the frog retina. Adapting one region of the field to light raised the threshold of other areas not illuminated and spectral sensitivities were altered in a manner similar to the Purkinje shift that occurs with light and dark adaptation in the human eye (see Burkhardt and Berntson (1972), for further studies on the frog; Easter (1968), for a similar study on the goldfish retina, and Cleland and Enroth-Cugell (1968, 1970), for related studies on the cat).

In addition to these short-term changes with light and dark adaptation, some long-term changes in receptive fields of retinal ganglion cells may be expected to take place as an animal grows and develops. This expectation has been borne out in some experiments by Reuter (1969).

He found that the relative numbers of various types of ganglion cells change – with metamorphosis – as the tadpole develops into a frog. Such changes may well be related to the completely different feeding behavior of the young animals and the adults. Information provided by retinal ganglion cells that respond to small dark spots appear to initiate feeding responses in the adult frog, which feeds on lively, small invertebrates, and not to be essential for the feeding behavior of the tadpole, which feeds mainly on algae and microscopic or dead animals. Such units, Reuter found, appear to be numerous in the adult frog and rare in the tadpole. The results suggest that the simply organized types of receptive fields occur in about the same proportions in both young and adult forms, whereas the proportions of the more complicated types, which respond best to specific stimuli, change during metamorphosis of the animal, as does its feeding behavior.

Technique and Temperament. The apparent nature of the receptive field of a retinal ganglion cell depends not only upon intrinsic properties of the retina itself; in the measurements of a receptive field the techniques used in the experiment and the temperament of the experimenter using those techniques are often revealed, too. That is to say, the characteristics of a receptive field depend upon the characteristics of the stimuli used to map it, and the choice of those stimuli frequently depends upon the particular interests of the experimenter and the particular objectives of his experiment. As a result of these untoward influences the various functions of retinal ganglion cells that are described in the literature are frequently much less clear cut than their names and classifications might suggest. Indeed, when viewed from several different standpoints, many turn out to fit equally well into several different classifications, and there is sufficient overlap of many supposedly specialized functions to indicate that all may be but variations on a single theme: the integration – over both space and time – of opposed excitatory and inhibitory influences. In short, the various special properties of different retinal networks do not appear to depend upon special or unique underlying neural mechanisms; rather, they seem to depend on nothing more complicated than a few simple variations in the spatial and temporal configurations of the opposed fields of excitation and inhibition. Therefore, when we achieve a better understanding of the few basic general principles governing these integrative processes we will, at the same time, achieve a better and broader understanding of the many 'special' functions that nature has constructed out of them.

REFERENCES

Barlow, H. B. (1953), 'Summation and Inhibition in the Frog's Retina', *J. Physiol.*, **119**, 69–88.

Barlow, H. B., FitzHugh, R., and Kuffler, S. W. (1957), 'Dark Adaptation, Absolute Threshold and Purkinje Shift in Single Units of the Cat's Retina', *J. Physiol.*, **137**, 327–337.

Barlow, H. B., FitzHugh, R., and Kuffler, S. (1957), 'Change of Organization in the Receptive Fields of the Cat's Retina during Dark Adaptation', *J. Physiol.*, **137**, 338–354.

Barlow, H. B., Hill R. M., and Levick, W. R. (1964), 'Retinal Ganglion Cells of the Rabbit Responding Selectively to Direction and Speed of Image Motion', *J. Physiol.*, **173**, 377–407.

Barlow, H. B., and Levick, W. R. (1965), 'The Mechanism of Directionally Selective Units in the Rabbit's Retina', *J. Physiol.* (Lond.), **178**, 477–504.

Baumgartner, G. (1961), 'Kontrastlichteffekte an retinalen Ganglienzellen: Ableitungen vom Tractus opticus der Katze', In *Neurophysiologie und Psychophysik des visuellen Systems*, R. Jung and H. Kornhuber, eds., Springer Verlag, Berlin, 45–53.

Bicking, L. A. (1965), *Some Quantitative Studies on Retinal Ganglion Cells*, Thesis, The Johns Hopkins University.

Bishop, P. O., and Rodieck, R. W. (1965), 'Discharge Patterns of Cat Retinal Ganglion Cells', in *Proceedings of the Symposium on Information Processing in Sight Sensory Systems*, Caltech, 116–127.

Burkhardt, D. A., and Berntson, G. C. (1972), 'Light adaptation and excitation: lateral spread of signals within the frog retina', *Vision Research*, **12**, 1095–1112.

Cleland, B. G., and Enroth-Cugell, C. (1968), 'Quantitative aspects of sensitivity and summation in the cat retina', *J. Physiol.* (Lond.), **198**, 17–38.

Cleland, B. G., and Enroth-Cugell, C. (1970), 'Quantitative aspects of gain and latency in the cat retina', *J. Physiol* (Lond.), **206**, 73–82.

Cooper, G. F., and Robson, J. G. (1966), 'Directionally Selective Movement Detectors in the Retina of the Grey Squirrel', *J. Physiol.*, **186**, 116–117 P.

Daw, N. W. (1968), 'Colour-Coded Ganglion Cells in the Goldfish Retina: Extension of their Receptive Fields by Means of New Stimuli', *J. Physiol.*, **197**, 567–592.

De Valois, R. L., Smith, C. J., Kitai, S. T., and Karoly, A. J. (1958),

'Response of Single Cells in Monkey Lateral Geniculate Nucleus to Monochromatic Light', *Science*, **127**, 238–239.

Donner, K. O., and Rushton, W. A. H. (1959), 'Rod-Cone Interaction in the Frog's Retina Analysed by the Stiles-Crawford Effect and by Dark Adaptation', *J. Physiol.*, **149**, 303–317.

Dowling, J. E. (1967), 'The Site of Visual Adaptation', *Science*, **155**, 273–279.

Dowling, J. E. (1970), 'Organization of vertebrate retinas', *Invest. Ophthal.*, **9**, 655–680.

Dowling, J. E., and Ripps, H. (1970), 'Visual adaptation in the retina of the skate', *J. Gen. Physiol.*, **56**, 491.

Dowling, J. E., and Ripps, H. (1971), 'S-potentials in the skate retina. Intracellular recordings during light and dark adaptation', *J. Gen. Physiol.*, **58**, 163.

Dowling, J. E., and Ripps, H. (1972), 'Adaptation in skate photo-receptors', *J. Gen. Physiol.*, **60**, 698–719.

Dowling, J. E., and Werblin, F. S. (1971), 'Synaptic organization of the vertebrate retina', *Vision Research Suppl.* **No. 3**, 1–15.

Easter, S. S. (1968), 'Adaptation in the Goldfish Retina', *J. Physiol.*, **195**, 273–281.

Enroth-Cugell, C., and Robson, J. G. (1966), 'The Constrast Sensitivity of the Retinal Ganglion Cells of the Cat', *J. Physiol*, **187**, 517–552.

Gaze, R. M., and Jacobson, M. (1963), ' "Convexity Detectors" in the Frog's Visual System', *J. Physiol.*, **169**, 1–3 P.

Gordon, J. (1969), *Edge Accentuation in the Frog Retina*, Thesis, Brown University.

Grüsser-Cornehls, U., Grüsser, O.-J., and Bullock, T. H. (1963), 'Unit Responses in the Frog's Tectum to Moving and Nonmoving Visual Stimuli', *Science*, **141**, 820–822.

Hubel, D. H., and Wiesel, T. N. (1960), 'Receptive Fields of Optic Nerve Fibres in the Spider Monkey', *J. Physiol.*, **154**, 572–580.

Kaneko, A. (1971), 'Physiological studies of single retinal cells and their morphological identification', *Vision Research Suppl.* **No. 3**, 17–26.

Kuffler, S. W. (1952), 'Neurons in the Retina: Organization, Inhibition, and Excitation Problems', *Cold Spr. Harb. Symp. Quant. Biol.*, **17**, 281–292.

Kuffler, S. W. (1953), 'Discharge Patterns and Functional Organization of Mammalian Retina', *J. Neurophysiol.*, **16**, 37–68.

Levick, W. R. (1967), 'Receptive fields and trigger features of ganglion cells in the visual streak of the rabbit's retina', *J. Physiol.*, **188**, 285–307.

Lipetz, L. E. (1961), 'A Mechanism of Light Adaptation', *Science*, **133**, 639–640.

Lipetz, L. E. (1962), 'A Neural Mechanism of the Purkinje Shift', *Amer. J. Optom. Arch. Amer. Acad. Optom.*, **299**, 1–8.

MacNichol, E. F. (1966), 'Retinal Processing of Visual Data', *Proc. Nat. Acad. Sci.*, **55**, 1331–1344.

Maffei, L., Fiorentini, A., and Cervetto, L. (1971), 'Homeostasis in retinal receptive fields', *J. Neurophysiol.*, **34**, 579–587.

Maturana, H. R., Lettvin, J. Y., McCulloch, W. S., and Pitts, W. H. (1960), 'Anatomy and Physiology of Vision in the Frog (*Rana Pipiens*)', *J. Gen. Physiol.*, **43**, 129–175.

Maturana, H. R., and Frenk, S. (1963), 'Directional Movement and Horizontal Edge Detectors in the Pigeon Retina', *Science*, **142**, 977–979.

Michael, C. R. (1968), 'Receptive Fields of Single Optic Nerve Fibers in a Mammal with an All-Cone Retina. I: Contrast-Sensitive Units, II: Directional Selective Units, III: Opponent Color Units', *J. Neurophysiol.*, **31**, 249–282.

Patel, A. S. (1966), 'Spatial Resolution by the Human Visual System. The Effect of Mean Retinal Illuminance', *J. Opt. Soc. Amer.*, **56**, 689–694.

Ratliff, F. (1965), *Mach Bands: Quantitative Studies on Neural Networks in the Retina*, Holden-Day, San Francisco.

Reichardt, W., and MacGinitie, G. (1962), 'Zur Theorie der lateralen Inhibition', *Kybernetik*, **1**, 155–165.

Reuter, T. (1969), 'Visual Pigments and Ganglion Cell Activity in the Retinae of Tadpoles and Adult Frogs (*Rana Temporaria L.*)', *Acta Zool. Fennica*, **122**, 1–64.

Rodieck, R. W. (1965), 'Quantitative Analysis of Cat Retinal Ganglion Cell Response to Visual Stimuli', *Vision Res.*, **5**, 583–601.

Rodieck, R. W., and Stone, J. (1965), 'Response of Cat Retinal Ganglion Cells to Moving Visual Patterns', *J. Neurophysiol.*, **28**, 819–832.

Rodieck, R. W., and Stone, J. (1965), 'Analysis of Receptive Fields of Cat Retinal Ganglion Cells', *J. Neurophysiol.*, **28**, 833–849.

Spekreijse, H., Wagner, H. G., and Wolbarsht, M. L. (1972), 'Spectral and spatial coding of ganglion cell responses in goldfish retina', *J. Neurophysiol.*, **35**, 73–86.

Taylor, W. K. (1956), 'Electrical Simulation of Some Nervous System Functional Activities', in *Information Theory*, Colin Cherry, ed., Academic Press, New York.

Varju, D. (1969), 'Functional Classification and receptive field organization of retinal ganglion cells in the frog', in *Proceedings of the International School of Physics 'Enrico Fermi'*, Course **XLIII,** Editor W. Reichardt, Academic Press, New York, pp. 366–383.

Wagner, H. G., MacNichol, E. F., and Wolbarsht, M. L. (1960), 'The Response Properties of Single Ganglion Cells in the Goldfish Retina', *J. Gen. Physiol.*, **43,** 45–62.

Wagner, H. G., MacNichol, E. F., and Wolbarsht, M. L. (1963), 'Functional Basis for "On"-Center and "Off"-Center Receptive Fields in the Retina', *J. Opt. Soc. Amer.*, **53,** 66–70.

Werblin, F. S., and Dowling, J. E. (1969), 'Organization of the Retina of the Mudpuppy, *Necturus Maculosus*. II. Intracellular Recording', *J. Neurophysiol.*, **32,** 339–355.

Werblin, F. S. (1971), 'Adaptation in a vertebrate retina: intracellular recording in *Necturus*', *J. Neurophysiol.*, **34,** 228.

The response of single optic nerve fibers of the vertebrate eye to illumination of the retina

H. KEFFER HARTLINE

Eldridge Reeves Johnson Foundation for Medical Physics,
University of Pennsylvania

Reprinted from the AMERICAN JOURNAL OF PHYSIOLOGY,
Vol. 121, no. 2, pp. 400–415, February 1938

In a series of three papers Adrian and Matthews (1927, 1928) presented a study of the discharge of impulses in the optic nerve of the eel's eye, and so opened a new approach to problems of visual physiology. In those papers the simultaneous activity of large numbers of optic nerve fibers was recorded. The possibility of extending that work to an analysis of the activity in single optic nerve fibers was suggested by the subsequent investigation of Hartline and Graham (1932) on the optic nerve fibers of a primitive arthropod eye (*Limulus*). The present paper describes the discharge of impulses in single optic nerve fibers of the cold-blooded vertebrate eye, in response to illumination of the retina.

METHOD. The usual methods for obtaining action potentials from only one fiber in a nerve trunk have not succeeded when applied to the vertebrate optic nerve. It is therefore necessary to utilize the intra-ocular portion of the optic nerve fibers, by exposing the fundus of the eye and dissecting small bundles of fibers from the anterior (vitreous) surface of the retina, where they converge to the head of the optic nerve.

From a freshly pithed animal (in most of these experiments large bull-frogs (*Rana catesbiana*) were used) an eye is excised, pinned fundus down in a moist chamber, and its anterior half (cornea, lens, choroid body) removed. A wide V-shaped cut extending almost to the nerve head gives access to the fundus and permits the vitreous humor to be drained away. It is then possible to dissect free small bundles of nerve fibers for a length of 1 to 2 mm., and these may be further dissected until only one fiber remains active. A bundle is severed where it enters the nerve head and the cut end lifted up onto one of the electrode wicks; the second electrode is diffuse, touching the surface of the retina. The action potentials from such bundles of nerve fibers are amplified and recorded by means of an oscillograph. The preparation is mounted in a light-tight, electrically shielded box, in the hollow walls of which water at constant temperature (*ca.* 20°C.) is circulated.

157

Prepared in this manner the retinas of most cold blooded vertebrate eyes survive for 4–8 hours, as evidenced both by the normal type of retinal action potentials which can be obtained from them (*cf.* Chaffee, Bovie and Hampson, 1923) and by the normal responses and lack of spontaneous activity in nerve fiber bundles freshly dissected from the retina. Fine bundles themselves, after having been lifted away from the retina, rarely remain conducting for more than an hour or two, and usually fail to show action potentials in a much shorter time. Attempts to obtain single fibers are successful in only a very small percentage of trials.

Light from a concentrated tungsten filament lamp is focussed by a condensing lens 12 mm. in diameter upon an objective lens, which in turn forms an image ($\frac{1}{3}$ size) of the illuminated condensing lens upon the retina. A 45° prism close to the objective lens reflects the light downward onto the retina; it can be rotated so as to project the rays at approximately normal incidence onto that portion of the retina from which the nerve fibers in any particular bundle come. At the condensing lens can be placed a suitable diaphragm to limit the size and shape of the illuminated area; this diaphragm is carried on crossed micrometers controlling its position to within 0.01 mm., and its image is accurately focussed on the retina by micrometer movements carrying the preparation itself. The intensity of illumination upon the retina can be reduced by known amounts with Wratten Neutral Tint filters; the full intensity (no filters in the beam) is $2 \cdot 10^4$ meter candles.

RESULTS. The discharge of impulses in any moderately large bundle of intraocular optic nerve fibers of the vertebrate eye is similar to that previously described for the whole optic nerve. Beginning several hundredths of a second after the light is turned on, there is a strong, brief outburst of impulses. Impulses continue to be discharged at a low rate as long as light continues to shine, and when it is turned off there is a renewed vigorous outburst which subsides gradually. Such responses were initially described by Adrian and Matthews (1927) in the eel's optic nerve and subsequently recorded by Granit (1933) from the mammalian optic nerve. It is not until the bundles have been dissected down until only one, or at most only a few, fibers remain active that a new and striking property of the vertebrate optic response is revealed. For such experiments show conclusively that not all of the optic nerve fibers give the same kind of response to light. This diversity of response among fibers from closely adjacent regions of the same retina is extreme and unmistakable; it does not depend upon local conditions of stimulation or adaptation, but appears to be an inherent property of the individual ganglion cells themselves.

Types of response. In figure 1 are records of the action potentials in single optic nerve fibers of the frog's retina. Figure 1A shows a response in which the initial burst of impulses, at high frequency, is followed by a steady discharge at much lower frequency which lasts throughout the duration of illumination. When the light is turned off this discharge stops. Such a response is similar to that from a simple photoreceptor, observed in *Limulus* optic nerve fibers, even to the short pause following the initial burst. But while *Limulus* optic nerve fibers invariably show this type of response, in the frog's retina it is obtained in less than 20 per cent of the fibers. The other fibers show strikingly different types of response. At least 50 per cent respond (fig. 1B) with a short burst of impulses at high frequency when the light is turned on, but show no im-

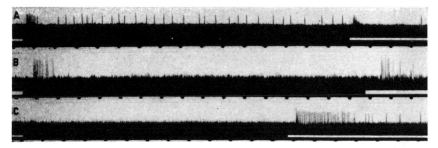

Fig. 1. Oscillographic records of the action potentials in three single intraocular optic nerve fibers of the frog's eye, showing three characteristic response types.

A. Response to illumination of the retina consisting of an initial burst of impulses, followed by a maintained discharge lasting throughout illumination. There is no response to cessation of illumination in this fiber (the off response in this record is partly due to retinal potential, partly to another fiber which discharged several small impulses). See also figure 6.

B. Response only to onset and cessation of light. See also figure 2, figure 5A and C.

C. Response only to cessation of illumination. See also figure 5B, D and E.

In this and subsequent records, the time is marked in ⅕ second, and the signal marking the period of illumination fills the white line immediately above the time marker.

pulses as long as it continues to shine steadily; when the light is turned off there is another brief outburst of impulses. Such responses constitute the most prominent feature of the vertebrate optic response—bursts of impulses occurring only when the conditions of illumination on the retina are changed abruptly. In a third type of response, occurring in about 30 per cent of the fibers, no impulses appear at all during illumination, but there is a vigorous discharge of impulses when the light is turned off (fig. 1C). This discharge may last many seconds, and usually subsides gradually. It is undoubtedly responsible for most of the "off" response obtained from the whole optic nerve.

Most of the optic nerve fibers in the vertebrate eye give responses similar to one or another of the above described types. These categories, how-ever, are not absolutely rigid, and it would be a mistake to ignore the occasional fiber whose response is intermediate in character. Thus it is not infrequently found that a fiber whose response is of the first type has a maintained level of discharge of a low and irregular frequency, which tends to adapt out after several seconds. No clear-cut cases have been found in which a fiber giving an initial burst followed by a maintained discharge has shown an "off" response; the doubtful cases which have been recorded could have been due to a second fiber, as is the case in figure 1A (see fig. 6A for a clear-cut case, where there is no additional fiber giv-ing an "off" effect). Fibers have been found, however, whose response lacks the initial burst; in these rare cases the discharge builds up slowly (in 2–3 sec.) to a steady level of *ca.* 20 to 30 per sec. When the light is turned off these fibers do show an "off" effect—a distinct increase in fre-quency for several tenths of a second before the discharge subsides. It is true that fibers which respond predominantly to a change in intensity with "on" and "off" bursts may occasionally show very irregularly scat-tered impulses or bursts of two or three impulses every few seconds during steady illumination. This, however, is quite different from the regular discharge of figure 1A, and may be regarded as an atypical, intermediate variety of response. Furthermore, fibers showing predominantly an "off" response are occasionally found in which a few scattered impulses "escape" during prolonged illumination.

From these observations it follows that the responses of the entire optic nerve are complex, containing different contributions from different fibers. An analysis of the optic response must therefore take up the properties of the different types of single fiber response separately.

Effect of intensity. Chief among the factors governing the response in any single fiber is the intensity of illumination with which the retina is stimulated. In figure 2 is shown a series of records of the responses to lights of different intensity of a single fiber of the "on-off" response type. With higher intensities of light the responses show shorter latent periods, higher maximum frequencies of discharge and greater numbers of impulses in both the "on" and the "off" bursts. This holds from threshold to intensities 4–5 logarithmic units above it. In figure 3 are plotted, on the left, the reciprocals of the latent periods and, on the right, the frequencies of the discharges (measured from the first six impulses) for both the "on" and the "off" bursts in this same fiber. In this fiber the threshold in-tensity was the same for both the "on" and the "off" bursts; frequently, however, one or the other of the bursts may have a somewhat lower thres-hold (usually within one logarithmic unit). It is to be noted that the curves rise abruptly from threshold—frequently the weakest response obtainable has a fairly large number of impulses, at a fairly high frequency.

While the threshold is sharp, it is not always reliable, and may fluctuate in spite of carefully controlled conditions.

The experiment of figure 2 and figure 3 shows the very considerable range over which intensity is effective in speeding up the discharge. This might be expected in view of the wide range which is covered by single

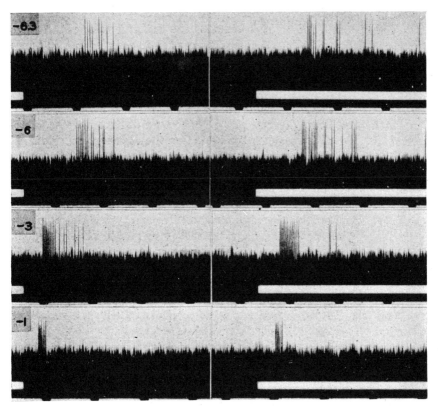

Fig. 2. Effect of intensity of retinal illumination upon the discharge of impulses in a single optic nerve fiber of the frog's eye. Logarithm of the intensity indicated on each record (unit intensity $= 2 \cdot 10^4$ meter candles, in this and subsequent figures). Diameter of the spot of light $= 0.10$ mm. Portions of the records, representing 2 to 3 seconds in each case, have been removed. They contained no impulses, except for the -6 record, which showed four impulses scattered over 2.5 seconds.

visual sense cells in the *Limulus* eye (Hartline and Graham, 1932). This experiment also shows the characteristic effect of very high intensity in reducing the number of impulses and often the frequency of discharge in the bursts. This is especially pronounced for the "off" burst, which may be entirely missing at the highest intensities available.

Similar effects of intensity can be shown for the other types of response.

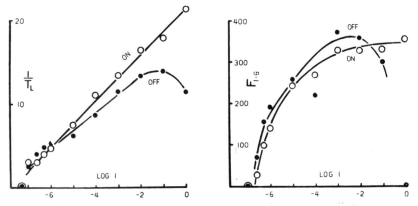

Fig. 3. The relation between intensity of stimulating light and response in a single optic nerve fiber of the frog's eye. Data from experiment of figure 2. On left the ordinates give reciprocal latent period (T_L, secs.); circles give values for "on" burst, dots for "off" burst. On right, ordinates give frequency (impulses per sec.) for the first six impulses of the bursts; circles give values for "on" burst, dots for "off" burst. Abscissae, in both graphs, give the logarithms (base 10) of the stimulating intensity. When no response appears, $1/T_L$ is assigned a value of zero; if fewer than 6 impulses are discharged, F_{1-6} is given a value of zero.

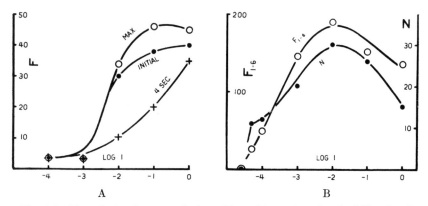

Fig. 4 A. The relation between the logarithm of intensity of retinal illumination (abscissae) and frequency of response (ordinates) in a single optic nerve fiber of the frog's eye. This fiber gave a response consisting of an initial burst followed by a discharge which was maintained throughout illumination. Dots and circles give, respectively, initial and maximum frequencies (three impulses) of initial burst; crosses give the frequency attained after four seconds of steady illumination.

Fig. 4 B. The relation between intensity and response of a single optic nerve fiber in the frog's eye. This fiber gave a response only upon cessation of illumination. Abscissae give the logarithms of the intensity of light. Ordinates (F_{1-6}, on the left) for the circles give the frequency (impulses per second) for the first six impulses; ordinates (N, on the right) for the dots give the total number of impulses in the burst.

In figure 4A are plotted the frequencies of various parts of the discharge in a fiber giving an initial burst followed by a maintained discharge. The initial frequency (first three impulses) and maximum frequency (usually between the 5th to 8th impulse) of the initial burst are given, together with the final level of frequency attained after four seconds of steady illumination. This graph may be compared with a similar plot for the *Limulus* single optic nerve fiber (Hartline and Graham, 1932, fig. 6). At low intensities, near threshold, the maintained discharge usually adapts out completely after a second or two, and often only the initial burst can be obtained.

The degree of activity in a fiber giving only an "off" response is also dependent upon the intensity of the light. In figure 4B are plotted the initial frequencies of the discharge from such a fiber, in response to cessation of lights of different intensities. The sharp threshold, and the diminshed values at high intensities are similar to the corresponding plot of the "off" burst of figure 3. This particular fiber gave a rather short, sharply defined burst not unlike the "off" response in a typical "on-off" fiber. This enabled a reliable count to be made of the total numbers of impulses in the bursts, also plotted in figure 4B. Usually, however, as has been said, the discharge in a fiber giving only an "off" response is prolonged, and dies down very gradually. (Compare fig. 1B with C; fig. 5A and C with B, D and E.) The higher the intensity the longer does the discharge last; at very high intensities the initial part of it may be reduced to a few impulses, but after several seconds it is gradually resumed, and may persist for many minutes at a frequency which may be as high as twenty or thirty impulses per second. Several instances have been observed where such a discharge broke up into rhythmic bursts, coming at about 3 to 5 per second.

Change in intensity. The amount of change in intensity also affects the magnitude of the responses. Fibers which discharge a brief burst of impulses in response to the onset and cessation of illumination also respond to a sudden increase or decrease in its intensity (fig. 5A); the bursts, however, have fewer impulses at a lower frequency. Likewise the "off" fibers will respond, though less strongly, if the illumination is partially reduced (fig. 5B) but not if it is increased in intensity. The frequency of the maintained discharge in those fibers which show such a response is of course determined only by the level of the steady illumination—an increase or decrease in intensity results in a corresponding rise or fall in frequency (fig. 7C).

Light and dark adaptation. A given intensity of light is effectively weaker in the light adapted retina than after dark adaptation. As dark adaptation proceeds the response to a given intensity increases, and correspondingly the threshold falls, rapidly at first and then more gradually.

After one half hour in the dark a fiber may respond to light 1/100 to 1/1000 the intensity of that necessary to elicit a response in the light adapted condition. The essential character of the response in any given fiber, however, is unchanged by adaptation. Reliable quantitative meas-

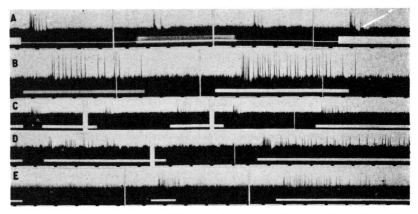

Fig. 5. Records of the impulse discharge in single optic nerve fibers of vertebrate eyes. Record B is from an alligator, the rest are from frogs. Recording as in figure 1.

A. Response to a partial reduction and to an increase in intensity of an "on-off" fiber. Left to right: Onset of light (log I = −2.0); intensity reduced by 0.5 log unit; intensity increased to original value; light turned off.

B. Response to partial reduction in intensity in a fiber giving only "off" responses. Left to right: light of an intensity log I = −2.0 reduced in intensity by 0.7 log unit; (a length of record equivalent to ½ sec., showing a gradually decreasing discharge, has been removed) light increased to original intensity; (a length of record equivalent to 1 sec., showing no impulses, has been removed) light turned off; (a length of record equivalent to 1 sec., showing a steadily decreasing discharge, has been removed) light turned on again.

C. (Time scale same as in the other records.) Effect of exposure in producing an "off" burst in an "on-off" fiber. Left to right: exposures, to a constant intensity, of 0.18 sec., 0.70 sec., 3.0 sec. Exposures made successively within about 10 seconds of each other, hence the "on" bursts in last two records are somewhat weaker than in first record, taken in the completely dark adapted condition.

D. Same as C for a fiber giving only an "off" response. Left to right: exposure to a constant intensity of 0.20 sec. and of 2.2 sec.

E. Inhibition of "off" discharge by re-illumination. (See also B of this fig.). After an interruption of 0.23 sec. light is turned on again (middle section of record); full "off" response shown in last section of record.

urements of the effect of adaptation in these experiments are difficult to obtain, owing to the comparatively short time fibers stay alive in a dissected bundle.

Duration of exposure. The strength of an "off" response at a given intensity depends on the length of time the preceding light has been allowed to shine. It is entirely absent following short flashes, and in general is stronger the longer the exposure. This is true for the fibers giving both "on" and "off" bursts (fig. 5C) as well as for fibers giving only "off" responses (fig. 5D). Similarly the "on" burst will be absent or weak unless there has been a sufficiently long period of darkness preceding (fig. 7B). The exact time requirements for the development of the "on" and "off" bursts vary widely with different fibers.

Inhibition of the "off" response. The presence, in the vertebrate eye, of a fair percentage of fibers responding only when the light is turned off or reduced in intensity is one of the somewhat surprising findings of the present study. Although no impulses appear in such fibers during illumination, it is to be emphasized that the "off" discharge depends upon the preceding period of illumination for its excitation. The effect of this excitation does not appear until after the stimulating agent has been removed. Indeed, if the retina be re-illuminated before an "off" response has subsided, the discharge is abruptly suppressed. This may be seen in figure 5E, by comparing the effect of the brief interruption of the illumination with the fully developed "off" response following permanent cessation of the light. A very brief interruption (shorter than the latent period of the "off" response) will still give rise to a burst of impulses, but one which is very short and with considerably reduced impulse frequency. The prolonged "off" discharge following intense and prolonged illumination can always be stopped by re-illumination, even at considerably lower intensity. Following such a period of low illumination the discharge re-appears, augmented by the "off" response caused by cessation of the weak light.

This inhibitory action of light on the "off" discharge is one of the most striking features of the vertebrate optic response. Most of its effects which have been noted here have already been described in responses from the whole optic nerve (Granit and Therman, 1935; Granit and Riddell, 1934). The present results clarify the analysis considerably, by showing the rôles played by different fibers. Thus the latency of the suppression of the "off" discharge is usually very short—shorter than the latency of the "on" bursts in other fibers, especially under the conditions of light adaptation which necessarily exist. Hence in bundles containing many active fibers a brief pause occurs, shortly following re-illumination, during which no impulses are discharged (fig. 7B). This interval between the time when the activity in the "off" response fibers has been suppressed and the moment of appearance of the "on" bursts in other fibers probably corresponds to the "A" wave of the retinal action potential. As shown by Granit and Therman (1935), the principal effect of the "A" wave is to remove what "off" effect may be present; it is large when there is still a strong discharge in the "off" response fibers. When the discharge has subsided in most of these fibers, after dark adaptation, and the "on" bursts in other fibers are stronger and have a shorter latency, the "A" wave is correspondingly small.

Stability of response types. a. *Conditions of stimulation.* It is to be seen from the preceding sections that the various types of response which are obtained in different fibers are characteristic of the particular fibers in question, rather than being due to the conditions of stimulation. Thus fibers giving "on" and "off" bursts, or only "off" responses do so over the entire range of intensities to which they respond; and fibers in which a discharge is maintained during steady illumination show this response for all intensities except near threshold. Likewise during light and dark adaptation of the eye, the type of response in any given fiber does not change. Frogs kept in bright sunlight for as long as 4–6 hours show no essential differences in the types of responses from those which have been kept in complete darkness for 48 hours, have had their eyes removed and prepared in red light, and the nerve bundles rapidly dissected in the weakest possible white light.

b. *External factors.* In order to test the possible influence of some of the more obvious external factors which might affect the retina, the following experiments were done. While not extensive, they do indicate a considerable stability in the essential features of the various response types. *Asphyxia:* if hydrogen is passed through the moist chamber, responses quickly become feeble and soon fail; they return to their former strength if oxygen is promptly readmitted. But at no time do they change their essential character during asphyxia. *pH and CO_2:* changing the pH of the Ringer's solution between 6.8 and 8.5 (phosphate buffers) with which the retina was then bathed for a few minutes produced no very apparent change in the responses, in one experiment. Two per cent CO_2 mixed with the air passed into the moist chamber causes reversible failure, with no change in the character of the responses. *Ion unbalance:* bathing the retina for a few minutes with Ringer's solution containing no calcium brings about a great increase in spontaneous activity, and tends to prolong the bursts of both the "on-off" and "off" types, with possibly some tendency to show "escape" of scattered impulses during illumination. Ringer's solution containing no potassium, on the other hand, abolishes even that spontaneous activity which may be present normally, and reduces the number of impulses in the bursts caused by change in illumination. In fibers which normally show a maintained discharge the response is not abolished, although its frequency may be reduced. These changes with unbalanced Ringer's solution are all reversible. *Temperature:* between 18° and 24°C. there is a marked speeding up of the responses with higher temperature, but there is no essential change in their character. *Season:* over a period of three years these experiments have shown no differences that could be correlated with the season of the year, or whether the animals were freshly caught or had been kept in the laboratory.

Thus external agents which definitely affect the degree of response do not, however, change its essential character. That seems to be a fixed attribute of each particular ganglion cell.

Responses in other vertebrates. Responses in optic nerve fibers have been recorded in a variety of cold blooded vertebrates other than the frog. These experiments include one shark, one *Necturus*, a number of turtles and alligators, one iguana and several varieties of snakes. While not extensive, they show unmistakably the same general result that is found in the experiments on frogs. In the eyes of all these animals there are fibers which maintain a discharge as long as the retina is illuminated (or at least for the first several minutes), other fibers which give bursts of impulses only in response to changing the intensity of light, and still others which respond only when the illumination is reduced. Minor differences have, however, been found, and a more exhaustive comparative study might even reveal significant variation in optic function among different vertebrates. Thus in the experiment on *Necturus* the maintained discharge disappeared completely after a half minute exposure to light, and the "off" responses were feeble and required at least ten or more seconds' exposure before they could be elicited. And in both the turtle and alligator eyes fibers are not infrequently found giving only a brief burst when light is turned on, with neither maintained discharge nor "off" response. On the other hand, where one might expect to find striking differences, as in the pure cone retina of the snake, neither the actual types of response nor the relative frequency with which they were obtained differed notably from those in the mixed, though predominantly rod retina of the frog. (Only four satisfactory experiments have been done on the snake eye, since it is a difficult preparation.)

Spatial effects. No description of the optic responses in single fibers would be complete without a description of the region of the retina which must be illuminated in order to obtain a response in any given fiber. This region will be termed the receptive field of the fiber. The location of the receptive field of a given fiber is fixed; its extent, however, depends upon the intensity and size of the spot of light used to explore it, and upon the condition of adaptation; these factors must therefore be specified in describing it. For moderate intensities (less than *ca.* 4 logarithmic units above threshold) and small spots (of the order of 0.1 mm.) the receptive fields of most of the fibers of the frog's retina are roughly circular, with a diameter of the order of 1 mm. in the dark adapted condition. Even at threshold a small spot of light 0.05 mm. in diameter will usually elicit a response in most fibers anywhere within an area of *ca.* 0.5 mm. diameter. At higher intensities the size of this region from which a response can be obtained is larger, but the strongest response is always obtained from the central portion of the receptive field; from the margins the response is usually of the threshold type (fig. 6). Thus the results of illumination of different points within a restricted region of the retina converge upon a given ganglion cell, and cause responses in its axone. This convergence extends over greater distances the stronger the stimulus; and for a given intensity the effects are strongest in the center of the region of convergence. Of particular importance to the present discussion is that, no matter what part of the receptive field is stimulated, the response in any given fiber is always essentially of the same type. This holds true for all types of response, and applies to stimulation anywhere within the receptive field. A few apparent exceptions have been observed, in which the type of response was different for different positions on the retina of the stimulating

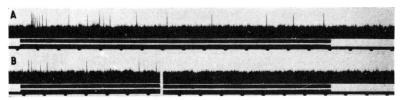

Fig. 6. Records of the impulse discharge in a single optic nerve fiber of the frog's eye, showing stronger response upon illumination in center of receptive field of the fiber than that obtained near margin.

A. Spot of light (log I = −2.0) 0.05 mm. in diameter carefully centered on most sensitive portion of the retina for this fiber.

B. Spot placed 0.22 mm. from this position (a portion of this record corresponding to 0.66 sec., and containing one impulse 0.45 sec. from the last one in the record, has been removed). Responses to this spot could be obtained anywhere within a radius of *ca*. 0.4 mm. of the position giving record A; the discharge was maintained throughout the entire period of illumination, however, only for positions very close to the central one (within ca. 0.05 mm.).

spot of light. In those cases where opportunity permitted a closer investigation, however, they proved to be either anomalous effects near threshold, or else due to two active fibers whose action potentials were so nearly similar as to be confused.[1] If true exceptions do exist, they must be quite rare; nevertheless they would be of considerable significance in explaining the diversity of the response types.

No correlation has been noted between the type of response given by a fiber and the location in the retina of its receptive field; all response types

[1] Such confusion does not arise very often, and when it does there is usually adequate opportunity to recognize the impulses due to separate fibers when the bundle begins to die, since it is very unlikely that different fibers will fail to conduct at the same time and show the same changes in the form and magnitude of their action potentials.

can be obtained from any part of the retina. (Whether this holds true for the foveal region in animals possessing a well-defined rod-free area needs to be determined.) Indeed, the receptive fields of different fibers picked up in the same bundle frequently overlap considerably, and in fortunate preparations, where impulses in different fibers can be clearly distinguished by differences in the form and magnitude of their action potentials, it is easy to show that fibers with different types of response

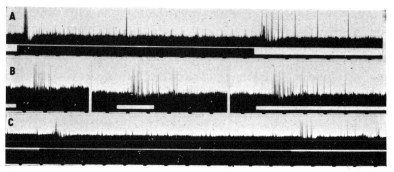

Fig. 7. Records of the discharge of impulses in bundles of optic nerve fibers of vertebrate eyes, each showing different types of responses in different fibers from the same region of the retina.

A. Bundle from turtle's eye, showing one fiber giving "on" and "off" bursts (large impulses); another discharging impulses throughout whole period of illumination (small impulses); and a third giving only a brief "off" response (medium sized impulses).

B. Bundle from frog's eye, showing two active fibers, one giving typical "on" and "off" bursts (large impulses), the other responding only to turning light off. Re-illumination after 0.36 sec. (middle part of record) stopped the discharge in fiber giving only the "off" response (compare with last part of record, where light was left off) and produced a very weak "on" response in the "on-off" fiber.

C. Bundle from frog's eye, showing a fiber (small impulses) which maintained its discharge at a low frequency during period of illumination at beginning of record Intensity doubled, this fiber gave an initial burst and then maintained its discharge at a higher level of frequency. Intensity reduced to its former value; frequency in this fiber dropped, and another fiber responded with a vigorous "off" response, (large, thin impulses). A third fiber (medium sized, thin impulses) gave a short burst in response to the increase, and very few impulses (difficult to distinguish) in response to the decrease.

are usually present and are stimulated simultaneously by a small spot of light (fig. 7). Such observations constitute good evidence for the distinctness of the response types, for they are obtained under identical conditions of adaptation, stimulation, and external environment.

DISCUSSION. From this experimental study it is apparent that each individual ganglion cell has a relatively fixed character of response, which, with few exceptions, falls under one of three distinct types. Concerning the explanation of this rather unexpected result one can only speculate. The retina, of course, does not possess a homogeneous population of end-organs, and it is possible that the different types of response originate in different types of visual sense cells, merely being relayed through the ganglion cells unaltered. Thus the rods and cones might give rise to responses of different types. Ignoring for the moment the presence of all three types of response in the pure cone retina of the snake, it is still difficult to fit three response types into a duplicity theory, and evidence is still lacking that would associate any of the response types with either rod or cone function. But different forms of both rods and cones are present in most cold-blooded vertebrate retinas, and different sense cells show adaptation of their responses in different degrees. It is not unreasonable to assume that certain of either the rods or cones, or both, might adapt completely following their initial discharge of impulses. Even pure "off" responses might be supposed to originate in certain cells excited by a shift in their equilibrium in the sense opposite to that which usually gives rise to the discharge of impulses.

The diversity of response might, on the other hand, originate in the layers of the retina between the rod and cone layer and the ganglion cells. Thus a given ganglion cell may be subject to diverse and rival influences, and its response determined by the relative amounts of each. This, in turn, may be fixed in large measure by the anatomical connections between the ganglion cell and its underlying neurones. This study in fact has shown clearly that the excitation produced by light may be subject to modification by an influence which may justifiably be termed inhibitory. Thus the relative amounts, and rates of rise and fall of excitatory and inhibitory influences upon a ganglion cell might determine its response. The "off" effect may then be due to a post-inhibitory release of the effects of an excitation which are all the greater for having been suppressed during the actual period of illumination. Granit and his co-workers have urged the use of these concepts in the interpretation of optic response.

Still another explanation to be considered is the possibility that functional differences may exist among the ganglion cells. While subject to essentially the same influences from the underlying retinal layers, different ganglion cells may respond differently to shifts in their equilibrium. The further consideration of these and other possibilities must wait upon the results of further experiments.

SUMMARY

1. Action potentials in single optic nerve fibers of cold-blooded vertebrate eyes may be obtained from small intraocular bundles dissected off the anterior surface of the retina of excised, opened bulbs.

2. Responses in different single fibers from the same retina show differ-

ent types of response. In about 20 per cent of the fibers response to illumination of the retina begins with a burst of impulses at high frequency, followed by a steady discharge at lower frequency which is maintained throughout illumination, and stops when the light is turned off. About 50 per cent of the fibers show only a burst of impulses in response to the onset of illumination, and another in response to its cessation; no impulses are discharged during steady illumination of the retina. The third type of response, obtained from about 30 per cent of the fibers, shows no discharge either at the onset of illumination, or throughout its duration, but gives a vigorous and prolonged discharge when the light is turned off.

3. In general the higher the intensity of retinal illumination the shorter is the latent period of the response, the higher its frequency of discharge, and the greater the number of impulses in a burst.

4. Fibers which give a response to the onset and cessation of light also respond, though less strongly, to an increase or a reduction in its intensity. Fibers giving only an "off" response respond, though less strongly, to a reduction in intensity; they give no response to an increase.

5. As dark adaptation of the eye progresses, the discharge which can be obtained from any fiber in response to a given intensity increases; the threshold of response correspondingly falls, rapidly at first and then more gradually, for half an hour or more.

6. "Off" responses are weak or absent following short periods of illumination; similarly "on" responses require a sufficiently long preceding period of darkness for their full development.

7. The discharge in fibers giving only an "off" response is promptly suppressed by re-illumination of the retina.

8. The type of response in any given fiber does not depend upon conditions of stimulation or adaptation of the eye. Even certain external agents (asphyxia, CO_2, ion unbalance, temperature), while affecting the responses do not alter their essential character.

9. Experiments on fish, amphibian and reptilian eyes give essentially the same results as regards the types of response found.

10. Responses can be obtained in a given optic nerve fiber only upon illumination of a certain restricted region of the retina, termed the receptive field of the fiber.

11. The location on the retina of the receptive field of a fiber is fixed. Its extent depends upon the size and intensity of the spot of light used to explore it, and upon the state of adaptation of the eye.

12. With possible rare exceptions the type of response in any fiber does not depend upon the portion of its receptive field which is illuminated.

13. The type of response in a fiber is not correlated with the location of its receptive field in the retina.

14. The question is discussed as to whether the diversity in types of

response is due to different types of sensory cells, whether it arises in the intermediate layers of the retina, or whether it is the result of functional differences among the ganglion cells.

REFERENCES

ADRIAN, E. D. AND R. MATTHEWS. J. Physiol. **63**: 378, 1927.

　　　J. Physiol. **64**: 279, 1927.

　　　J. Physiol. **65**: 273, 1928.

CHAFFEE, E. L., W. T. BOVIE AND A. HAMPSON. J. Opt. Soc. Am. **7**: 1, 1923.

HARTLINE, H. K. AND C. H. GRAHAM. J. Cell. and Comp. Physiol. **1**: 277, 1932.

GRANIT, R. J. Physiol. **77**: 207, 1933.

GRANIT, R. AND L. A. RIDDELL. J. Physiol. **81**: 1, 1934.

GRANIT, R. AND P. O. THERMAN. J. Physiol. **83**: 359, 1935.

The receptive fields of optic nerve fibers

H. KEFFER HARTLINE

*Eldridge Reeves Johnson Research Foundation, University of Pennsylvania,
Philadelphia*

Reprinted from the AMERICAN JOURNAL OF PHYSIOLOGY
Vol. 130, no. 4, pp. 690–699, October 1940

Appreciation of the form of the retinal image depends upon a correspondence between the distribution of light on the retina and the distribution of activity among the fibers of the optic nerve. This correspondence may be studied directly by recording the activity in single optic nerve
fibers in response to illuminating various parts of the retina.

A given optic nerve fiber responds to light only if a particular region of
the retina receives illumination. This region is termed the receptive field
of that fiber. In a previous paper describing the responses in single optic
nerve fibers from the cold-blooded vertebrate eye (Hartline, 1938) it
was noted that the receptive fields of the optic nerve fibers are of small but
appreciable extent, and that their locations on the retina are fixed. It is
the purpose of the present paper to describe further the characteristics
of receptive fields, and to discuss some of the spatial factors involved in
the excitation of the fibers of the optic nerve.

METHOD. The method for recording the activity in single optic nerve
fibers from the eyes of cold-blooded vertebrates has been described in
the previous paper (loc. cit.). An eye is excised, cut open, and small
bundles of optic nerve fibers are dissected from the anterior surface of the
exposed retina. The action potentials in these bundles are amplified and
recorded with an oscillograph. When such a bundle has been split successfully, until only a single active fiber remains, the retina must be
searched with a small spot of light to determine the region supplying that
fiber. This search is aided by noting the direction, on the retina, from
which the nerve fibers in the small bundle come, and by using large spots
of light at first to locate the approximate position of the sensitive region.

The optical system employed in these experiments has likewise been
described. A spot of light of suitable size is projected upon the exposed
retina; the coördinates of its position, referred to an arbitrary point of
origin on the retina, are obtained from readings of crossed micrometers
which control its location. The micrometer readings are reduced to millimeters on the retina by multiplying them by the magnification of the
optical system (0.32 or 0.15). Sharpness of focus of the spot on the retina

173

is checked in every experiment by direct observation through a dissecting microscope.[1] This optical system can provide a maximum intensity of illumination on the retina of $2 \cdot 10^4$ meter candles, which may be reduced to any desired value by means of Wratten "Neutral Tint" filters.

Eyes from large frogs (R. catesbiana), and from a few alligators, were used in the present study. In none of these experiments did the receptive fields of the fibers lie in or near the *area acuta* of the retina; this paper is therefore concerned only with properties of the peripheral retina. The preparations were always allowed 20 to 30 minutes for dark adaptation (at 25°C.), and observations were checked whenever possible to guard against slow changes in sensitivity.

RESULTS. The sensitivity of different regions of the retina to light must be defined with respect to the particular optic nerve fiber which is under observation. A spot of light in one location on the retina may elicit a vigorous discharge of impulses in an optic nerve fiber, but in a different location may produce no responses at all in this particular fiber. The distribution of sensitivity over the receptive field of a fiber may be determined by systematic exploration with a small spot of light, noting the responses elicited at various locations, and charting the boundaries of the region over which the spot is effective, at different intensities.

In figure 1 are given two examples. Figure 1a was obtained with a fiber whose responses consisted of a burst of impulses when the light was turned on, and another burst upon turning it off.[2] At the highest intensity (log I = 0.0) the exploring spot (50 μ in diameter) would elicit responses if located anywhere within the outermost closed curve. The

[1] Although sharply focussed, such a spot of light on the retina is always surrounded by a faint halo of scattered light. This is due chiefly to Tyndall scattering in the layers of the retina overlying the rods and cones (diffraction, and reflection and scatter from the surfaces of the optical system contribute only a small amount). The relative intensity of this halo has been estimated by direct observation in several fresh preparations. A piece of gelatin neutral-tint filter was placed in the eye-piece of the dissecting microscope, just covering the image of the spot of light on the retina. With a large spot of light (1 mm. square), filters of densities between 2.0 and 3.0 were necessary to reduce the intensity of the spot, seen through the filter, to match approximately the intensity of the halo of scattered light, seen over the edge of the filter. Thus in nearly all cases the intensity of the halo, within a few microns of the edge of the spot, is 1 per cent or less of the spot intensity, and falls off rapidly with increasing distance from the edge of the spot.

[2] It has been shown previously that different optic nerve fibers of the vertebrate eye give different kinds of discharges in response to illumination of the retina. In some of the fibers impulses are discharged steadily as long as the light shines; others give only a brief burst of impulses when the light is turned on, and again when it is turned off; still others respond only to turning the light off. The general characteristics of the receptive fields of different fibers, however, are essentially the same, regardless of their type of response.

dots mark locations at which the spot could just elicit a response, at this intensity. For such locations on the boundary, both the "on" and the "off" bursts consisted of only one or two impulses, but locations inside the boundary gave rise to stronger discharges, and when the spot was located in the center of the region, vigorous bursts were obtained. At a lower intensity (1/100 of the former: log I = −2.0) responses could be obtained only when the spot was located within the much smaller region enclosed by the innermost curve, and at this intensity the discharges

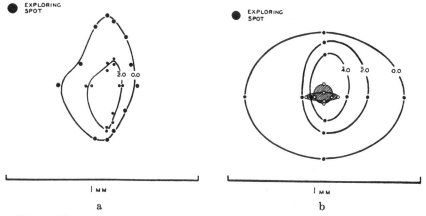

Fig. 1. Charts of the retinal regions supplying single optic nerve fibers (eye of the frog). a. Determination of the contours of the receptive field of a fiber at two levels of intensity of exploring spot. Dots mark positions at which exploring spot (50 μ diameter) would just elicit discharges of impulses, at the intensity whose logarithm is given on the respective curve (unit intensity = 2.10⁴ meter candles). No responses at log I = −3.0, for any location of exploring spot. This fiber responded only at "on" and "off." b. Contours (determined by four points on perpendicular diameters) of receptive field of a fiber, at three levels of intensity (value of log I given on respective contours). In this fiber steady illumination (log I = 0.0 and −2.0) produced a maintained discharge of impulses for locations of exploring spot within central shaded area; elsewhere discharge subsided in 1–2 seconds. No maintained discharge in response to intensities less than log I = −2.0; no responses at all to an intensity log I = −4.6.

were very weak even when the spot was located in the center of the region. At a tenth of this intensity, log I = −3.0, no responses could be obtained for any location of the exploring spot whatever.

Figure 1b is a chart of the receptive field of another fiber, which in this case was capable of a steady discharge of impulses, maintained as long as illumination lasted. As in the previous experiment, the brighter the exploring spot, the larger was the region over which it would elicit responses, and, at any given intensity, the responses were stronger the more nearly central the location of the exploring spot. Indeed, it was only for locations in the very center (cross-hatched region in fig. 1b) that the discharge would be maintained throughout an indefinitely long period of illumination. Elsewhere it would subside and finally stop in a second or two (cf. Hartline, loc. cit., fig. 6). At the lowest intensity represented in the figure (log I = −4.0) no maintained discharge could be obtained at all; the responses consisted of only a few impulses, and at $\frac{1}{4}$ of this intensity (log I = −4.6) no responses whatever could be elicited.

These experiments show that the sensitivity to light, referred to a particular optic nerve fiber, is not uniform over the fiber's receptive field. The central portion of the receptive field has a lower threshold and, at intensities above threshold, gives rise to stronger responses than the outlying areas. The sensitivity is thus maximal in the center, and falls off steadily with increasing distance from this center, to become inappreciable outside an area approximately one millimeter in diameter. Charts such as those of figure 1 are contour maps of this distribution of sensitivity. The faint halo of scattered light surrounding the exploring spot is a source of error in the construction of these charts. However, at relatively low intensities (100 or even 1000 times the minimum threshold) this scattered light is of little consequence, and a map obtained at these intensities must closely approximate the actual distribution of sensitivity over the receptive field of the fiber under observation.

Factors other than the absolute intensity of the exploring spot affect the extent of the region from which responses in a given fiber can be elicited. If the exploring spot is made smaller, its intensity must be increased if it is to be effective over as large an area. But with this smaller spot the threshold measured in the most sensitive central region is correspondingly increased. It is the intensity relative to this minimum threshold which is significant in charting the distribution of sensitivity. Similarly, if the retina is not completely dark adapted, its level of sensitivity is decreased, and for a particular fiber the thresholds in the center and on all the contours of its receptive field are increased proportionately. Receptive fields of different fibers must likewise be compared with due regard to their minimum thresholds, which may differ considerably.

The vertebrate retina responds vigorously to small, sudden movements of the retinal image (Ishihara, 1904; Adrian and Matthews, 1927). This may be observed in the responses of single optic nerve fibers, and is helpful in determining the distribution of sensitivity in their receptive fields. Figure 2 shows records of the discharge in a fiber responding at "on" and "off." Although no impulses were discharged while the spot of light was shining steadily, a slight movement of it, of only a few microns in any direction, produced a short burst of impulses. Responses to movement are stronger, within limits, the larger and more intense the moving spot, and the greater and the more rapid its displacement. Responses to a slight movement of a spot of light of given size and intensity can be elicited anywhere within the region over which this spot is effective in producing discharges when it is turned on or off. They are weak when the spot is near the boundary of this region, and stronger the more nearly central its location in the receptive field. Figure 3 shows the contour

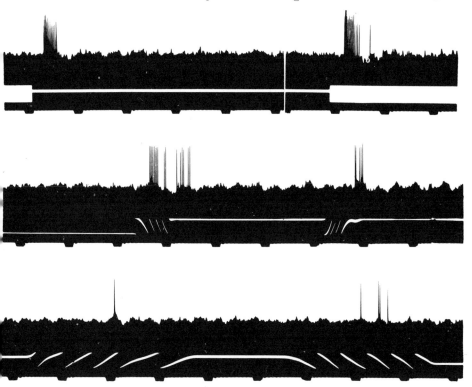

Fig. 2. Oscillograms of action potentials in a single optic nerve fiber (frog), showing responses to slight movements of small spot of light (50 μ diameter) on the retina. Fiber responded only at "on" and "off"; no discharge during steady illumination if stimulus spot was stationary (upper record; signal marking period of illumination blackens the white strip above time marker). Slight movements of stimulus spot elicited short bursts of impulses (middle and lower records). Movements of spot on retina are signalled by narrow white lines appearing above time marker; these are shadows of spokes attached to head of micrometer screw controlling position of stimulus spot. Each spoke corresponds to 7 μ on the retina. Time in ⅕ second.

within which a spot of light 50 μ in diameter, about 100 times the minimum threshold, produced responses in a fiber responding to "off" only. The arrows show the limits, on two diameters, between which slight movements of this spot (ca. 20 μ in ca. 0.05 sec.) would elicit bursts of impulses. Outside of these limits no responses to movement could be obtained, no matter how great or how rapid the displacements. It is characteristic of a fiber which responds only to "off" that it also responds only to movements of the spot away from the center of its receptive field.

Bursts of impulses are also elicited in response to movement of a shadow on the uniformly illuminated retina. A slight, sudden movement of a narrow band of shadow produces responses if it falls across the receptive field of the fiber under observation, and these responses can be elicited over a region many times wider than the shadow itself. To show this, all diaphragms were removed from the optical system, and a fine wire

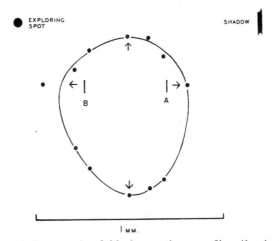

Fig. 3. Chart of the receptive field of an optic nerve fiber (frog), showing limits within which responses were elicited by movements of an illuminated spot, and of a narrow band of shadow. Dots mark locations at which exploring spot produced responses when turned off (fiber responded only to "off"). Spot 50 μ in diameter, intensity 100 times minimum threshold. Arrows mark the limits (on two diameters) between which slight movements of illuminated spot elicited bursts of impulses. With large area of retina illuminated (4 mm. diameter) a band of shadow 20 μ wide produced discharges of impulses when moved slightly, if it crossed the receptive field within the limits marked by the vertical lines *A* and *B*. Shadow extended across entire illuminated area, in direction lengthwise of page; movements were crosswise. See figure 4 for records of responses to moving shadow.

was stretched across the beam. This yielded a circular patch of light on the retina, 4 mm. in diameter, across which was a band of shadow 20 μ wide. In the experiment of figure 3 the limits within which slight movements of this shadow produced responses are indicated by the vertical lines, A and B. If the shadow was near either of these limits the responses to its movement were weak, as shown in the upper and the lower records of figure 4, while if it fell across the center of the sensitive region the same amount of displacement elicited stronger bursts of impulses (middle record of fig. 4). Responses to movement of a shadow are elicited regardless of the direction of the motion, both in the fibers responding to "on" and "off" and in those responding to "off" only.

From these experiments it is evident that the receptive field of an optic nerve fiber from the peripheral retina covers an area much greater than

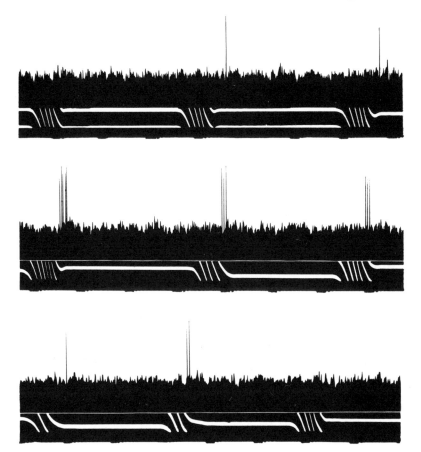

Fig. 4. Records of the impulses discharged in an optic nerve fiber in response to movement of a shadow on the retina. Experiment of figure 3. Narrow band of shadow, on uniformly illuminated retina, was moved from right to left (chart of fig. 3) in a series of short, quick jerks. First response (upper record) occurred at position A in figure 3; responses elicited to every succeeding movement until position B was reached (lower record shows last response). Responses were strongest midway between (middle record). Signal of movement as in figure 2. Time in $\frac{1}{5}$ second.

that occupied by a single receptor cell. The receptor elements are small, even compared to the exploring spot used in these experiments; consequently, if illumination of but one rod or cone gave rise to the responses in a given optic nerve fiber, charts such as figure 1 would be faithful representations of the distribution of light associated with the exploring spot. Direct observation of this spot on the retina showed that it was small and sharply focussed, with a halo of scattered light at most only $\frac{1}{100}$ as intense as the spot itself. Yet this spot, at intensities only 4 to 10 times the minimum thresholds for the various fibers, elicited responses over regions many times its own diameter. The observed distributions of sensitivity, with broad maxima several tenths of a millimeter in diameter, in no way resembled the minute exploring spot, only 50 μ in diameter, as they would have if only a single receptor cell had been responsible for the excitation of each optic nerve fiber. Likewise, high sensitivity to slight movement of the spot was not found to be restricted to regions as small as the stimulus spot itself. Finally, the use of the narrow band of shadow upon the uniformly illuminated retina definitely rules out possible effects of scattered light. The sensitivity to slight movements of this shadow, over a region many times its width, offers conclusive proof that many receptor cells are concerned in the excitation of a single optic nerve fiber.

A retinal ganglion cell, therefore, can receive excitatory influences over many convergent pathways; its axon is the final common path for nervous activity originating in many sensory elements. This, of course, is in keeping with the known anatomical organization of the vertebrate retina. It furnishes the functional basis for the spatial effects in the vertebrate retina, observed in experiments on the whole optic nerve by Adrian and Matthews (1927, 1928). They found that the latency of the optic discharge was shorter the greater the area of the retina illuminated, and attributed this to summation of the excitatory effects due to activity in convergent retinal pathways. It is worthy of note that this spatial summation was limited to retinal distances of approximately 1 mm., which is the order of magnitude of the diameter of the receptive fields of the single optic nerve fibers. Moreover, the spatial effects were smaller the greater the retinal distances, in keeping with the diminished effectiveness of the outlying regions of the receptive fields. This diminished effectiveness may be ascribed to a smaller number of receptor elements in a unit area that are in connection with a given retinal ganglion cell, or to a less effective transfer of nervous activity over the longer and less direct pathways from the margins of the receptive field.

The receptive fields of different fibers may overlap considerably (Hartline, loc. cit.). Consequently, illumination of a single point on the retina can produce activity in many different fibers, and illumination of two discrete points may produce activity in many fibers in common. It is for this reason that fine detail cannot be resolved by the peripheral retina. From the standpoint of visual function, it is necessary to consider the distribution of activity among the different fibers of the optic nerve, elicited by illumination of a particular small element of area on the retina.

A bundle containing a number of active optic nerve fibers may be used to sample this distribution. If not too many fibers are present, it is possible to distinguish the activity in the different ones by means of the loud speaker and the cathode ray oscilloscope. When the responses in such a bundle are tested it is at once apparent that many fibers are excited by a small spot of light (50 μ in diameter), even at intensities close to threshold. Certain of the fibers respond vigorously to the light; these are the ones whose receptive fields are centered close to the stimulus spot. Others give only feeble responses; these either have higher thresholds, or are fibers whose receptive fields are centered at some distance from the stimulus spot, which consequently falls in the less sensitive peripheries of their fields. When the spot of light is tested in a slightly different location on the retina, it is strikingly evident that the composition of the response is changed. Fibers which had been active cease responding, new fibers come into play, fibers which had given strong responses give weak ones, and some of those which had only given slight discharges dominate the response.

It is evident that illumination of a given element of area on the retina results in a specific pattern of activity in a specific group of optic nerve fibers. The particular fibers involved, and the distribution of activity among them, are characteristic of the location on the retina of the particular element of area illuminated. Corresponding to different points on the retina are different patterns of nerve activity; even two closely adjacent points do not produce quite the same distribution of activity, although they may excite many fibers in common. The more widely two illuminated spots are separated the fewer fibers will be involved in common, but it is reasonable to suppose that it is only necessary to have two recognizable maxima of activity in order to resolve the separate spots. It is this spatial specificity of groups of optic nerve fibers, and of the distribution of activity among them, that furnishes the basis for distinguishing the form of the retinal image.

SUMMARY

The region of the retina which must receive illumination in order to elicit a discharge of impulses in a particular optic nerve fiber is termed the receptive field of that fiber. Characteristics of the receptive fields of individual optic nerve fibers from the peripheral retinas of cold-blooded vertebrates (frog, alligator) have been investigated by recording the action potentials in single fibers in response to illuminating various parts of the retina. In several experiments the distribution of sensitivity over the receptive field of a particular fiber has been determined by systematic exploration of the retina with a small spot of light, noting the responses elicited in the fiber at various locations, and charting the boundaries of the region over which the spot is effective, at various intensities.

The sensitivity to light, referred to a particular optic nerve fiber, is maximal over the central portion of the fiber's receptive field, where the threshold is lower than in the outlying areas, and where intensities above threshold give rise to the strongest responses. The sensitivity is less the greater the distance from this central region, and is usually inappreciable outside an area about one millimeter in diameter. Contour maps of the distribution of sensitivity are given for two examples.

Single optic nerve fibers (of the types responding to "on" and "off," and to "off" only) respond to sudden, slight movements of an illuminated spot, or of a band of shadow on the uniformly illuminated retina, if the moving spot or shadow falls within the receptive field of the fiber. Movements of only a few micra of a small spot or a narrow shadow can elicit responses in a particular optic nerve fiber over a retinal region several tenths of a millimeter in diameter—many times the width of the spot or shadow.

These experiments prove that the receptive field of an optic nerve fiber from the peripheral retina covers an area much greater than that occupied by a single rod or cone. A retinal ganglion cell, therefore, can receive excitatory influences over many convergent pathways; its axon is the final common path for nervous activity originating in many sensory elements. This finding furnishes the functional basis for the spatial effects observed in the peripheral vertebrate retina.

Action potentials recorded from small bundles containing many active optic nerve fibers show that a single small spot of light excites many fibers: the receptive fields of different fibers overlap considerably. The particular fibers activated, and the distribution of activity among them, is characteristic of the location on the retina of the particular element of area illuminated. This spatial specificity of groups of optic nerve fibers, and of their patterns of activity, furnishes the basis for distinguishing the form of the retinal image.

REFERENCES

ADRIAN, E. D. AND R. MATTHEWS. J. Physiol. **63:** 378; **64:** 279, 1927; **65:** 273, 1928.
HARTLINE, H. K. This Journal **121:** 400, 1938.
ISHIHARA, M. Pflüger's Arch. **114:** 569, 1904.

The effects of spatial summation in the retina on the excitation of the fibers of the optic nerve

H. KEFFER HARTLINE

Eldridge Reeves Johnson Research Foundation, University of Pennsylvania, Philadelphia

Reprinted from the AMERICAN JOURNAL OF PHYSIOLOGY
Vol. 130, no. 4, pp. 700–711, October 1940

In a previous paper (Hartline, 1940) it was shown that a ganglion cell in the peripheral retina of the vertebrate eye is excited by activity in many convergent pathways, from sensory elements distributed over a receptive field covering approximately a square millimeter of retinal area. Illumination of any portion of the receptive field of a retinal ganglion cell will accordingly produce a discharge of impulses in its axon, the strength of the response to illumination of a fixed retinal area usually being greater the higher the intensity of the stimulating light. The present paper will show that the discharge of impulses in a single optic nerve fiber also depends upon the size of the illuminated area. The excitation of a ganglion cell is therefore controlled by the number of active pathways which converge upon it, as well as by the degree of activity in the individual pathways.

Spatial summation in the vertebrate retina has previously been demonstrated by Adrian and Matthews (1927–1928). They showed that the latency of the discharge of impulses in the whole optic nerve of the eel was shorter the larger the area of the retina illuminated, and the latency of the response to four spots of light was shorter than the shortest latency obtained with any of the spots singly. This summation was enhanced by the application of strychnine, indicating that it depended upon the nervous interconnections within the retina. The study of the activity in single optic nerve fibers has now furnished more direct evidence for the convergence of excitatory effects within the retina; the present paper is concerned with the extension of this study to an analysis of spatial summation, in terms of the activity of the individual units of the retina.

METHOD. The method for studying the activity of single optic nerve fibers in the retinas of cold-blooded vertebrates, and for determining the location and extent of their receptive fields has been described in previous papers (Hartline, 1938, 1940). In the present experiments the eyes from

---

[1] With the support of a grant from the American Philosophical Society.

large frogs (R. catesbiana) were used. None of the receptive fields of the fibers studied lay within or near the *area acuta* of the retina; the properties here reported are those of the peripheral retina.

The apparatus for illuminating the retina has likewise been described previously. It provided a beam of light which could be directed upon any part of the exposed retina, more than large enough to cover the region under investigation. The illumination was restricted to any desired area within this beam by means of diaphragms, with apertures of suitable size and shape imaged on the retina. Sharpness of focus was assured, in every experiment, by direct observation of the patterns of light on the retina by means of a dissecting microscope ($\times 32$). The diaphragms were readily interchangeable, and slipped into place against mechanical stops in a holder. The accuracy and reproducibility of their alignment in the beam was checked by exposing photographic plates in the place of the retina. Fine adjustments on the diaphragm holder enabled it to be shifted slightly, within the limits of the beam, so that the patterns of illumination could be accurately centered upon the receptive field of the fiber under observation.

RESULTS. In figure 1 are shown oscillograms of the amplified action potentials in a single optic nerve fiber, obtained in response to illumination of the retina with patches of light of various sizes. The areas illumi-nated, which were circular in shape, had been carefully centered upon the most sensitive portion of the fiber's receptive field, and fell well within its limits. The larger the area of the stimulus patch, the shorter was the latency of response, and, for moderate degrees of stimulation, the higher was the frequency and the greater the number of impulses in the discharge. The fiber used in this experiment was one responding with a burst of impulses at the onset of illumination, and again when the light was turned off (no discharge during steady illumination). Fibers giving other types of response (cf. Hartline, 1938) show a similar dependence of the discharge upon the area illuminated.

Varying the area of the retina illuminated by a fixed intensity thus affects the response in a single optic nerve fiber: this effect, moreover, is exactly similar to that obtained by varying the intensity of illumination upon a fixed retinal area (cf. Hartline, 1938). To permit a comparison, two series of records are shown in figure 1, obtained at two different intensities of illumination. The responses in the right hand column were obtained with an intensity ten times that used in the left. It is to be noted that responses at the higher intensity are comparable to those obtained with areas approximately ten times larger, at the lower intensity. Only the total luminous flux falling upon the retina (area $\times$ intensity) is of significance in determining the response of the ganglion cell. This rule has been found to hold, except for very strong stimulation, to within the limits of accuracy of this method. It applies only to illumination falling well within the receptive field of the fiber under observation.

A simple demonstration of this reciprocal relation between the area and intensity necessary to produce a constant effect in an optic nerve fiber is furnished by the determination of the threshold intensity, $I_{thresh.}$,

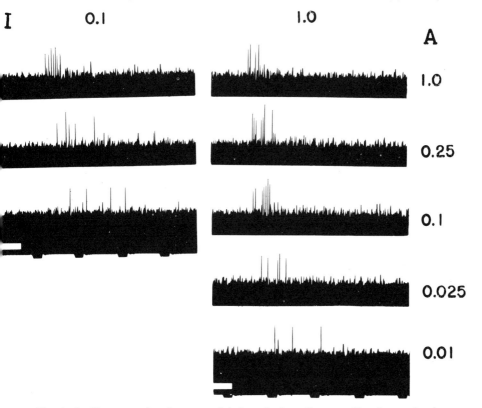

Fig. 1. Oscillograms of action potentials in a single optic nerve fiber from a frog's retina, showing effect of size of stimulus patch upon the discharge of impulses. Retina illuminated with circular patches of light, centered on receptive field of the fiber; relative areas (A) given on right (A = 1 corresponds to 0.006 mm.^{2}). For the responses in the left hand column the intensity of illumination was $\frac{1}{10}$ that used for the right hand column. (I = 1 equivalent to 3.10^5 meter candles). Fiber was one responding with bursts of impulses at "on" and at "off" with no impulses discharged during steady illumination. Only "on" burst shown here. Signal of illumination blackens white line above time marker (only shown in bottom records). Time in $\frac{1}{5}$ second.

for various areas, A, of retinal illumination, plotted in figure 2. The line through the experimental points has a slope of -1, representing, on this double logarithmic plot, the relation

$$A \cdot I_{thresh.} = \text{constant.}$$

This relation was demonstrated by Adrian and Matthews (1927–1928) in the optic discharge of the eel's eye; the present experiments show it to be a property of the individual retinal ganglion cells. Its limitation to retinal distances less than 1 mm., as reported by Adrian and Matthews, is due to the fact that the diameter of the receptive field of a ganglion cell is, on the average, of this order of magnitude.

Measurements of the reciprocal of the latent period and of the initial frequency of the discharge of impulses (in the same fiber whose responses are shown in fig. 1) are plotted, in figure 3, as functions of the area of illumination, for various levels of intensity. For moderate degrees of stimulation, these measures of the response increase steadily and approximately linearly with the logarithm of the area illuminated. Curves ob-

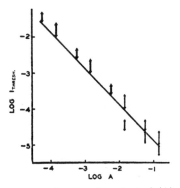

Fig. 2. Relation between area of retina illuminated (A) and threshold intensity, $I_{thresh.}$ for stimulation of a single optic nerve fiber. For each arrow, upper point gives lowest intensity which elicited one or two impulses; lower point gives highest intensity which failed to elicit any response (determinations made to nearest 0.3 or 0.4 log unit). Where duplicate determinations coincided, arrows are drawn heavier. Line drawn through points has slope of −1. (Log I = 0 equivalent to 3.10^5 meter candles; area in mm.^{2}.)

tained at different levels of intensity are separated, parallel to the axis of abscissae, by amounts roughly equal to the logarithms of the ratios of their intensities, in accordance with the reciprocity relation discussed above.

Figure 3 shows that the responses increase with increasing area only up to a certain point. Beyond this point the responses actually decrease with increasing size of stimulus area, although these areas are well within the limits of the receptive field of the fiber. It is furthermore to be noted that the higher the intensity the smaller is the area at which this decrease begins. This effect may also be seen in the right hand column of figure 1, where the response to the largest area contains fewer impulses than the response to the area one-fourth as large. A similar depressing effect on the response has been reported, when the intensity of retinal illumination on a fixed retinal area is increased above an optimal value (Hartline, 1938). It is as though the ganglion cell can be "overloaded," and the fact that this can be accomplished by increasing the area of the retina illuminated, as well as by increasing the intensity of the light, serves to emphasize the principle that the final response of the ganglion cell is determined by the sum total of activity reaching it over many convergent pathways.

It has been pointed out previously that in these experiments the sensitivity to light of any point on the retina must be defined with respect to the particular optic nerve fiber under observation. The sensitivity, thus defined, is not uniform over the receptive field of a fiber; the outlying portions are less effective in producing responses than is the central region (Hartline, 1940). It is reasonable to suppose that the outlying portions of the receptive field also contribute less to the total summed excitation

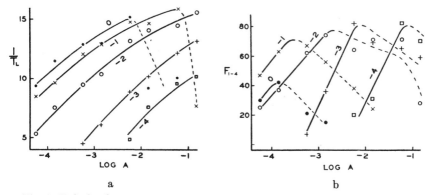

a   b

Fig. 3. Relation between area of retina illuminated (A) and response in a single optic nerve fiber, at five levels of intensity. (Measurements of the complete experiment from which the records shown in fig. 1 were selected.) a. Reciprocal of latent period in seconds, T_L, of "on" burst vs. log A (in mm.²). The number on each curve gives the logarithm of the intensity of illumination for that curve (log I = 0 equivalent to 3.10^5 meter candles). b. Initial frequency of discharge of "on" burst (F_{1-4}; 1st 4 impulses) vs. log A. Numbers on curves give respective values of log I.

of the ganglion cell. To test this point, and to study the relative contributions from the component portions of an illuminated area under different conditions, the following series of experiments have been performed.

A square area, large enough to cover nearly all of the receptive field of a fiber under observation, was subdivided into 25 small squares by means of diaphragms with appropriate apertures. Each of these small areas could be illuminated separately and the response to it compared with the response to illumination of the entire area, or of areas comprising several of the small subdivisions.

The requirements for threshold excitation of a fiber responding at "on" and "off" (only the "on" response recorded) are given in figure 4. The minimal intensity necessary to produce a response was determined for each small square illuminated alone, and also for areas covered by 4, 9 and 25 of these small squares, as indicated in the figure. The reciprocals of these threshold intensities are entered in the respective squares, so that the greater the number in a particular square the more effective was that

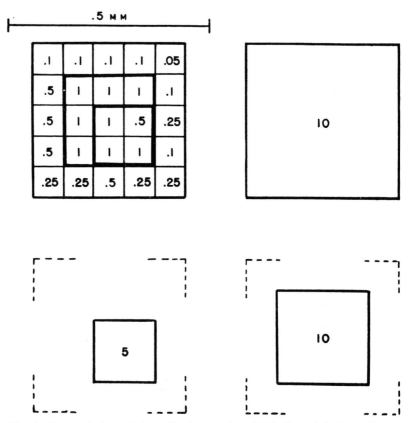

Fig. 4. Chart of the relative effectivness, in stimulating a single optic nerve fiber, of different portions of the fiber's receptive field. "Effectiveness" of a region of the retina defined as reciprocal of threshold intensity for that region. Upper left: numerical values of effectiveness of 25 subdivisions of large square area tested individually. (Comparative scale of retinal distance given above.) Threshold intensity of the most effective subdivisions set equal to 1 (equivalent to 8.10^{-3} meter candles) Lower left: effectiveness of area covering 4 of the central subdivisions (heaviest outline in upper left). Lower right: effectiveness of area covering the 9 central subdivisions (heavy outline in upper left). Upper right: effectiveness of entire large square. Fiber gave "on" and "off" bursts. "Threshold" taken as the lowest intensity (within 0.3 or 0.4 log unit) which would reliably produce an "on" burst of one or two impulses.

area in producing excitation of the ganglion cell. It is to be seen that the region of maximum sensitivity of the receptive field of this fiber was covered by eight of the nine central squares; the 16 border subdivisions

were all considerably less effective. When the larger area covered by
four of the central squares was illuminated, the threshold intensity was
one-fifth that of any of its subdivisions alone; when the still larger area
covered by the nine central squares was exposed the threshold was still
lower—only one-tenth of the threshold of the most sensitive subdivision.
Thus, for the central portion of the receptive field, large illuminated areas
were more effective in exciting the ganglion cell than any of their subdivisions. However, when the entire area covered by the 25 small squares
was illuminated, the threshold intensity was not measurably lower than
the threshold of the central region covered by only nine squares. Adding
the 16 border subdivisions did not appreciably increase the effectiveness of
the illumination, in this experiment. To judge from other experiments,
the outlying portions of the receptive field do contribute somewhat to
the total effect, and this might have been observed in the present experiment, had the thresholds been determined more closely. Nevertheless,
the inclusion of less sensitive regions of the receptive field contributes
correspondingly little to the summed effect; illumination of areas entirely
outside the receptive field contributes nothing at all to the excitation of
the ganglion cell.

Spatial summation in the vertebrate retina is thus limited to the receptive field of the retinal ganglion cell, and its effects are most readily
observable in the more sensitive central portion of that field. A series
of experiments has been performed, designed to analyze the contributions
from component subdivisions of an illuminated area, which in every case
lay well within the receptive field of the fiber under observation.

The experiment of figure 4, just cited, furnishes evidence of the summation of subliminal excitation. Thus illumination of any single square
at an intensity $1/I = 10$ failed to produce a response, yet this illumination
must have produced some degree of activity in the pathways converging
upon the ganglion cell, for when the nine central squares were illuminated
together, at this intensity, impulses were discharged in the optic nerve
fiber. Another example is furnished by an experiment on a fiber responding only to the cessation of illumination. At a suitable intensity, illumination of any one of four small squares singly produced no responses, but
when all four were illuminated together "off" responses were regularly
elicited, consisting of at least 7 impulses, at frequencies of 45 to 60 per
second. Evidently, weak light can produce effects in the individual
subdivisions of an area which are subliminal when they act alone, but
which sum to reach the threshold of the ganglion cell when all act together.
Since the activity in the retinal pathways presumably involves nerve impulses, we must conclude that more than one impulse must reach the
retinal ganglion cell in order to excite a response in its axon.

The experiment of figure 1 shows that spatial summation not only affects the threshold intensity to which a ganglion cell will respond, but also determines the magnitude of response at intensities above threshold. By testing different subdivisions of an area separately it can be shown, first, that the responses to illumination of a given area may be augmented by subliminal excitation from adjacent regions of the receptive field, and second, that illumination strong enough to elicit responses from each single

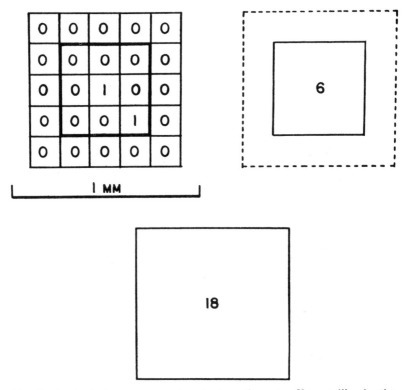

Fig. 5. Chart of the responses of a single optic nerve fiber to illumination of different portions of its receptive field, at a fixed intensity (2.10⁻³ meter candles). Upper left: number of impulses in response to each of 25 subdivisions of large square, tested individually (comparative scale given below). Upper right: response to illumination of area covered by 9 central subdivisions (heavy outline in upper left). Below: response to illumination of entire square. Fiber responded only to "off." Duration of exposure for each test *ca.* 5 sec.

subdivision of an area produces still greater excitation when the total area is exposed.

In an experiment (fig. 5) on a fiber responding only to cessation of illumination, only two of the central squares, out of the 25, would elicit a response (one impulse) when illuminated singly. However, when the area covered by the nine central squares was exposed, at this same intensity, responses of 6 to 10 impulses, at average frequencies of 10 to 20 per second, were elicited. And when the 16 border subdivisions were added, the response increased to 18 impulses, at 53 per second, although none of these border squares alone could produce any response at this intensity. While

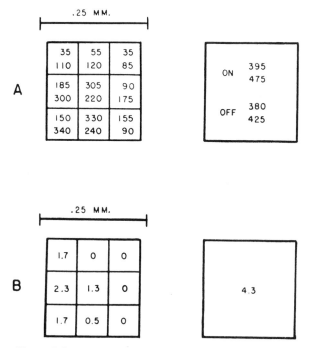

Fig. 6. a. Chart of the responses of a single optic nerve fiber (responding at "on" and at "off") to illumination of different portions of its receptive field, at a fixed intensity (0.3 meter candles). Left: frequencies of discharge (1st 6 impulses) of "on" and "off" bursts (upper and lower numbers, respectively) for each of 9 small squares tested individually (scale of distance given above). Right: frequencies of discharge of the "on" and "off" bursts (upper and lower pairs of numbers, respectively) in response to illumination of entire area covered by the 9 small squares. Upper member of each pair of numbers gives value obtained before testing the small squares, lower member the value afterwards. b. Chart of the frequencies of maintained discharge (13th to 15th second of continuous illumination) of single optic nerve fiber, in response to illumination of each of 9 small squares (left) compared with response to illumination of entire area covered by these squares (right). Scale given above. Intensity 300 meter candles.

it has been shown that border subdivisions contribute less to the summed effect of the illumination than do the more central ones, this experiment shows that their contribution nevertheless may be quite appreciable. This is especially true at low levels of excitation, where a slight increase in the stimulus usually causes a considerable increase in the response.

At an intensity moderately above threshold, the response to illumination of a large area is greater than the greatest response to illumination of any subdivision of this area at this same intensity. Illumination of nine small squares individually at an intensity above threshold resulted in the responses tabulated in figure 6a. When the entire area covered by these nine squares was exposed, at this same intensity, the frequency of the discharge was greater than in the responses of even the most effective subdivision illuminated alone. With fibers of this kind, responding to a change in illumination, both the "on" and the "off" bursts show the effects of spatial summation. A similar result, with a fiber whose discharge was maintained during steady illumination, is shown in figures 6b and 7. The frequency of the steady discharge resulting from illumination of each

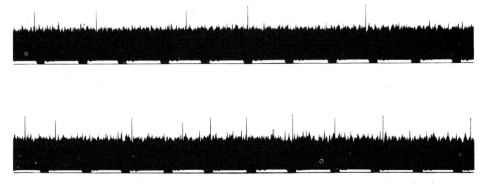

Fig. 7. Records of the maintained discharge of impulses in a single optic nerve fiber, showing effects of spatial summation. Top: response to illumination of most effective one of 9 subdivisions of an area of the retina (small square labelled 2.3 in fig. 6, b). Bottom: response to illumination of entire area covered by the 9 subdivisions (labelled 4.3 in fig. 6, b). Records include the 13th to 15th seconds of steady illumination. Intensity 300 meter candles. Time marked in $\frac{1}{5}$ second.

of the subdivisions singly is given in the respective square in figure 6b. When the entire area was illuminated, the frequency of the resulting discharge exceeded the highest frequency obtained from any of the small squares alone. Figure 7 shows the records of the responses to illuminating the entire area and to illuminating its most effective subdivision at the same intensity.

As noted previously, excitation above an optimal limit results in diminished responses in an optic nerve fiber. Thus it can happen that the response to the total area is actually less than that to any of its component subdivisions. The fiber, cited above, whose "off" responses illustrated the summation of subliminal effects from four subdivisions of an area, gave the following responses when tested at an intensity 100 times higher. The individual squares, illuminated singly, gave "off" bursts having initial frequencies of 265, 230, 205 and 195 impulses per second. In response to illuminating the whole area covered by these four squares, at the same intensity, the initial frequency of impulses in the burst was only 175. That this diminished response was due to the excessively high total excitation was shown by reducing the intensity of the light to $\frac{1}{4}$ its previous value; illumination of the whole area then gave a response whose initial frequency was 240 impulses per second. Summation of excitation due to activity in convergent pathways takes place over the entire range of the response of the retinal ganglion cell.

Spatial summation can take place, of course, only where there is convergence of the effects of stimulation. In the more simple eye of *Limulus*, there is no convergence, and the response in a given optic nerve fiber depends only upon the illumination of the sensory cell giving rise to that fiber. Illumination of adjacent areas of the eye has no effect upon this response (Graham, 1932). But where there is convergence there need not be summation; the response in the final common path might be determined solely by the most strongly excited component. This is not so in the vertebrate retina, as was originally evident from the studies of Adrian and Matthews. The present experimental study furnishes direct evidence that the excitation of a single retinal ganglion cell is determined by the summated effects of activity in the pathways converging upon it.

SUMMARY

A study has been made of the action potentials of single optic nerve fibers of the frog's retina, in response to illuminating areas of the retina of various sizes. In these experiments the fibers used were from the peripheral retina, where many receptor elements are connected with each retinal ganglion cell.

The discharge of impulses in a single optic nerve fiber is stronger the larger the area of the retina illuminated, within the limits of the fiber's receptive field. Except for very strong illumination, the responses have a shorter latency and a higher frequency the greater the number of receptors illuminated. The threshold intensity is also lower the larger the area of the stimulating patch of light.

Varying the area of the retina illuminated by a fixed intensity affects the discharge of impulses in a single optic nerve fiber in the same way as varying the intensity of illumination of a fixed area. For threshold excitation and for levels of response above threshold, only the total quantity of light (A·I) determines the response, provided the illumination is confined to the central portion of the fiber's receptive field.

Excitation of a retinal ganglion cell above an optimal limit results in diminished responses in its optic nerve fiber: this effect can be produced by increasing either the intensity or the area of the retinal illumination.

The discharge of impulses in response to illumination of a given area within the receptive field of an optic nerve fiber has been compared with the responses to illumination of subdivisions of this same area. 1. Illumination of the less effective subdivisions in the margins of the receptive field contributes correspondingly little to the summed effect upon the ganglion cell. Illumination of areas entirely outside the receptive field has no effect upon the discharge of impulses. 2. Subliminal effects from the subdivisions of an area can sum to reach the threshold of the ganglion cell when all the subdivisions are illuminated together. From this it is concluded that more than one nerve impulse must reach the retinal ganglion cell, over the pathways converging upon it, in order to excite a discharge in its optic nerve fiber. 3. The discharge of impulses in response to illumination of a given area is stronger than the strongest response from any subdivision of this area, illuminated at the same intensity. This is true provided the ganglion cell is not stimulated too strongly; at very high levels of excitation the response to illumination of the entire area is diminished.

An optic nerve fiber is the final common path for nervous activity originating in many receptor elements of the retina; excitation due to the activity in the retinal pathways converging upon a single ganglion cell summates to determine the response in its optic nerve fiber.

REFERENCES

ADRIAN, E. D. AND R. MATTHEWS. J. Physiol. **63**: 378; **64**: 279, 1927; **65**: 273, 1928.
GRAHAM, C. H. J. Cell. and Comp. Physiol. **2**: 295, 1932.
HARTLINE, H. K. This Journal **121**: 400, 1938; **130**: 690, 1940.

The neural mechanisms of vision

H. KEFFER HARTLINE

Eldridge Reeves Johnson Research Foundation, University of Pennsylvania
Philadelphia

Reprinted from 'The Harvey Lectures, 1941–1942', Series XXXVII, pp. 39–68
The Science Press Printing Company, Lancaster, Pennsylvania

OUR awareness of conditions in the external environment depends on the activity of our sense organs. These outposts of the nervous system signal the external conditions which affect the organism, translating environmental change into activity in sensory nerve fibers. It is then the function of the central nervous system to interpret this sensory information, integrating it into an appropriate pattern of behavior. The analysis of these complicated receptor and neural processes is the aim of sensory physiology.

A direct attack upon the problem of sensory mechanisms has been made possible by physical instruments for recording the minute and rapid electrical changes which accompany nervous activity. Thus the nerve messages from the sense organs can be intercepted. Furthermore, methods devised by Adrian and Bronk (1) for isolating single units from nerve trunks make it possible to record the activity in individual sensory nerve fibers. The analysis of visual mechanisms by these methods is the subject of this lecture.

The isolation of single fibers from the optic nerve, and the recording of their activity in response to illumination of the eye are accomplished by procedures now well known in electrophysiology. Small bundles of fibers dissected from the optic nerve are placed across electrodes in the input of an amplifier and their amplified action potentials recorded with an oscillograph. These bundles may be teased apart into fine strands, to the point where illumination of the eye elicits a regular sequence of uniform spike potentials, such as is recorded in Fig. 1. Such action potentials, it has been proved (1, 6, 33) are characteristic of the activity of single nerve fibers; they are the electrical sign of the

¹ Lecture delivered October 30, 1941.

regular trains of uniform impulses which constitute the nerve messages of the functional units of the nervous system.

The initiation of trains of nerve impulses by the action of light on the visual receptor cells is the first problem to be investigated by these methods. By the choice of a sufficiently primitive eye, in which the optic nerve fibers arise directly from visual sense cells, it has been possible to investigate the properties of the receptor mechanism in terms of the nervous activity it generates. The lateral eye of the horse-shoe crab, *Limulus*, provides a suitable preparation for this purpose (25), since the optic nerve fibers in this animal are the axones of the visual receptor elements themselves. The use of this preparation thus avoids the com-

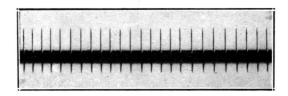

FIG. 1. Oscillogram of the amplified action potentials in a single optic nerve fiber (eye of *Limulus*) in response to steady illumination of the eye. Magnitude of deflection ca. 1 mv. Full length of record equals 1 second.

plexities introduced by the ganglionic structure of the vertebrate retina.

The simple sensory discharges recorded from the optic nerve fibers of *Limulus* resemble in their general properties nervous activity initiated by other kinds of receptors. The manner in which intensity of stimulation affects the discharge of nerve impulses provides an example. The relation between the intensity of illumination of the receptor and the resulting sensory discharge is shown in the records of Fig. 2. The higher the intensity of light falling upon this receptor cell, the greater was the frequency of impulses discharged in its optic nerve fiber. The individual nerve impulses, of course, were not graded in size (in keeping with the well known "all-or-nothing" property of nerve fibers); nevertheless, the receptor cell was able to signal different intensities of illumination by different frequencies of its sensory

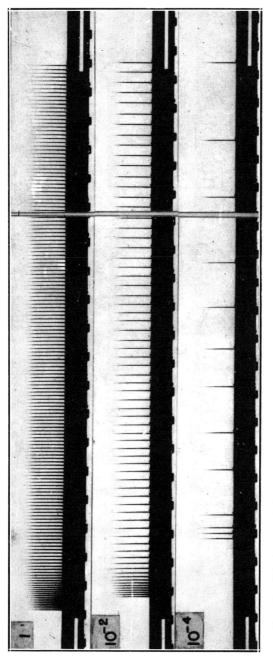

Fig. 2. Discharge of impulses in an optic nerve fiber (eye of *Limulus*) in response to illumination of the eye at three different intensities (relative values given at left). Eye partially light adapted. Signal of exposure to light blackens out white line above time marker. Time marked in 1/5 sec.

discharge. This is how intensity of stimulus is mediated by the individual sensory elements. Not only the visual receptor cells, but all the other sensory endings which have been studied by of stimulus by altering the frequency of the sensory discharge these methods show this same mechanism of signaling intensity (5, 6, 10, 32, 33, 34, 35).

Another property of the visual sense cell which it shares with other kinds of receptors is also shown in Fig. 2. At the onset of illumination of each intensity, the discharge of impulses began

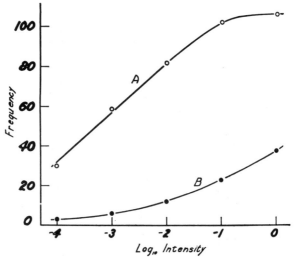

FIG. 3. Relation between frequency of impulses (number per record) and logarithm of intensity of stimulating light for the discharge in a single optic nerve fiber (eye of *Limulus*). Curve A, frequency of initial maximal discharge. Curve B, frequency of discharge 3.5 sec. after onset of illumination (Hartline and Graham (25)).

at a high frequency which declined, at first rapidly, then more slowly, approaching a steady level which was maintained as long as the light continued to shine. Such sensory adaptation is exhibited to a greater or less degree by all kinds of receptors thus far studied. Subjectively, it is common experience that a light when first turned on appears considerably brighter than after it has been shining several seconds. We have no absolute gauge of the intensity of a light, and this we may ascribe directly to the property of sensory adaptation of the receptor elements of our retinas, which furnish no fixed single value of impulse frequency corresponding to a particular absolute intensity of illumination.

Adaptation of the visual receptor, nevertheless, has useful functions. Not only does it serve to emphasize sudden changes in conditions of illumination, but it extends the range of intensities which a single receptor can mediate. Fig. 3 shows graphically the variation of frequency of discharge in a single optic nerve fiber with intensity of illumination. Curve A gives the values for the initial maxima of the sensory discharges, Curve B the values of the frequencies after 3 sec. of continuous illumination. At high intensities curve A tends to flatten out, and would ultimately be limited by the inability of the receptor to generate such high frequencies, or of the nerve fiber to follow; after adaptation to these high intensities, however, the receptor, as shown by Curve B, is able to give a significant variation of frequency with intensity. Thus each individual visual sense cell combines a high sensitivity with a wide range of response.

The mechanism whereby light energy is translated by the receptor cell into nervous activity is as yet far from being understood. However, it is clear that the initial step in this process must be the absorption of light by a photosensitive substance in the sensory cell. The resulting photochemical reaction is then the first step in the excitation of the receptor. Only light that is absorbed can be effective in initiating a photochemical reaction, and since photosensitive substances do not in general absorb all wavelengths equally, it follows that different wavelengths will have different effectiveness in exciting the visual sense cell. In Fig. 4 are shown records of the activity of a single optic nerve fiber whose receptor was stimulated by brief flashes of light of various wavelengths. The different spectral lights were not equally effective, and in order to produce equal responses of the sense cell (measured in terms of number of impulses discharged in its optic nerve fiber) it was necessary to adjust the relative energies of the flashes of different wavelengths to the values given in the figure. The receptor was less sensitive to red and

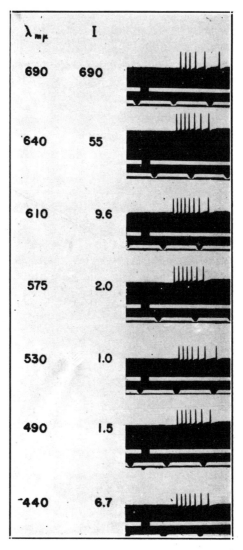

$\lambda_{m\mu}$	I
690	690
640	55
610	9.6
575	2.0
530	1.0
490	1.5
440	6.7

FIG. 4. Discharges of impulses in a single optic nerve fiber (*Limulus*) in response to lights of different wavelengths (λ), showing that responses can be made practically identical by suitable adjustment of the incident intensities (I). Values of I (thermopile determinations) are given relative to its value at $\lambda = 530$ mμ. Duration of stimulus flash 0.04 sec., signaled in the white line above time marker. Time in 1/5 sec. (Graham and Hartline (14)).

violet light than to green; the "visibility curve" plotted from these measurements (Fig. 5) may be simply interpreted as the absorption spectrum of the photosensitive substance of the visual sense cell (14, 15, 18, 30).

The comparatively simple nature of the primary photochemical reaction in the visual sense cell is indicated by the responses to short flashes of light of various intensities and durations (19).

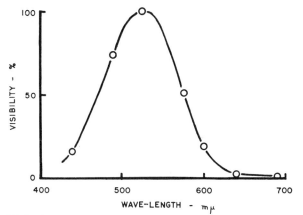

FIG. 5. Visibility curve for a single visual sense cell (*Limulus*). "Visibility" at each wavelength is the reciprocal of the relative intensity necessary to produce a specified burst of impulses (cf. Fig. 4) (data from Graham and Hartline (14)).

Fig. 6 is an array of records of the responses of a single optic nerve fiber, showing that both the intensity and the duration of the stimulating flash affect the latency of the response, the number of impulses discharged and the frequency of the discharge. These two parameters of the stimulus indeed affect the response of the sense cell to the same degree quantitatively, as may be seen by an inspection of the figure. The recorded responses which stand in any given diagonal of this array (upper left to lower right) are very closely equal; for each of these responses the energy of the stimulating flash (product of intensity by duration) was the same. Apparently the photochemical reaction which is the first step in the excitation of the receptor is sufficiently simple so that the reciprocity law of photochemistry applies to it, provided only short durations of exposure are considered.

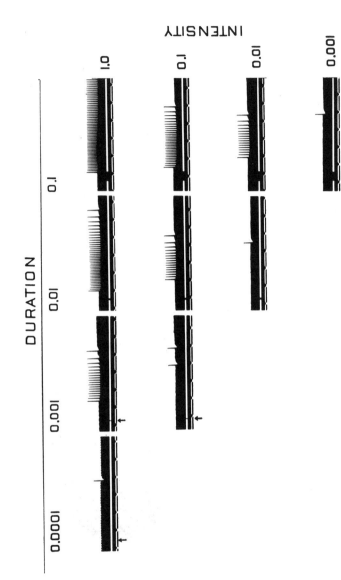

FIG. 6. Discharges of impulses in a single optic nerve fiber (*Limulus*) in response to short flashes of light of various intensities and durations. Relative intensity for each horizontal row given on right. Duration of flash (in seconds) for each vertical column given at top. Signal of light flash blackens the white line above time marker (arrows mark position of signal for very short flashes). Time in ½ sec. (Hartline (19)).

The photochemical change produced by light necessarily results in a depletion of the photosensory substance of the sensory
cell, with a consequent fall in its sensitivity. This undoubtedly

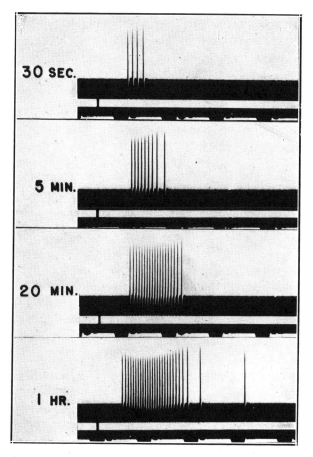

FIG. 7. Dark adaptation of a visual sense cell. Discharges of impulses
in an optic nerve fiber (*Limulus*) in response to a test flash of light (0.01
sec., fixed intensity) at various times (given at left) following an adapting
exposure. Signal of flash appears in white line above time marker. Time
in 1/5 sec. (Hartline and McDonald, in preparation).

is the explanation, in part, of the "sensory adaptation" described
above. It is to be noted, however, that the discharge (Fig. 2)
does not subside completely, but reaches a steady level at which

impulses continue to be discharged as long as light shines on the eye. Evidently there are restorative processes in the sense cell which can maintain the supply of photosensitive material even in the face of active photolysis. A stationary state is reached when the rate of the restorative reaction equals that of photolysis (28); its level depends upon the intensity of illumination, and in turn determines the frequency of the discharge of impulses in the nerve fiber.

Following a period of exposure to light the restorative reaction proceeds unopposed by photolysis, and as the photosensitive material accumulates the receptor cell recovers its original sensitivity in the process of dark adaptation. This may be measured by recording the discharge of impulses in response to a test flash of constant intensity thrown upon the eye at various times following exposure to an adapting light (26). Records from such an experiment are shown in Fig. 7. Immediately after the adapting exposure the flash could elicit only a few impulses, but as dark adaptation proceeded, the responses to the flash became greater and greater, until the receptor had completely recovered its original sensitivity. The course of dark adaptation following various amounts of preceding light adaptation is shown graphically in Fig. 8. The greater the intensity of the pre-adapting exposure, the greater was the initial depression of sensitivity, and the slower the subsequent recovery. Curves revealing similar changes in sensitivity are characteristically obtained in studies of human dark adaptation (27, 31, 37).

These reactions of photolysis and regeneration of photosensitive materials are not purely hypothetical; chemical studies of photosensitive substances which can be extracted from the eyes of vertebrates furnish a sound basis for our understanding of the photochemical mechanism of the visual receptor. Not only can the photosensitive substances and their photoproducts be identified chemically, in some cases, but the photochemical reactions and the recombination of the photoproducts may be observed *in vitro* (12, 29, 36). Thus the first step in the excitation of the visual sense cell is beginning to be understood. On the other hand, very little is known about the processes intermediate between the initial reaction and the final discharge of nerve impulses (20). This problem, however, is not confined to the visual sense cell; it is part of more fundamental questions concerning the excitation of nerve cells of any kind, and the mechanisms whereby they initiate trains of impulses in their fibers (9, 11). It is to be hoped that recent studies on the origin of trains of impulses from chemically treated regions of peripheral nerve fibers will aid in the understanding of this fundamental mechanism of the sense cell (7, 8, 13).

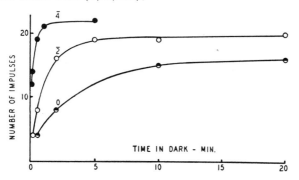

FIG. 8. Recovery of sensitivity of a single visual sense cell (*Limulus*) during the dark adaptation following various intensities of light adaptation. Ordinates give number of impulses discharged in response to test flash of fixed energy; abscissae give time in minutes after the end of the 10 sec. period of exposure to light. Numbers on the curves gives the logarithm of the relative intensities of the adapting light. (Hartline and McDonald, in preparation).

In a study of visual mechanisms it is not enough to limit one's attention to the properties of the isolated visual sense cells. The eye comprises many sensory elements, differing in their individual properties and varying in their responses with the degree and kind of illumination upon them. It is the aggregate of the diverse sensory messages arising from all the receptor elements that the visual centers must integrate. Thus the sensory elements of our retinas are spread in a mosaic to receive the retinal images of different external objects. In *Limulus,* different facets point in different directions to accomplish, crudely, a similar effect. Fig. 9 shows records obtained from a preparation in which the nerve strand happened to contain two active fibers, coming from receptor cells in different facets of the eye. Because of local differences under the recording electrodes the different fibers gave rise to spike potentials of different heights; it is consequently easy to distinguish activity in the separate fibers. The figure shows how illumination of one or the other or both facets resulted in corresponding activity in one or the other or both nerve fibers (25). This is so elementary as to be almost

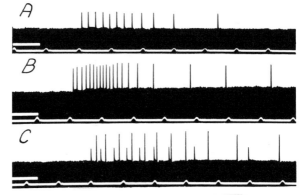

FIG. 9. Action potentials of two optic nerve fibers from two separate facets of the eye of *Limulus*. A. Discharge in response to illumination of the first facet alone. B. Discharge in response to illumination of the second facet alone. C. Discharge in response to illumination of both facets together. Signal of illumination above time marker. Time in 1/5 sec. (Hartline and Graham (25)).

trivial, yet it is the basic sensory information which enables the animal to distinguish visual form and pattern.

Not only can the distribution of light and shade in the retinal image be recognized but many of the higher animals can distinguish the color of light as well. It was pointed out above that lights of different wavelengths have different degrees of effectiveness in exciting the visual sense cell of *Limulus*. However, once the energy of the incident light is adjusted to compensate for this difference in effectiveness, the responses to different colored lights are identical; there is nothing in the discharge of impulses by an individual sense cell to distinguish what wavelength is used to excite it. It is not known whether *Limulus* can distinguish colors, but even in animals known to possess color vision we would hardly expect any other result from a study of their isolated receptor cells. Different qualities of the stimulus are probably mediated not by individual sensory elements, but by the aggregate of them. Different receptor cells, possessing different spectral distributions of sensitivity, are usually supposed to furnish the peripheral basis for color discrimination. It is in-

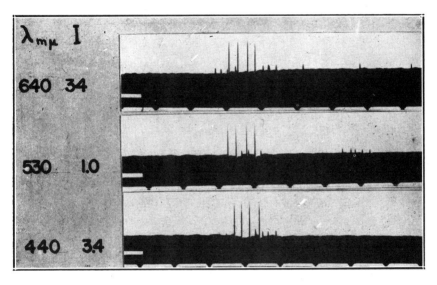

Fig. 10. Action potentials of two optic nerve fibers (*Limulus*) in response to lights of different wavelengths (λ). Relative intensities (I) adjusted to elicit 4 impulses in fiber giving large spikes; these intensities are not equally effective for the fiber giving the small spikes. Signal of illumination above time marker. Time in 1/5 sec. (Graham and Hartline (14)).

teresting that even the primitive eye of *Limulus* possesses this much of a possible color vision mechanism. In Fig. 10 the activity in two optic nerve fibers from two sensory elements, closely adjacent in the eye, can be recognized by characteristic differences in height of the spike potentials. The three spectral lights used were adjusted to produce equal responses (4 impulses) in the fiber yielding the large impulses. It is seen that this does not constitute a match for the other fiber, whose receptor cell was relatively more sensitive to the red end of the spectrum. While neither sense cell, acting alone, could signal the wavelength of the light, it is evident that the information provided by both together could be used by the animal to distinguish one end of the spectrum from the other (14). To make use of this sensory information the animal must possess the adequate central mechanisms for integrating this kind of pattern of nerve fiber activity. Recent studies by Granit (16, 17) on neurons of the vertebrate retina have shown that differential sensitivity to lights of different wavelengths is well developed in animals possessing the ability to discriminate color.

The properties of the higher neurons in the visual pathway, whose function it is to integrate the various patterns of receptor activity, may be analyzed ultimately by methods similar to those we have just described. To make a beginning in this analysis the vertebrate eye has been chosen since the axons of the retinal ganglion cells are accessible as the fibers of the optic nerve. The retinal ganglion cells are the third neurons in the chain, counting the receptor elements (rods and cones) as the first, and it is not surprising to find that their activity is considerably more complicated than the simple sensory discharges of the visual sense cells of *Limulus*. The discharge of impulses in the vertebrate optic nerve was first studied by Adrian and Matthews (2, 3, 4); the experiments to be described are an extension of their studies to an investigation of the properties of the individual retinal neurons.

A slightly different procedure is necessary to record the discharge of impulses in single optic nerve fibers from the vertebrate eye (21). The eye of a frog or other cold-blooded vertebrate is removed and opened, and its cornea, lens and vitreous humor are removed, exposing the retina. The optic nerve fibers form a thin layer on the surface of the retina, and small bundles of them may be dissected from the retina in the region where they converge to the head of the optic nerve. Such a bundle, split until only a single nerve fiber remains active, may be placed on electrodes and its electrical activity recorded in the usual manner. The retina is then explored with a small spot of light to determine the region which must be illuminated in order to elicit a discharge of impulses in the fiber. Recently micro-electrodes have been devised which when inserted in the retina record the activity from a very few retinal neurons, and records have been published which show clearly the activity from single ganglion cells (16, 18, 38, 39; cf. also Fig. 12). This method has made it possible to extend these studies to the mammalian retina.

The most striking feature of the activity of vertebrate optic nerve fibers wherein they differ from simple sensory discharges, is the wide diversity of the responses of different fibers. Fig. 11 shows the three principal types of response observed in single optic nerve fibers from the eye of the frog. In some of the fibers (Fig. 11 A) the discharge is similar to that from a simple receptor cell: impulses are discharged regularly as long as the light shines. Other fibers (Fig. 11 B) discharge impulses only briefly, when the light is turned on and again when it is turned off, showing no activity whatever as long as the light shines steadily. The "off" responses in these fibers are a marked departure from simple sense-organ activity. Even more remarkable are the fibers whose only response occurs when the light is turned off (Fig. 11 C). These different kinds of response are not due to different conditions of stimulation or adaptation of the retina; a given optic nerve fiber has its fixed pattern of response, and fibers with different types of response can be found in the same bundle of fibers, coming from closely adjacent regions of the retina. These same types of response are commonly met in all the cold-blood vertebrates that have been studied and have also been reported from the retinas of mammals (16, 39).

There is no certain explanation for this diversity of response among the optic nerve fibers of the vertebrate eye. It does seem reasonable, however, to ascribe it to the complex ganglionic structures of the retina intervening between the sensory receptors and the axons of the retinal ganglion cells. Moreover, direct evidence has been obtained that ganglionic structures are capable of

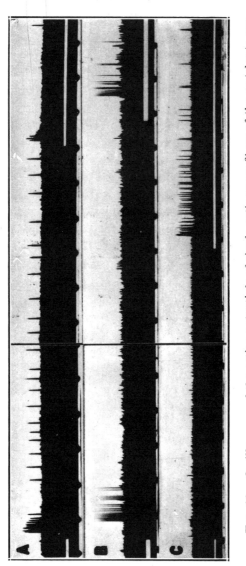

FIG. 11. Oscillograms of the action potentials of single optic nerve fibers of the vertebrate eye (frog) illustrating the three most common types of response to illumination of the retina. Signal of the retinal illumination blackens the white line above the time marker. Time in 1/5 sec. (Hartline (21)).

modifying the simple sensory discharge, and so give rise to quite different patterns of response. This has been shown in the optic ganglion of *Limulus,* by the use of micro-electrodes for recording the activity of single neurons (40). We have already described the activity in the optic nerve fibers of *Limulus,* and in the hundreds of preparations we have studied not a single case has been found of anything but the simple discharge of impulses during illumination of the eye. When the optic lobe of the central ganglion is explored, however, activity of neurons has been recorded in which the discharge of impulses occurs only in response to cessation of illumination upon the eye (Fig. 12).

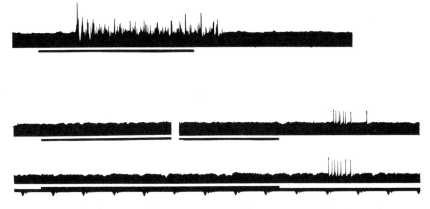

FIG. 12.   Action potentials recorded by micro-electrodes in the optic ganglion of *Limulus.*   Upper record, responses to illumination of the eye recorded by a large electrode inserted in the ganglion at the point of entrance of the optic nerve.   Lower record, responses to illumination of the eye recorded by a small electrode inserted in the same ganglion approximately 2 mm. posterior to the point of entrance of the optic nerve.   Signal of illumination above time marker.   Time in 1/5 sec.   (Hartline and Wilska, in preparation).

These responses can be elicited equally well by electrical stimulation of the central end of the optic nerve, and occur only upon the cessation of stimulation.   In all their properties these "off" responses found in the *Limulus* optic ganglion resemble the pure "off" discharges observed in the vertebrate retina (Record C of Fig. 11).

The same factors which have been shown to determine the

responses of the visual sense cells in the eye of *Limulus* likewise affect the discharge of impulses in the vertebrate optic nerve fibers. Thus the frequency of the discharge is greater the higher the intensity of the retinal illumination; likewise the sensitivity of the retina is diminished by light adaptation and recovers as the eye is allowed to remain in darkness. In addition, certain new properties emerge. The fibers responding with short bursts of impulses at the onset and cessation of illumination also respond even to slight changes in intensity—the greater the change the stronger the response. These fibers are also extremely sensitive to movements of the retinal image, whether it be a spot of light or a small shadow on the uniformly illuminated retina (Fig. 13). The higher the intensity, and the more rapid and extensive the movement, the greater the number of impulses discharged in response. The importance of this type of discharge to the animal is obvious.

The discharge of impulses in fibers which respond only to turning the light off usually subsides in a second or two; the initial frequency and the duration of this discharge are greater the higher the intensity and the longer the duration of the preceding exposure. Thus the "off" responses are strictly dependent on the preceding illumination, although these ganglion cells discharge no impulses during the period when their excitation is being built up. Indeed, the discharge in these fibers can be abruptly suppressed at any time merely by re-illumination of the retina (Fig. 14). The "off" responses from the *Limulus* ganglion have these same properties. Thus in the visual system there are neurons whose activity is governed by inhibitory as well as excitatory influences, and the interplay of excitation and inhibition which is characteristic of central nervous activity is a prominent feature of retinal function.

The detailed analysis of the integration of sense cell activity by the higher neurons is a formidable problem, and one that may be more suitably attacked elsewhere than in the visual pathway. Nevertheless it is possible to show how some of the fundamental principles of central nervous function govern the activity of neurons in the visual system.

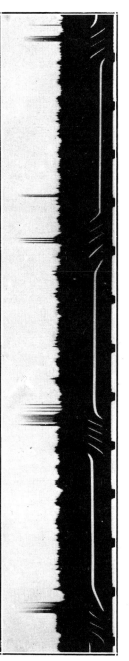

Fig. 13. Bursts of impulses discharged in an optic nerve fiber (frog) in response to movement of a small spot of light (50 μ diameter) on the retina. White lines above time marker signal the movement; each stroke corresponds to a movement of 7 μ on the retina. Time in 1/5 sec. (Hartline (23)).

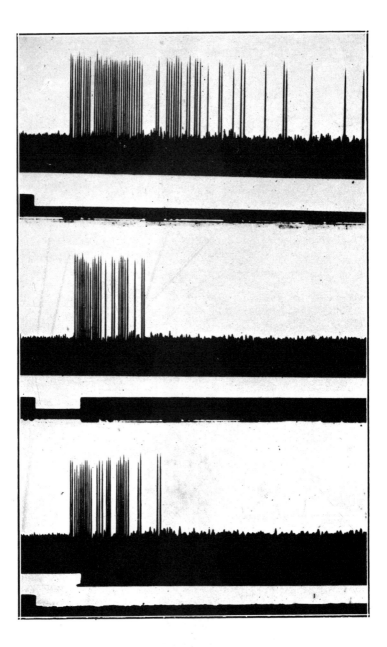

It is well known that the receptor elements of the vertebrate eye greatly outnumber the retinal ganglion cells, and that each ganglion cell in the peripheral retina makes connection with many retinal rods (through the intermediate bipolar cells). It is therefore not surprising to find that a single retinal ganglion cell can be excited by light falling anywhere within a retinal area which, although small, has appreciable extent, and must comprise many receptor elements (23). The retinal region occupied by visual sense cells whose connections converge upon a given retinal ganglion cell shall be termed the receptive field of that ganglion cell. The extent and the distribution of sensitivity within the receptive fields of ganglion cells has been charted by exploring the retina with a small spot of light while recording the activity in single optic nerve fibers. In Fig. 15 a are plotted the contours of the area within which a spot of light elicited a discharge of impulses in an optic nerve fiber from the peripheral retina of a frog's eye. Two intensities of exploring spot were used; the less intense one could elicit responses only when it fell within the more sensitive central portion of the fiber's receptive field. Fig. 15 b shows, in another experiment, the contours for three different intensities of exploring spot. These experiments show that sensitivity to light, for a particular ganglion cell, is not uniformly distributed over the whole retina. The region of maximal sensitivity is usually at least several tenths of a millimeter in diameter, but responses to light can be elicited over a considerably larger region; appreciable sensitivity generally extends over an area of approximately one square millimeter.

FIG. 14. Inhibition of the ''off response'' (frog optic nerve fiber) by re-illumination of the retina. Upper record: discharge of impulses in response to cessation of illumination (cf. Fig. 11 C). Short black strip appearing on lower edge of white band (above time marker) signals the retinal illumination by the spot of light giving rise to this off response. Middle record: ''Off response'' cut short by re-illumination of the same spot of light (black strip is interrupted during the brief interval of darkness). Lower record: ''Off response'' is cut short by illumination of an adjacent spot of light (0.2 mm. removed), signalled by black strip on upper edge of white band. Time in 1/5 sec. (Hartline, in preparation).

Not only do excitatory influences converge upon each ganglion cell from different parts of its receptive field, but in the case of ganglion cells giving pure "off" responses, inhibitory influences converge as well. Fig. 14 shows "off" responses which have been abruptly cut short by re-illumination of the retina. In the middle record the re-illumination was applied to the same retinal area as the initial (exciting) illumination; in the lower record

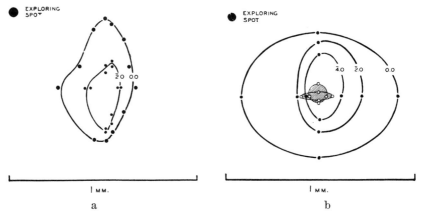

a   b

Fig 15. Charts of the retinal regions supplying single optic nerve fibers (eye of the frog). a. Determination of the contours of the receptive field of a fiber at two levels of intensity of exploring spot. Dots mark positions at which exploring spot (50 μ in diameter) would just elicit discharges of impulses, at the intensity whose logarithm is given on the respective curve (unit intensity = 2.10⁴ meter candles). No responses at log I = – 3.0, for any location of exploring spot. This fiber responded only at "on" and "off." b. Contours (determined by four points on perpendicular diameters) of receptive field of a fiber, at three levels of intensity (value of log I given on respective contours). In this fiber steady illumination (log I = 0.0 and – 2.0) produced a maintained discharge of impulses for locations of exploring spot within central shaded area; elsewhere discharge subsided in 1–2 seconds. No maintained discharge in response to intensities less than log I = – 2.0; no response at all to an intensity log I = – 4.6. (Hartline (23)).

it was applied to an area 0.2 mm. away from the initial spot, but still within the receptive field of the fiber. The efficacy of a spot of light in inhibiting an "off" discharge is greatest if it falls in the center of the receptive field; the less sensitive margins require more intense illumination to produce the same degree of inhibition (22).

Where there is convergence of neural pathways it is not surprising to find spatial summation. This is a property of the vertebrate retina which has been clearly demonstrated by the work of Adrian and Matthews (2, 3, 4). Spatial summation of excitatory effects is most simply shown in the influence of the area of the retinal illumination upon the discharge of impulses in a single optic nerve fiber (24). Fig. 16 shows the responses to

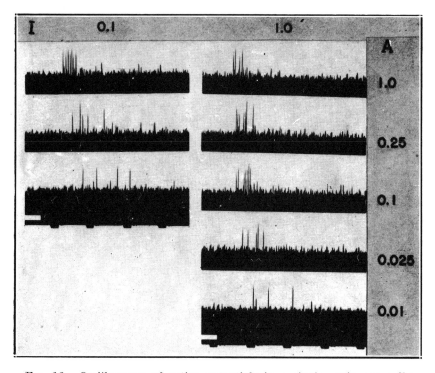

FIG. 16. Oscillograms of action potentials in a single optic nerve fiber from a frog's retina, showing effect of size of stimulus patch upon the discharge of impulses. Retina illuminated with circular patches of light, centered on receptive field of the fiber; relative areas (A) given on right (A = 1 corresponds to 0.006 mm.^{2}). For the responses in the left hand column the intensity of illumination was 1/10 that used for the right hand column. (I = 1 equivalent to 3.10^5 meter candles). Fiber was one responding with bursts of impulses at "on" and at "off" with no impulses discharged during steady illumination. Only "on" burst shown here. Signal of illumination blackens white line above time marker (only shown in bottom records). Time in 1/5 sec. (Hartline (24)).

illumination of the retina with patches of light of various sizes falling well within the limits of the fiber's receptive field. The larger the area illuminated by a stimulus patch of fixed intensity the shorter was the latency of the response, and, for moderate degrees of stimulation, the higher was the frequency and the greater the number of impulses in the discharge. These effects are similar to those obtained by increasing the intensity of a

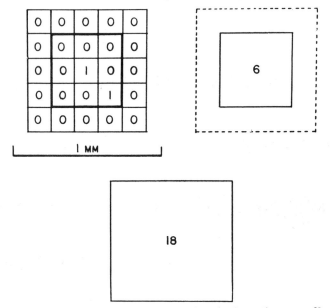

FIG. 17. Chart showing the responses of a single optic nerve fiber (frog eye) to illumination of different portions of its receptive field, at a fixed intensity (2.10^{-3} meter candles). Upper left: number of impulses in response to each of 25 subdivisions of large square, tested individually (comparative scale given below). Upper right: response to illumination of area covered by 9 central subdivisions (heavy outline in upper left). Below: response to illumination of entire square. Fiber responded only to "off." Duration of exposure for each test ca. 5 sec. (Hartline (24)).

patch of light of fixed area, as may be seen from a comparison of the responses in the two columns of Fig. 16 (obtained at two different intensities). Indeed, it is only the total amount of luminous flux (area × intensity) that determines the response of the ganglion cell. This relation holds only provided the area illuminated does not include the less sensitive marginal regions of the fiber's receptive field, which can contribute only a little to the excitation of the ganglion cell. With large areas which exceed the size of the receptive field only the intensity of illumination determines the response.

To show the relative contributions of different elements of area to the total excitation of the ganglion cell the responses to illumination of subdivisions of a retinal region may be compared with each other and with the responses to illumination of the entire area. Such experiments show that the threshold intensity for a given area is lower than the threshold for its most sensitive subdivision; it is the total number of convergent pathways activated that determines the response in the final common pathway. Fig. 17 shows a chart of the number of impulses obtained in response to illumination of a retinal area and its subdivisions. The intensity was so chosen that none of the smallest subdivisions when illuminated alone could elicit a response in the optic nerve fiber with the exception of two, each of which could elicit only one impulse. Yet when the nine most central subdivisions were illuminated together at this same intensity the ganglion cell responded with six impulses, and when all 25 subdivisions were illuminated a burst of 18 impulses resulted. Evidently the separate retinal pathways can be excited to a degree which is subliminal for the ganglion cell, but when several convergent pathways act together their effects can sum to produce a discharge of nerve impulses. The summation of subliminal effects indicates that more than one nerve impulse in the retinal pathways must impinge upon the retinal ganglion cell to produce even a single impulse in its axon.

If the retinal illumination is made intense enough even a very small subdivision of the receptive field of a fiber will elicit a discharge of impulses. When several such subdivisions are illuminated together, spatial summation takes place and the excitation of the ganglion cell is greater than that produced by the most effective subdivision acting alone. Fig. 18 is a chart showing the frequencies of discharge in a fiber in which activity was maintained throughout a steady illumination. The frequency of discharge in response to illumination of the large area was higher than the highest frequency obtained by illumination of any one of the nine subdivisions of this area. Fig. 19 shows the records of the discharge due to illumination of the total area and that due to its most effective subdivision. The retinal ganglion cell is the final common path for sensory activity originating in many receptor elements; its excitation is determined by the summation of all the excitatory influences reaching it over the pathways which converge upon it.

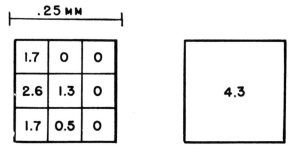

FIG. 18. Chart showing the response of a single optic nerve fiber (frog eye) to illumination of different areas in its receptive field. Discharge in this fiber was maintained during steady illumination; numbers give the frequency of this discharge in response to illumination of each of the 9 small squares (left) compared with the response to illumination of the entire area covered by these squares (right). Scale of retinal distances given above. (Hartline (24)).

Because of the spatial summation taking place in the peripheral retina we are enabled to see dimly illuminated objects which would otherwise be invisible, provided they are large enough. This sensitivity, however, is achieved at the expense of visual resolution; we cannot distinguish fine detail in the periphery of our visual field. It is recognized that this poor resolution is due to the large number of sensory elements corresponding to each ganglion cell in the peripheral retina. These experiments have shown how illumination falling anywhere within the receptive field of a single ganglion cell can cause its excitation. Moreover, the receptive fields of different ganglion cells overlap, so that

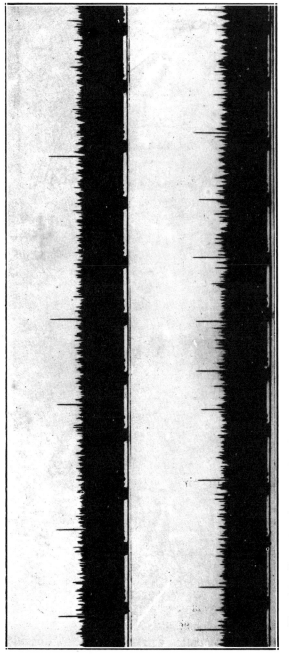

FIG. 19. Records of the maintained discharge of impulses in a single optic nerve fiber, showing effect of spatial summation. Top: response to illumination of most effective one of 9 subdivisions of an area of the retina (small square labelled 2.6 in Fig. 18). Bottom: response to illumination of entire area covered by the 9 subdivisions (labelled 4.3 in Fig. 18). Time marked in 1/5 sec. (Hartline (24)).

illumination of a given small area on the retina can excite several optic nerve fibers. This may be observed experimentally in bundles which have not been split by dissection, so that many optic nerve fibers remain active (23). Usually the activity in the various fibers can be distinguished (if there are not too many of them) by slight differences in their impulses, as observed with the aid of an oscilloscope. From such experiments it is possible to reconstruct the representation in the optic nerve of an illuminated point on the retina. A given element of retinal area lies within the central, most sensitive region of the receptive fields of certain retinal ganglion cells. The axons of these cells will be stimulated effectively by illumination of this element of area. For other cells this point lies in the less sensitive margins of their receptive fields; these cells will be activated less strongly by illumination of this particular element of retinal area. Illumination of a particular point on the retina therefore elicits a specific pattern of activity among the fibers of the optic nerve. The specific fibers involved, and the relative strengths of the discharges of nerve impulses they transmit, are characteristic of this particular point. Corresponding to other points are different patterns of activity; even two closely adjacent points do not produce quite the same distribution of activity, although they may excite many fibers in common. This may be observed directly, by watching on the oscilloscope the altered pattern of electrical activity resulting as a small spot of light is tested at different positions on the retina. For two points of the retinal image to be resolved, they need not necessarily be separated so widely that they activate entirely different groups of optic nerve fibers; it might suffice if two discrete maxima of activity are produced among the fibers involved. Nevertheless, one can hardly expect the resolution of detail to be as good as in the fovea, where each optic nerve fiber probably corresponds to only one receptor element.

The experiments reviewed in this lecture constitute the first steps in the unitary analysis of the mechanism of vision. They have shown that the visual sense cells initiate trains of nerve impulses closely resembling the sensory discharges from other kinds of receptors. Evidence for the photochemical basis of the sensitivity to light of the visual receptor cell has been provided, but the processes intervening between the initial action of light and the final discharge of nerve impulses are not yet understood. The sensory information from receptor elements acts in turn upon higher neurons in the visual pathway. The early part of this process has been studied by recording the responses of the gang-lion cells of the vertebrate retina. Their activity has been found to be governed by principles of nervous action well known from studies of the central nervous system. The study of these retinal neurons has emphasized the necessity for considering patterns of activity in the nervous system. Individual nerve cells never act independently; it is the integrated action of all the units of the visual system that gives rise to vision.

A part of the experimental work reported here was supported by generous grants from the American Philosophical Society and from the John and Mary Markle Foundation.

REFERENCES

1. Adrian, E. D., and Bronk, D. W., *J. Physiol.*, 1928, **66**, 81.
2. Adrian, E. D., and Matthews, R., *J. Physiol.*, 1927, **63**, 378.
3. Adrian, E. D., and Matthews, R., *J. Physiol.*, 1927, **64**, 279.
4. Adrian, E. D., and Matthews, R., *J. Physiol.*, 1928, **65**, 273.
5. Adrian, E. D., and Umrath, K., *J. Physiol.*, 1929, **68**, 139.
6. Adrian, E. D., and Zotterman, Y., *J. Physiol.*, 1926, **61**, 151.
7. Arvanitaki, A., *Arch. intern. Physiol.*, 1939, **49**, 209.
8. Brink, F., and Bronk, D. W., *Am. J. Physiol.*, 1941, **133**, P222.
9. Bronk, D. W., *Trans. and Studies, College of Physicians of Philadelphia*, 1938, (4) **6**, 102.
10. Bronk, D. W., and Stella, G., *Am. J. Physiol.*, 1935, **110**, 708.
11. Bronk, D. W., and Brink, F., *Ann. Rev. Physiol.*, 1939, **1**, 385.
12. Chase, A. M., and Smith, E. L., *J. Gen. Physiol.*, 1939, **23**, 21.
13. Fessard, A., L'Activité rythmique des nerfs isolés, Paris, Hermann et Cie, 1926.
14. Graham, C. H., and Hartline, H. K., *J. Gen. Physiol.*, 1935, **18**, 917.
15. Graham, C. H., and Riggs, L., *J. Gen. Psychol.*, 1935, **12**, 279.
16. Granit, R. *Acta Physiol. Scand.*, 1941, **2**, 93.
17. Granit, R., *J. Opt. Soc. Am.*, 1941, **31**, 570.

18. Granit, R. and Svaetichin, G., *Upsala Lakaref. Forhandl.*, 1939, **45**, 161.

19. Hartline, H. K., *J. Cell. and Comp. Physiol.*, 1934, **5**, 229.

20. Hartline, H. K., *Cold Spring Harbor Symposia*, 1935, **3**, 245.

21. Hartline, H. K., *Am. J. Physiol.*, 1938, **121**, 400.

22. Hartline, H. K., *Am. J. Physiol.*, 1939, **126**, P527.

23. Hartline, H. K., *Am. J. Physiol.*, 1940, **130**, 690.

24. Hartline, H. K., *Am. J. Physiol.*, 1940, **130**, 700.

25. Hartline, H. K., and Graham, C. H., *J. Cell. and Comp. Physiol.*, 1932, **1**, 277.

26. Hartline, H. K., and McDonald, R., *Am. J. Physiol.*, 1941, **133**, P321.

27. Haig, C., *J. Gen. Physiol.*, 1941, **24**, 735.

28. Hecht, S., *Physiol. Rev.*, 1937, **17**, 239.

29. Hecht, S., Chase, A. M., Shlaer, S., and Haig, C., *Science*, 1936, **84**, 331.

30. Hecht, S., and Williams, R. E., *J. Gen. Physiol.*, 1922, **5**, 1.

31. Hecht, S., Haig, C., and Chase, A. M., *J. Gen. Physiol.*, 1937, **20**, 831.

32. Lowenstein, O., and Sand, A., *Proc. Roy. Soc. (London)*, ser B., 1940, **129**, 256.

33. Matthews, B. H. C., *J. Physiol.*, 1931, **71**, 64.

34. Pfaffmann, C., *J. Cell. and Comp. Physiol.*, 1941, **17**, 243.

35. Pumphrey, R. J., *J. Cell. and Comp. Physiol.*, 1935, **6**, 457.

36. Wald, G., *J. Gen. Physiol.*, 1935, **19**, 351.

37. Wald, G., and Clark, A.-B., *J. Gen. Physiol.*, 1937, **21**, 93.

38. Wilska, A., *Acta Soc. Med. Fenn.* ''Duodecim,'' 1939, **22**, 63.

39. Wilska, A., *Acta Soc. Med. Fenn.* ''Duodecim,'' 1939, **22**, 63.

40. Wilska, A., and Hartline, H. K., *Am. J. Physiol.*, 1941, **133**, P491.

Part Three

The Double Retina of the Eye of
the Scallop, *Pecten*

INTRODUCTION by F. Ratliff

'*Let us place side by side the eye of a vertebrate and that of a mollusk such as the common* Pecten. *We find the same essential parts in each, composed of analogous elements.
The eye of the* Pecten *presents a retina, a cornea, a lens of cellular structure like our
own. There is even that peculiar inversion of retinal elements which is not met with, in
general, in the retina of the invertebrates. Now, the origin of the mollusks may be a
debated question, but, whatever opinion we hold, all are agreed that mollusks and vertebrates separated from their common parent-stem long before the appearance of an eye so
complex as that of the* Pecten. *Whence, then, the structural analogy?*'
Henri Bergson, *Creative Evolution*, 1911.

The scallop has always been a source of wonder and delight to man.
The beautiful symmetry of its shell, enhanced rather than spoiled by the
slight asymmetry at the hinge, is most pleasing to the eye. The scallop
shell also has a certain mystique about it, as well as an undeniable
beauty (see Cox, 1957). In addition to its many purely decorative uses,
it has served variously – throughout the centuries – as the cradle of
Venus in art and mythology, as the badge of St. James in religion, as an
heraldic bearing in numerous coats of arms, and – presently – as the
emblem of the Manhattan Philosophical Society.

The living animal itself is no less a delight to the naturalist. Its
prowess as a swimmer is most remarkable – the vigorous clapping together of the two valves of the shell can send it flying here and there
through the water like a butterfly through the air. But this flight is by
no means erratic or haphazard – by proper control of the muscular
edges of the mantles hanging from the two valves of the shell, nozzles
can be formed at any point, and the sudden ejection of water as the
valves are closed will cause the scallop to twist or turn, or to move
forward or backward according to the location of the resulting jets.

The Eyes of the Scallop. The hundred or so eyes of the scallop, set
like tiny emeralds around the upper and lower mantles, are perhaps the
most remarkable of all the many remarkable features of this animal.
Not content with a mere hundred eyes, the scallop has a double retina
in every eye, with each of the two retinas served by a separate optic
nerve. The eyes are extremely small, of course, being only about one

millimeter in diameter. The two retinas and their optic nerves, which are located on the outer end of a tentacle-like structure, appear to be easily accessible – in anatomical drawings. In actual practice, however, the flexible tentacle is most difficult to dissect. Nevertheless, Hartline was able to isolate single fibers in each of the two optic nerves and to obtain oscillographic records of their activity. He found that the proximal retina gave a simple maintained discharge of impulses much like that of the *Limulus* optic nerve. But, in conformity with the scallop's vigorous 'shadow reaction', the distal retina gave pure 'off' responses, much like those of some vertebrate retinal ganglion cells. Indeed, if we place two sets of oscillographic records of such 'off' responses side by side, one can scarcely be distinguished from the other.

The course of light and dark adaptation in the scallop eye is about the same as in the vertebrate eye. It has been measured by recording the discharge of impulses in the optic nerve (Hartline 1938, Land 1966) and by observing the amplitude of the retinal action potential (Ratliff 1956). The spectral sensitivity of the eye of the scallop, *Pecten maximus*, has been determined by finding the intensity at various wavelengths just sufficient to elicit a 'shadow reaction' when the light was turned off (Cronly-Dillon, 1966) and, in the eye of *Aequipecten irradians*, by measurements of the retinal action potential (Wald and Seldin, 1968). Cronly-Dillon found two peaks, a main one at 475 mμ and a smaller one at 540 mμ. Wald and Seldin found only one simple curve with a peak at about 490–495 mμ. It is uncertain, however, whether these action spectra represent the primary photochemical processes – direct spectrophotometric measurements of the photopigments have yet to be made.

Types of Receptors. The structural and functional analogy between the eyes of vertebrates and mollusks is impressive, indeed. But the differences are just as striking. The double retina of *Pecten* seems to be unique. Miller (1958, 1960) found that the photoreceptor cells of the distal retina are layered structures that appear to be derived from cilia (as are rods and cones in the vertebrate retina) while the cells of the proximal retina have microvillous borders and appear not to be derived from cilia (as are typical invertebrate photoreceptors). See also Barber, Evans, and Land (1967). The axons of the optic nerve are first-order, that is, they arise directly from the photoreceptors. This is quite unlike the vertebrate eye in which the optic nerve is made up of third-order neurones.

Optics. Although superficially similar, the optical system of the *Pecten* eye actually differs markedly from that of the vertebrate eye.

According to Land (1965) the lens by itself does not produce a retinal image in the scallop eye. The image visible in microscopic examination is produced by the combined effects of the lens and the curved multi-layer interference reflector formed by the tapetum at the back of the eye (Land, 1966). The reflected image is formed on the distal retina in much the same way that an image is formed by a reflecting telescope. There is no sharp image formed on the proximal retina. The distal 'off' retina therefore can signal information about the spatial distribution of light in the environment, whereas the proximal 'on' retina, on which the illumination is diffuse, can signal only changes in intensity.

Intraretinal Activity. A recent review by Land (1968) of the optical and functional organization of the mollusk eye assesses the behavioral, anatomical, and physiological evidence for distinct 'on' and 'off' types of photoreceptors in gastropod and bivalve mollusks. Land's experiments on the scallop (1966) indicate that the distal cells may be pure 'off' receptors, functioning independently of the proximal cells. But whether opposed excitatory and inhibitory influences interacting within the distal retina, or between the two retinas, contribute to the 'off' response can best be determined by direct intraretinal observations. Only two such experiments have been carried out, as yet. In some preliminary investigations, Toyoda and Shapley (1967) recorded intra-retinal activity in the eye of *Aequipecten irradians* with fine micropipettes and found evidence of hyperpolarizing (inhibitory) potentials (cf. Tomita, 1970). An extension of this work by Gorman and McReynolds (1969) and McReynolds and Gorman (1970a and 1970b) has since revealed both depolarizing (excitatory) and hyperpolarizing (inhibitory) potentials. The two potentials appear to originate in the proximal ('on') and distal ('off') layers of the retina, respectively. These findings therefore suggest (but do not yet prove) that the two retinas are independent and that the photoreceptors in them give opposite primary responses to light. It would probably be a mistake, however, to conclude that the receptors in the distal retina are purely inhibitory. While no impulses may be discharged by the distal retina during illumination, excitation is nevertheless building up during that time; the 'off' discharge depends strictly upon the duration and intensity of the preceding illumination.

REFERENCES

Barber, V. C., Evans, E. M., and Land, M. F. (1967), 'The Fine Structure of the Eye of the Mollusc *Pecten Maximus*', *Z. Zellforsch. mikrosk. Anat.*, **76**, 295–312.

Cox, I., ed. (1957), *The Scallop*, The 'Shell' Transport and Trading Co., London.

Cronly-Dillon, J. R. (1966), 'Spectral Sensitivity of the Scallop *Pecten Maximus*', *Science*, **151**, 345–346.

Gorman, A. L. F., and McReynolds, J. S. (1969), 'Hyperpolarizing and Depolarizing Receptor Potentials in the Scallop Eye', *Science*, **165**, 309–310.

Hartline, H. K. (1938), 'The Discharge of Impulses in the Optic Nerve of Pecten in Response to Illumination of the Eye', *J. Cell. Comp. Physiol.*, **11**, 465–478.

Land, M. F. (1965), 'Image Formation by a Concave Reflector in the Eye of the Scallop, *Pecten Maximus*', *J. Physiol.* (Lond.), **179**, 138–153.

Land, M. F. (1966), 'Activity in the Optic Nerves of *Pecten Maximus* in Response to Changes in Light Intensity, and to Pattern and Movement in the Optical Environment', *J. Exp. Biol.*, **45**, 83–99.

Land, M. F. (1966), 'A Multilayer Interference Reflector in the Eye of the Scallop, *Pecten Maximus*', *J. Exp. Biol.*, **45**, 433–447.

Land, M. F. (1968), 'Functional Aspects of the Optical and Retinal Organization of the Mollusc Eye', in *Invertebrate Receptors*, J. D. Carthy and G. E. Newell, eds., Academic Press, London, 75–96.

McReynolds, J. S., and Gorman, A. L. F. (1970a), Photoreceptor potentials of opposite polarity in the eye of the scallop, *Pecten irradians*', *J. Gen. Physiol.*, **56**, No. 3, 376–391.

McReynolds, J. S., and Gorman, A. L. F. (1970b), 'Membrane conductances and spectral sensitivities of *Pecten* photoreceptors', *J. Gen. Physiol.*, **56**, No. 3, 392–406.

Miller, W. H. (1958), 'Derivatives of Cilia in the Distal Sense Cells of the Retina of *Pecten*', *J. Biophys. Biochem. Cytol.*, **4**, 227–228.

Miller, W. H. (1958), 'Fine Structure of Some Invertebrate Photoreceptors', *Ann. N.Y. Acad. Sci.*, **74**, 204–209.

Miller, W. H. (1960), 'Visual Photoreceptor Structures', in *The Cell*, J. Brachet and A. E. Mirsky, eds., Academic Press, London, **4**, 325–364.

Ratliff, F. (1956), 'Retinal Action Potentials in the Eye of the Scallop', *Biol. Bull.*, **111**, 310.

Tomita, T. (1970), 'Electrical activity of vertebrate photoreceptors', *Quarterly Reviews of Biophysics*, **3,** No. 2, 179–222.

Toyoda, J., and Shapley, R. M. (1967), 'The Intracellularly Recorded Response in the Scallop Eye', *Biol. Bull.*, **133,** 490.

Wald, G., and Seldin, E. B. (1968), 'The Electroretinogram and Spectral Sensitivity of the Common Scallop', *Biol. Bull.*, **135,** 441–442.

The discharge of impulses in the optic nerve of *Pecten* in response to illumination of the eye

H. K. HARTLINE

Eldridge Reeves Johnson Foundation, University of Pennsylvania, Philadelphia, and
Marine Biological Laboratory, Woods Hole, Massachusetts

Reprinted from the JOURNAL OF CELLULAR AND
COMPARATIVE PHYSIOLOGY, Vol. II, no. 3, pp. 465-478, June 1938

Responses of animals to light include not only reactions elicited during actual illumination, but also responses to the cessation, or sudden diminution in intensity, of a steadily shining light. Many of the lower animals exhibit vigorous 'shadow reactions' in response to shading their photoreceptors. In the vertebrate eye response to a decrease in intensity of retinal illumination is a prominent feature both of the retinal action potential and of the discharge of impulses in the optic nerve (Adrian and Matthews, '27; Granit, '33). It has recently been shown (Hartline, '38) that these 'off' responses in the vertebrate optic nerve are largely contributed by a certain group of fibers in which no impulses are discharged at all either in response to the onset of illumination or while light shines steadily on the retina, but which respond vigorously as soon as it is turned off. The complexity of the vertebrate retina, however, renders obscure the mechanism of the 'off' response, and for this reason it has seemed desirable to look for 'off' responses from simpler photoreceptors among the invertebrates.

The scallop, Pecten irradians, gives a vigorous 'shadow reaction' and hence might be expected to show an 'off' response in its optic discharge. Its eyes, moreover, possess two apparently independent layers of visual cells, quite different

231

from each other morphologically. The possibility that these two layers respond differently to light can be tested experimentally, since each gives rise to a separate branch of the optic nerve.

The structure of the Pecten eye (Dakin, '10, '28; Küpfer, '16) with its two layers of visual cells, is shown schematically in figure 1. The cells in the proximal layer (prox. c.) are long and rod-like, with their free ends pointed toward the back of the eye. Their axones pass to the margins of the

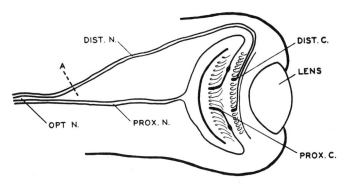

Fig. 1 Diagram of the eye of Pecten (modified after Dakin) showing schematically the two layers of visual cells and their innervation. The cells of the proximal layer (prox. c.) give rise to axones which form the proximal branch of the optic nerve (prox. n.); the cells of the distal layer (dist. c.) give rise to axones which form the distal branch of the optic nerve (dist. n.). The two nerve branches unite to form the common optic nerve (opt. n.) 1 to 2 mm. back of the eye. Severing the distal branch at the point A enables separate records to be obtained of the activity from either layer, in response to illumination of the eye. The eyes used were usually 1 to 1.5 mm. in diameter.

retina and curve closely around the back of the eye to the center of the eye stalk, where they form the proximal branch of the optic nerve (prox. n.). The cells in the distal layer (dist. c.) are short and rounded, and like the proximal cells have their free ends pointed toward the back of the eye. Their axones collect at the margin of the retina on the side of the eye stalk next the shell, and form the distal branch of the optic nerve (dist. n.). The proximal and distal branches of the optic nerve remain separate for 1 to 2 mm. before uniting, back of the eye, to form the common optic nerve (opt. n.).

This, in turn, has a length of 1 to 2 mm. before reaching the circumpallial nerve, which it crosses to become one of the pallial nerves in the mantle.

Histologically it seems well established that there are no additional neurones in or near the eye, and no synapses intervening between retinal cells and optic fibers.[1] All workers are agreed that the rod-like proximal cells are primary visual sense cells, and the later workers state that the distal cells are likewise primary sense cells. This identification seems to rest primarily on the appearance of these cells, and on the fact that no connections have been observed between them and the cells of the proximal layer.[2] (Compare Dakin, '28; Küpfer, loc. cit.; Roche, '25; Schoepfle and Young, '36).

METHOD

Activity in the optic nerve fibers, in response to illumination of the eye, is detected by oscillographic recording of their amplified action potentials. A small piece of the mantle fringe containing one of the larger eyes (1 to 1.5 mm. in diameter) is mounted in a moist chamber, the common optic nerve is identified at the point where it leaves the circumpallial nerve, and is dissected free to its point of branching. Further dissection frees the distal branch for 1 to 2 mm. almost to the point where it leaves the margin of the retina. Cutting this branch close to the point of juncture with the proximal branch (fig. 1, A) enables one to record the activity either in the fibers from the distal cell layer only (distal branch), or in those from the proximal cell layer only (common optic nerve, connected only by the proximal branch). Records from single fibers are most easily obtained by dissecting the common optic nerve (usually the pallial portion), and identifying the layer of origin at the end of the experiment by

[1] Contrary findings by Hyde ('03) are expressly denied by Dakin ('10) and have received no confirmation from other workers.

[2] From the standpoint of the dioptric system, it is worth noting that one or the other of the layers, if both are sensory, must be useless for acute vision of distant objects. In view of the minute dimensions of the eye this probably comprises all objects beyond 2 or 3 cm.

cutting the distal branch, and noting whether the response is abolished.

The eye is illuminated through the glass front of the moist chamber by an incandescent concentrated tungsten filament imaged on the lens of the eye by microscopic objective. This results in an even illumination of practically the entire retina. The intensity of light on the lens is 10^5 meter candles; on the retina it is probably 0.1 to 0.01 of this. The light can be reduced to any desired intensity by inserting Wratten 'Neutral Tint' filters in the beam.

The moist chamber is filled with sea water to a level which is sufficient to immerse the eye but which still permits the short nerve twigs to be brought out and suspended on fine wick electrodes. Leads are taken from two points on the nerve, or from the cut end and a diffuse electrode in the sea water bath. The action potentials are amplified and recorded by means of a General Electric Company loop oscillograph.

RESULTS

A record of action potentials in the common optic nerve, with both branches intact, is shown in figure 2 A. Following the onset of illumination of the eye there is a vigorous discharge of nerve impulses, strongest at the very beginning and diminishing gradually during the next few seconds. The discharge continues as long as the light shines, but at a considerably reduced frequency. When the light is turned off there is a renewed outburst of nerve impulses, which gradually diminishes and eventually dies out completely.

These responses in the common optic nerve are composed of quite different contributions from the proximal and distal branches. From the proximal fibers (fig. 2 B) responses are obtained only during illumination of the eye; when the light is turned off the discharge stops abruptly. The distal branch (fig. 2 C) on the other hand gives no response at all during the actual period of illumination; when the light is turned off there is a vigorous discharge of impulses, which subsides gradually. There is thus a marked difference in optic function between the two layers of cells of the Pecten retina.

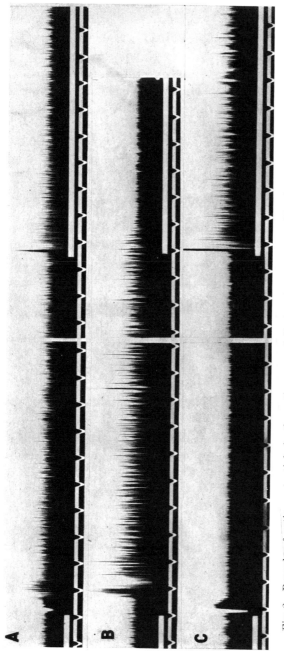

Fig. 2 Records of action potentials in the optic nerve of Pecten, in response to illumination of the eye. Successive records taken in the course of one experiment on the same eye. A, response in the common optic nerve, both branches intact; B, response in the proximal optic fibers, leads from the common optic nerve, after severing the distal branch from it at the point A, fig. 1); C, response in the distal optic fibers, leads from the distal branch. Time (lowest line) in ½ second; signal marking illumination of the eye fills the white line immediately above the time marker.

The responses from the proximal cells are typical of sense organ activity. Beginning (after a short latent period) at a high frequency, the discharge subsides to a considerably lower level of frequency, which then continues throughout illumination. The more intense the stimulating light, and the more completely dark adapted the eye, the shorter is the latent period and the higher the frequency of discharge. In figure 3 are records of responses of a single fiber from the proximal layer, showing the nature of the discharge and the effects of intensity. During prolonged illumination the frequency of discharge in these fibers falls slowly but steadily, even at moderate intensities; at very high intensities the discharge may disappear entirely after 10 or 20 seconds. A short period of dark adaptation must then be allowed before a response can again be obtained. The discharge in these fibers usually stops abruptly upon the cessation of the light. However, at high intensities, especially following rather short exposures (few seconds), it may persist for several seconds afterward, and die out gradually. There is, however, never any true 'off' response in the proximal nerve fibers, in the form of a renewed outburst of activity following the end of the period of illumination. These responses are closely similar to those obtained from the optic nerve fibers from the eye of Limulus (Hartline and Graham, '32). In Limulus, as in the present case, the optic nerve fibers are axones of the primary sense cells in the eye. In the vertebrate eye a similar type of response is also observed in about 20% of the optic nerve fibers (Hartline, '38).

In complete contrast to the proximal cell responses, the distal nerve fibers of the Pecten eye show no activity, as a rule,[3] during illumination of the retina. Their responses are

---

[3] Occasional preparations of the distal nerve have shown, in addition to the normal 'off' response, a weak discharge of impulses during illumination at high intensities. This discharge begins gradually, several seconds after the onset of illumination, and frequently dies out several seconds later. It apparently involves only a few fibers. Single fiber preparations in such cases may show a feeble discharge of irregularly scattered impulses during illumination. These cases, however, are exceptional; as a rule no impulses at all appear during the actual period of illumination.

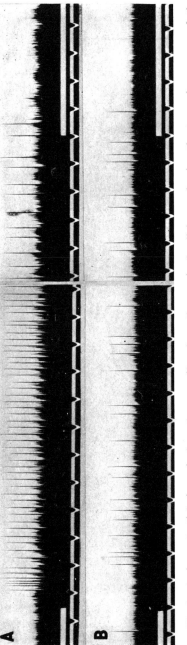

Fig. 3 Action potentials in a single optic nerve fiber from the proximal cell layer, showing the type of response and the effect of intensity. Intensity for record A, 100 times that for B. (Amplification in B slightly less than in A.) Illumination ends 30 seconds after onset. Recording as in figure 2.

elicited upon the cessation of light, or following a sudden reduction in its intensity. Figure 4 A shows a typical response in a single fiber from the distal cell layer. The discharge begins $\frac{1}{10}$ or $\frac{2}{10}$ second ofter the cessation of illumination, at a frequency which is initially high, but which falls, rapidly at first, then more gradually, and usually dies away entirely after many seconds. These 'off' responses are strictly dependent on the preceding period of illumination for their generation. To produce an 'off' response in a given distal nerve fiber, the preceding illumination must be above a definite threshold of intensity, and must last a minimum time (of the order of 1 second, more or less, depending on the intensity). The higher the intensity of the preceding period of illumination, and the longer its duration (up to 1 minute or 2), the shorter is the latent period of the 'off' response, the higher its frequency, and the longer does it last. Following prolonged exposure to a bright light it may require $\frac{1}{2}$ hour to subside completely. If the eye is re-illuminated before the response in one of these fibers has disappeared, the discharge stops abruptly. Even if the re-illumination occurs at the height of the 'off' response, it nevertheless cuts it short abruptly (fig. 4 B).

In the vertebrate retina, approximately 30% of the optic fibers show responses only upon the cessation, or sudden reduction in intensity, of illumination (Hartline, '38). A close comparison shows that these pure 'off' responses from the vertebrate eye are practically indistinguishable in their properties from the responses of the distal fibers of the Pecten eye. Thus two of the three chief types of response found in vertebrate optic nerve fibers are also observed in this much simpler invertebrate eye, in which, moreover, it has been possible to identify the two different kinds of elements giving rise to the respective responses.

The distal cells of the Pecten retina have been identified, in all of the recent anatomical studies, as primary sense cells. If this interpretation is correct, the present findings establish them as a new kind of sensory cell, capable of being stimulated

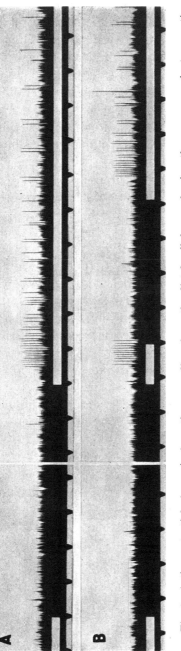

Fig. 4 Action potentials in a single optic nerve fiber from the distal cell layer, showing the response only to cessation of illumination, and in B the effect of re-illumination of the eye at the height of the 'off' response. Illumination ends 20 seconds after onset. Recording as in figure 2.

only by the removal of an environmental agent. It is perhaps not entirely unreasonable that certain kinds of nerve cells should be thrown into activity by a shift in their equilibrium in the direction opposite to that which causes excitation in other nerve cells. And this is especially so among photoreceptor cells, where there is a 'back' reaction which restores the photosensitive substance (Hecht, '34), and which, when unopposed by light, manifests itself as dark adaptation. This reaction is stronger the more intense and more prolonged the preceding illumination; it has a high velocity initially which diminishes steadily until completion, and its course is instantly reversed by re-illumination. It is possible that this unopposed 'back' reaction might, in certain types of sensory cells, initiate their response.

If this view is correct, it becomes necessary to consider seriously the possibility that in the vertebrate retina the different types of response originate in functionally different sensory cells in the rod-cone layer (Hartline, '38). The alternative possibility, that the 'off' responses arise in the ganglionic layers of the retina, could apply to the case of Pecten only if it can be shown that the two layers of retinal cells are not independent of one another. Thus there might be anatomical interconnections which have escaped observation, or the closely adjacent layers might influence each other by chemical or electrical means, and so function analogously to the more complex vertebrate retina.

That some sort of interaction may take place, at least between the individual cells of the distal layer, is suggested by the appearance, under suitable conditions, of synchronized rhythmic bursts of impulses in the discharge from the distal nerve (fig. 5). In the occasional preparation in which this type of activity has been seen (possibly associated with temperatures above 24°C.) the 'off' discharge following intense and prolonged illumination breaks up into a series of rhythmic bursts of impulses, occurring at about 3 to 10 per second. Like the normal 'off' discharge, this activity is promptly suppressed by re-illumination of the eye; when the light is again turned off the ensuing 'off' response is at first a normal steady discharge, but the rhythmic bursts usually reappear within the first second. Initially, moreover, the bursts in the various fibers are asynchronous, but get into step within 1 second or so. Such synchronized rhythmic activity has never been observed in the proximal branch, even in preparations whose distal branch shows it very markedly.

Similar synchronous activity has been observed by Adrian and Matthews ('28) during illumination of the eel's eye, and

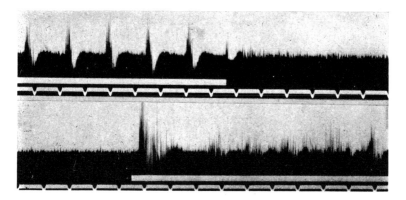

Fig. 5 Action potentials in the optic nerve in a preparation showing synchronized rhythmic activity in the distal fibers. Record begins about 1 minute after cessation of previous prolonged and intense illumination. Recording as in figure 2 (signal has been retouched).

Granit and Therman ('35) have recorded synchronized rhythmic bursts of impulses in the 'off' response of the whole vertebrate optic nerve which are very similar to the present records from Pecten. Recently Adrian ('37) has described synchronous activity in the optic ganglion of Dytiscus, both during intense illumination (bright rhythm) and in the complete absence of light (dark rhythm). Moderate intensities produce no rhythmic activity, and indeed suppress any dark rhythm which may be present, just as illumination suppresses the synchronous bursts in Pecten.

The occasional presence of synchronized activity in the cells of the distal layer of the Pecten retina raises some doubt as to the pure receptor nature of these cells, for synchronized activity is usually taken as evidence of ganglionic interaction.[4] Indeed, the function of this layer might find a more acceptable explanation if it could be shown that its cells are not primary sense cells at all, but ganglion cells (second order neurones) connected functionally with the sense cells of the proximal layer and depending on them as the source of their excitation. The dioptric system of the eye would then be more reasonable; it would not be necessary to postulate a new kind of sensory cell which responds only to cessation of a stimulating agent, and the synchronous activity of the distal cells could be ascribed to ganglionic interaction. The origin of the 'off' response would then be ascribed to neurones central to the sensory cell and to properties of ganglionic organization, both in Pecten and in the vertebrate retina. This probably does not alter essentially the problem of the origin of the 'off' response; it is still necessary to determine the mechanism whereby certain visual cells, whether receptor cells or ganglion cells, discharge nerve impulses only in response to cessation of the stimulating light. That such visual cells do exist in a comparatively simple invertebrate eye has been definitely established by this investigation; diversity of optic function among different cells of the visual system is not confined to the vertebrate retina.

SUMMARY

The retina of the Pecten eye possesses two layers of visual cells, each giving rise to a separate branch of the optic nerve. Fibers from the proximal layer of sensory cells show a discharge of impulses during illumination of the eye, with properties characteristic of simple visual end organs. These

---

[4] This does not necessarily follow, as synchronization can occur in injured peripheral nerve (Adrian, '30). As Adrian points out, under suitable conditions very weak influences may be sufficient to bring rhythmically acting elements into step.

responses are similar in all respects to those obtained from the visual sense cells of Limulus; they also resemble responses obtained in about 20% of the optic fibers of the vertebrate retina. Fibers from the distal layer respond only to cessation of illumination, or a reduction in its intensity. No impulses at all (as a rule) are discharged during illumination, but the 'off' response is nevertheless strictly dependent for its excitation upon the preceding period of illumination. Reillumination promptly suppresses the discharge in these fibers. In several experiments following intense illumination the discharge in the distal fibers broke up into rhythmic bursts of impulses, and the bursts in all the fibers became synchronous. These 'off' responses are similar in all respects to the discharges of impulses in the 'off' response fibers of the vertebrate retina. The distal cells in the Pecten retina have been described as primary sense cells completely independent of the proximal layer of sense cells. If this be correct, the present experiments establish the existence of a new kind of sensory cell, capable of being excited only by the removal of a stimulating agent. The possible presence of similar sensory cells in the vertebrate retina would then need to be considered seriously in any discussion of the origin of the 'off' response in this eye. A somewhat more acceptable interpretation, however, might be made on the assumption, contrary to anatomical opinion, that the distal cells of Pecten are ganglion cells (second order neurones), depending upon the proximal cells as the source of their excitation.

LITERATURE CITED

ADRIAN, E. D. 1930 Effect of injury on mammalian nerve fibers. Proc. Roy. Soc. Ser. B., vol. 106, p. 596.

———— 1937 Synchronized reactions in the optic ganglion of Dytiscus. J. Physiol., vol. 91, p. 66.

ADRIAN, E. D., AND R. MATTHEWS 1927 Action of light on the eye. Part I. J. Physiol., vol. 63, p. 378.

———— 1928 Action of light on the eye. Part II. J. Physiol., vol. 65, p. 274.

DAKIN, W. J. 1910 The eye of Pecten. Quart. J. Micros. Sci., vol. 55, p. 49.

———— 1928 Eyes of Pecten and allied lamellibranchs. Proc. Roy. Soc. Ser. B., vol. 103, p. 355.

GRANIT, R. 1933 Components of retinal action potentials in mammals and their relation to the discharge in the optic nerve. J. Physiol., vol. 77, p. 207.

GRANIT, R., AND P. O. THERMAN 1935 Excitation and inhibition in the retina and optic nerve. J. Physiol., vol. 83, p. 359.

HARTLINE, H. K. 1938 Response of single optic nerve fibers of the vertebrate eye to illumination of the retina. Am. J. Physiol., vol. 121, p. 400.

HARTLINE, H. K., AND C. H. GRAHAM 1932 Nerve impulses from single receptors in the eye. J. Cell. and Comp. Physiol., vol. 1, p. 277.

HECHT, S. 1934 Vision: II. The nature of the photoreceptor process. A handbook of general experimental psychology, Clark University Press, Worcester, p. 704.

HYDE, IDA H. 1903 Nerve distribution in the eye of Pecten irradians. Mark Anniversary Volume: New York.

KÜPFER, M. 1916 Die Sehorgane am Mantelrande der Pecten-Arten. Gustav Fischer: Jena.

ROCHE 1925 The distal retina of Pecten. J. Roy. Micros. Soc., June, p. 145.

SCHOEPFLE, G., AND J. Z. YOUNG 1936 The structure of the eye of Pecten. Biol. Bull., vol. 71, p. 403.

Part Four

Inhibitory Interaction in the Lateral Eye of *Limulus*: the Steady State

INTRODUCTION by F. Ratliff

> *Since every retinal point perceives itself, so to speak, as above or below the average of its neighbors, there results a characteristic type of perception. Whatever is near the mean of the surroundings becomes effaced, whatever is above or below is disproportionately brought into prominence. One could say that the retina schematizes and caricatures. The teleological significance of this process is clear in itself. It is an analog of abstraction and of the formation of concepts.'*
> Ernst Mach, *Kaiserliche Akademie der Wissenschaften*, Wien, 1868.

The deduction by Mach, 100 years ago, that the processing of visual information begins in the retina has since been verified innumerable times. And so has his conception that the underlying neural mechanisms are the opposed influences of excitation and inhibition. It is now evident that many of the extremely complex functions performed at all levels of the visual pathways – indeed, throughout the entire nervous system – are the resultant of the simple interaction and integration of these opposite, and yet complementary influences. In a very real sense excitation and inhibition are the *yang* and *yin* of the nervous system.

In a continuing series of investigations the retina of the compound eye of *Limulus* has proven to be an especially well-suited neural network for research on inhibitory interaction; the lateral influences in it appear to be almost purely inhibitory. To introduce the first part of those investigations (on the steady state) let us consider a few aspects of the phenomenon of simultaneous contrast – the most obvious and most widely known of the many specific visual effects of inhibition – and then discuss briefly the more general significance of inhibitory interaction, with special reference to contrast-like effects elsewhere in the nervous system.

Contrast. The effects of lateral inhibition can be seen directly in the familiar phenomenon of brightness contrast; and from these effects numerous fundamental principles of inhibitory interaction can easily be deduced. Indeed, the so-called Mach bands (bright and dark lines seen at the bright and dark edges of a penumbra), upon which Mach based most of his ideas about interactions in the retina, are simply a special case of brightness contrast. It is easy to see how such contrast effects at or near boundaries between brightly illuminated and dimly illuminated

245

areas of a retinal image, can be brought about by lateral inhibition. Fields of inhibitory influence that extend for some distance are all that is required. Because of these extended fields, a unit in the retinal network within the dimly illuminated region, but near the boundary, will be inhibited not only by dimly illuminated neighbors, but also by brightly illuminated ones. The total inhibition exerted on such a unit will be greater, therefore, than that exerted on other dimly illuminated elements that are farther from the boundary; consequently, its response will be less than theirs. Similarly, a unit within, but near the boundary of, the brightly illuminated field will have a greater response than other equally illuminated units that are located well within the bright field, for they are subject to stronger inhibition there since all their immediate neighbors are also brightly illuminated. Because of these differential effects, maxima and minima appear in the responses of units in the network on bright and dim sides of boundaries even though there are no such maxima and minima in the distribution of the stimulus itself. Changes in the pattern of illumination are thus accentuated in the corresponding changes in the pattern of the neural response. Such effects can be observed directly in the retina of the compound eye of *Limulus*. For similar experiments on the vertebrate visual system, see Baumgartner (1961), Enroth-Cugell and Robson (1966), Gordon (1969), and De Valois and Pease (1971).

It might appear that the effect of inhibition must actually be detrimental in the end, because it can only suppress information, not restore it. Indeed, because the direct effect of inhibition is to suppress neural responses, it has generally been assumed that the magnitude of a response to a step, for example, can only be less with inhibition than without. An important question that has arisen, therefore, in the study of contrast effects in the retina, and elsewhere in the nervous system, is: In what sense, if at all, can inhibition improve, or 'sharpen', a response?

Sharpening. There are no perfect transducers. In the transmission of information from one place to another or from one form to another – as by a receptor organ – there is always some loss. In the visual system, for example, the chromatic and spherical aberrations and other optical imperfections of the eye degrade the retinal image somewhat. Mach suggested, in 1865, that the apparent sharpness of the image perceived might result, in part, from contrast effects occurring at the concave and convex parts of the blurred intensity distribution. (For a translation of Mach's papers on vision, see Ratliff, 1965.) Since that time the notion has been generally accepted and the same kind of explanation proposed for 'sharpening' in other sensory systems.

It is evident, however, from both direct experimental observations and from theoretical calculations that not only is the sharpness of the original distribution of the energy in the stimulus inevitably degraded by the receptor mechanism, the transformation of an optical image on the retina to a 'neural image' in the optic nerve just as inevitably loses more information. But, although information once lost cannot be recovered, the important point is that the loss can be selective. In short, by selectively suppressing less significant information, inhibition can enhance the more significant information that remains.

This notion is easier to understand, perhaps, when the various components of the visual system are considered as filters. As Mach pointed out in 1866, a complex spatial pattern of illumination may be analyzed into component sinusoidal frequencies in much the same way that a complex sound wave may be analyzed into its component sinusoidal frequencies. Therefore, lenses may be regarded as devices which 'transfer' spatial frequencies from object space to image space. In the same way, the retina transfers spatial frequencies from the optical image on the receptor mosaic to a neural image in the optic nerve. Neither the optical nor the neural component is perfect, therefore each acts as a filter, and – depending on the characteristics of each filter – some spatial frequencies may be transmitted through the whole system almost perfectly, others may only be attenuated somewhat, and still others may be filtered out almost entirely.

In search of a more general and more rigorous quantitative description of various visual systems many investigators have begun to consider them as a series of optical filters in cascade. Analysis in these terms is facilitated by the use of sinusoidal stimuli; for analysis of spatial properties, the so called sine-wave gratings that vary in one dimension only are generally used. By observing the relative amplitudes of the sinusoidal responses elicited by such stimuli, a function analogous to the so-called transfer function of a linear system of optical or electrical filters can be determined.

All visual systems analyzed in this way thus far, including the human eye, are similar in that they transmit low spatial frequencies poorly, intermediate frequencies relatively well, and high frequencies poorly or not at all. These findings are in accord with our own everyday visual experience: gradual changes (low spatial frequencies) in a spatial distribution of illumination are seen as nearly uniform, if at all; moderate amounts of change (intermediate spatial frequencies) are seen distinctly; and very sharp features (containing very high spatial frequencies) cannot be fully resolved. For surveys of some of the work on the human visual system using psychophysical measures, see Campbell (1968), Fry (1969), and Cornsweet (1970). Analogous electrophysiological experiments have been done on the cat retina (Enroth-Cugell and Robson, 1966), and theoretical calculations on the lateral eye of *Limulus* by Kirschfeld and Reichardt (1964) and by Ratliff, Knight, and Graham (1969).

How do opposed influences of excitation and inhibition bring about the observed effects? First, let us consider the excitatory component. This includes optical blur – which is somewhat less than early measurements and calculations had indicated (see Campbell and Gubisch, 1966) but which is considerable, nevertheless – and the limitations imposed by the grian of the receptor mosaic (see Ohzu, Enoch, and O'Hair, 1972, and Ohzu and Enoch, 1972) and by any lateral spread of excitation within the retina (Fry, 1969). The width of this total spread of excitation is such that high spatial frequencies (above about one or two cycles per minute of visual angle) are transmitted very poorly – if at all; that is, the excitatory component is a low pass filter. The characteristics of the inhibitory network are similarly determined by its spatial dimensions. Having considerable width, the inhibitory network is a low pass filter, too, as far as its transformation of excitatory influences into inhibitory influences is concerned. But since the ultimate effect of the network is *inhibitory* (negative) this means that it diminishes responses to low frequencies and does not significantly affect the amplitudes of responses to high frequencies. In the end, therefore, the inhibitory network is a high pass filter.

Thus, the opposite influences – the one (excitatory) cutting off high frequencies and the other (inhibitory) cutting off low frequencies – 'tune' the eye to respond best to intermediate frequencies. The inhibition cannot, by some magic, restore information already lost; but what it can and does do is accentuate certain aspects of the remaining information. Indeed, particular spatial distributions of these influences can lead to an 'amplification' of the response (Ratliff, Knight, and Graham, 1969). As a result of this amplification, the amplitude of the inhibited response to a *change* in the level of illumination can actually be greater than the uninhibited response, but this is achieved at the expense of information about the absolute level. In general, the information that is accentuated by this 'tuning' and 'amplification' is that about changes in the stimulus. It is in this sense that inhibition can be said to improve or sharpen an image.

Is Contrast an Epiphenomenon? The emphasis that has been placed on relatively simple spatial contrast effects has detracted attention from other more subtle, and possibly more important, roles played by inhibition. For example, in the balance of excitation and inhibition that gives rise to the complex responses of vertebrate retinal ganglion cells, and which is the basis for the many and diverse 'special' functions that they have, such as sensitivity to motion, orientation, configuration, color, etc., a certain lateral spread of inhibition is generally required. Contrast enhancement is an almost inevitable consequence of this spread. One might be tempted to conclude, therefore, that evolution has shaped the inhibitory mechanisms to serve these other more complex purposes and that contrast is simply a more noticeable, but actually rather insignificant by-product – a mere epiphenomenon. Another possibility is that these simpler contrast mechanisms and effects were nature's first approximations to the more complex ones, and that they still play elementary but vital roles in vision.

The Influence of Contour on Surrounds. The pronounced influence of neighboring areas on borders and contours, described above, is well known. But even more striking are the less familiar effects of borders and contours on neighboring areas (see Craik, 1966). O'Brien (1958) has described some remarkable phenomena of this sort. For example, it is possible to construct the common border of a bipartite distribution of illumination in such a way that one half of the field with a higher luminance appears dimmer than the other half with a lower luminance. Although a recent scientific discovery, these effects have been known to oriental artists since the Sung dynasty in China (Ratliff, 1971, 1972). Similar effects have been described by Cornsweet (for an illustration see Ratliff, 1965, page 75). This latter effect has been investigated further by Thomas and Kovar (1965), by Thomas (1966), by Hood and Whiteside (1968), and by Arend, Buehler, and Lockhead (1971). The effects are not restricted to brightness; Kanizsa (1957) has shown that the nature of the gradient at the border of an extended field of color has a similar pronounced effect on the chromatic quality of that field. See also, Krauskopf (1963). A tentative explanation of effects of contour on contrast in terms of lateral inhibition has been proposed by Ratliff (1971, 1972).

These experiments bring into question the notion that the stimulus image, the 'neural image' and the perceived image are, or must be, simply isomorphic. Only a small part of the information in the retinal image is abstracted from the whole, and that small part undergoes many complex transformations as it is transmitted from one point to another in the visual system. What is ultimately seen depends, of course, upon the retinal image – but the relation between the optical image and the image perceived, as these contrast and contour effects show, is not a simple isomorphism.

The Ubiquity of Contrast. Lateral inhibition and contrast phenomena are not unique to the visual system. Similar processes and effects are not only common in other sensory systems (see Békésy, 1967), they are found throughout the entire nervous system (see Brooks 1959), for a short review, and for more details, the two international symposia on inhibition: Florey (1961), and Euler, Skoglund, and Söderberg (1968). Also, strikingly similar contrast effects are found in electronic, photochemical, and other non-living systems (Ratliff, 1965, 1971, 1972).

The phenomenon of disinhibition, which occurs in many different situations, illustrates how widespread even the more subtle contrast effects are. It is a 'second-order' effect; if one process is inhibited by another, and this second process is itself subsequently inhibited by a third one, then the first is released from inhibition. The end result resembles direct facilitation, and sometimes – when the underlying inhibitory mechanisms cannot be observed – cannot easily be distinguished from it. The concept of disinhibition was first formulated by Pavlov to explain, in quasi-neurophysiological terms, some effects that he saw in his experiments on animal behavior. It was not until several decades later that disinhibition was actually observed in a neural network – the lateral eye of *Limulus* (Hartline and Ratliff, 1957). Subsequently, Wilson and Burgess (1962) found that disinhibition was the explanation for some paradoxical 'facilitation' in the spinal cord; Ito *et al.* (1968) have observed a similar disinhibition in the cerebellar system. The concept of disinhibition – which originated in the study of behavior – has finally gone full circle, and now, along with the more general concept of contrast, is applied in behavioral studies once more. (See, for example, Catania and Gill (1964), Hinrichs (1968), and Singh and Wickens (1968)).

Contrast-like effects are not restricted to the nervous system, they can and do occur in any interacting system in which the necessary fields of opposed positive (excitatory) and negative (inhibitory) influences exist. Whether the system is neural, physical, electrical, chemical, mathematical – or what have you – is irrelevant; all that is required are certain distributions of the opposed influences (for several non-neural examples see Ratliff, 1965). The resemblance of the contrast effects in such diverse systems is not a trivial coincidence. It is instead, an indication of a 'universal' that transcends certain particulars: contrast depends upon the relations among interacting elements in a system, not upon the particular mechanisms that achieve those relations.

REFERENCES

Arend, L. E., Buehler, J. N., and Lockhead, G. R. (1971), 'Difference information in brightness perception', *Perception and Psychophysics*, **9** (3B), 367–370.

Baumgartner, G. (1961), 'Kontrastlichteffekte an retinalen Ganglienzellen: Ableitungen vom Tractus opticus der Katze', in *Neurophysiologie und Psychophysik des visuellen Systems*, R. Jung and H. Kornhuber, eds. Springer-Verlag, Berlin, 45–53.

Békésy, G. von (1967), *Sensory Inhibition*. Princeton University Press, New Jersey.

Brooks, V. B. (1959), 'Contrast and Stability in the Nervous System', *Trans. N.Y. Acad. Sci.*, **21**, 387–394.

Campbell, F. W., and Gubisch, R. W. (1966), 'Optical Quality of the Human Eye', *J. Physiol.*, **186**, 558–578.

Campbell, F. W. (1968), 'The Human Eye as an Optical Filter', *Proc. of the IEEE*, **56**, 1009–1014.

Catania, A. C., and Gill, C. A. (1964), 'Inhibition and Behavioral Contrast', *Psychonomic Science*, **1**, 257–258.

Cornsweet, T. N. (1970), *Visual Perception*, Academic Press, New York.

Craik, K. J. W. (1966), *The Nature of Psychology*, in A Selection of Papers, Essays and Other Writings, Stephen L. Sherwood, editor, Cambridge University Press, Cambridge, pp. 94–97.

De Valois, R. L., and Pease, P. L. (1971), 'Contours and contrast: responses of monkey and lateral geniculate nucleus cells to luminance and color figures', *Science*, **171**, 694–696.

Eccles, J. C., Llinás, R., and Sasaki, K. (1965), 'The Inhibitory Interneurones Within the Cerebellar Cortex', *Exp. Brain Res.*, **1**, 1–16.

Enroth-Cugell, C., and Robson, J. G. (1966), 'The Contrast Sensitivity of Retinal Ganglion Cells of the Cat', *J. Physiol.*, **187**, 517–552.

Euler, C. von, Skoglund, S., and Söderberg, U., eds. (1968), *Structure and Function of Inhibitory Neuronal Mechanisms*. Pergamon Press, Oxford.

Florey, E. ed. (1961), *Nervous Inhibition*, Pergamon Press, New York.

Fry, G. A. (1969), 'Visibility of Sine-Wave Gratings', *J. Opt. Soc. Amer.*, **59**, 610–617.

Gordon, J. (1969), *Edge Accentuation in the Frog Retina*, Thesis, Brown University.

Hartline, H. K., and Ratliff, F. (1957), 'Inhibitory Interaction of Receptor Units in the Eye of *Limulus*', *J. Gen. Physiol.*, **40**, 357–376.

Hood, D. C., and Whiteside, J. A. (1968), 'Brightness of Ramp Stimuli as a Function of Plateau and Gradient Widths', *J. Opt. Soc. Amer.*, **58**, 1310–1311.

Hinrichs, J. V. (1968), 'Disinhibition of Delay in Fixed-Interval Instrumental Conditioning', *Psychonomic Science*, **12**, 313–314.

Ito, M., Kawai, N., Udo, M. and Sato, N. (1968), 'Cerebellar-evoked disinhibition in dorsal Deiters neurones', *Exp. Brain Res.*, **6**, 247–264.

Kanizsa, G. (1957), 'Gradient Marginal et Perception Chromatique', in *Problèmes de la Couleur*, I. Meyerson, ed., S.E.V.P.E.N., Paris, pp. 107–113.

Kirschfeld, K., and Reichardt, W. (1964), 'Die Verarbeitung stationärer optischer Nachrichten im Komplexauge von Limulus', *Kybernetik*, **2**, 43–61.

Krauskopf, J. (1963), 'Effect of Retinal Image Stabilization on the Appearance of Heterochromatic Targets', *J. Opt. Soc. Amer.*, **53**, 741–744.

O'Brien, U. (1958), 'Contour Perception, Illusion and Reality', *I. Opt. Soc. Amer.*, **48**, 112–119.

Ohzu, H., Enoch, J. M., and O'Hair, J. C. (1972), 'Optical modulation by the isolated retina and retinal receptors', *Vision Research*, **12**, 231–244.

Ohzu, H., and Enoch, J. M. (1972), 'Optical modulation by the isolated human fovea', *Vision Research*, **12**, 245–251.

Ratliff, F. (1965), *Mach Bands: Quantitative Studies on Neural Networks in the Retina*, Holden-Day Inc., San Francisco.

Ratliff, F. (1971), 'Contour and contrast', *Proceedings of the American Philosophical Society*, **115**, No. 2, 150–163.

Ratliff, F. (1972), 'Contour and contrast', *Scientific American*, **226**, 90–103.

Ratliff, F., Knight, B. W., and Graham, N. (1969), 'On Tuning and Amplification by Lateral Inhibition', *Proc. Nat. Acad. Sci.*, **62**, 733–740.

Singh, D., and Wickens, D. D. (1968), 'Disinhibition in Instrumental Conditioning', *J. Comp. and Physiol. Psych.*, **66**, 557–559.

Thomas, J. P., and Kovar, C. W. (1965), 'The Effect of Contour Sharpness on Perceived Brightness', *Vis. Res.*, **5**, 559–564.

Thomas, J. P. (1966), Brightness Variations in Stimuli With Ramp-Like Contours', *J. Opt. Soc. Amer.*, **56**, 238–242.

Wilson, V. J., and Burgess, P. R. (1962), 'Disinhibition in the Cat Spinal Cord', *J. Neurophysiol.*, **25**, 392–404.

Inhibition of activity of visual receptors by illuminating nearby retinal areas in the *Limulus* eye

H. KEFFER HARTLINE

Department of Biophysics, Johns Hopkins University, Baltimore, Md., and the Johnson Research Foundation, University of Pennsylvania, Philadelphia, Penna.

Reprinted from FEDERATION PROCEEDINGS, Vol. 8, no. 1, p. 69, March 1949

A discharge of impulses in a given single optic nerve fiber from the eye of *Limulus* can be elicited only by the illumination of some one particular facet of the eye, containing the receptor that gives rise to that nerve fiber. It has been found that illumination of neighboring areas of the eye, while unable to initiate activity in a given fiber, can nevertheless affect the responses to illumination of its receptor. A steady discharge of impulses was obtained by a small spot of light confined to the appropriate facet; illuminating nearby facets then caused a slowing of the discharge. The frequency dropped markedly at first (after a latency of 0·2–0·4 sec.), then rose somewhat; on turning off the adjacent illumination, the frequency increased and within 0·4 sec. had recovered its original value. This inhibitory effect was greater the higher the intensity and the greater the area illuminated; it decreased with increasing distance between the particular facet and the neighboring area illuminated. The role of this effect in enhancing visual contrast is obvious: brightly illuminated areas inhibit the activity from dimly lighted regions more than the latter inhibit the activity from the former. In *Limulus*, axons of the receptor cells enter a non-ganglionic plexus before leaving the eye via the optic nerve; by recording from fibers between the receptors and the plexus, it could be shown that the inhibitory effect of adjacent illumination depended on the integrity of the nervous connection between the receptor and the plexus.

Inhibition in the eye of *Limulus*

H. KEFFER HARTLINE, HENRY G. WAGNER, AND
FLOYD RATLIFF*

*The Rockefeller Institute for Medical Research, New York, and the
Naval Medical Research Institute, Bethesada‡*

Reprinted from the JOURNAL OF GENERAL PHYSIOLOGY,
20 May 1956, Vol. 39, no. 5, pp. 651–673

The integration of nervous activity in sensory systems often begins in the receptor organs themselves. Numerous electrophysiological studies of the vertebrate visual system, in particular, have shown that in the eye the activity of elements in one region of the retina may be affected by illumination of other regions. Both excitatory and inhibitory interactions have been demonstrated. Granit's extensive researches, especially, have shown the importance of these retinal processes in visual physiology. (For reviews, see Granit, 1947, sections I and II, and 1955, chapter 2.) Interaction in the vertebrate eye may be ascribed to the complex organization of the retina, which is indeed a "nervous center."

In the lateral eye of the horseshoe crab, *Limulus polyphemus* (L.), the histological organization is much simpler than in the vertebrate retina. Nevertheless, the sensory elements in this eye do exert an influence upon one another (Hartline, 1949). The interaction is inhibitory: the frequency of the discharge of impulses in a single optic nerve fiber is decreased and may even be stopped by illuminating areas of the eye in the neighborhood of the sensory element from which the fiber arises. The occurrence of a purely inhibitory action in a relatively simple eye is of general interest; the role that may be played by inhibitory interaction in enhancing contrast gives it an importance to visual physiology. It is the purpose of this paper to report in detail our experiments on this inhibitory phenomenon in the eye of *Limulus*.

Material

The lateral eye of *Limulus* is a coarsely faceted compound eye containing, on the average, some 800 ommatidia. In a medium sized adult (25 cm. broad) each eye forms an ellipsoidal bulge on the side of the carapace, about 12 mm. long by 6 mm.

* National Research Council Fellow in the Biological Sciences during part of the period covered by this research (1950–51).

‡ Much of the experimental work in this study was done in the Jenkins Laboratories of Biophysics, Johns Hopkins University, Baltimore, supported by contract Nonr248(11) with the Office of Naval Research. Reproduction in whole or in part is permitted for any purpose of the United States Government.

255

wide. Each ommatidium has an optical aperture about 0.1 mm. in diameter; the facets are spaced approximately 0.3 mm. apart, center to center, on the surface of the eye. Each ommatidium has a "visual field" subtending a few square degrees of solid angle about its optical axis. Light coming from within this solid angle reaches the sensory component of the ommatidium directly through the transparent cornea and the crystalline cone of the ommatidium. The optical axes of the ommatidia diverge, so that the visual fields of all those in one eye (each one overlapping somewhat those of its neighbors) cover approximately a hemisphere. The location of the visual field of each ommatidium within the visual field of the entire eye is correlated in a more or less regular manner with the position of that ommatidium on the surface of the eye (*cf*. Waterman, 1954, for a recent study of the directional sensitivity of the ommatidia of the lateral eye of *Limulus*).

The sensory component of each ommatidium consists of a cluster of cells that give rise to nerve fibers (*cf*. Hartline, Wagner, and MacNichol, 1952). There are two kinds: 10 to 20 retinula cells arranged radially about the axis of the ommatidium, and one eccentric cell (occasionally two). The axons of these cells leave the heavily pigmented envelope of the ommatidium as a small bundle, and most, perhaps all, of them proceed more or less directly and apparently without interruption to become fibers of the optic nerve.

Immediately after emerging from the ommatidia the axons of the retinula and eccentric cells become associated with an extensive system of cross-connecting strands of nerve fibers, to form a three dimensional network about 1 mm. thick (Fig. 1). The organization of this "plexus" (Watase, 1890) is not fully understood. No nerve cell bodies have been observed within it and it has not yet been possible to determine with certainty the origins and terminations of the fibers that make up the cross-connecting strands. However, it has been observed that the plexus fibers come into close association with the axons of the eccentric cells where they emerge from the proximal ends of the ommatidia. The plexus clearly furnishes numerous anatomical interconnections among the ommatidia.

Each ommatidium apparently functions as a single "receptor unit" in the discharge of optic nerve impulses. The action potentials recorded from a large bundle of fibers dissected from the optic nerve give evidence of the activity of many fibers when a large area of the eye is illuminated, but when the illumination is carefully confined to one ommatidium, a regular train of uniform action potential spikes is elicited, typical of the activity of just one single fiber (see also Waterman and Wiersma, 1954). If the bundle is dissected until but a single active fiber is left, a discharge of impulses can be elicited in it by illumination of one, and only one, particular ommatidium. The strand of optic nerve containing such a single active fiber can be followed in the peripheral direction through the plexus by dissecting it free of surrounding tissue, all the way to the ommatidium in which its activity originates.

The discharge of impulses may be recorded directly from an ommatidium by means of a micropipette electrode, but only from a sharply localized region within the receptor structure (Hartline, Wagner, and MacNichol, 1952). In recent experiments, done in collaboration with Dr. MacNichol, we have been able to see the living eccentric cells in exposed ommatidia; upon thrusting a micropipette electrode into one of them, large action potential spikes have been observed, and from no other structure in the ommatidium could such spikes be recorded. Apparently the discharge of impulses recorded in a single fiber of the optic nerve originates in the eccentric cell of the ommatidium from which that fiber comes. Waterman and Wiersma (1954) have reached the same conclusion. The function of the retinula cells and their associated fibers is still unknown.

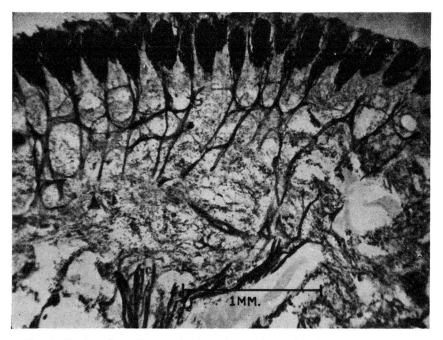

FIG. 1. Section through part of a lateral eye of an adult *Limulus*, perpendicular to the cornea, showing the heavily pigmented portions of the ommatidia (upper border of the section), the bundles of nerve fibers emerging from them, the plexus of interconnecting fibers, and a portion of the optic nerve (bottom of figure). The chitinous cornea with the attached crystalline cones of the ommatidia had been stripped away prior to fixation. Samuel's silver stain. (Prepared by W. H. Miller.)

The axons of the eccentric cells apparently traverse the plexus without interruption by one way synapses, for Prof. T. Tomita, working in our laboratory, observed that antidromic impulses elicited by electrical stimulation of a single fiber dissected from the optic nerve could be recorded by a microelectrode placed on the ommatidium in which that fiber originated.

Methods

In most of the experiments reported in this paper, we recorded the action potentials of single fibers dissected from the optic nerve. A lateral eye was excised with 1 to 2 cm. of optic nerve and mounted in a chamber maintained at 18°C. A small strand containing only a single active fiber was separated from the nerve. Its proximal end was lifted out of the sea water or blood bathing the back of the eye, placed over wick electrodes, and its action potentials amplified and recorded oscillographically (Hartline and Graham, 1932). The ommatidium from which this fiber arose was stimulated by focussing a small spot of light directly upon its facet; receptors in other regions of the eye were then illuminated to determine the effect of their activity upon the responses of this particular ommatidium.

In a few experiments (specifically indicated) we recorded action potentials within an ommatidium by means of a microelectrode. A glass pipette electrode (tip $\frac{1}{2}$ μ to 3 μ), filled with sea water, was thrust into one of the ommatidia to record the nerve impulses at the site of their origin in the receptor unit. This was done either by stripping away the cornea of the eye and thrusting the electrode axially into the exposed distal end of an ommatidium (method devised in collaboration with Mr. M. Wolbarsht), or by cutting the eye in a plane perpendicular to the cornea, and thrusting the electrode into the side of one of the ommatidia lying near the cut edge (Hartline, Wagner, and MacNichol, 1952).

The apparatus for illuminating the eye (cf. Hartline and McDonald, 1947) provided two independently controllable beams of light from a common source (incandescent tungsten filament). The intensities of these beams could be varied by optical wedges of neutral density calibrated in place; the exposures were controlled by electromagnetic shutters operated by electronic timing devices. In most experiments the pattern of illumination of each beam was formed by an aperture in a diaphragm, an image of which was focussed on the corneal surface of the eye by a photographic objective lens. The preparation was mounted upon a horizontal turntable, and the beams were directed upon it by adjustable mirrors, so that the light could be made to fall upon the eye from any direction necessary to produce an optimum effect.

Several arrangements of the beams were required. In many of the experiments the two beams were combined by means of a semireflecting mirror so that their fields of illumination were superimposed. The beams then could illuminate, in common, a circular region of the eye 5 mm. in diameter; diaphragms in each beam were used to limit the illumination to the desired receptors within this region. Thus, for example, a small spot of light 0.1 to 0.2 mm. in diameter, formed by a diaphragm in one beam, could be centered on the corneal facet of an ommatidium from which a discharge of nerve impulses was to be recorded; a diaphragm in the other beam could then be adjusted to form another spot of light on a nearby region of the eye to inhibit this discharge. The size and shape of this second spot and its location with respect to the first one could be varied as desired within the limits imposed by the 5 mm. field available to the two beams.

In some experiments it was necessary to illuminate regions of the eye separated by more than 5 mm. or to control independently the angles of incidence of the beams. We then directed the beams through separate mirror systems, thus enabling each one to be brought onto any part of the eye from the appropriate direction for maximal stimulating effectiveness of the ommatidia it illuminated. In addition to the main optical system just described, a small accessory light source and projector were sometimes used in special experiments.

RESULTS

1. General Properties of the Inhibition

Illumination of regions of a *Limulus* lateral eye in the vicinity of any particular ommatidium reduces the ability of that receptor unit to discharge impulses in response to light. During such illumination, the threshold of the receptor unit is raised, the number of impulses it discharges in response to a suprathreshold flash of light is diminished, and the frequency with which it discharges impulses during steady illumination is reduced. The latter effect is especially convenient for demonstrating the properties of the inhibition.

In an illustrative experiment, an ommatidium from which discharges of impulses were recorded was illuminated steadily by a small spot of light focussed upon its facet. After this exciting light had been shining for several seconds, to permit the frequency of the discharge to reach a steady level, a region of the eye surrounding the selected ommatidium was illuminated. The effect on the discharge is shown in Fig. 2, upper record. When the surrounding light was turned on, the discharge suddenly underwent a drop in frequency (from 65 impulses per second), then recovered partially and continued at a lower rate (approximately 30 per second) as long as the region surrounding the ommatidium was illuminated. When this inhibiting light was turned off, the frequency rose to its original value. At the onset of the inhibiting illumination, there was a latency of 0.14 second before the frequency began to fall; at the end of the illumination it took about 0.3 second to recover its original value.

This record shows the typical features of the inhibition of nervous activity of a receptor unit that results from stimulation of other sensory elements near it in the eye. A sudden onset of the inhibition after an appreciable latency, a deep initial minimum in frequency, a steady maintenance of a depressed rate of discharge, and a prompt though not instantaneous recovery after turning off an inhibiting light are characteristic. During inhibition the discharge is neither more nor less regular, as a rule, than the discharge at a comparable frequency obtained in response to a weaker stimulating light in the absence of inhibition. The level of frequency can be graded smoothly by varying the factors that affect the degree of inhibition; there is no suggestion that the depression of frequency is brought about by the dropping out of impulses from the regular series of an uninhibited discharge. The return of the frequency to the uninhibited level usually takes place directly, although in some preparations a slight "overshoot" has been observed (*cf.* Fig. 2, lower record, and Fig. 4, "0.0").

Inhibition is exhibited not only when the activity is recorded from the fibers of the optic nerve but also when the impulses are recorded close to their point of origin in the ommatidium. Fig. 2, lower record, is an oscillo-gram obtained in a typical experiment in which a microelectrode was thrust into an ommatidium to record the action potential spikes from its eccentric cell. This ommatidium was excited by shining a small beam of light into it; illumination of a region of the eye close to it then produced a slowing of the

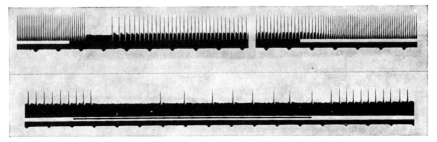

FIG. 2. Oscillograms of electrical activity of single receptor units in the lateral eye of *Limulus*, showing the reduction in frequency that occurred when regions of the eye were illuminated near these units.

In each of the two experiments shown, a small spot of light, projected on the facet of the ommatidium in which the activity originated, had been turned on sev-eral seconds before the beginning of the record. During the interval marked by the signal (blackening of the white band above the time marks) a region of the eye was illuminated near the ommatidium under observation. Amplifier time constant 0.1 second. Time in one-fifth seconds.

Upper record: Action potentials from a single fiber dissected from the optic nerve. The inhibiting illumination covered an annular region surrounding the facet of the ommatidium in which that optic nerve fiber originated. The inner boundary of the annulus was approximately 2 mm. in diameter, the outer boundary approximately 4 mm. in diameter.

Lower record: Action potentials recorded by a microelectrode thrust into the distal end of an ommatidium after removal of the cornea and crystalline cone. The inhibiting illumination was a spot of light approximately 2 mm. in diameter, centered about 2 mm. from the ommatidium in which the activity was being recorded.

discharge rate, similar to that observed when the sensory discharge was re-corded from a fiber dissected from the optic nerve. The inhibitory influence is evidently exerted within the ommatidium itself, upon some process that determines the rate of discharge of nerve impulses.

Illumination of regions of the eye in the neighborhood of any particular ommatidium not only reduces the ability of that receptor unit to discharge impulses in direct response to light but also inhibits activity that can occur when it is in complete darkness. The after-discharge following intense stim-ulation by light, the spontaneous activity exhibited by some preparations in complete darkness, and activity that can be induced by an excess of K^+ in the solution bathing the eye have all been observed to be inhibited by illuminating a region of the eye close to the discharging ommatidium, even though that receptor unit was in darkness when the inhibiting light was turned on.

In any one eye in which marked inhibition was observed, it was our experience that every single fiber picked at random from the optic nerve showed some degree of reduction in the frequency of its discharge when an appropriate region of the eye was illuminated near the ommatidium from which it originated. We have often prepared three or four, sometimes even more, single fibers in the course of an experiment on one eye, coming from ommatidia in different regions of the eye, all of which showed typical inhibitory effects. The same has been found with a microelectrode, testing many ommatidia in succession.

Simultaneous observation of the responses from two receptor units has shown that nearby ommatidia often inhibit one another mutually. An example is given in Fig. 3. In this experiment the discharges of impulses in two optic nerve fibers were recorded at the same time; the responses may be distinguished in the records by differences in the size and shape of the action potential spikes. Fibers were chosen that came from two ommatidia close together in the eye, each illuminated by a separate spot of light confined to its facet. To obtain the upper record one ommatidium (giving rise to the large spikes) was illuminated for several seconds until its discharge had reached a steady frequency. The second ommatidium was then illuminated, initiating a train of impulses (small spikes) in its fiber, and at the same time slowing the discharge from the first receptor unit. To obtain the lower record, the roles of the two ommatidia were interchanged; inhibition of the discharge from the second ommatidium resulted when the first one was illuminated. It is evident that these two individual receptor units in the eye inhibited each other mutually. Many other experiments have shown that mutual inhibition is common between ommatidia that are close together in an eye, although it has been observed that the effects are not always equally strong in the two directions. The consequences of such interaction are complex, and we will defer their treatment to a later communication (*cf.* Hartline, Wagner, and Tomita, 1953, and Hartline and Ratliff, 1954).

The inhibitory influence appears to be mediated by the plexus of fibers that lies behind the layer of ommatidia. In many experiments a single fiber was picked up from the optic nerve and then isolated by dissection all the way up to the ommatidium in which it originated (the isolated fiber was always kept immersed in the blood bathing the preparation, except for its proximal end, which was placed on the electrodes). During the course of such dissection, the inhibitory effect diminished progressively as the fiber bundle was cut away from its connections within the plexus. Sometimes cutting a prominent cross-connection seemed to be especially effective in reducing the inhibitory effect that could be obtained. When the dissection had been extended up to and completely around the pigmented body of the ommatidium, no inhibition could ever be obtained by illuminating adjacent

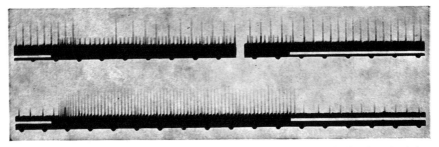

FIG. 3. Mutual inhibition of two receptor units in the eye of *Limulus*. Activity was recorded from an optic nerve strand containing two active fibers. The responses of the two fibers may be distinguished by the different sizes of their action potential spikes. The ommatidia from which these fibers arose were 0.7 mm. apart; each was illuminated independently of the other by a small spot of light confined to its facet. For the upper record, the ommatidium whose optic nerve fiber gave the large spikes was illuminated steadily, beginning 5 seconds before the start of the record; the signal marks the period of illumination of the other ommatidium, whose fiber gave the small spikes. The record shows the slowing of the rate of discharge of the large spikes, shortly after the onset of the discharge of small ones, and recovery to the original frequency after the small ones stop.

For the bottom record the roles of the two units were interchanged: the frequency of the small spikes was decreased during the discharge of the large ones. (Two small spikes were discharged during the first 0.2 second of the discharge of large ones; there followed a gap of 0.5 second, after which the discharge of small spikes was renewed at a frequency lower than that which occurred before and after the discharge of large ones.)

regions of the eye. These observations strongly suggest that the inhibitory effect depends on the integrity of nervous pathways in the plexus. Nevertheless, more extensive experimentation on this crucial point is still desirable.

The inhibitory effects that we have described are typical of those observed in most of several hundred lateral eyes[1] of *Limulus* that we have studied. Occasionally preparations were found that showed only weak inhibition. In a very few preparations the inhibitory effect diminished, became sluggish,

[1] Dr. W. H. Miller, in our laboratory, has observed similar inhibitory effects in the median eyes of this animal.

and sometimes became imperceptible several hours after excision of the eye, even though the optic nerve discharges in response to light were undiminished.

Effects that might be attributed to the physiological spread of excitatory influences in the eye of *Limulus* have never been observed. However, the physical scatter of light in the optical system and within the cornea of the eye itself sometimes complicates the manifestation of inhibition caused by illuminating regions close to an ommatidium. In some preparations the sudden gap in the discharge that marked the onset of inhibition was preceded by a very brief rise in frequency—two or three intervals between impulses that were shorter than the preceding ones in the regular series. Correspondingly, when the inhibiting spot of light was turned off, a very brief drop in frequency occurred before the recovery from the inhibition began. These fluctuations could be traced to the direct excitatory effects of stray light from the inhibiting beam scattered into the ommatidium under observation, which provided an increment to its stimulus, and which acted with a short latency (*cf.* MacNichol and Hartline, 1948). Such effects could always be reduced, and often completely abolished, by using a separate optical system for the inhibiting beam. Sometimes it was necessary to shave away as much as possible of the chitinous cornea to reduce light scatter within the eye. When the effects produced by stray light had been abolished by such procedures, no evidence for excitatory interaction could be observed. We believe that the physiological interaction in the eye of *Limulus* is purely inhibitory.

2. Factors Affecting the Magnitude of the Inhibition

The degree of inhibition of the response of a receptor unit by illumination of regions of the eye in its neighborhood may be measured by taking the difference between the frequency of impulses discharged during a period of inhibiting illumination and the frequency during a comparable interval of time in a control exposure, when no light is shining on the neighboring region. The magnitude of the inhibition depends upon a number of factors. Those that we will describe in this paper are (*a*) the intensity of the inhibiting illumination; (*b*) the area of the region covered by the inhibiting illumination; (*c*) the location of this region with respect to the ommatidium under observation, and (*d*) the level of excitation of this ommatidium.

(*a*) *Effect of Intensity of Inhibiting Illumination.*—The degree to which the activity of an ommatidium is inhibited by illumination of regions of the eye near it is greater the higher the intensity of that illumination.

This is shown in the experiment illustrated in Fig. 4, in which each graph shows the time-course of the frequency change when an inhibiting light was turned on during steady illumination of an ommatidium. The different graphs are from records taken with different intensities of inhibiting illumination.

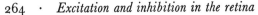

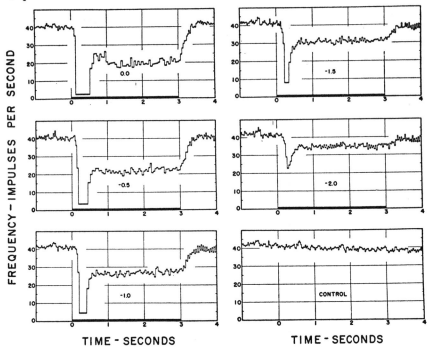

FIG. 4. Inhibition of the discharge of impulses in a single optic nerve fiber by various intensities of illumination on a region of the eye near the ommatidium from which the fiber arose. Frequency of impulse discharge is plotted as ordinate *vs.* time as abscissa. The graphs were prepared from oscillograms similar to those of Fig. 2: a horizontal line has been plotted for each interval between successive impulses, beginning at the abscissa of one impulse and ending at that of the next, having an ordinate equal to the reciprocal of the time interval between the two impulses. The ommatidium from which the fiber arose was illuminated steadily for 10 seconds by a small spot (0.2 mm. diameter) of light of fixed intensity (0.2 lumen/cm.² on the eye), starting 4 seconds before the onset of the inhibiting light, which illuminated a region of the eye 1 mm. in diameter, centered approximately 1.5 mm. from the ommatidium. The inhibiting light was turned on for a period of 3 seconds, as indicated by the heavy line at the base of each graph. The intensity of the inhibiting illumination is indicated on the respective graphs by the numbers, which are logarithms of relative intensity values. The most intense illumination (log $I_{inhib.}$ = 0.0) was 0.5 lumen/cm.² on the surface of the eye. The "control" was taken from a comparable record, for which no inhibiting light was turned on. Temperature 18°C.

The more intense the inhibiting illumination, the deeper and longer was the initial depression of the frequency of the discharge and the greater was the depression of the steady level that was reached after the inhibiting light had been shining for a second or more. The quantitative relation between

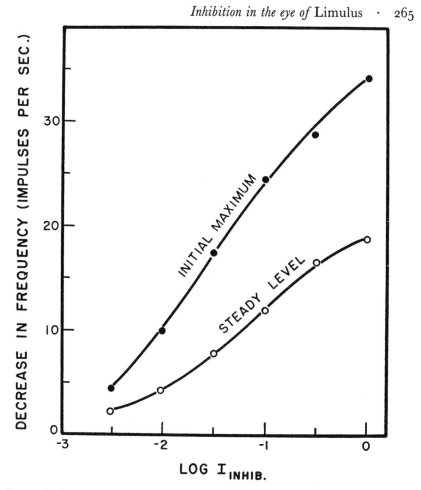

Fɪɢ. 5. Relations between intensity of inhibiting illumination and the magnitude of initial maximum and subsequent steady level of inhibition. From the experiment of Fig. 4. The lower curve (open circles) shows the decrease in average frequency measured over the second and third seconds of inhibiting illumination (determined by subtracting the frequency of the inhibited discharge from the average frequency measured over a comparable control period). The upper curve (solid circles) shows the decrease similarly measured in each of the records over that half-second period which exhibited the lowest average frequency (*i.e.*, maximum decrease in frequency).

intensity of inhibiting light and depression of frequency it produced is shown in Fig. 5. The upper curve refers to the initial maximum depression, the lower curve to the steady level of the depression. The inhibiting effect, measured by the depression in frequency of a steadily excited receptor unit, varied approximately linearly with the logarithm of the intensity of the illumination on neighboring receptors.

(*b*) *Effect of Areal Extent of Inhibiting Illumination.*—The magnitude of the inhibition exerted upon the response of an ommatidium depends not only upon the intensity of illumination on a region of the eye near it, but also upon the number of facets covered by this illumination: the larger the area of the eye illuminated by the inhibiting beam, the greater is the slowing of the rate at which the ommatidium discharges nerve impulses.

This is shown in an experiment in which annular patterns of light of constant intensity were projected onto the surface of the eye, surrounding the facet of the ommatidium giving rise to the nerve fiber that was on the recording electrodes. Different areas of the annulus were obtained by enlarging its outer boundary. The greater the area, the greater was the depression of frequency of the discharge from this ommatidium, which was independently illuminated at a constant intensity (Fig. 6). It is clear that the receptors in the regions of the eye surrounding the ommatidium contributed inhibitory influences that were summed in determining the total inhibition of its response; the greater the number of neighboring receptors stimulated, the greater was their inhibitory effect.

As shown in Fig. 6, the reduction in frequency was not in a simple proportion to the area of the eye illuminated. Several factors probably influenced the quantitative relation in this experiment. As the outer diameter of the annulus was increased, the additional ommatidia illuminated probably exerted smaller inhibitory influences upon the central ommatidium because of their increased distance from it; also, these receptors were undoubtedly stimulated less effectively than were those at the inner border of the annulus because of the increased divergence of their optical axes with respect to the direction of the incident light. Perhaps the most important factor, however, was the mutual inhibitory interaction among the receptor units involved (*cf.* Hartline and Ratliff, 1954). We will defer the treatment of the exact law of spatial summation of the inhibitory influences to a later report.

(*c*) *Effect of Location of Inhibiting Illumination.*—The response of an ommatidium is most effectively inhibited by illumination of other ommatidia located close to it; the effectiveness diminishes with increasing distance. Usually, however, some degree of inhibition of an ommatidium can be produced by illumination anywhere within a region surrounding it that may cover as much as one-half of the total area of the eye.

The variation in the magnitude of inhibition produced by illumination of regions of the eye located at different distances from an ommatidium is illustrated in the following experiment. The discharge of impulses was recorded from an ommatidium situated near the center of the eye. This ommatidium was illuminated by a small accessory optical projector, adjusted for optimal stimulating effectiveness. This projector was mounted on the turntable that carried the preparation, so that once correctly adjusted it remained in a fixed position with respect to the eye. Another beam, for inhibiting the

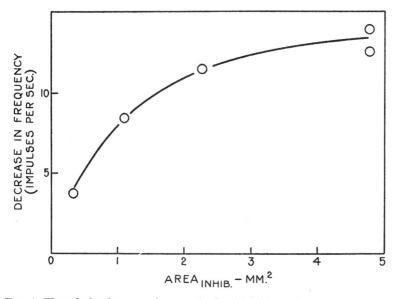

FIG. 6. The relation between the magnitude of inhibition (decrease in frequency) and the area (mm.²) of the region on the surface of the eye illuminated by an inhibiting beam of fixed intensity. Records were obtained of the action potential spikes in a single optic nerve fiber from an ommatidium illuminated for 10 seconds by a small spot of light (0.25 mm. diameter and of fixed intensity) focussed on its facet. The inhibiting light illuminated an annular region concentric with the small spot. Four annular patterns having different areas were tested. The inner diameter of the annulus was kept at 0.38 mm.; its outer diameter was 0.75, 1.25, 1.75, or 2.50 mm. The inhibiting light was turned on for 3 seconds, beginning 4 seconds after the onset of the illumination on the ommatidium from which responses were recorded. The decrease in frequency was determined by measuring the average frequency of discharge over the second and third seconds of inhibiting illumination and subtracting this value from the estimated control frequency. The latter was obtained by interpolation between the average frequency of the uninhibited discharge occurring just before and that occurring just after the inhibiting illumination. (Illumination on the surface of the eye was approximately 20 lumens/cm.² for the small central spot, 2 lumens/cm.² for the annulus.)

activity of the ommatidium, was directed onto the eye from the main optical system. The spot formed by this beam could be moved to various locations on the surface of the eye, and the direction of incidence adjusted for maximum inhibiting effect at each location. This inhibiting spot was 1 mm.

in diameter and of fixed intensity. The stimulating light was turned on for a period of 8 seconds; during the last 5 seconds of this exposure the inhibiting light was turned on and the impulses discharged during this 5 second interval were counted. This count was compared with the number of impulses discharged in a comparable interval during a control exposure, when only the stimulating light was shining.

When the inhibiting spot was centered at a distance of 1 mm. from the ommatidium, it decreased the number of impulses discharged in 5 seconds by 50 (from 110 to 60); after it had been moved to a location 3 mm. away, the maximum effect it could produce at the intensity employed was to decrease the number of impulses discharged in 5 seconds by only 8. Moved to a distance of 5 mm., it had no perceptible effect at this intensity, no matter how the direction of incidence of the beam was adjusted. The regions tested in this part of the experiment were located on a line extending lengthwise of the eye (antero-posterior). At right angles to this direction (dorso-ventral) the inhibitory effectiveness diminished more rapidly with increasing distance, no measurable effect being produced when the spot was only 2.8 mm. from the ommatidium under observation.

It would be difficult by this method to map the distribution of the inhibitory effectiveness in the entire region surrounding an ommatidium. Therefore, in another experiment we modified our method, utilizing the directional sensitivity and small visual fields of the ommatidia (*cf.* section on *Material*) to localize the stimulation. Instead of focussing spots of light on restricted regions of the eye, sources of light were presented in different positions in front of the eye. Although these sources illuminated the whole eye, they stimulated only those ommatidia in whose visual fields they were located. One very small source, for exciting the ommatidium from which responses were recorded, was the filament of a bare ophthalmoscope bulb mounted 6 cm. in front of the eye on the turntable that carried the preparation: its position, once having been adjusted to yield the maximum discharge of impulses, thereafter remained fixed with respect to the eye. The second light source, for inhibiting the activity of this ommatidium, was furnished by the main optical system. The objective lens ordinarily used was removed, resulting in the formation of a virtual source of light 2 cm. in diameter, located 30 cm. in front of the eye. This source could be made to appear in any desired position in the visual field of the eye by rotating the horizontal turntable carrying the preparation and by rotating in a vertical plane the mirror system that directed the light onto the eye. The eye was located at the intersection of the axes of rotation of the turntable and mirror system; protractors centered on each axis permitted the angular coordinates of the source to be specified with respect to arbitrary reference planes through the eye.

This arrangement enabled us to determine contours on a map of the visual field of the eye for several intensities of inhibiting illumination, giving the angular positions of the virtual source at which a certain constant inhibitory effect was exerted upon the selected ommatidium. The criterion effect was arbitrarily chosen to be a transient reduction of the frequency of dis· charge by just one-half, measured at the minimum frequency in the initial depression immediately following the onset of the inhibiting light. (Fig. 4, "−2.0" shows an effect of approximately this magnitude.) In making these determinations the ommatidium was excited by steady illumination for several minutes at a time; after the discharge of impulses had reached a steady rate, the inhibiting light was flashed on for exposures of 1 second duration at intervals of 4 seconds. Setting the intensity of the inhibiting light at a fixed value, we then adjusted its position in the visual field by rotating the mirror system or the turntable, or both, until the criterion effect was obtained. This position, read from the protractors, gave one point on a contour for that particular intensity. The preparation was then allowed to rest for several minutes (exciting light turned off), and the process repeated to determine another point on this same contour. Contours obtained for two values of inhibiting intensity are shown in Fig. 7. These results are typical of those found in other similar but less extensive experiments.

These measurements of inhibitory effectiveness of a light in various positions in the visual field were compared with the results of the previous experiment in which a spot of light was projected directly upon the surface of the eye in various locations. To do this, an approximate correlation was made between the angular position of the inhibiting light source in the visual field of the eye and the location on the surface of the eye of the group of ommatidia it stimulated. This correlation was made by noting the location of the pseudo-pupil[2] seen from different directions of view. The correlation was then used to transform the contours on the map of the visual field into contours on a map of the surface of the eye (insert of Fig. 7). Although different methods were used, the conclusions to be drawn from the two experiments are in essential agreement: in each case, the activity of the selected ommatidium could be inhibited by the stimulation of other ommatidia separated from it by as much as several millimeters; the inhibition diminished with increasing distance, and the diminution was more rapid in the dorso-ventral direction than in the antero-posterior.

Thus the activity of any one ommatidium is inhibited by illumination

---

[2] The pseudo-pupil is a black spot usually about 2 mm. in diameter, that is observed in a fresh eye; it is caused by the failure of those ommatidia that are pointed in the direction of the observer to reflect to his eye any light that falls on them. Light from a given direction can penetrate and stimulate efficiently only those ommatidia that lie within the confines of the pseudo-pupil that is observed from that direction. The size of the pseudo-pupil varies considerably from one part of the eye to another; consequently the stimulus conditions in the two experiments that are being discussed in this section were not strictly comparable.

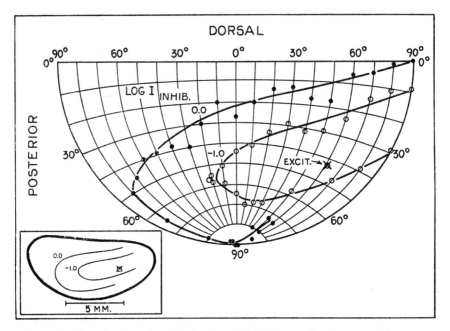

Fig. 7. Map showing the distribution of inhibitory effectiveness, with respect to a particular ommatidium, of light in the visual field of the eye. Contours are plotted for two intensities of a light source giving the locations at which it produced a constant inhibitory effect upon the ommatidium. A small incandescent lamp was mounted in front of the eye at the position (labelled "Excit.") that produced the most effective excitation of the particular ommatidium selected. The light source used to produce the inhibitory effect was tested in various positions in front of the eye to determine those positions at which it produced a certain constant magnitude of inhibition of the discharge in the optic nerve fiber from the ommatidium (transient reduction of the steady frequency to one-half its value, measured at the minimum frequency in the initial depression immediately following the onset of the inhibiting light). Each of the positions thus determined furnished one point on the contour corresponding to the particular value of inhibiting intensity employed. The highest intensity employed (log $I_{inhib.}$ = 0.0) illuminated the surface of the eye with approximately 0.1 lumen/cm.^{2}; points indicated by solid circles. For the points indicated by open circles the intensity was one-tenth this value (log $I_{inhib.}$ = −1.0). The source was circular; its diameter subtended a visual angle of 4°. In this map (a globular projection representing approximately one-half of the total visual field of the eye) the plane of the equator is inclined approximately 20° above the horizontal plane of the animal's body; the 0° meridian lies approximately in a transverse plane.

The insert, lower left, is a sketch of the eye (heavy outline) showing contours drawn on its surface corresponding to the contours shown in the main figure (see text).

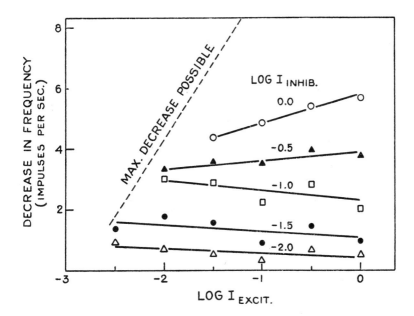

Fig. 8. Relation between the intensity of the exciting light illuminating an ommatidium and the magnitude of the inhibition exerted upon that ommatidium as a result of illuminating a nearby region of the eye at fixed intensity, for five different values of such inhibiting intensity. The abscissae give the intensities of the spot of light (0.25 mm. diameter) focussed on the ommatidium to excite a steady discharge of impulses in its optic nerve fiber (log $I_{excit.}$ = 0.0 corresponds to an illumination of approximately 0.5 lumen/cm.²). The ordinates give the depression of frequency averaged over a 3 second period of inhibiting illumination, starting 3 seconds after the onset of the exciting light. This depression was measured by subtracting the value of the frequency during the exposure to inhibiting illumination from its value during similar control periods, when no inhibiting light was shining. Each point was determined from two experimental periods and three control periods. The region of the eye that was illuminated to produce the inhibition was 1 mm. in diameter, centered approximately 1 mm. from the ommatidium from which the responses were recorded. Each graph is for a fixed intensity of the inhibiting light (numbers give the logarithms of the relative intensities; log $I_{inhib.}$ = 0.0 corresponds to an illumination of approximately 0.5 lumen/cm.² on the surface of the eye).

The dotted line (points omitted) labelled "Max. decrease possible" is a plot, to the same coordinates, of the frequency of the discharge (impulses per second) from the ommatidium as a function of the intensity of its exciting light. It is the locus that points would have if there had been inhibition sufficient to reduce the frequency of the discharge to zero.

anywhere within a region that covers an extensive area of the eye. Conversely, illumination of any given region of an eye inhibits the activity of many ommatidia in its vicinity, for the distributions of inhibitory effectiveness for most of the ommatidia of an eye overlap one another considerably.

(d) *Effect of Level of Excitation.*—If a fixed region of the eye is illuminated at a constant intensity, the frequency of discharge of a nearby ommatidium is depressed by an amount that is approximately constant irrespective of the level of excitation of the ommatidium.

We have performed several experiments in which we varied the intensity of the light exciting an ommatidium from which the optic nerve discharge was being recorded, while holding constant the intensity, area, and location of an inhibiting spot of light on a nearby region of the eye. The results of the most extensive of these experiments are shown in Fig. 8. The inhibitory effect was measured by the reduction in the frequency of discharge averaged over the entire period (3 seconds) of exposure to inhibiting light. It has been plotted as a function of the intensity of the light exciting the ommatidium, for five different intensities of inhibiting illumination. At all intensities of the inhibiting illumination, the reduction in frequency that was produced changed by only a small amount with change in the level of excitation of the receptor unit. For the two highest intensities of the inhibiting light, the depression of frequency became somewhat greater as the exciting intensity was increased, but we have not found this in other experiments. On the other hand the slight negative slope shown by each of the three lower lines has been observed in several other experiments; it probably resulted from the mutual interaction between that ommatidium from which activity was recorded and those in the region illuminated by the inhibiting beam. These deviations from constancy, it should be emphasized, were not very great, compared to the changes that were produced by varying the intensity of the inhibiting light over an equal range. To a first approximation, the reduction of the frequency of discharge from an ommatidium caused by a constant inhibitory stimulus in its neighborhood has been found to be independent of its level of excitation.

DISCUSSION

Our study has shown that the lateral eye of *Limulus* is more than an aggregation of independent receptors; it has a simple functional organization. Activity in any one optic nerve fiber, although it can be elicited by illumination of only the one specific receptor unit (ommatidium) from which the fiber arises, nevertheless may be affected by illumination of other ommatidia of the eye. The influence exerted upon a receptor unit by the activity of its neighbors appears to be purely inhibitory; it is of interest to consider how this action may take place and what its role may be in the physiology of vision.

Our present investigations provide a first step in the analysis of the mechanism of inhibition in the eye of *Limulus*, and suggest the direction that future studies may take. Some possible mechanisms can be eliminated immediately.

Activity of receptor units might release chemical agents, which on diffusion through the tissues of the eye could affect the responses of neighboring elements. The inhibitory action, however, is so rapid that this seems out of the question; slowing of the discharge of a receptor unit begins suddenly in a few tenths of a second following illumination of a region of the eye several millimeters distant. Moreover, preliminary measurements that we have made show that the latency of the inhibition does not change markedly with changing the distance from the inhibiting area to the affected receptor element: transmission time for the effect seems to be only a small fraction of the latent period.

Electric currents generated by the retinal action potentials of receptors and flowing in the volume-conducting mass of the eye tissue could presumably affect the activity of nearby retinal elements. However, it is unlikely that the inhibition we are dealing with is produced in this way, for, in *Limulus*, the retinal action potentials that are recorded by electrodes in tissue external to the receptor elements are small and are transient, subsiding almost to zero in the first few tenths of a second of steady illumination (Hartline, Wagner, and MacNichol, 1952). The inhibition, we have shown, although exhibiting an initial maximum, remains quite strong for many seconds, as long as the inhibitory light continues to shine. Moreover, isolation of the nerve strand by dissection up to its ommatidium was shown to abolish the inhibitory effect, although the preparation was always kept immersed in blood (or sea water). Such dissection could hardly have altered, to any great extent, the gross electrical current flow in the volume-conducting medium.

The inhibitory effect apparently depends on the integrity of the nervous interconnections in the plexus of fibers just behind the layer of ommatidia. It would appear, then, that the search for an explanation of the inhibitory action can be narrowed to an investigation of the nature of the influence transmitted in the plexus and its mode of action on the sensory discharge.

Histological studies of the *Limulus* eye have failed to show any ganglion cells within the plexus, and functional studies have shown that nerve impulses can traverse the fiber pathways from ommatidia to optic nerve in either direction, apparently without interference. Still, some neural relay in the plexus may have escaped notice, and the inhibitory influence might be exerted upon it, or in some other way modify the sensory discharge as it traverses the plexus. However, this could not explain the slowing of the rate of discharge that was observed when the impulses were recorded by a micro-electrode within an ommatidium. Evidently the inhibitory action is exerted within the ommatidium itself, where the conducted impulses originate. This direct action upon an ommatidium does not operate by inducing some re-action within it that interferes with the access of light to the sensory struc-ture (as by some unknown pigment migration or other retinomechanical effect). This is shown by the inhibition exerted upon an after-discharge or other form of activity that may occur in darkness.

We have been unsuccessful as yet in attempts to record impulses in the cross-connections of the plexus or to demonstrate nervous activity, clearly associated with inhibitory effects, in fibers that run between the ommatidia in the plexus. However, we have noted the occurrence of prominent elec-trotonic potentials in fiber bundles in the *Limulus* eye (*cf.* Hartline, Wagner and MacNichol, 1952), and these may be significant in the inhibitory process.

A search for slow potential changes that might be recorded by microelec-trodes in the ommatidia during inhibition, measurement of the changes in threshold for electrical stimulation of the ommatidia, exploration of the inhibiting effects produced by antidromic stimulation of the optic nerve (*cf.* Hartline, Wagner, and Tomita, 1953), and a survey of the action of phar-macological agents[3] are among the lines being pursued in further studies to elucidate the mechanism of the inhibitory effect.

Interaction in the eye is an example of an integrative process in a sensory system that takes place in the receptor organ itself. Mutual inhibition among the receptor units in the eye of *Limulus* is an important factor in determin-ing the over-all patterns of nervous activity in the visual pathways of this animal. The discharge of impulses in any one optic nerve fiber, in response to steady illumination of the eye, depends not only upon the stimulus to the specific receptor unit from which that nerve fiber arises but also upon the spatial distribution of the stimulation over the entire population of mutually interacting elements. Furthermore, when the illumination changes, the tran-sient component of the inhibitory influence modifies the temporal patterns of the responses of the individual receptor units. Thus a relatively simple, purely inhibitory interaction results in the generation of patterns of activity in the optic tract that are more than mere copies of the spatial and temporal pat-terns of stimulation on the sensory mosaic. In the vertebrate retina inter-action has even more complex effects, for it comprises both excitatory and inhibitory influences. Indeed, the diversity of the responses of various optic nerve fibers in the vertebrate eye is probably the result of a complex interplay

---

[3] Dr. E. F. MacNichol (personal communication) found that 5 per cent ethyl alcohol in sea water reversibly abolished the inhibitory effect in the *Limulus* eye, without affecting the responses to light to any great extent.

of excitatory and inhibitory components of interaction in the retina (Hartline, 1941–42; Kuffler, 1953; Granit, 1952, and 1955, chapter 2, section 5).

The inhibitory component of the interaction in the vertebrate retina[4] is similar, in many respects, to the purely inhibitory interaction that we have found in the eye of *Limulus*. In the frog (Hartline, 1939) and in the cat (Kuffler, 1953) it has been shown that illumination of some parts of the receptive field of a retinal ganglion cell may inhibit responses generated by illuminating other parts of the same receptive field. Even more analogous to our observations on *Limulus* is Barlow's finding (1953) that the responses of a retinal ganglion cell in the frog may be inhibited by illumination of retinal regions entirely outside of its receptive field. (Recently one of us, HGW, has confirmed this observation.)

Inhibitory interaction by itself can achieve important visual effects. One of its consequences is the enhancement of visual contrast. In an animal's normal environment different receptors of the eye are usually subjected to unequal intensities of illumination from different parts of the visual field. In *Limulus* we have shown that the more intensely illuminated receptor units exert a stronger inhibition upon the less intensely illuminated units than the latter exert upon the former, especially if they are close together. As a result, differences in activity from differently lighted retinal regions are exaggerated; thus the contrast is enhanced (Hartline, 1949). In human vision, many of the familiar properties of simultaneous brightness contrast can be explained by postulating a similar inhibitory interaction in the visual pathways (Fry, 1948); if the inhibitory influence is assumed to decrease with increasing distance between retinal regions, border contrast and related effects may find an explanation.

SUMMARY

In the compound lateral eye of *Limulus* each ommatidium functions as a single receptor unit in the discharge of impulses in the optic nerve. Impulses originate in the eccentric cell of each ommatidium and are conducted in its axon, which runs without interruption through an extensive plexus of nerve fibers to become a fiber of the optic nerve. The plexus makes interconnections among the ommatidia, but its exact organization is not understood.

The ability of an ommatidium to discharge impulses in the axon of its eccentric cell is reduced by illumination of other ommatidia in its neighborhood: the threshold to light is raised, the number of impulses discharged in response to a suprathreshold flash of light is diminished, and the frequency

---

[4] In the auditory system of the cat, Galambos and Davis (1944) observed that the activity of single elements could be inhibited by tones that presumably excited other parts of the organ of Corti than those concerned in the excitation of the elements in question.

with which impulses are discharged during steady illumination is decreased. Also, the activity that can be elicited under certain conditions when an ommatidium is in darkness can be inhibited similarly. There is no evidence for the spread of excitatory influences in the eye of *Limulus*.

The inhibitory influence exerted upon an ommatidium that is discharging impulses at a steady rate begins, shortly after the onset of the illumination on neighboring ommatidia, with a sudden deep minimum in the frequency of discharge. After partial recovery, the frequency is maintained at a depressed level until the illumination on the neighboring receptors is turned off, following which there is prompt, though not instantaneous recovery to the original frequency.

The inhibition is exerted directly upon the sensitive structure within the ommatidium: it has been observed when the impulses were recorded by a microelectrode thrust into an ommatidium, as well as when they were recorded more proximally in single fibers dissected from the optic nerve.

Receptor units of the eye often inhibit one another mutually. This has been observed by recording the activity of two optic nerve fibers simultaneously.

The mediation of the inhibitory influence appears to depend upon the integrity of nervous interconnections in the plexus: cutting the lateral connections to an ommatidium abolishes the inhibition exerted upon it. The nature of the influence that is mediated by the plexus and the mechanism whereby it exerts its inhibitory action on the receptor units are not known.

The depression of the frequency of the discharge of nerve impulses from an ommatidium increases approximately linearly with the logarithm of the intensity of illumination on receptors in its vicinity.

Inhibition of the discharge from an ommatidium is greater the larger the area of the eye illuminated in its vicinity. However, equal increments of area become less effective as the total area is increased.

The response of an ommatidium is most effectively inhibited by the illumination of ommatidia that are close to it; the effectiveness diminishes with increasing distance, but may extend for several millimeters.

Illumination of a fixed region of the eye at constant intensity produces a depression of the frequency of discharge of impulses from a nearby ommatidium that is approximately constant, irrespective of the level of excitation of the ommatidium.

The inhibitory interaction in the eye of *Limulus* is an integrative process that is important in determining the patterns of nervous activity in the visual system. It is analogous to the inhibitory component of the interaction that takes place in the vertebrate retina. Inhibitory interaction results in the exaggeration of differences in sensory activity from different regions of the eye illuminated at different intensities, thus enhancing visual contrast.

BIBLIOGRAPHY

Barlow, H. B., Summation and inhibition in the frog's retina, *J. Physiol.*, 1953, **119**, 69.

Fry, G. A., Mechanisms subserving simultaneous brightness contrast, *Am. J. Optom. and Arch. Am. Acad. Optom.*, 1948, **25**, 162.

Galambos, R., and Davis, H., Inhibition of activity in single auditory nerve fibers by acoustic stimulation, *J. Neurophysiol.*, 1944, **7**, 287.

Granit, R., Sensory Mechanisms of the Retina, London, Oxford University Press, 1947.

Granit, R., Aspects of excitation and inhibition in the retina, *Proc. Roy. Soc. London, Series B*, 1952, **140**, 191.

Granit, R., Receptors and Sensory Perception, New Haven, Yale University Press, 1955.

Hartline, H. K., Excitation and inhibition of the "off" response in vertebrate optic nerve fibers (abstract), *Am. J. Physiol.*, 1939, **126**, 527.

Hartline, H. K., The neural mechanisms of vision, *Harvey Lectures*, 1941–42, **37**, 39.

Hartline, H. K., Inhibition of activity of visual receptors by illuminating nearby retinal areas in the *Limulus* eye (abstract), *Fed. Proc.*, 1949, **8**, 69.

Hartline, H. K., and Graham, C. H., Nerve impulses from single receptors in the eye, *J. Cell. and Comp. Physiol.*, 1932, **1**, 277.

Hartline, H. K., and McDonald, P. R., Light and dark adaptation of single photoreceptor elements in the eye of *Limulus*, *J. Cell. and Comp. Physiol.*, 1947, **30**, 225.

Hartline, H. K., and Ratliff, F., Spatial summation of inhibitory influences in the eye of *Limulus* (abstract), *Science*, 1954, **120**, 781.

Hartline, H. K., Wagner, H. G., and MacNichol, E. F., The peripheral origin of nervous activity in the visual system, *Cold Spring Harbor Symp. Quant. Biol.*, 1952, **17**, 125.

Hartline, H. K., Wagner, H. G., and Tomita, T., Mutual inhibition among the receptors of the eye of *Limulus*, *XIX Internat. Physiol. Congr., Abstr. of Communications*, 1953, 441.

Kuffler, S. W., Discharge patterns and functional organization of mammalian retina, *J. Neurophysiol.*, 1953, **6**, 37.

MacNichol, E. F., and Hartline, H. K., Responses to small changes of light intensity by the light-adapted photoreceptor (abstract), *Fed. Proc.*, 1948, **7**, 76.

Watase, S., On the morphology of the compound eye of arthropods, *Studies Biol. Lab., Johns Hopkins Univ.*, 1890, **4**, (6), 287.

Waterman, T. H., Directional sensitivity of single ommatidia in the compound eye of *Limulus*, *Proc. Nat. Acad. Sc.*, 1954, **40**, 252.

Waterman, T. H., and Wiersma, C. A. G., The functional relation between retinal cells and optic nerve in *Limulus*, *J. Exp. Zool.*, 1954, **126**, 59.

Inhibitory interaction of receptor units in the eye of *Limulus* *

H. KEFFER HARTLINE AND FLOYD RATLIFF

The Rockefeller Institute for Medical Research

Reprinted from the JOURNAL OF GENERAL PHYSIOLOGY,
20 January 1957, Vol. 40, no. 3, pp. 357-376

In the lateral eye of the horseshoe crab, *Limulus*, the visual receptor units exert an inhibitory influence mutually upon one another. The discharge of impulses in any one optic nerve fiber, generated in the sensory structure of the particular ommatidium from which that fiber arises, is determined principally by the intensity of the light stimulus to the ommatidium and the state of adaptation of this receptor unit. However, the ability of an ommatidium to discharge impulses is reduced by illumination of the ommatidia in neighboring regions of the eye: its threshold to light is raised, and the frequency of the discharge that it can maintain in response to steady suprathreshold illumination is decreased. This inhibitory action is exerted reciprocally between any two ommatidia in the eye that are separated by no more than a few millimeters. As a result of inhibitory interaction among neighboring receptors, patterns of optic nerve activity are generated which are not direct copies of the patterns of external stimulation, but are modified by this integrative action that takes place in the eye itself.

These basic features of inhibition in the eye of *Limulus* have been described in detail in a recent paper (Hartline, Wagner, and Ratliff, 1956). In that paper it was shown that the anatomical basis for the inhibitory interaction is a plexus of nerve fibers lying just back of the layer of ommatidia, connecting them together. Furthermore, a direct experiment demonstrated mutual inhibitory action between two ommatidia whose respective optic nerve fibers were placed on the recording electrodes together. It is the purpose of the present paper to analyze the inhibitory interaction of receptor units in the eye of *Limulus*, and to describe quantitative properties of receptor activity that arise as a consequence of this interaction.

Method

The experiments reported in the present study are based on the measurement of the frequency of the discharge of nerve impulses from two receptor units simultane-

---

* This investigation was supported by a research grant (B864) from the National Institute of Neurological Diseases and Blindness, Public Health Service, and by Contract Nonr 1442(00) with the Office of Naval Research. Reproduction in whole or in part is permitted for any purpose of the United States government.

ously, enabling the exact description of their interaction. In each experiment, a lateral eye of an adult *Limulus* was excised with 1 to 2 cm. of optic nerve and mounted in a moist chamber (maintained at 18°C.). Two small strands were dissected from the optic nerve and each placed over a pair of wick electrodes connected to its own separate amplifier and recording system. In some experiments we dissected each strand until only a single fiber remained, as evidenced by the uniformity and regularity of the action potential spikes elicited in response to illumination of the eye. In other experiments, bundles containing many active fibers were used and the isolation of single units was accomplished by coating the eye with opaque wax (a heavy suspension of lampblack in paraffin wax) and then removing the coating carefully from a very small region, exposing the corneal facet of just that one ommatidium from which it was desired to record impulses. The black wax evidently prevents internal reflections inside the cornea of the eye, for by this method perfect isolation of single units can often be obtained,—a result rarely achieved merely by focussing a small spot of light on the facet by means of a lens.

The receptors of the eye were illuminated by the same optical system that was described in the paper mentioned above. Small spots of light were projected on the eye, their sizes controlled by diaphragms and their intensities by neutral wedges. The direction of incidence of each beam could be adjusted for maximal effectiveness by a system of mirrors. A separate system was employed for each spot of light, to avoid scatter in a common optical path.

Oscillograms of the amplified action potentials in the nerve fibers were recorded photographically in some experiments. Often, however, it was preferable to measure directly the frequency with which impulses were discharged in each nerve fiber. This was done by leading the output of each amplifier through a pulse-shaper into an electronic counter. The threshold of the pulse-shaper was calibrated, and could be set to discriminate between the action potential spikes and amplifier noise with perfect reliability (in *Limulus* optic fibers, spikes can usually be obtained that are many times greater than any fluctuations of potential due to noise); the uniform output of the pulse-shaper insured perfect operation of the counting circuits. Each counter was "gated" by an electronic timer, so that only those nerve impulses occurring within a specified interval of time (usually several seconds) were registered. The gating timer was activated by a delaying timer, which permitted the counting period to be started at any desired time (usually 1 or 2 seconds) after the onset of illumination to the eye.

To obtain maximum precision in the measurement of frequency of discharge, we displayed the gating voltages and the pulses to the counter from both recording channels on a dual trace oscilloscope. We then estimated for each channel that fraction of an interval between impulses that occupied the time between the onset of the counting period and the occurrence of the first counted impulse, at the beginning of the counting period, and the corresponding fraction between the last counted impulse and the cessation of the counting period. These fractions were added to the total number of intervals registered. For greater convenience in some experiments the delaying timer, instead of activating the counter gate directly, was arranged to sensitize an electronic "trigger" which, upon the occurrence of the next nerve impulse, activated the gate to the counter. Thus the counting period always started at the occurrence of an impulse, and only the fractional interval at the end of the gated counting period needed to be estimated. The precision gained by these methods was necessary when the counting period was short (1 or 2 seconds), and was desirable for the longer periods usually employed (7 to 10 seconds). Measurement to within about one-quarter interval was warranted by the regularity of the discharge found in many preparations, and the reproducibility of the frequencies observed.

In the experiments reported in this paper, we have confined our attention to the frequency of the discharge of impulses that is maintained at a more or less steady level during steady prolonged illumination of the eye. The transient changes in frequency that occur during the first second or two after light is turned on or off were excluded from the measurements. Exposures were fixed in duration (usually less than 10 seconds), and were repeated at fixed intervals of 2 to 5 minutes, with longer periods of rest interspersed, to minimize cumulative effects of light adaptation.

RESULTS

In the recent paper to which we have referred, direct evidence was given that receptor units in the *Limulus* eye may inhibit one another mutually. Recording the action potentials in a nerve strand containing two active fibers, it was shown that the discharge of impulses in either of the fibers was slowed when the other was brought into activity by illuminating the ommatidium from which it arose. A similar experiment is illustrated in Fig. 1, in which two strands dissected from the optic nerve, each containing a single active fiber, were placed on separate recording electrodes so that the action potentials of each of them were recorded separately. A small spot of light was centered on each of the ommatidia (designated "A" and "B") in which the fibers originated. The oscillograms show the effects of illuminating each of these small regions of the eye separately and together. The steady frequency of discharge of impulses in each fiber was less when both receptor units were active than when they were stimulated singly.

In the experiment shown in Fig. 1 the spots of light centered on the respective ommatidia were each made large enough to illuminate several receptors immediately adjacent to them in order to make the slowing of the discharges large enough to be apparent at a glance. Strictly mutual inhibition of the individual units, however, was exerted by these receptors, for similar (though less pronounced) slowing of the discharge was produced when each was illuminated by a spot so small as to be confined to the facet of its ommatidium, except for slight amounts of light that may have been scattered in the eye. In many of the experiments to be reported below, we took precautions to ensure that we were dealing with the mutual interaction of only two ommatidia by using opaque wax to effect complete optical isolation, as described in the section on Method.

From our previous study, we know that the inhibition of a receptor unit, measured by the decrease in the frequency of its discharge, is greater the

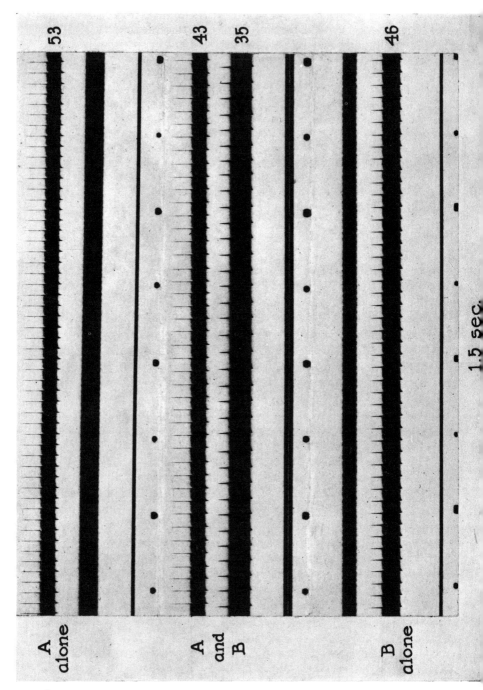

FIG. 1. Oscillograms of action potentials recorded simultaneously from two optic nerve fibers of a lateral eye of *Limulus*, showing the discharge of nerve impulses when the respective ommatidia in which these fibers originated were illuminated singly and together. In the top record, one ommatidium ("A," nerve fiber activity recorded by upper oscillographic trace) was illuminated by itself at an intensity that elicited the discharge of 53 impulses (as indicated at the right) in the period of 1.5 seconds covered by the records. In the bottom record, the other ommatidium ("B," activity recorded by lower trace) was illuminated by itself at an intensity that elicited the discharge of 46 impulses in 1.5 seconds. In the middle record, both ommatidia were illuminated together, each at the same intensity as before; ommatidium A discharged 43 impulses, ommatidium B 35 impulses, in 1.5 seconds. For A, the decrease in frequency of 10 impulses per 1.5 seconds is taken as the magnitude of the inhibition exerted upon it while B was discharging at the rate of 35 impulses per 1.5 seconds; for B, the decrease of 11 impulses per 1.5 seconds measures the inhibition exerted upon it while A was discharging at the rate of 43 impulses per 1.5 seconds. Two separate optical systems were used, each focusing a small spot of light (approximately 0.5 mm. in diameter) on the eye, one centered on ommatidium A, the other centered on ommatidium B. The spots were 1 mm. apart, center to center. Each spot illuminated about 5 ommatidia in addition to A and B. For each record, the light had been turned on 7 seconds before the start of that portion of the record shown in the figure. Time marked in one-fifth seconds; black bands above time marks are the signals of the stimulating illumination.

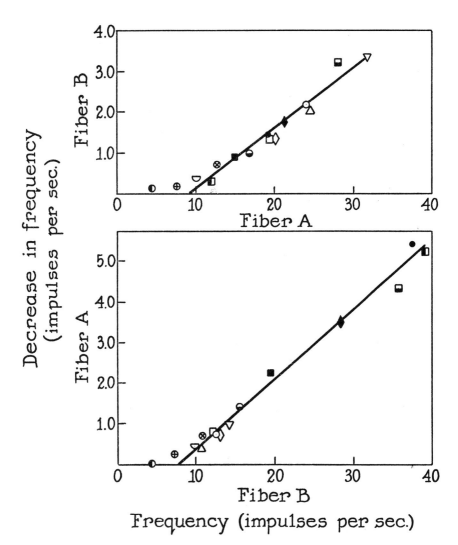

FIG. 2. Graphs showing mutual inhibition of two receptor units in the lateral eye of *Limulus*. In each graph the magnitude of the inhibition of one of the ommatidia is plotted (ordinate) as a function of the degree of concurrent activity of the other (abscissa). Sets of optic nerve fiber responses similar to those shown in Fig. 1 were analyzed as explained in the legend of that figure, each set yielding a point in the upper graph (inhibition of ommatidium B by ommatidium A) and a corresponding point (designated by the same symbol) in the lower graph (inhibition of ommatidium A by ommatidium B). The different points were obtained by using various intensities of illumination on ommatidia A and B, in various combinations.

Frequencies were determined by counting the number of impulse intervals during

stronger the stimulus to receptors that inhibit it. Experiments similar to that illustrated in Fig. 1 make it possible to show quantitatively how the amount of inhibition exerted on a receptor varies with the degree of activity of a nearby receptor unit that exerts this inhibition; the mutual interaction of two receptors can be analyzed by stimulating each of them at different intensities singly and in combination. The result of such an experiment is shown in Fig. 2. In this experiment, the frequencies of discharge of each of two ommatidia were measured, for various intensities of illumination, when each was illuminated alone and when both were illuminated together. The decrease in the frequency of discharge of each has been plotted as ordinate against the frequency of the concurrent discharge of the other as abscissa. The upper graph shows the amount of inhibition exerted upon ommatidium B by ommatidium A, as a function of the degree of activity of A; the lower graph shows the converse effect upon A of the activity of B. Both sets of points are adequately fitted by straight lines. In each case there was a fairly distinct threshold for the inhibition; each ommatidium had to be brought to a level of activity of 8 or 9 impulses per second before it began to affect the discharge of the other. Above this threshold, the frequency of discharge of B was decreased by 0.15 impulse per second for each increment of 1 impulse per second in the level of activity of A; the corresponding coefficient of the inhibitory action in the reverse direction (A acted on by B) was 0.17.

We have performed many similar experiments. Six of them, including the one just described, were done with "optical isolation," employing large nerve bundles that had exhibited activity of many fibers before the application of

---

the last 5 seconds of a 7 second exposure to light (so that only the steady discharge was measured). To obtain each pair of points in the two graphs two such counts were made for each of the following conditions of illumination: A alone, B alone, A and B together, presented in an order designed to minimize systematic errors. The averages of such duplicate determinations of the magnitude of the inhibition are the values plotted in the graph. From the distribution of the differences between the individual measurements in each duplicate determination the standard error of the points in the graph was calculated to be 0.12 impulse per second. The straight lines were fitted by the method of least squares. In the upper graph the line has a slope of 0.15, which is the value of the "inhibitory coefficient" $K_{B,A}$ (effect of A on B); in the lower graph the slope is 0.17 (= $K_{A,B}$, the coefficient of the effect of B on A). The intercept of the line on the axis of abscissae is 9.3 impulses per second for the upper graph, 7.8 for the lower. Disregarding a possible "toe" at the bottom of each plot, these give the values, respectively, of the thresholds of the inhibitory effect of A acting on B, designated later in the text as $r_A{}^0$, and of B acting on A ($r_B{}^0$).

In this experiment illumination was restricted to the two ommatidia from which activity was recorded by masking the rest of the eye with opaque wax (see text). These ommatidia were 1 mm. apart.

opaque wax to the eye to mask all but those two receptor units singled out for observation. In such experiments we could be quite certain that not any of the receptors adjacent to those under observation were excited by scattered light (since no nerve impulses from them were observed). In these experiments, therefore, the observed inhibitory effects were entirely those exerted mutually by the two receptor units upon one another. In other experiments we could be less certain about possible contributions from adjacent receptors excited by scattered light, although the scattered light was never very strong, and its effects were probably below threshold in most cases. All these experiments have shown features similar to those exhibited in Fig. 2. All showed a linear relation between the magnitude of the inhibition of one receptor (measured by the decrease in its frequency) and the degree of concurrent activity of the other (measured by its frequency). Nearly all experiments showed a "threshold" frequency below which no inhibitory effect was detected. The threshold was usually about as distinct as that shown in Fig. 2—a slight "toe" at the bottom of the curve was often noted. Although the values of the two thresholds were nearly identical in the experiment of Fig. 2, in other experiments they were not always the same for both members of an interacting pair. Likewise the slopes of the two curves often differed more than was the case in the experiment we have figured, sometimes by as much as a factor of 2.

The key to the analysis of the mutual interaction in the eye of *Limulus* lies in the correlation between the magnitude of the inhibition of a receptor and the degree of concurrent activity of the receptors that inhibit it. The degree of activity of any one of these receptors, however, depends not only on the stimulus to it but also on whatever inhibitory influences it may be subjected to in turn. It is the resultant level of activity of a receptor unit that determines the strength of the inhibition it exerts on a neighboring receptor. We have direct experimental evidence for this. Fig. 3 shows a small portion of the upper graph of Fig. 2; the points plotted as open symbols are measurements of the inhibition of ommatidium B produced by illuminating ommatidium A at two different intensities (two points at each intensity), with B illuminated at a low intensity. At the higher of the two intensities on A, which elicited a discharge in fiber A of approximately 24 impulses per second, the response of B was decreased by a little more than 2.0 impulses per second; at the lower intensity (A discharging at the rate of approximately 20 impulses per second) the discharge of B was reduced by about 1.3 impulses per second, following the trend of the solid line, which is a portion of that drawn through all the experimental points in the upper graph of Fig. 2. For these points plotted as open symbols, the activity of B itself was small (11 to 12 impulses per second); consequently the inhibition that B exerted back on A was also small (a little less than 1 impulse per second). This is indicated by the short dotted arrows; the "tails" of these arrows are plotted at the abscissae that represent the values of the frequency obtained when ommatidium A was illuminated alone. The two points marked by the solid symbols, on the other hand, were obtained with B illuminated at higher in-

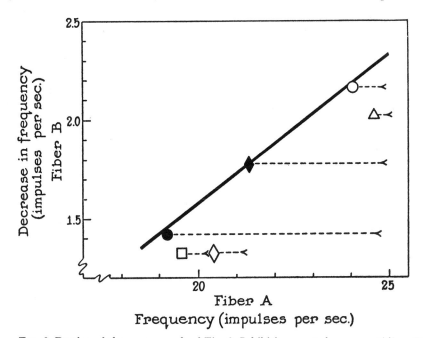

FIG. 3. Portion of the upper graph of Fig. 2. Inhibition exerted on ommatidium B is correlated with the degree of activity of ommatidium A. For the open symbols, B was illuminated at low intensity and exerted very little inhibition back on A. This is shown by the short lengths of the dotted lines, the right hand ends of which are plotted at the abscissae which give the frequency of A when it was illuminated alone. For the solid symbols, B was illuminated at high intensity and exerted strong inhibition back on A, as shown by the long lengths of the dotted lines associated with these points. For the solid symbols, ommatidium A was illuminated at the higher of the two intensities used for the open symbols. The solid line is a portion of that plotted in Fig. 2. The symbols are the same as those used for these same points in Fig. 2.

tensities. As a consequence of the resulting higher levels of activity of B (28 and 37 impulses per second), the discharge rates of ommatidium A (which for these points was illuminated at the higher of the two intensities used before) were much reduced, as can be seen by the lengths of the dotted arrows associated with these points. Corresponding to the reduced activity of A, the magnitude of the inhibition it exerted on B was smaller. This also followed the trend of the solid line. Thus any change in the frequency of A, whether brought about directly by changing the intensity of its stimulating light, or indirectly by changing the amount of inhibition exerted upon it as a consequence of altering the level of activity of B, resulted in comparable changes in the amount of inhibition it in turn exerted upon ommatidium B. Other sets of points can be found illustrating this same principle, both in other parts of this same graph, and in the other graph of this same experiment (effect of ommatidium B on the response of A). We have performed other experiments as well, that verify this principle for the interaction of a pair of receptor units. All the observations show that an alteration in the activity of a receptor unit, whether produced by changing the intensity of light shining on it, or by changing the inhibition exerted upon it by the other member of the pair (by changing the degree of activity of the latter), results equally in an alteration of the amount of inhibition it in turn exerts upon the other member of the pair. This result sometimes has been obscured by the scatter of the points, but usually there has been good agreement (as in Fig. 3), and we have never observed a case in which this principle was violated.

In the analysis we have just made we assumed that when the intensity on ommatidium B was increased, so that it discharged impulses at a higher rate, the ensuing diminution of the inhibition on this receptor unit was solely the result of the lowered discharge rate of ommatidium A. Our interpretation is based on the experimental finding described in the previous paper (Hartline, Wagner, and Ratliff, 1956) that the magnitude of the inhibition of a receptor unit, when measured by the absolute decrease in its frequency of impulse discharge, is independent of its own level of activity. This basic result, however, was established only as an approximation; indeed, it was noted in that paper that as the level of excitation of a "test" receptor was raised, the reduction in its frequency resulting from a fixed illumination of nearby ommatidia did in fact decrease slightly but significantly, in most experiments. This was attributed to an appreciable inhibition of the nearby ommatidia by the test receptor, just as we have done in the present case. But it might be argued alternatively that the measure of inhibition we have adopted has the inherent property that it yields a smaller value as the frequency of discharge of the test receptor is increased, and that the quantitative correlation of this measure of inhibition of one receptor unit with degree of activity of the other is only fortuitous in the present experiments. Independent experimental evidence is required to establish our interpretation more firmly.

Such independent evidence is furnished by experiments in which a third spot of light has been introduced to provide additional inhibitory influences that could be controlled independently of the two interacting receptor units whose activity was being measured. We have made use of the fact that the

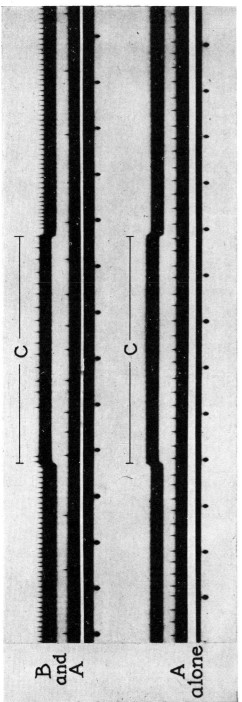

FIG. 4. Oscillograms of the electrical activity of two optic nerve fibers, showing disinhibition. In each record, the lower oscillographic trace records the discharge of impulses from ommatidium A, stimulated by a spot of light 0.1 mm. in diameter confined to its facet. The upper trace records the activity of ommatidium B, located 3 mm. from A, stimulated by a spot of light 1 mm. in diameter, centered on the facet of B, but that also illuminated approximately 8 to 10 ommatidia in addition to B. A third spot of light ("C"), 2 mm. in diameter, was directed onto a region of the eye centered 2.5 mm. from B and 5.5 mm. from A (B approximately midway between A and C); exposure of C was signalled by the upward offset of the upper trace. Lower record; activity of ommatidium A in the absence of illumination on B, showing that illumination of C had no perceptible effect under this condition. Upper record; activity of ommatidia A and B together, showing (1) lower frequency of discharge of A (as compared with lower record) resulting from activity of B, and (2) effect of illumination of C, causing a drop in the frequency of discharge of B and concomitantly an increase in the frequency of discharge of A, as A was partially released from the inhibition exerted by B.

Time marked in one-fifth seconds. The black band above the time marks is the signal of the illumination of A and B, thin when A was shining alone, thick when A and B were shining together.

inhibitory influence becomes weaker with increased separation between an affected receptor and the region of the eye used to inhibit it (Hartline, Wagner, and Ratliff, 1956). Consequently, it is often possible to find a region on the eye that is too far from the first of the two receptor units under observation to affect that one directly by an appreciable amount, but that is near enough to the second to inhibit it markedly. We then observe the effect that the altered frequency of discharge from this inhibited receptor has on the response of the first ommatidium. Fig. 4 shows oscillograms of the activity recorded simultaneously from two receptor units, showing the effects of illuminating regions of the eye in the manner just described. When one of these receptor units (A) was illuminated alone (lower trace, lower record) its activity was not appreciably affected by illuminating a distant region of the eye (C) (signalled by the upward displacement of the upper trace). When ommatidium A was illuminated together with a small region centered on ommatidium B, which was intermediate in position between A and C, the discharge of impulses by A was markedly slower than when A was illuminated alone (lower trace, upper record). This result is attributable to the vigorous activity of ommatidium B and the receptors stimulated with it, evidenced by the discharge of impulses in B's optic nerve fiber (upper trace, upper record). Then when C was turned on, the discharge rate of A actually increased, concomitantly with a decrease in frequency of discharge from B. When C was turned off, the discharge rate of B rose again and that of A fell. We interpret this result to mean that as the receptors in the region that included ommatidium B were inhibited by illumination of region C, the decrease in their activity partially released ommatidium A from the inhibition they exerted upon it. The amount of inhibition exerted on A by region B, measured by the difference in frequency of A between the lower record (A alone) and the upper (A with B) was less when C was being illuminated than when it was not; this diminished inhibition paralleled the lessened degree of activity recorded in fiber B.

The parallelism between the degree of activity of a receptor subjected to inhibition and the inhibition it in turn exerts on its neighbors is quantitative. This is shown in Fig. 5, drawn from data obtained from the same experiment as Fig. 4, except that the spot of light centered on ommatidium B was reduced in size, so that it was confined to that ommatidium. Consequently, the inhibition exerted by B may be correlated strictly with the activity recorded in its axon. In Fig. 5, the inhibition (decrease in frequency) of ommatidium A is plotted as a function of the frequency of discharge of ommatidium B; the open symbols are for two different values of light intensity on ommatidium B with no illumination on region C. The solid symbols are for a high intensity on B, but with the addition of light on the region C. The effect that C had on the discharge of B is represented by the length of the

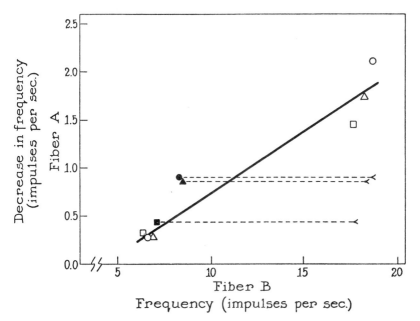

FIG. 5. Decrease of the inhibition exerted on one receptor unit (A) by another (B), as a result of inhibiting the activity of the second by illuminating a region of the eye (C) close to it. From the same experiment as that of Fig. 4 (see legend), but with the spot of light on ommatidium B reduced to 0.2 mm. diameter. The inhibition of ommatidium A was measured by the difference between its frequency when illuminated alone and when it was illuminated together with ommatidium B; this has been plotted as ordinate against the frequency of B as abscissa (as in Figs. 2 and 3). Three points were determined for a high intensity and three for a low intensity on B, when there was no illumination on C (open symbols). Three points were similarly determined for a high intensity on B when the nearby region of the eye, C, was illuminated (see legend of Fig. 4). These points are designated by the solid symbols. The lengths of the dotted lines associated with these points show the amount of reduction in the frequency of discharge of ommatidium B, as a result of the inhibition exerted upon it by C. Corresponding to this reduction in the activity of B, the inhibitory effect it in turn exerted on A was reduced, by an amount that is in quantitative agreement with the reduction obtained by lowering the intensity on B, as given by the solid line drawn through the open symbols. Illumination of the region C with no light shining on ommatidium B had very little effect on the activity of A: a reduction in frequency of 0.3 impulse per second was the maximum observed (the region C must have contributed even less than this amount to the total inhibition, since the receptors in it were also subject to inhibition by the activity of B).

Determination of the frequencies was made as described in the legend of Fig. 2.

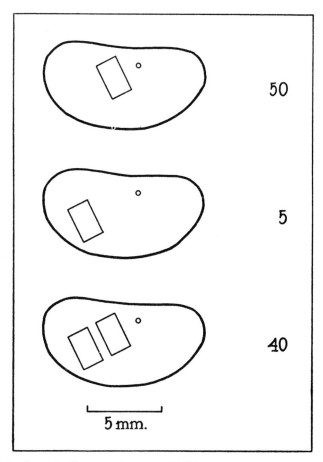

50

5

40

5 mm.

FIG. 6. A schematic diagram of patterns of light on a lateral eye of *Limulus* in an experiment illustrating disinhibition. The heavy lines are sketches of the outer margins of the eye. A small spot of light marked "o" was centered on the facet of a "test" ommatidium whose activity was measured by recording the action potentials in the optic nerve fiber arising from it. This spot was small enough to illuminate only the ommatidium on which it was centered. For each measurement the small spot of illumination was turned on for 12 seconds at a constant intensity. The number of impulses discharged by the test ommatidium in the last 10 seconds of such exposure was determined when the ommatidium was illuminated alone, and again when it was illuminated together with rectangular patches of light on other regions of the eye, as shown in the three sketches. The difference in the counts (decrease in frequency, in impulses per 10 seconds) measures the magnitude of the inhibition exerted on the test ommatidium by the receptors in the regions illuminated by the rectangular patches of light; these differences are given at the right for the respective parts of the experiment. Upper sketch, a rectangular patch of light near the test omma-

dotted lines. This experiment shows that the diminution in activity of ommatidium B had the same effect in reducing the inhibition exerted on A, whether that diminution was the result of inhibition of B by illumination of region C, or the result of reduction in the intensity of the light stimulus to B. Thus the degree of activity of a receptor unit does indeed determine, quantitatively, the strength of the inhibition it exerts on another receptor unit. Our analysis of the interaction between two receptor units illuminated together is therefore substantiated.

The release of a receptor unit from the inhibiting effects of others, by causing those others to be inhibited by yet a third group of receptors, is interesting physiologically. Such "disinhibition" is not difficult to obtain, though it may require some pains to show a strong effect. We have performed one other experiment similar to that of Figs. 4 and 5, recording from two fibers and using a third spot of light to inhibit one and disinhibit the other. It is considerably easier to show disinhibition when recording from only one receptor, for then it is possible to choose a favorable combination of locations for the spots of light that serve to inhibit and to disinhibit this test receptor. We have done many such experiments. An example is given in Fig. 6; the experiment is explained in its legend. Instead of focussing spots of light in various locations on the surface of the eye, disinhibition can also be demonstrated by using sources of light in various places in the external visual field, where the directional sensitivity of the ommatidia determines the location in the eye of the groups of receptors stimulated by the respective light sources. Dr. William Miller, in our laboratory, has also demonstrated disinhibition of receptors in the median eye of *Limulus* (a simple eye), using light sources in the external visual field.

Disinhibition simulates facilitation: illumination of a distant region of the eye results in an increase in the activity of the test receptor. In the *Limulus* eye the dependence of such an effect on the stimulation of receptors in an intermediate region of the eye (to produce the original inhibition) makes it

---

tidium produced a decrement of 50 impulses in 10 seconds. Middle sketch, a similar rectangular patch of light farther away from the test ommatidium produced a decrement of 5 impulses in 10 seconds. Lower sketch, both patches of light shining together produced a decrement of only 40 impulses in 10 seconds.

Thus in the last case the distant patch, rather than adding to the inhibition exerted by the near one, caused a disinhibition of 10 impulses per 10 seconds. As established by the experiments of Figs. 4 and 5, this was the result of the inhibition of the receptors in the near patch by the activity of those in the distant one, with the consequence that they in turn exerted less inhibition on the test ommatidium. This release of the test ommatidium from the inhibition exerted by the receptors in the near patch was greater than the slight inhibitory effect exerted directly on the test ommatidium by the receptors in the distant patch.

easy to recognize the mechanism involved. But if such a group of intermediate inhibiting elements were active spontaneously, or through uncontrolled
influences, it might be difficult to recognize the true nature of a disinhibiting
action. Perhaps the most significant aspect of these experiments showing
disinhibition is the principle that they reveal, that indirect effects may extend considerably beyond the limit of the direct inhibitory connections among
the receptors of the eye. Indeed, no member of the population of receptors
is completely independent, under every condition, of the activity in any
part of the eye. This is a direct consequence of the principle of interaction
that we have established: the inhibiting influence exerted by a receptor depends on its activity, which is the resultant of the excitatory stimulus to it
and whatever inhibitory influences may in turn be exerted upon it.

The principles that we have established experimentally may be conveniently summarized in a simple algebraic expression. The activity of a receptor unit—its response (r)—is to be measured in the present case by the frequency of the discharge of impulses in its axon. This response is determined
by the excitation (e) supplied by the external stimulus to the receptor, diminished by whatever inhibitory influences may be acting upon the receptor
as a result of the activity of neighboring receptors. The excitation of a given
receptor is to be measured by its response when it is illuminated by itself,
thus lumping together the physical parameters of the stimulus and the characteristics of the photoexcitatory mechanism of the receptor. Each of two
interacting receptor units inhibits the other to a degree that depends (linearly) on its own activity. The responses of two such units are therefore given by a pair of simultaneous equations:

$$r_A = e_A - K_{A,B}(r_B - r_B{}^0)$$

$$r_B = e_B - K_{B,A}(r_A - r_A{}^0)$$

in which the subscripts are used to label the respective receptor units. In
each of these equations, the magnitude of the inhibitory influence is given
by the last term, written in accordance with the experimental findings as a
simple linear expression. The "threshold" frequency that must be exceeded
before a receptor can exert any inhibition is represented by r^0. The "inhibitory coefficient," K, in each equation is labelled to identify the direction of
the action: $K_{A,B}$ is the coefficient of the action of receptor B on receptor
A; $K_{B,A}$ *vice versa*. It is to be clearly understood that the equations do not
apply in the ranges of responses for $r < r^0$ in either case: negative values of
inhibition must be excluded since they are never observed. Also, r and e, by
their nature (being measured by frequencies), cannot be negative. Appropriate changes must be made in the equations in those ranges of the variables where these restrictions apply: if, for example, $r_B < r_B{}^0$, the first equation must be replaced by $r_A = e_A$; if, to choose another example, r_B is

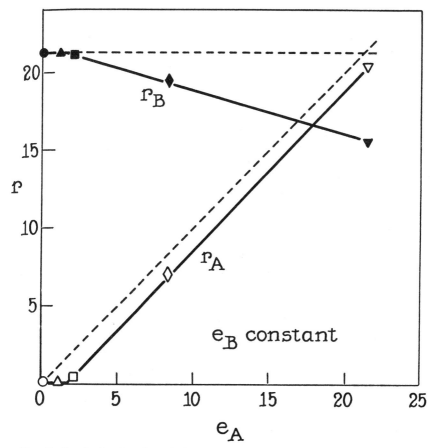

FIG. 7. Graph showing the relation of the responses of two interacting receptor units. One ommatidium (B) was illuminated at a fixed intensity; the intensity on the other (A) was varied. Responses (r) were measured by the frequency of the steady discharge of nerve impulses (last 7 seconds of a 10 second exposure to light). When both A and B were illuminated together, r_A refers to the response of ommatidium A (open symbols), r_B refers to the response of ommatidium B (solid symbols). The excitation of A, designated by e_A, is measured by the response of this ommatidium when it was illuminated alone; the excitation of B, designated by e_B, is measured by the response of B when it was illuminated alone. For each set of exposures (A alone, B alone, A and B together) with a given intensity for ommatidium A, the values of r_A and r_B obtained have been plotted (ordinates) against the value of e_A (abscissa). Values obtained for e_B were consistent within 0.1 impulse per second for all the sets of exposures; their average (21.2 impulses per second, shown by the horizontal dotted line) has been used in the calculations. The solid lines are the solutions of the simultaneous equations given in the text; the calculations and values of the constants are given there. The vertical distance from each dotted line ($r = e_A$, and $r = e_B$) to the corresponding solid line beneath it shows the amount of the inhibition for each receptor at that value of e_A.

so great that $e_A < K_{A, B} (r_B - r_B^0)$, then the first equation must be replaced by $r_A = 0$.

In Fig. 7 we give the results of an experiment using two receptor units to illustrate the solutions of the simultaneous equations governing their responses. A small spot of light centered on ommatidium B was maintained at a fixed intensity, such as to give a frequency of discharge (when it was shining alone) of 21.2 impulses per second in the optic nerve fiber from this receptor unit. This is the value of e_B. Another small spot, centered on ommatidium A, was set at various intensities of illumination; at each intensity the steady frequency of discharge of this receptor unit was determined when the spot illuminating it was shining alone. These measurements give the value of e_A, for the corresponding stimulus intensities. The frequencies of the discharges obtained when the two receptor units were illuminated together are plotted for each one (r_A and r_B) as functions of e_A. On another graph (not shown) similar to Fig. 2 we plotted the decrease in frequency ($e - r$) for each unit as a function of the corresponding frequency (r) of the other, obtaining plots which, when fitted by straight lines, gave values of the intercepts $r_A^0 = 0$ (an unusual value, in our experience), $r_B^0 = 4.0$, and slopes $K_{A, B} = 0.09$, $K_{B, A} = 0.26$. The solid lines of Fig. 7 are drawn as determined by these values of the constants in the solutions of the simultaneous equations given above. For low intensities of illumination on ommatidium A (small values of e_A), activity of this receptor was prevented ($r_A = 0$) by the strong inhibition exerted by the activity produced by illumination of ommatidium B, and therefore, since no inhibition was exerted on B, the activity of B was the same as when it was illuminated alone ($r_B = e_B$). At the intensity for which the excitation e_A just overcame the effects of the inhibition exerted by B ($e_A = K_{A, B} [e_B - r_B^0] = 1.6$), receptor A began to respond; as e_A increased, the frequency of its discharge increased linearly with

a slope of 1.024 $\left(= \dfrac{1}{1 - K_{A,B} K_{B,A}} \right)$. At this same value of e_A (since $r_A^0 =$

0), the inhibition by A on B began to be exerted, and r_B decreased linearly

with increasing e_A, the slope being $-0.27 \left(= \dfrac{-K_{B,A}}{1 - K_{A,B} K_{B,A}} \right)$. (The dotted

lines show the form the graphs would have taken had there been no inhibition.) In this experiment each spot of light actually illuminated about 8 or 9 other ommatidia in the immediate vicinity of the one on which it was centered and from which activity was recorded. For purposes of illustration, it is permissible to treat the results as though individual units were interacting, although in actuality it was each small group. That the principles involved hold rigorously when only two single receptor units are actually used is inherent in the treatment, for these principles were derived from the experiment of Fig. 2 (and those like it), in which strict optical isolation of individual ommatidia was employed.

The mutual interdependence of two receptor units responding to steady illumination is thus concisely and accurately described by a pair of simultaneous equations. Similar equations hold for the responses of any two ommatidia that are close enough together in the eye to interact. When more than two interacting elements are activated, similar relations apply simultaneously to the responses of all of them. In addition, however, each receptor unit is subjected to inhibitory influences from all the others, and the degree to which its response is decreased is known to be greater, the greater the number of neighboring ommatidia that are stimulated (Hartline, Wagner, and Ratliff, 1956). The simultaneous equations governing the responses of more than two ommatidia therefore must contain terms expressing the inhibition contributed from all the active elements, combined according to some law of spatial summation. Experiment shows that simple arithmetic addition of such terms is adequate to describe spatial summation of inhibitory influences in the eye of *Limulus*. In a paper that will follow (see also Hartline and Ratliff, 1954 and Ratliff and Hartline, 1956) we will describe the experiments that establish this law of spatial summation and will illustrate some of the effects that are obtained when more than two receptor units in the eye inhibit one another mutually.

SUMMARY

The inhibition that is exerted mutually among the receptor units (ommatidia) in the lateral eye of *Limulus* has been analyzed by recording oscillographically the discharge of nerve impulses in single optic nerve fibers. The discharges from two ommatidia were recorded simultaneously by connecting the bundles containing their optic nerve fibers to separate amplifiers and recording systems. Ommatidia were chosen that were separated by no more than a few millimeters in the eye; they were illuminated independently by separate optical systems.

The frequency of the maintained discharge of impulses from each of two ommatidia illuminated steadily is lower when both are illuminated together than when each is illuminated by itself. When only two ommatidia are illuminated, the magnitude of the inhibition of each one depends only on the degree of activity of the other; the activity of each, in turn, is the resultant of the excitation from its respective light stimulus and the inhibition exerted on it by the other.

When additional receptors are illuminated in the vicinity of an interacting pair too far from one ommatidium to affect it directly, but near enough to the second to inhibit it, the frequency of discharge of the first increases as it is partially released from the inhibition exerted on it by the second (disinhibition).

Disinhibition simulates facilitation; it is an example of indirect effects of interaction taking place over greater distances in the eye than are covered by direct inhibitory interconnections.

When only two interacting ommatidia are illuminated, the inhibition exerted on each (decrease of its frequency of discharge) is a linear function of the degree of activity (frequency of discharge) of the other. Below a certain frequency (often different for different receptors) no inhibition is exerted by a receptor. Above this threshold, the rate of increase of inhibition of one receptor with increasing frequency of discharge of the other is constant, and may be at least as high as 0.2 impulse inhibited in one receptor per impulse discharged by the other. For a given pair of interacting receptors, the inhibitory coefficients are not always the same in the two directions of action. The responses to steady illumination of two receptor units that inhibit each other mutually are described quantitatively by two simultaneous linear equations that express concisely all the features discussed above. These equations may be extended and their number supplemented to describe the responses of more than two interacting elements.

BIBLIOGRAPHY

Hartline, H. K., and Ratliff, F., Spatial summation of inhibitory influences in the eye of *Limulus, Science,* 1954 **120,** 781 (abstract).

Hartline, H. K., Wagner, H. G., and Ratliff, F., Inhibition in the eye of *Limulus, J. Gen. Physiol.,* 1956, **39,** 651.

Ratliff, F., and Hartline, H. K., Inhibitory interaction in the eye of *Limulus, Fed. Proc.,* 1956, **15,** 148 (abstract).

Spatial summation of inhibitory influences in the eye of *Limulus*, and the mutual interaction of receptor units*

H. KEFFER HARTLINE AND FLOYD RATLIFF

The Rockefeller Institue for Medical Research

Reprinted from the JOURNAL OF GENERAL PHYSIOLOGY,
20 May 1958, Vol. 41, no. 5, pp. 1049–1066

The inhibitory influences exerted mutually among the receptor units (ommatidia) of the lateral eye of *Limulus* are additive. If two groups of receptors are illuminated together the total inhibition they exert on a "test receptor" near them (decrease in the frequency of its nerve impulse discharge in response to light) depends on the combined inhibitory influences exerted by the two groups. If the two groups are widely separated in the eye, their total inhibitory effect on the test receptor equals the sum of the inhibitory effects they each produce separately. If they are close enough together to interact, their effect when acting together is usually less than the sum of their separate effects, since each group inhibits the activity of the other and hence reduces its inhibitory influence. However, the test receptor, or a small group illuminated with it, may interact with the two groups and affect the net inhibitory action. A variety of quantitative effects have been observed for different configurations of three such groups of receptors. The activity of a population of n interacting elements is described by a set of n simultaneous equations, linear in the frequencies of the receptor elements involved. Applied to three interacting receptors or receptor groups equations are derived that account quantitatively for the variety of effects observed in the various experimental configurations of retinal illumination used.

The inhibition that is exerted mutually among the ommatidia of the lateral eye of *Limulus* depends on the degree of activity of each of these receptor units. It also depends on the number and location of units interacting: the discharge of nerve impulses by a given ommatidium is slowed to an extent that is greater the larger the number of other ommatidia that are illuminated in its vicinity and the closer they are to the ommatidium in question (Hartline, Wagner, and Ratliff, 1956). When many receptor units are active in an eye—each one affecting and affected by its neighbors—the resulting pattern of activity is determined by a set of simultaneous relationships that expresses not only

* This investigation was supported by a research grant (B864) from the National Institute of Neurological Diseases and Blindness, Public Health Service, and by Contract Nonr 1442(00) with the Office of Naval Research. Reproduction in whole or in part is permitted for any purpose of the United States government.

299

the distribution of external stimulating light over these elements, but also the magnitudes of the inhibitory influences exerted mutually among them and the way in which the influences from many elements combine to affect the activity of each one.

In a preceding paper (Hartline and Ratliff, 1957) we dealt specifically with interaction between pairs of receptor units. We showed that a pair of simultaneous linear equations is required to describe the frequency of the discharge of nerve impulses from two ommatidia in the eye, illuminated independently of one another. When more than two interacting receptor units are activated simultaneously, so that each is subjected to inhibition from more than one other, the set of simultaneous equations must also describe how the inhibitory influences from several receptor units combine in exerting their net inhibition upon any given receptor unit. It is the purpose of this paper to present experimental results establishing the law of spatial summation of inhibitory influences in the eye of *Limulus*, to proceed with the construction of the set of simultaneous equations governing the action of a number of interacting ommatidia, and to show some of the consequences of the mutual inhibitory interaction when more than two receptors are illuminated simultaneously at various intensities.

Method

In each of the experiments reported here, we recorded the discharge of impulses in a single optic nerve fiber from the lateral eye of *Limulus* when the ommatidium in which it originated was illuminated. We then determined the inhibitory effects of illuminating nearby regions of the eye. The ommatidium from which activity was recorded was stimulated by a spot of light of constant intensity, usually so small as to be confined to its facet. The inhibitory effect on this "test receptor," when other receptor units in its vicinity were being illuminated, was measured by taking the difference between the frequency of discharge of the test receptor when it was illuminated by itself and its frequency when it was illuminated together with the other receptors. It has already been shown that the magnitude of the decrease in frequency produced by a constant inhibitory influence is independent of the level of activity of the test receptor (Hartline, Wagner, and Ratliff, 1956).

The receptors whose inhibitory influences were to be studied were illuminated by patches of light, usually circular and about 1 to 2 mm. in diameter, centered several millimeters from the facet of the test ommatidium. Approximately 10 to 20 ommatidia would be illuminated uniformly by such patches of light. The several groups of receptors and the test receptor were illuminated through separate optical systems to minimize the effects of scattered light. The amplified action potential spikes were either recorded oscillographically or registered by an electronic counter suitably "gated" for a desired interval of time. Frequency determinations were always made 2 or 3 seconds after the onset of any illumination to permit the transient changes in frequency to subside before impulses were counted; the counting intervals were 5 to 10 seconds long. Thus the present paper, like the preceding one, deals only with the steady levels of the receptor discharge and the steady inhibition exerted upon it. The exposures were made at regular intervals, usually 2 minutes or more, to minimize cumulative effects of light adaptation. All measurements required for each determination of an inhibitory effect were made at least in duplicate, in an order designed to minimize systematic errors. Details of our method are described in the previous papers already cited.

RESULTS

We have analyzed the spatial summation of inhibitory influences by measuring the inhibition exerted on a test receptor separately by each of two small groups of ommatidia near it, and then by these two groups together. Since ommatidia close to each other in the eye inhibit one another mutually it may be anticipated that in general the results of such an experiment will depend on the amount of interaction between the two groups. We will begin with a case in which there was little or no interaction. This could easily be achieved experimentally, since the interaction between ommatidia is less the greater their separation (Hartline, Wagner, and Ratliff, 1956; Ratliff and Hartline, 1957); consequently it was possible to choose two regions of the eye, on either side of the test receptor, that were too far apart to affect each other appreciably, but that still were close enough to the test receptor to inhibit it significantly.

The results of such an experiment were quite simple, as shown in Fig. 1: the inhibitory effect on the test receptor produced by the groups of receptors on either side of it, when both were acting together, was equal to the sum of the inhibitory effects produced by these groups acting separately. Measurements of the discharge frequency of the test receptor were made for several different intensities of light on the inhibiting receptor groups, in various combinations. For the points at the upper end of the graph, both receptor groups were illuminated at high intensity; for those at the lower end, both were illuminated at low intensity. For the intermediate points, some were obtained by equal illumination of the two groups of receptors at intermediate intensities, others by illuminating one group at high intensity and the other at low intensity, and still others with these unequal intensity relations interchanged. A line has been drawn through the origin with a slope of unity, representing equality between ordinates and abscissae. Most of the points lie as close to this line as is in accord with the reproducibility of the measurements. The fact that some of them fall slightly above the line will be discussed below. No systematic effects of different combinations of intensities were noted in the data. Many other less extensive experiments gave similar results; some of these will appear below.

It is our suggestion that the experiment of Fig. 1, and those like it, establish the law of spatial summation of inhibitory influences in the lateral eye of *Limulus*, for the steady levels of response to steady illumination: the total

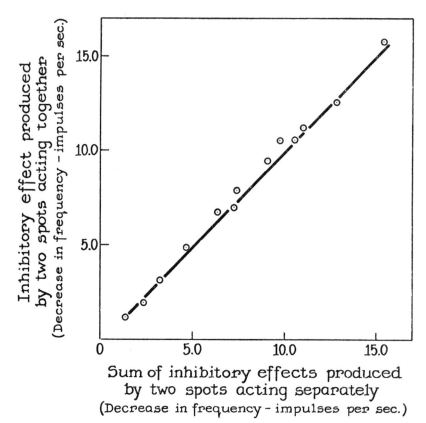

Inhibitory effect produced by two spots acting together (Decrease in frequency – impulses per sec.)

Sum of inhibitory effects produced by two spots acting separately
(Decrease in frequency – impulses per sec.)

FIG. 1. The summation of inhibitory effects produced by two widely separated groups of receptors. The sum of the inhibitory effects on a test receptor produced by each group acting separately is plotted as abscissa; the effect produced by the two groups of receptors acting simultaneously is plotted as ordinate. The solid line is not fitted to the experimental points, but instead is drawn through the origin with a slope of 1.0 (equality of ordinates and abscissae); a line fitted to the points by the method of least squares would have the equation $y = 1.030x - 0.11$.

The two spots of light used to stimulate the two groups of receptors were each 1.0 mm. in diameter, each illuminating about a dozen receptors, and were 4.6 mm. apart on the eye. The test receptor, located midway between these two spots of light, was illuminated by a third small spot of light of constant intensity confined to its facet. Several intensities of illumination were used for the two larger spots, in various combinations (see text).

Exposures were for a period of 8 seconds; 2 seconds after onset, the counter registering the number of impulses from the test receptor was gated for a period of 5 seconds. Frequency measurements obtained when the test receptor was exposed alone were interspersed between measurements obtained when it was illuminated together with one or the other or both of the inhibiting spots. Two such series of measurements were made for each combination of intensities on the inhibiting regions, and the corresponding frequencies averaged.

inhibitory influence exerted by more than one group of receptor units is equal to the sum of the inhibitory influences exerted by each group. We will show how this simple law can explain a variety of experimental results.

When the regions illuminated to inhibit a test receptor were not widely separated, their combined influences produced an effect that was no longer equal to the sum of their separate effects. An example is shown in Fig. 2. Spots of light were projected onto the eye in three different locations near a test receptor, singly and in combination. The locations of these small regions were chosen to produce inhibitory effects that were nearly the same for each when illuminated singly. Two of these locations were close together, the third was some distance away from these two. Each panel of Fig. 2 is a map of the region of the eye in the vicinity of the test receptor (marked X) showing the locations of the spots of light and the decrease their exposure produced in the number of impulses discharged by the test receptor in 8 seconds (numbers at the right). The three panels on the left show the inhibitory effects of each of the three spots exposed singly, the three on the right show the effects when they were exposed in pairs. For the upper two panels on the right, the most widely separated pairs of spots were used. These two cases resemble the experiment of Fig. 1, just described. In each of these cases the decrease in frequency produced by the two spots together was almost equal to the sum of the decreases produced by each one of them alone (40 compared with 22 + 22, and 42 compared with 22 + 23). The bottom panel on the right shows that the two spots close to each other together produced an inhibitory effect (35) considerably less than the sum of the effects they produced singly (22 + 23). This experiment illustrates results we have obtained invariably in many experiments: simultaneous illumination of receptor groups that were close together produced an inhibitory effect on a test receptor in their neighborhood that was less than the sum of the separate effects produced by illumination of each group singly.

Our interpretation of this experimental result is based on the fact that the inhibitory influence exerted by a receptor unit depends on its activity, which is the resultant of the excitation provided by the stimulating light and whatever inhibition may in turn be exerted upon it by other receptor units in its neighborhood (Hartline and Ratliff, 1957). In the experiment of Fig. 2, the spots of light to the right of the test receptor illuminated receptor groups that were close enough together to inhibit one another. As a result, the amount of receptor activity produced in each group, and hence the inhibitory influence exerted by each group, must have been less when both groups were illuminated together than when each was illuminated separately. Consequently, the inhibitory effect produced by the combined influences of these two groups on the test receptor when both spots of light were shining should have been less than the sum of the inhibitory effects produced by each receptor group illuminated alone. This is what was observed.

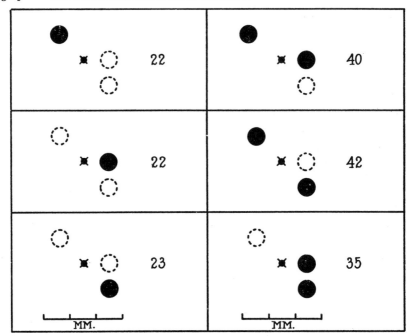

FIG. 2. The summation of inhibitory influences exerted by two widely separated groups of receptors and by two groups of receptors close together. Each panel in the figure is a map of the same small portion of the eye. The test receptor, location indicated by the symbol X, was illuminated steadily by a small spot of light confined to its facet. Larger spots of light could be placed singly in any of three locations, as shown in the three panels on the left side of the figure, or in pairs, as shown in the three panels on the right. The filled circles indicate the spots actually illuminated in each case; the other locations (not illuminated) are indicated in dotted outline merely for purposes of orientation. The number of impulses discharged from the test receptor in a period of 8 seconds was decreased upon illumination of the neighboring spot or spots by the amount shown at the right in each panel. Thus for the upper left hand panel, the test receptor when illuminated alone discharged 252 impulses in an 8 second period beginning 2 seconds after the onset of steady illumination on its facet. This is the mean of 39 determinations taken over a 2 hour period (σ_m = 0.4). When the test receptor was illuminated together with the group of receptors indicated in the panel as being above it and to its left, it discharged 230 impulses in a correspondingly timed period. This is the mean of 6 determinations, ranging from 228 to 232, interspersed among the above controls and the determinations recorded in the other panels. The other determinations were made similarly. See text for discussion of results.

It is the essential feature of this interpretation that the law of spatial summation itself is not called into question; indeed, it is assumed that the inhibitory influences exerted on any given receptor by other receptors in its neighborhood always add according to the simple law stated above. The mutual inhibition among receptors, however, affects the quantitative outcome in any configuration of interacting elements. This interpretation is supported by the analysis of the following experiments.

We have made quantitative determinations of the inhibitory effects produced by the combined influences from two interacting regions of the eye, exerted on a test receptor (X) near them, for various intensities of illumination upon them. For these experiments we have considered it sufficient to vary the intensity on only one of the regions (A), holding constant the intensity on the other (B). We have presented the results in terms of A's effects on the response of X when A was illuminated together with B, expressed as a function of the amount of inhibition exerted on X by A alone.

These determinations were made by measuring the frequency of discharge of nerve impulses from the test receptor, over the last 10 seconds of a 15 second exposure, in response to illuminating it alone and again when it was illuminated together with region A. The difference between the two frequencies is the measure of the inhibition exerted on X by A alone; we designate it $I_{X(A)}$ and have used it as the abscissa of the point to be plotted. The frequency of discharge was next measured when the test receptor was illuminated together with region B; the difference between this frequency and the frequency of the test receptor illuminated alone is designated $I_{X(B)}$. Finally, the frequency of X was measured with A and B illuminated together, yielding $I_{X(A + B)}$. The difference between these last two measurements, $(I_{X(A + B)} - I_{X(B)})$, is the amount of inhibitory effect produced by A and B together in excess of the amount produced by B alone. This difference has been plotted as ordinate (y) at the abscissa already determined. This procedure yielded graphs with coordinates similar to Fig. 1, but with the origin shifted to the point at which both ordinate and abscissa equal the inhibitory effect of B alone (effect of A equal to zero). Regions between which there was no interaction would yield points lying on a line of slope +1, as in Fig. 1 (provided the influence of the test receptor's activity is negligible). This line has been dotted in the graphs we will show.

Fig. 3 shows the results of several experiments of the kind just described; points from a particular experiment are identified by the same symbol. All the points in Fig. 3 fall below the diagonal (dotted) line; *i.e.*, in all cases the total inhibitory effect of A and B acting together was less than the sum of their separate effects. In the experiment designated by the open circles, the points are only slightly below the dotted line; in this experiment the regions A and B were on opposite sides of the test receptor, about 4.0 mm. apart, and, as was the case in the experiment of Fig. 1, evidently interacted very little. The other experiments showed varying degrees of failure of the total effect to equal the sum of the separate effects. For the most part, the degree of such failure could be correlated with the separation on the eye of the regions A and B in the various experiments: the less the separation the farther the points fell below the diagonal line. But, as we shall see, the spatial relations of all three illuminated regions affect the graphs.

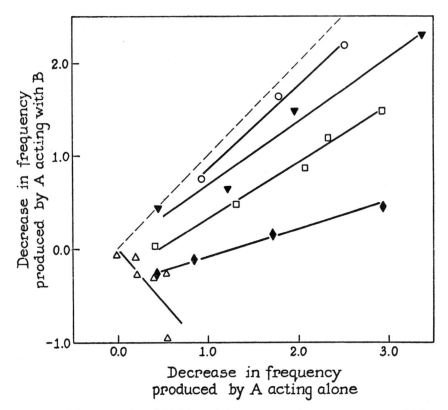

FIG. 3. The summation of inhibitory influences exerted on a test receptor (X) by two groups of receptors at various distances from one another and from X. Each of the graphs was obtained from an experiment on a different preparation. In each case B refers to a spot held at fixed intensity and A refers to a spot illuminated at various intensities. As abscissa is plotted the magnitude of the inhibition (decrease in frequency of response of the test receptor in impulses per second) resulting from illumination of A alone. In the text this quantity is designated $I_{X(A)}$. As ordinate, y, is plotted the change in frequency produced by A when it acted with B; that is, the decrease in frequency produced by illumination of spots A and B together less the decrease produced by illumination of spot B alone. In the text this quantity is designated $(I_{X(A + B)} - I_{X(B)})$.

For each frequency measurement the impulses in the discharges were counted over the last 10 seconds of a 15 second exposure; these measurements were made in duplicate and averaged for each determination of both ordinate and abscissa of each point. The standard error of the determination was of the order of 0.1 impulse per second for each point (see the legend of Fig. 2 in our previous paper for description of the procedure comparable to that used in these experiments).

The upper graph (open circles) was obtained in an experiment in which the two spots A and B were each centered 2 mm. from the test receptor, one on either side.

The results of any one experiment in Fig. 3 are adequately described by a linear relation between the variables that have been used. This relation is a consequence of two factors. The first is the linearity of the inhibitory influence exerted by each receptor as a function of its degree of activity, established in our preceding paper; the second is the simple law of spatial summation of inhibitory influences from more than one receptor, established by the experiment of Fig. 1 and those like it. We will show this in a theoretical section to be given below. We will also show that usually the stronger the interaction between two regions, the greater should be the depression of the line below the diagonal of the graph, and the smaller its slope, as is shown experimentally in Fig. 3.

In one of the experiments of Fig. 3 (points marked by open triangles), region A was located on the opposite side of region B from the test receptor, so far away from the latter that it exerted only slight inhibition on it when acting alone. In this case illumination of A together with B resulted in a decrease instead of an increase in the net inhibitory effect—the ordinates of these points on the graph are all negative. This is a case of disinhibition, discussed in our preceding paper, and is in fact taken from the experiment described in Fig. 6 of that paper. Disinhibition illustrates with especial force the need to consider the mutual interaction of the receptors in analyzing the effects of inhibitory influences in the eye.

Up to this point we have considered only how the inhibition of a test receptor by groups of receptors in its neighborhood is modified by the inhibitory interaction between these groups. We have neglected the influence that

------

A was 1 mm., B 1.5 mm. in diameter. The average value of $I_{X(B)}$ was 2.55. The equation of the line is: $y = 0.903 I_{X(A)} - 0.057$. For the second graph (filled triangles), A and B were on the same side of the test receptor, equidistant from it (centered 1.25 mm. from X, 1.9 mm. apart); they were each 1.75 mm. in diameter. Average $I_{X(B)} = 2.72$. Equation of line: $y = 0.670 I_{X(A)} + 0.043$. For the third graph (open squares) A and B were rectangular patches of light 2.5 mm. long, 0.75 mm. wide long edges parallel, the adjacent edges being 0.2 mm. apart. The test receptor was 0.75 mm. from one end of B, on the prolongation of its center line. Average $I_{X(B)} = 2.72$. Equation of line: $y = 0.588 I_{X(A)} - 0.253$. For the fourth graph (filled diamonds), B was a spot 1.1 mm. in diameter centered 1.0 mm. from the test receptor; A was a rectangular patch (approximately 2 mm. × 3.5 mm.) on the opposite side of B from the test receptor, centered 2 mm. from the center of B. Average $I_{X(B)} = 2.66$. Equation of line: $y = 0.288 I_{X(A)} - 0.359$. The fifth graph (open triangles) was obtained from the experiment described in Fig. 6 of our previous paper (Hartline and Ratliff, 1957). As in the fourth graph, A was on the opposite side of B from the test receptor, but the patches of light were more widely separated. Average $I_{X(B)} = 4.97$. Equation of line: $y = -1.12 I_{X(A)} + 0.05$. All lines were fitted to the points by the method of least squares. For all cases, the frequency of discharge of the test receptor when illuminated alone (e_X) was of the order of 20 impulses per second.

the test receptor itself may have on the activity of these groups, and how this might be reflected in the inhibition they exert. It is true that this influence must have been comparatively small in the experiments we have

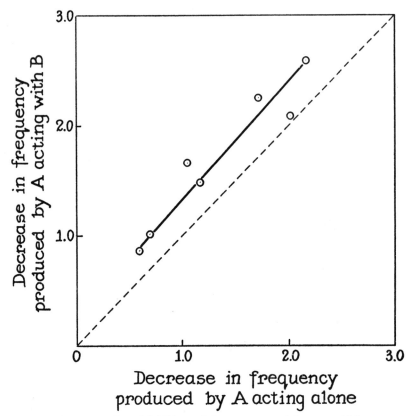

FIG. 4. The summation of inhibitory influences exerted by two widely separated groups of receptors upon a test receptor within a third active group of receptors. Spots A and B were located on either side of the test receptor. They were each approximately 1.0 mm. in diameter and were centered about 2.0 mm. from the test receptor. Unlike the previous experiments, the illumination on the test receptor was not confined to its facet: the spot of light used was about 1.0 mm. in diameter and illuminated some 8 or 9 receptors in addition to the one in the center of the group from which the discharge of impulses was recorded. Abscissae and ordinates as in Fig. 3. The positions of the points above the dotted diagonal reflect the influence of the test receptor group, as discussed in the text. Because of the variability of the points in this experiment the slope of the line that should be drawn through them cannot be determined with precision. The line that has been drawn is in accordance with plausible assumptions concerning the constants of the interacting system as given in the text of the section on Theory. Average $I_{X(B)} = 1.55$. The equation of this line is: $y = 1.13 \ I_{X(A)} + 0.20$.

reported thus far, for the test receptor region was illuminated by a spot of light confined to just that one ommatidium from which impulses were recorded, while the illumination on each of the adjacent regions usually covered 10 to 20 ommatidia. Nevertheless, the test receptor is a member of the interacting system and its influence on the other receptor units must be included in a complete description of this system.

The influences exerted by the test receptor region can be augmented be enlarging the spot of light projected on it, so that several other ommatidia are illuminated in addition to the one from which impulses are recorded. The effects of this group that includes the test receptor are most clearly seen in experiments in which the other two regions, A and B, are widely separated, so that they do not interact with one another. It is easy to predict the result of such an experiment: the activity of the ommatidia in groups A and B will be reduced by the inhibitory action of the group containing the test receptor; consequently the amount of inhibition they in turn exert back on the test receptor group will be less than if no such action took place. Since the activity of the test receptor and the others in its group will be less when both the region A and the region B are illuminated together than when only one of them is illuminated, the receptors in each of these regions will be subject to less inhibition from the test receptor group when they act together than when one or the other of them acts alone. Consequently, the inhibitory effect of A and B together will actually be greater than the sum of their separate effects.

Fig. 4 confirms this expectation; the experimental points fall above the diagonal line of the graph by a significant amount. Likewise, in Fig. 1 some of the points fell above the diagonal of the graph; evidently the test receptor had an effect in this experiment even though we had confined the spot of light to its facet alone. It should be realized, of course, that the test receptor also must have exerted its influences in the other experiments we have described (Fig. 3), affecting the positions and slopes of the lines. The theoretical treatment developed in the next section will clarify and render more exact the understanding of the diverse effects that result from the interaction of all three receptor groups under different experimental conditions.

THEORY

In our preceding paper, we showed that the activity of two interacting receptor units may be described by a pair of simultaneous linear equations:

$$r_A = e_A - [K_{AB} (r_B - r_{AB}^0)]$$
$$r_B = e_B - [K_{BA} (r_A - r_{BA}^0)]$$

(1)

In each equation, the response (r) of the receptor to which that equation applied was put equal to the excitation (e) of the receptor minus a term representing the inhibition exerted on it by the other receptor. This inhibitory term was written in accordance with the experimental findings, as a linear function of the response of the other receptor.

When three receptors (A, B, and X) are active, three simultaneous equations will be required. Each equation will contain two inhibitory terms similar to those just mentioned, combined by simple addition as required by the law of spatial summation that we have established experimentally in the present paper. These equations are:

$$r_A = e_A - [K_{AB} (r_B - r^0_{AB}) + K_{AX} (r_X - r^0_{AX})]$$

$$r_B = e_B - [K_{BX} (r_X - r^0_{BX}) + K_{BA} (r_A - r^0_{BA})]$$ (2)

$$r_X = e_X - [K_{XA} (r_A - r^0_{XA}) + K_{XB} (r_B - r^0_{XB})]$$

In these equations, the notation is that adopted in our preceding paper. The response, r, of a particular receptor unit, designated by an appropriate subscript, is measured by the steady frequency of the discharge of impulses in its optic nerve fiber, elicited by steady illumination of its corneal facet at a specified intensity, under whatever conditions of neighboring illumination may also be specified. The excitation, e, of this unit is defined as the receptor's response to this same intensity when it is illuminated by itself. The subscripts serve to identify the respective receptor units: r_A is the response of ommatidium A, etc. Each inhibitory term is written to express the experimental facts, established in our preceding paper, that for each receptor unit there is a "threshold" frequency (represented by the constant r^0) below which it exerts no inhibition on a particular neighboring unit, and that the magnitude of inhibitory influence it exerts on that particular neighbor is directly proportional to the amount by which its frequency exceeds this threshold. The constant of proportionality, K, in each term is labelled with subscripts to identify the receptor units interacting. These subscripts are ordered to indicate the element acted upon and the element exerting the influence. Thus K_{AB} is the coefficient of the inhibitory action exerted on ommatidium A by ommatidium B.

Unfortunately for the simplicity of the treatment, the threshold constants as well as the Ks must also be labelled so as to distinguish the receptor units involved in the inhibitory action. For it has turned out (experiments not yet published) that the threshold frequency for the action of one receptor on a second is not necessarily the same as the threshold for the action of the first receptor on a third (e.g., $r^0_{BA} \neq r^0_{XA}$), and in our previous paper we showed that thresholds for the mutual inhibition of two receptors are often different for the two directions of action (e.g., $r^0_{AB} \neq r^0_{BA}$).

Equations (2) apply only in the range of conditions for which their solutions yield values of r such that none of the quantities $(r - r^0)$ is less than zero.

The above equations are meant to apply strictly to individual interacting receptor units; however, it is reasonable to extend their meaning to apply to small groups of receptors, such as have been studied in the present experiments. This extension can be made rigorously if it is assumed that every receptor in a given group has the same properties and that each is subject to equal influences from every other member of that group, and furthermore that each receptor within a given group is subject to equal influences from every receptor in any other particular group. Even if the properties of the receptors and the influences exerted are not exactly uniform in this sense, it is plausible to assume that this extension of the equations will yield a useful approximation.

With this extension understood, a response, r, in any equation of a given set refers to the frequency of discharge of a typical receptor in the group specified by the subscript attached to r when that group was illuminated together with the other groups in the given experimental configuration. Similarly an excitation, e, will be understood to refer to the response of a typical receptor in the group specified by the attached subscript when that group was illuminated alone. Each coefficient, K, will be understood to refer to the coefficient of the inhibitory action exerted on each receptor in the group specified by the first subscript of K, by the receptors acting together in the group specified by the second subscript. Thus K_{AB} would be given by the decrease in frequency of a typical receptor in group A per unit increment in frequency of a typical receptor in group B.

In any given configuration of illumination on the receptor mosaic the total inhibition exerted on a receptor in a particular group by the other groups or receptors will be given by one of the expressions in square brackets in the set of equations appropriate to the configuration. It is convenient to designate it by a single term, I, labelled so as to identify the interacting groups. Thus the entire expression in the square brackets of the third equation of (2) will be designated $I_{X(A + B)}$. It represents the total inhibition exerted on the test receptor (one of the group X) by groups A and B acting together. For the measurements in which the test receptor group was illuminated together with A alone, and for those with B alone, two pairs of equations similar to (1) are required, appropriately labelled. The inhibition measured in these two cases will be designated respectively $I_{X(A)}$ and $I_{X(B)}$. It is these quantities, I $(= e - r)$, that are needed in the discussion of the experiments, for they are determined from measurements of frequencies for the uninhibited and inhibited conditions taken in such order as to minimize effects of drift and systematic errors on their averages.

In the experiments we are discussing in this paper each experimental point is obtained from determinations of $I_{X(A)}$, $I_{X(B)}$, and $I_{X(A + B)}$ (see section on Results). The three sets of equations yielding these quantities can be solved for them in terms of the es, the Ks, and the r^0s. The solutions can be combined, and after appropriate eliminations yield $I_{X(A + B)}$ as a linear function of $I_{X(A)}$ and $I_{X(B)}$:

$$I_{X(A+B)} = MI_{X(A)} + NI_{X(B)} + R \tag{3}$$

in which $\qquad M \equiv (1/D) (1 - K_{XA}K_{AX}) (1 - K_{BA}K_{XB}/K_{XA})$

$$N \equiv (1/D) (1 - K_{XB}K_{BX}) (1 - K_{AB}K_{XA}/K_{XB})$$

$$R \equiv (1/D) [K_{BA} (K_{XB} - K_{XA}K_{AB}) (r^0_{BA} - r^0_{XA}) + K_{AB} (K_{XA} - K_{XB}K_{BA}) (r^0_{AB} - r^0_{XB})]$$

$$D \equiv 1 - K_{XA}K_{AX} - K_{XB}K_{BX} - K_{AB}K_{BA} + K_{AX}K_{XB}K_{BA} + K_{XA}K_{BX}K_{AB}$$

In the experiments that were described in Fig. 3, we varied the intensity on only one of the spots of light (A), holding that on B constant, and found it convenient to plot as ordinate (y) the quantity $(I_{X(A + B)} - I_{X(B)})$. This may be described as A's effect in the presence of B. (This practice permits several experiments, for which $I_{X(B)}$ had widely different values, to be represented in a single figure.)

Equation (3) thus accounts for the linearity of the graphs in Fig. 3. The slope and position of each graph yield an experimentally determined value of M and of the intercept y_0. The kind of experiments reported in this paper cannot provide enough information to evaluate separately the six coefficients, K, and the four thresholds, r^0, that occur in equation (3). Therefore, the particular values of these constants that occur in combination in the expressions for M and y_0 may be chosen with considerable latitude, although consideration of the sizes and separations of the interacting groups narrows this choice. We will show, for each experiment in Figs. 3 and 4, that plausible choices of the constants can be made to account for the observed values of the slopes and positions of the graphs. The theory may thus be used to account for the diverse effects obtained by various configurations of interacting groups of receptors. Special cases for which simplifying assumptions can be made will be considered first.

In most experiments the group (X) contained the "test" receptor alone; the influence of a single receptor on larger groups is comparatively small, and may be neglected in a first approximation (K_{AX}, $K_{BX} \cong 0$). To begin with, we may note that if the groups of receptors A and B exert no inhibition on each other ($K_{AB} = K_{BA} = 0$), then $I_{X(A + B)} = I_{X(A)} + I_{X(B)}$. This was essentially the situation in the experiment of Fig. 1, when A and B were on opposite sides of X, too far apart to affect one another.

The consequence of interaction between A and B is clearly seen if we consider a symmetrical configuration in which these groups are of equal size, and are equally distant from X. Because of the symmetry, A and B may usually be assumed to have equal coefficients of action on each other, ($K_{AB} = K_{BA} \equiv \bar{K}$), and on X, ($K_{XA} = K_{XB}$). Equation (3) (neglecting R) then yields $I_{X(A + B)} = \dfrac{1}{1 + \bar{K}} (I_{X(A)} + I_{X(B)})$; the net effect of A and B acting together should thus be less than the sum of their separate effects, as experiments have shown. Moreover, the greater the interaction (the closer A and B are to one another) the greater should be the amount by which the net effect falls below this sum. In the experiments that provided the data for the upper three curves of Fig. 3 the configurations of the illuminated groups were approximately symmetrical. On the assumption that the inhibitory coefficients were indeed symmetrical, the slopes of these lines would be accounted for by values of $\overline{K}$ of 0.11, 0.50, and 0.70 (top to bottom, respectively).

If the influences are not exerted symmetrically by the groups A and B on the test receptor or on each other, the slope M of the line in a plot like Fig. 3 is affected. Thus, if the receptor group on which the intensity is being varied (A) has a smaller coefficient of action on the test receptor than the other group (B) (so that $K_{XB}/K_{XA} > 1$), the slope M may be much reduced, even though the interaction between A and B is only moderate (K_{AB} and K_{BA} small). This was the case in the experiment whose graph in Fig. 3 is next to the bottom (diamonds). The numerical value of the slope of this line can be accounted for by assuming that $K_{AB} = K_{BA} = 0.30$, but that $K_{XB} = 2.5\,K_{XA}$ (since B was closer to X than was A).

A closer consideration of the experiments represented by the upper three graphs of Fig. 3 suggests that in these experiments also the influences were probably not strictly symmetrical. For the uppermost graph (open circles) the spot B was about twice the size of A; if the influences each exerted on the other and on X were in this ratio, the observed value of the slope M could be accounted for by the assumptions $2K_{BA} = K_{AB} = 0.10$; $2K_{XA} = K_{XB}$. For the third graph from the top (squares) A and B were equal in size but B was closer to X than was A, and might be expected to have affected X more strongly than did A. The assumptions $K_{BA} = K_{AB} = 0.27$; $K_{XB} = 1.7\,K_{XA}$ yield the observed value of M. For the second graph from the top (solid triangles) there is some reason to prefer the assumption that the coefficients of the action on X were also unequal even though the geometrical configuration was symmetrical. The assumptions $K_{BA} = K_{AB} = 0.15$; $K_{XB} = 2.3\,K_{XA}$ yield the observed value of M for this experiment.

A sufficiently great inequality of coefficients, with A exerting comparatively little direct influence on X, can even result in a negative slope ($K_{BA}K_{XB}/K_{XA} > 1$), as in the lower graph of Fig. 3 (open triangles). This is the case of disinhibition, which we have already discussed. The set of assumptions $K_{BA} = K_{AB} = 0.30$; $K_{XB} = 6.7\,K_{XA}$ is not implausible and yields the numerical value of M that was observed.

If the inequality of the coefficients of the inhibitory action exerted on the test receptor is in the opposite direction, so that $K_{XA} > K_{XB}$, the slope of the line will be greater than if the coefficients are equal: it can equal or even exceed 1 even though A and B interact ($K_{XB}/K_{XA} < K_{AB}$). We have performed one experiment in which A (the spot whose intensity was varied) was closer to the test receptor than was B, and exerted a stronger inhibition on it. This experiment yielded a line with a slope of 0.97.

To account for the position of each line of Fig. 3, an appropriate value of R (Equation 3) is required. Values of the individual constants that appear in the expression for R may be assumed with some latitude, to yield the value required to fit the data. However, consideration of the known properties of the thresholds of inhibitory effects restricts this choice, and these properties may manifest themselves directly in the experimental results. One example is the graph in Fig. 3 next to the lowest (diamonds). In the experiment that provided the data for this graph, the region A was closer to the region B than to the test receptor. Consequently, it might be expected (on the basis of experiments reported elsewhere, Ratliff and Hartline, 1957) to have reached the threshold of its inhibitory action on B at a lower level of activity than that at which it began to inhibit X. At low levels, therefore, A would first produce an indirect effect on X, releasing it partially from B's inhibition before its direct inhibitory action on X began. The graph should therefore begin at a negative value of y, as is indeed the case. The value of R we have given for this graph is negative (-0.26), reflecting the condition $r_{BA}^0 < r_{XA}^0$ (one may assume $r_{AB}^0 \cong r_{XB}^0$, since B was roughly equidistant from A and X). It should be added that the necessity to find a suitable value of R affected the choice of the particular values of the Ks needed to account for the slope M. Similar considerations applied to the other experiments but the details need not be pursued here, for the principles are better illustrated by more informative experiments in which representative receptor activity is recorded simultaneously from more than one of the interacting groups.

We may now turn to a consideration of the effect that the test receptor itself (or the group X including it) has on these relations. The simplest case to consider is a symmetrical configuration in which the two spots A and B are on opposite sides of the test receptor, too far apart to interact ($K_{AB} = K_{BA} = 0$; from the symmetry, $K_{XA} = K_{XB}$; $K_{AX} = K_{BX}$). Then $M = N = \dfrac{1 - K_{XA}K_{AX}}{1 - 2K_{XA}K_{AX}}$. Thus in this case the slope of the line relating $I_{X(A+B)}$ to $(I_{X(A)} + I_{X(B)})$ is greater than unity: the two regions together produce an inhibitory effect that is greater than the sum of their separate effects, as has already been explained (Fig. 4). The assumptions $K_{AX} = K_{BX} = K_{XA} = K_{XB} = 0.32$; $K_{AB} = 0$, $K_{BA} = 0$, account for the line that has been drawn through the points of Fig. 4. Turning to Fig 1, a reasonable value of $K_{XA} = K_{XB} = 0.5$ would require only the small value of $K_{AX} = K_{BX} = 0.06$ to account for the slope of a line fitted to the points by the method of least squares, which would be slightly greater than 1. It is evident that the effects of the test receptor, though small, probably never are entirely negligible, and must have been present in all the experiments of Fig. 3.

The theory presented in this section is a logical development based on the experiments reported in our previous paper, taken together with the experiments in this paper that demonstrate the additivity of inhibitory influences. These basic experiments dealt with the interaction of carefully isolated single receptor units, or at most with the interaction of small groups of receptors. To extend the theory to larger groups, we assumed a certain uniformity of action among the receptors of the groups. With this assumption the theory is successful in providing a quantitative interpretation of the responses of a "test receptor" subject to influences of two nearby groups of illuminated ommatidia in a variety of configural relations. If correct, the theory should be capable of interpreting fuller experiments than those reported here, such as can be done by measuring the responses of more than one receptor unit. Indeed, simultaneous measurements of the discharges of impulses in three optic nerve fibers, one from each of three small groups of receptors, could furnish a complete illustration of the principles that have been discussed, and should provide a crucial test of the theory. Preliminary attempts have shown that such experiments are feasible.

The establishment of the law of spatial summation of inhibitory influences permits the theory to be extended to describe the activity of any number of interacting elements. The set of simultaneous equations for n interacting receptors may be constructed by writing n equations, each with n-1 inhibitory terms combined by simple addition:

$$r_p = e_p - \sum_{j=1}^{n} K_{pj} (r_j - r_{pj}^0) \qquad \begin{matrix} p = 1, 2, \ldots n \\ j \neq p \\ r_j \lessdot r_{pj}^0 \end{matrix} \qquad (4)$$

The same restrictions apply to this set of equations that have been stated previously: only positive values of e, r, K, and r^0 are permitted; the terms in the summation for which $j = p$ are to be omitted; this set of equations applies only in the range of conditions for which no r is less than the associated r^0 in any term.

DISCUSSION

It is our basic interpretation of the experiments described in this paper that the inhibitory influences exerted on any ommatidium in the lateral eye of *Limulus* by other ommatidia always combine by simple addition. As we have shown, this does not mean that the net inhibitory effect produced by two ommatidia, or two groups of ommatidia, when they act simultaneously on a third, is necessarily equal to the sum of the effects which they each produce when acting alone. Indeed, we have shown that the net effect may range from values greater than the sum of the two separate effects to values less than that of one of the separate effects alone. Such results are entirely consistent with our basic interpretation, and reflect merely the consequences of the mutual interaction of the receptor units.

Such a variety of effects obtained with only a few small groups of interacting receptor units presages the complexity that would be encountered in analyzing the pattern of responses of a large population of interdependent elements. But in principle we now have available the theoretical means for expressing the simultaneous relations describing the activity of the entire population of receptors in the eye, and predicting how their mutual interactions would operate to affect the pattern of optic nerve activity for any configuration of interacting elements. Even when extended to a large number of elements, the theory should remain manageable, thanks to the linearity of the inhibitory terms in the equations, and the simple additive law of combination of the terms; different degrees of interaction are fully expressible by the different values of the inhibitory coefficients and the thresholds for the inhibitory effects.

In the mosaic of receptors that constitutes the sensory layer of the eye, the amount of inhibition exerted mutually between any two single receptor units is less the farther they are apart. We do not yet know the exact form of this dependence of the inhibitory influence on the separation of the interacting elements, or whether it can be expressed in any but statistical terms. Nevertheless, it is clear that this strong dependence of the inhibitory coefficients and the thresholds on distance introduces into the system a geometrical factor that must give to the inhibitory interaction special significance in retinal function. As a consequence, for example, the brightness contrast that retinal inhibition can engender must be accentuated in the neighborhood of sharp gradients and discontinuities of illumination in the retinal image.

Because of the inhibitory interaction and its dependence on the spatial relations of the stimulated elements of the retinal mosaic, the degree of activity of each element is affected by the responses of all the others and by their spatial distribution. The pattern of optic nerve activity is more than a reproduction of the pattern of the various stimulus intensities distributed over the receptor mosaic; it is modified by the inhibitory interaction so as to accentuate various significant features of the configuration of light and shade in the retinal image.

BIBLIOGRAPHY

Hartline, H. K., Wagner, H. G., and Ratliff, F., Inhibition in the eye of *Limulus*, *J. Gen. Physiol.*, 1956, **39**: 651.

Hartline, H. K., and Ratliff, F., Inhibitory interaction of receptor units in the eye of *Limulus*, *J. Gen. Physiol.*, 1957, **40,** 357.

Ratliff, F., and Hartline, H. K., Fields of inhibitory influence of single receptor units in the lateral eye of *Limulus* (abstract), *Science*, 1957, **126,** 1234.

The responses of *Limulus* optic nerve fibers to patterns of illumination on the receptor mosaic *

FLOYD RATLIFF AND H. KEFFER HARTLINE

The Rockefeller Institute

Reprinted from the JOURNAL OF GENERAL PHYSIOLOGY
20 July 1959, Vol. 42, no. 6, pp. 1241–1255

ABSTRACT

The inhibition that is exerted mutually among receptor units (ommatidia) of the compound eye of *Limulus* is less for units widely separated than for those close together. This diminution of inhibition with distance is the resultant of two factors: (1) the threshold of inhibitory action *increases* with increasing distance between the units involved; and (2) the coefficient of inhibitory action *decreases* with increasing distance.

The discharge of nerve impulses from ommatidia at various distances from one another may be described quantitatively by a set of simultaneous linear equations which express the excitatory effects of the illumination on each ommatidium and the inhibitory interactions between each ommatidium and its neighbors. The values of the thresholds and coefficients of inhibitory action, which appear as parameters in these equations, must be determined empirically: their dependence on distance is somewhat irregular and cannot yet be expressed in a~. exact general law. Nevertheless the diminution of inhibitory influences with distance is sufficiently uniform that patterns of neural response generated by various patterns of illumination on the receptor mosaic can be predicted qualitatively. Such predictions have been verified experimentally for two simple patterns of illumination: an abrupt step in intensity, and a simple gradient between two levels of intensity (the so-called Mach pattern). In each case, transitions in the pattern of illumination are accentuated in the corresponding pattern of neural response.

One of the significant features of the pattern of stimulation on the receptor mosaic of a sense organ is the locus of transitions from one level of intensity to another. Such transitions may be accentuated, in the patterns of neural activity generated by the sense organ, by neural interaction among the receptor units which make up the receptor mosaic. For example, in the lateral eye of *Limulus* the receptor units (ommatidia) are interdependent: the discharge of impulses

* This investigation was supported by a research grant (B864) from the National Institute of Neurological Diseases and Blindness, Public Health Service, and by Contract Nonr 1442 (00) with the Office of Naval Research. Reproduction in whole or in part is permitted for any purpose of the United States government.

from any one of them depends not only upon the stimulus to it, but also upon the activity of its neighbors. This interaction is purely inhibitory and is exerted mutually among the receptor units; each inhibits its neighbors and is, in turn, inhibited by them. The response of a receptor unit in the lateral eye of *Limulus* is most effectively inhibited by the illumination of other receptor units close to it; the effectiveness diminishes with increasing distance, although it may extend for several millimeters (Hartline, Wagner, and Ratliff, 1956). As we have briefly reported (Ratliff and Hartline, 1957; and Ratliff, Miller, and Hartline, 1958), the greater the separation between units, the higher are the thresholds and the smaller the inhibitory coefficients of their mutual interaction. It is the purpose of the present paper to describe, in detail, this dependence of the inhibitory action on distance and to demonstrate by experiment some of its consequences for pattern vision.

METHOD

The experiments to be reported are based on the measurement of the frequency of the discharge of nerve impulses in single optic nerve fibers. In each experiment, a lateral eye of an adult *Limulus* was excised with 1 to 2 cm. of optic nerve and mounted in a moist chamber maintained at 17.5°C. Small strands separated from the optic nerve were dissected until only a single active fiber remained in each, as evidenced by the uniformity and regularity of the action potential spikes observed and by the fact that they could be elicited only by illumination of a particular receptor unit (ommatidium). Each such small strand could be placed on a separate pair of wick electrodes connected to its own separate amplifying and recording system. In most of the experiments the frequencies of discharge of impulses in optic nerve fibers from two receptor units, or in some cases three, were measured simultaneously. In a few experiments we observed the discharge from a single receptor unit in response to some pattern of illumination, of a fixed configuration, in various positions on the receptor mosaic. Details of our method have been given in previous papers (Hartline, Wagner, and Ratliff, 1956; Hartline and Ratliff, 1957; and Hartline and Ratliff, 1958). As in those papers, we have confined our attention to the frequency of discharge of impulses that is maintained at a more or less steady level during steady illumination of the eye; the transient changes in frequency that occur during the first second or two after light is turned on or off were excluded from the measurements.

A typical measurement of the inhibitory effect was made as follows. A test receptor was illuminated alone at some fixed intensity for a period of 12 seconds. Beginning 3 seconds after the onset of this illumination the impulses discharged during the next 8 seconds were counted. After a 2 minute interval of rest, to minimize cumulative effects of light adaptation, the test receptor was again illuminated, together with a small group of adjacent receptor units, for 12 seconds. The activity of one of these adjacent units was recorded as representative of the activity of that group. As before, 3 seconds after the onset of illumination the impulses discharged from the test receptor were counted for a period of 8 seconds; simultaneously, the impulses discharged from the receptor in the adjacent group were counted separately. Two minutes later the test receptor was illuminated alone and the impulses discharged from it were counted, again for a period of 8 seconds. The frequency of impulses discharged by the test receptor when it and the neighboring group were illuminated together was substracted from the average of the two frequencies determined when the test receptor was illuminated alone. This difference was taken as the measure of the magnitude of the inhibition exerted upon the test receptor by the neighboring group of receptors. Modifications of this general technique, to suit particular experimental requirements, are described below.

RESULTS

We have analyzed the dependence of the inhibitory action on distance by measuring the inhibition exerted by a small group of receptors on two other receptor units located at different distances from it. The frequency of the discharge of impulses by one of the receptors in this small group (A) was taken as a measure of the level of activity of the whole group, and—in terms of this measure—the threshold and the inhibitory coefficient of the action of this group on the other two receptors (B and C) were determined.

The results of such an experiment are shown in Fig. 1. At low frequencies of discharge, the group of ommatidia (A) exerted no effect on either ommatidium B or ommatidium C. At successively higher frequencies of discharge from the group A, produced by higher intensities of illumination upon it, the threshold of its inhibitory effect on the nearest ommatidium (B) was reached (at 5.1 impulses/sec.), and the magnitude of the effect on this nearby element then increased with a large coefficient (0.17 impulse/sec. decrease in the discharge of B per impulse/sec. discharged in A). The threshold of the effect on the more distant ommatidium (C) was not reached until the frequency of discharge of A was much greater (18 impulses/sec.) and when reached it then increased with a much smaller coefficient (0.07) than did the effect on the nearer ommatidium (B).

Similar results have been obtained in a number of similar experiments, and—as a general rule—we have found that the threshold increases and that the inhibitory coefficient decreases with increasing distance between the unit inhibited and the unit or units inhibiting it. We have found, however, some minor exceptions to this rule. Occasionally the threshold of action was larger, and the inhibitory coefficient smaller, for a nearer element than for a more distant one. Such inversions are not observed when the difference in distance is very great, but they are sufficiently large and occur often enough so that it is apparent that any law relating magnitude of inhibition to distance must be of a statistical nature (see Discussion).

In the above experiment only the inhibitory action of one particular group of receptors (A) on two other receptors (B and C) at different distances from it was determined. In the following experiments we determined the effects of a number of different groups (A_1, A_2, etc.) on two such receptors (B and C) in various spatial configurations. Since it is not an easy technical matter to record from optic nerve fibers arising from each of these several groups we recorded from only the two receptors B and C and compared the effects exerted simul-

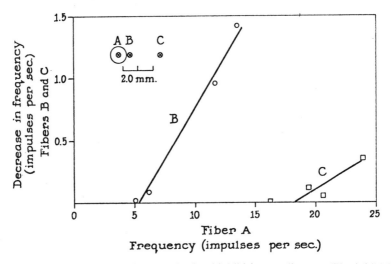

FIG. 1. The dependence of the magnitude of inhibition on distance. The inhibition (measured in terms of decrease in frequency) exerted by a small group of receptors (A) on two other receptors (B and C) is plotted as ordinate. As abscissa is plotted the concurrent frequency of the discharge of impulses of one of the receptors in the group A. The geometrical configuration of the pattern of illumination on the eye is shown in the insert. The locations of the facets of the receptors whose discharges were recorded are indicated by the symbol ⊗. The receptor A was at the center of a group of six or seven receptors illuminated by a spot of light 1 mm. in diameter. The illumina-on B and C was provided by spots of light 0.2 mm. in diameter and of fixed intensity. Measurements were made as described in the section on Method. The effects of the group A on B and on C were determined separately. Each point on the graph B is the average of three separate determinations; the points on the graph C are averages of from two to five separate determinations.

taneously on them by each of the several groups (A_1, A_2, etc.) in succession. It was possible, by this means, to determine the *relative* magnitudes of the inhibitory effects exerted on the two receptors by other groups of receptors at various distances from them without actually measuring the levels of activity of these groups of receptors.

The results of one such experiment are shown in Fig. 2. The group of receptors A_1, located equidistant from the receptor units B and C, exerted equal inhibitory effects on both. The group of receptors in the position A_2, closer to B than to C, exerted larger effects on B than on C. Although the responses of B and C were measured simultaneously, the conditions were such that they did not inhibit one another appreciably (tested by a separate experiment).

The results of a similar but more extensive experiment are shown in Fig. 3. The group of receptors, A_2, symmetrically located with respect to receptor units B and C, exerted nearly equal simultaneous effects upon them. The

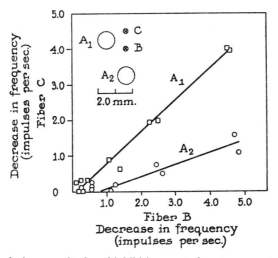

FIG. 2. The relative magnitudes of inhibition exerted on two receptors by a group of receptors equidistant from them, and by another group nearer to one than to the other. Records were obtained of the discharge of impulses from two receptors B and C, elicited by small spots of light 0.2 mm. in diameter and of fixed intensity confined to their facets. A third spot of light 1 mm. in diameter could be placed in either of two positions (A_1 or A_2) relative to B and C, as shown in the insert. In each of these positions the inhibitory effects exerted on B and C were determined simultaneously at various levels of intensity of A. For each point the decrease in the frequency of discharge of B is plotted as abscissa; the simultaneous decrease in frequency of discharge of C is plotted as ordinate.

group A_3, located near B, exerted a large effect on B and at the same time, practically no effect on C. A_1, on the other hand, was close to C and at a considerable distance from B; correspondingly there was a large inhibitory effect on C, and at the same time, a small effect on B.

The two experiments just described yield no direct information about the relation of the magnitude of the inhibitory effect to the level of activity of the receptor units exerting the inhibitory influence; they do show, however, that the relative magnitudes of the inhibitory effects are not the results of chance differences in the properties of the units that happened to have been chosen as test receptors. Since the effect on one unit may be changed relative to the effect on the other simply by changing the location of the inhibiting units, it is evident that these differences in the inhibition are attributable to the different distances between the inhibiting units and the test receptors. Consequently, the degree of inhibitory interaction among any set of receptor units in the lateral eye of *Limulus* must be determined, in part, by the locations of these units, relative to one another, in the receptor mosaic.

Theory —In our previous papers (Hartline and Ratliff, 1957, and Hartline and Ratliff, 1958) we showed that the activity of *n* interacting receptors may be described

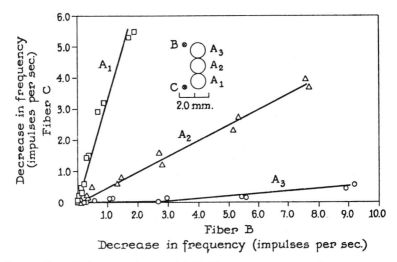

FIG. 3. The relative magnitudes of inhibition exerted on two receptors by other receptors in various positions with respect to them. The decrease in the frequency of discharge of B, for several intensities of A at each of three positions is plotted as abscissa; the simultaneous decrease in frequency of C, at each such position and intensity is plotted as ordinate. Same procedure as for the experiment of Fig. 2.

by a set of simultaneous linear equations, each with $n - 1$ inhibitory terms combined by simple addition:

$$r_p = e_p - \sum_{j=1}^{n} K_{pj}(r_j - r^0_{pj}) \qquad \begin{aligned} & p = 1, 2 \cdots n \\ & j \neq p \end{aligned}$$

The activity of a receptor unit—its response (r)—is measured by the frequency of discharge of impulses in its axon. This response is determined by the excitation (e) supplied by the external stimulus to the receptor, diminished by whatever inhibitory influences may be acting upon the receptor as a result of the activity of neighboring receptors. The excitation of a given receptor is measured by its response when it is illuminated by itself, thus lumping together the physical parameters of the stimulus and the characteristics of the photoexcitatory mechanism of the receptor. In each such equation, the magnitude of the inhibitory influence is given by the summated terms, written in accordance with the experimental findings as a simple linear expression. The "threshold" frequency that must be exceeded before a receptor can exert any inhibition is represented by r^0. It and the "inhibitory coefficient," K, in each term are labelled to identify the direction of the action: r^0_{pj} is the frequency of receptor j at which it begins to inhibit p; K_{pj} is the coefficient of the inhibitory action of receptor j on receptor p. Restrictions on these equations have been described elsewhere (Hartline and Ratliff, 1958).

The theoretical significance of the experiments reported in this paper is in the finding that the diminution of the inhibitory effect with increasing distance, which we observed earlier (Hartline, Wagner, and Ratliff, 1956), may now be ascribed more exactly to the combined effects of increasing thresholds (r^0_{pj}) and decreasing inhibitory coefficients (K_{pj}) which accompany increasing separation of the interacting elements p and j.

Although we can thus conveniently describe the activity of a system of interacting elements without making explicit reference to their relative locations in the receptor mosaic and to the spatial pattern of illumination (since the dependence of the inhibitory influences on distance is implicit in the values of the thresholds and inhibitory coefficients), it is nevertheless clear that the strong dependence of the inhibitory thresholds and coefficients on the separation of the elements introduces a topographic factor which must give to the inhibitory interaction its special significance in retinal function. Any complete description of the spatial characteristics of the inhibitory interaction must, therefore, provide an explicit statement of the relations between these inhibitory parameters and the corresponding distances on the receptor mosaic. At the present time, however, we are not prepared to state these relations in an exact quantitative form (see Discussion).

On the basis of the diminution of the inhibitory interaction with increasing distance one can predict the general form of the patterns of response which will be elicited from the elements of the receptor mosaic by various spatial patterns of illumination. Contrast effects, for example, may be expected to be greatest at or near the boundary between a dimly illuminated region and a brightly illuminated region of the retina. A unit which is within the dimly illuminated region, but which is near this boundary, will be inhibited not only by dimly illuminated neighbors but also by brightly illuminated ones. The total inhibition exerted on it will therefore be greater than that exerted upon other dimly illuminated elements that are farther from the boundary; consequently its frequency of response will be less than theirs. Similarly, a unit within but near the boundary of the brightly illuminated field will have a higher frequency of discharge than other equally illuminated units which are located well within the bright field but which are subject to stronger inhibition since all their immediate neighbors are also brightly illuminated. Thus the differences in the activity of elements on either side of the boundary will be exaggerated and the discontinuity in this pattern of illumination will be accentuated in the pattern of neural response.

The ideal experimental test of these qualitative predictions would be to record simultaneously the discharge of impulses from a great number of receptor units in many different positions with respect to a fixed pattern of illumination on the receptor mosaic. Such a procedure is impractical, so we measured, instead, the discharge of impulses from only one receptor unit near the center of the eye, and shifted the pattern of illumination between measurements so that this one receptor unit assumed successively a number of different positions with respect to the pattern.

The pattern of illumination was provided by focussing on the eye the demagnified image of a transilluminated photographic plate on which the desired

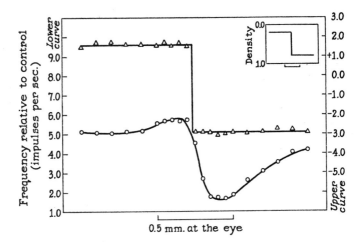

FIG. 4. The discharge of impulses from a single receptor unit in response to a simple "step" pattern of illumination in various positions on the retinal mosaic. The pattern of illumination was rectangular, covering an area 1.65 mm. × 1.65 mm. on the eye. It was obtained by projecting the demagnified image of a photographic plate on the surface of the eye. The insert shows the relative density of the plate along its length as measured, prior to the experiment, by means of a photomultiplier tube in the image plane where the eye was to be placed. The density of the plate was uniform across its entire width at every point. The measurements illustrated were made over the central 1.5 mm. of the image on the eye.

The upper (rectilinear) graph shows the frequency of discharge of the test receptor, when the illumination was occluded from the rest of the eye by a mask with a small aperture, minus the frequency of discharge elicited by a small "control" spot of light of constant intensity also confined to the facet of the test receptor. Scale of ordinate on the right.

The lower (curvilinear) graph is the frequency of discharge from the same test receptor, when the mask was removed and the entire pattern of illumination was projected on the eye in various positions, minus the frequency of discharge elicited

pattern of density had been developed. (This method permits more convenient control of the pattern of stimulation of the receptor mosaic than does the use of real illuminated objects in the visual field.) In the first experiment to be described the plate consisted of two contiguous rectangular areas, one of a uniform high density and the other of a uniform low density. The plate could be moved in a direction perpendicular to the boundary between the two areas, thus its image could be placed in a number of positions on the eye with respect to the ommatidium from which records were being obtained. In one part of the experiment, the entire eye, including the test receptor, was exposed to the pattern of illumination. For comparison, in another part of the same experiment, we exposed the test receptor alone to the same intensities of illumination. To do this, a mask with a small aperture was placed in a fixed position between the movable plate and the eye so that only the light passing through whatever area of the plate was imaged on the test receptor could reach the eye. A second channel of illumination, brought together with the first by means of a combining prism, could provide a second small beam of light of constant intensity, also confined to the facet of this same ommatidium. This provided the stimulus for control measurements with which the two sets of experimental measurements were subsequently compared. (This was necessary because we could not change quickly enough from the masked to the unmasked arrangement to make a direct comparison.)

The stimulus was turned on every 2 minutes for a period of 7.5 seconds. Beginning 2 seconds after the onset of this illumination the nerve impulses

---

by a small "control" spot of light of constant intensity confined to the facet of the receptor. Scale of ordinate on the left.

The image on the eye of the fixed aperture in the mask was made much smaller (0.05 mm. in diameter) than the facet of the test receptor (approximately 0.2 mm. in diameter) in order to insure that no light would reach adjacent receptors. Thus the absolute amount of light entering the receptor under this condition was considerably less than when the entire pattern was projected in the same position on the eye and the entire aperture of the test receptor was filled. (Use of the full aperture also produced a certain amount of "smoothing" of the lower curve.) In each case the intensity of the "control" spot of illumination was adjusted to produce a frequency of discharge in approximately the same range as the test measurements. The average control frequency for the upper curve was 12.8 impulses per second; for the lower curve, 9.0 impulses per second. The positions of the graphs on the ordinate were arbitrarily fixed by locating the point on the extreme right of the curvilinear graph one impulse per second below the corresponding point on the rectilinear graph. Such a displacement is in accordance with the common observation that, due to the inhibitory interaction, the frequency of discharge in a single optic nerve fiber is smaller when a large area of the eye is illuminated than when a small spot is used that just fills the entire aperture of that fiber's ommatidium. The principal point of comparison is the *form* of the curves rather than the absolute magnitudes of the frequencies.

discharged during the next 5 seconds were counted. Measurements were made of the discharge in response to the control stimulus of fixed intensity followed 2 minutes later by measurements of the discharge in response to light passing

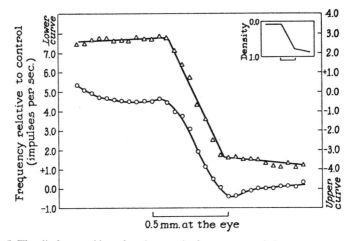

FIG. 5. The discharge of impulses from a single receptor unit in response to a pattern of illumination on the eye containing a simple gradient of intensity. The insert shows the relative density along the length of the photographic plate whose demagnified image (2.0 mm. × 2.0 mm.) was projected on the eye to provide the pattern of illumination. The density of the plate was uniform across its entire width at every point. The measurements illustrated were made over the central 1.5 mm. of the image on the eye.

The upper (rectilinear) graph shows the frequency of discharge of the test receptor, when the illumination was occluded from the rest of the eye, minus the frequency of discharge elicited by a small control spot of light of constant intensity confined to the facet of the test receptor. Scale of ordinate on the right.

The lower (curvilinear) graph is the frequency of discharge from the same test receptor, when the entire pattern was projected on the eye in various positions, minus the frequency of discharge elicited by a small control spot of light of constant intensity confined to the facet of the test receptor. Scale of ordinate on the left. Same procedure as for the experiment of Fig. 4. Average control frequency for the upper curve was 15.2 impulses per second; for the lower curve, 9.0 impulses per second.

through the plate with the mask in place followed again 2 minutes later by another control measurement. Following each such set of measurements the plate was shifted to a new position, with respect to the eye and the mask, at which the next set of measurements was made, and so on. The measurements made with the mask in place, and plotted relative to the control measurements, are analogous to physical measurements which might be made by scanning the plate with a densitometer of small aperture; that is, they show the response of a single photoreceptor unit to the illumination transmitted through the various portions of the plate. The resulting graph (Fig. 4, upper curve) is a rectilinear one closely resembling the distribution of density on the plate.

Next the mask was removed from the optical system so that the image of the entire plate was projected on the eye, illuminating all of the receptor mosaic in the neighborhood of the test receptor. The plate was again shifted in steps as before so that, in effect, the test receptor and its neighbors "scanned" in successive steps across the image of the plate. Since the response of the receptor unit was not, in this latter case, determined solely by the illumination on it, but also by the activity of the neighboring units, the response was no longer a simple function of the intensity of illumination on that receptor. As predicted above, the transition from the one level of intensity to the other was accentuated, with a maximum and a minimum appearing in the pattern of the response as a result of the inhibitory interaction among the neighboring receptors (Fig. 4, lower curve).

Particularly interesting among contrast phenomena are the dark and light bands seen at the edges of the penumbra of a shadow cast by an object placed in front of an extended source (first studied by Mach, 1865). To duplicate such a pattern in our experiments, a photographic plate was prepared, similar to the one described above, but with a more gradual linear gradation of density between the regions of uniform high and uniform low density. When the pattern of illumination thus obtained was moved across the eye of *Limulus*, utilizing the same general method as in the experiment just described, maxima and minima were found in the response of the test receptor even though there are no such maxima and minima in the distribution of intensity across the eye (Fig. 5). The explanation of this follows the same line of argument as that given above for a sharp step in the intensity.

DISCUSSION

It is evident from the results of the present experiments that each receptor unit exerts a field of inhibitory influence around itself. The extent and the magnitude of the field of inhibitory influence exerted by a particular ommatidium are not fixed, but depend upon the level of activity of that ommatidium. At low levels of activity only the thresholds of inhibitory action on nearby receptor units are reached; at higher levels more distant receptors are affected. Once the thresholds have been reached the magnitude of the inhibition exerted by an ommatidium on others near it increases rapidly with increases in its level of activity, while the inhibition it exerts on more distant ones increases only slowly.

This dependence of inhibition on distance between any two receptors in the mosaic cannot be expressed by simple mathematical functions relating the Ks and r^0s on the one hand to the separation between receptors on the other. One reason is that the thresholds and coefficients of the interaction between two receptor units are not always identical for both directions of action (Hartline and Ratliff, 1957). Furthermore, the inhibitory influences do not diminish uniformly in all directions from the receptors exerting the influence; they fall off more abruptly in dorso-ventral directions than in antero-posterior directions (Hartline, Wagner, and Ratliff, 1956). Also, in exceptional cases the threshold of action on a more distant element may be smaller, and the inhibitory coefficient greater than for a somewhat nearer element. However, such variability might be expected when the relationships are expressed in terms of direct distances across the surface of the receptor mosaic, for such distances are not necessarily equal to the distances over which the inhibitory influences may actually be transmitted in the plexus of lateral interconnections among the receptors. Such variability is relatively minor and yet it cannot be neglected; the general law relating inhibition to distance will ultimately have to be formulated in statistical terms. At present we do not have a sufficiently large number of measurements covering a wide variety of locations, directions, and distances such as will be required to formulate exactly such a law.

The physiological bases for the diminution of the inhibitory influence with distance are unknown. One possibility is that the effect may diminish with distance simply because of a decrement in transmission over the individual fibers of the plexus of lateral interconnections. Another possibility is that the effect may be transmitted without true decrement in the individual fibers and branchlets of the plexus, but that the magnitude of the total effect exerted on particular receptors may be greater the larger the number of active branchlets of the lateral connections terminating in neuropile around axons of the affected receptor units. Then if the branchlets of the lateral interconnections were more profuse near the units from which they arise than they are some distance away, the magnitude of the inhibition would diminish with distance even though conducted without decrement in the individual fibers. Since we have not, as yet, been able to record electrical activity in these lateral interconnections, nor to trace all their ramifications, any discussion of the matter must be speculative. (For details of the structure of the ommatidium, see Miller, 1957 and 1958; for the structure of the plexus and neuropile, see Ratliff, Miller, and Hartline, 1958.)

The physiological significance of the dependence of the inhibition on distance may be readily understood. Since intensely stimulated receptors exert stronger inhibition on less intensely stimulated ones than the latter exert on the former, and since these effects diminish with distance, contrast will be most strongly enhanced near the borders of differently stimulated regions of the receptor mosaic.

These consequences of inhibitory interaction could, in principle, be derived in exact mathematical form from the set of equations given above, once the law has been formulated giving the values of the Ks and r^0s as functions of distance between receptors. Until this formulation has been made, however, any mathematical model must remain largely speculative. Nevertheless, any hypothetical law that postulates the Ks decreasing and the r^0s increasing with increasing receptor separation (which experiment shows to be a fact, on the average) will predict, for appropriate intensity distributions similar to those we have used, maxima and minima in the patterns of receptor response that will be like those we have observed in the actual experiments of Figs. 4 and 5. We have investigated a few speculative models in which the inhibition was assumed to decrease with distance according to various laws. The set of simultaneous equations was written to describe the responses of receptors in a mosaic exposed to a step-function distribution of intensity; iterated substitution of successive numerical approximations converged to solutions that showed maxima and minima bordering the intensity step, resembling those in Fig. 4. The spatial distribution of the calculated "responses" did not differ greatly from that yielded by the theoretical model proposed by Fry (1948) to account for Mach's bands in human vision. Fry's postulates do not assume *mutual* inhibition of receptors. A mathematical model postulated by Taylor (1956) also yields maxima and minima of activity bordering a step-transition in intensity of stimulus to a mosaic of neural elements. His model provides for mutual interaction, and is similar to the one we have found by experiment to describe interaction in the *Limulus* eye. It differs in making no provision for varying thresholds of the inhibitory action, and the cases considered did not include graded inhibitory coefficients. These exercises are instructive, but it would be premature to try to fit the experimental data of this paper by a quantitative theory at the present time.

In human vision the pronounced brightness contrast near borders, the marked bright and dark lines known as Mach's bands (Mach, 1865), and the differing depressions of visual thresholds by adjacent illumination at different distances (Beitel, 1936) may all be explained by postulating such inhibitory influences in the visual pathways which decrease with distance (Fry, 1948). In addition to these "first order" effects, the phenomenon of *disinhibition* which we reported earlier (Hartline and Ratliff, 1957) also has its explanation in the dependence of the inhibitory effect on distance. Receptor units too far from another to affect it directly may nevertheless exert an indirect influence on it by inhibiting the activity of other intermediate receptors which do exert direct inhibitory influences upon it. Whether the disinhibition we have observed in the lateral eye of *Limulus* has a counterpart in human vision is not known. It seems probable that since some inhibitory effects in the human eye do diminish with distance the proper experimental arrangement might reveal disinhibition as well. It is also probable that various features of the organization of receptive fields in the vertebrate eye (Hartline, 1940; Kuffler, 1953; Barlow, 1953; Barlow,

FitzHugh, and Kuffler, 1957) are partly brought about by inhibitory influences which diminish with distance.

Similar inhibitory mechanisms are undoubtedly important in other sensory systems. For example, the possible role of inhibitory interaction as a "sharpening" mechanism in the auditory system was pointed out many years ago (Békésy, 1928); and, more recently, such inhibition has actually been observed in the auditory pathways (Galambos and Davis, 1944). In addition, contrast effects—similar to Mach's bands in vision—have been observed in skin sensations (Békésy, 1958).

In every instance cited it appears that the strong dependence of the inhibitory interaction on the separation of the elements in the receptor mosaic introduces a topographic factor which gives the inhibition its special significance in sensory function. As a consequence of this dependence, certain features of the spatial pattern of stimulation are enhanced in the pattern of sensory nerve response at the expense of accuracy of less significant information about intensity of stimulation on each receptor.

BIBLIOGRAPHY

Barlow, H. B., Summation and inhibition in the frog's retina, *J. Physiol.*, 1953, **119**, 69.

Barlow, H. B., FitzHugh, R., and Kuffler, S. W., Change of organization in the receptive fields of the cat's retina during dark adaptation, *J. Physiol.*, 1957, **137**, 338.

Beitel, R. J., Inhibition of threshold excitation in the human eye, *J. Gen. Psychol.*, 1936, **14**, 31.

Békésy, G. von, Zur Theorie des Hörens. Die Schwingungsform der Basilarmembran, *Physik. Z.*, 1928, **29**, 793.

Békésy, G. von, Funneling in the nervous system and its role in loudness and sensation intensity on the skin, *J. Acous. Soc. Am.*, 1958, **30**, 399.

Fry, G. A., Mechanisms subserving simultaneous brightness contrast, *Am. J. Optom. and Arch. Am. Acad. Optom.*, 1948, **25**, 162.

Galambos, R., and Davis, H., Inhibition of activity in single auditory nerve fibers by acoustic stimulation, *J. Neurophysiol.*, 1944, **7**, 287.

Hartline, H. K., The receptive fields of optic nerve fibers, *Am. J. Physiol.*, 1940, **130**, 690.

Hartline, H. K., and Ratliff, F., Inhibitory interaction of receptor units in the eye of *Limulus*, *J. Gen. Physiol.*, 1957, **40**, 357.

Hartline, H. K., and Ratliff, F., Spatial summation of inhibitory influences in the eye of *Limulus*, and the mutual interaction of receptor units, *J. Gen. Physiol.*, 1958, **41**, 1049.

Hartline, H. K., Wagner, H. G., and Ratliff, F., Inhibition in the eye of *Limulus*, *J. Gen. Physiol.*, 1956, **39**, 651.

Kuffler, S. W., Discharge patterns and functional organization of mammalian retina, *J. Neurophysiol.*, 1953, **16**, 37.

Mach, E., Über die Wirkung der räumlichen Verteilung des Lichtreizes auf die Netzhaut. I. *Sitzungsber. math.-naturwissensch. Cl., Wien,* 1865, II, **52,** 303.

Miller, W. H., Morphology of the ommatidia of the compound eye of *Limulus, J. Biophysic. and Biochem. Cytol.,* 1957, **3,** 421.

Miller, W. H., Fine structure of some invertebrate photoreceptors, *Ann. New York Acad. Sc.,* 1958, **74,** 204.

Ratliff, F., and Hartline, H. K., Fields of inhibitory influence of single receptor units in the lateral eye of *Limulus, Science,* 1957, **126,** 1234.

Ratliff, F., Miller, W. H., and Hartline, H. K., Neural interaction in the eye and the integration of receptor activity, *Ann. New York Acad. Sc.,* 1958, **74,** 210.

Taylor, W. K., Electrical simulation of some nervous system functional activities, *in* Information Theory, (C. Cherry, editor), New York, Academic Press, Inc., 1956, 314–327.

Mechanism of lateral inhibition in eye of *Limulus*[1]

TSUNEO TOMITA

Department of Physiology, Keio University School of Medicine.
Shinjuku-ku, Tokyo, Japan

Reprinted from JOURNAL OF NEUROPHYSIOLOGY
Vol. 21, no. 5, pp. 419–429, September 1958

IT HAS BEEN REPORTED by Hartline *et al.* (8, 9) that in the compound lateral eye of the horseshoe crab, *Limulus polyphemus*, activity in a single optic nerve fiber can be elicited by illumination of one, and only one, ommatidium but that, nevertheless, the discharge of impulses thus elicited is slowed by illumination of other regions of the eye. This inhibitory action is mediated by a plexus of nerve fibers that lies just back of the ommatidia. The present paper will deal with aspects of the mechanism underlying this lateral inhibition. Three experimental approaches were employed in the investigation of the inhibitory process. (i) Observations were made of inhibitory effects exerted on an ommatidium by antidromic stimulation of optic nerve fibers other than the one from that ommatidium. (ii) The amplitude of the action potential of a nerve fiber measured at a point close to its origin in the ommatidium was investigated as a function of inhibitory influences exerted as a result of activity in neighboring fibers. The amplitude of the action potential may be assumed to reflect the state of polarization of the nerve fiber. (iii) Measurements were made of the threshold to an electric shock delivered to a nerve fiber near its origin in the ommatidium; the effect of inhibition on this threshold was determined.

METHODS

The experiments described in this paper were performed on compound (lateral) eyes of *Limulus* excised with 1 cm. or more of optic nerve attached. Responses of single ommatidia were measured by recording the discharge of impulses in their nerve fibers. This was done by one of two methods. (i) With the eye intact, single fibers were dissected from the optic nerve and placed on wick-lead-off electrodes. (ii) After sectioning the eye with a sharp razor blade, in a plane perpendicular to the surface of the cornea, one of the ommatidia exposed near the cut surface was selected and a microelectrode pressed, within less than 0.5 mm. of its proximal end, on the small bundle of nerve fibers that can be seen emerging from it. This electrode, essentially the same as that described by Tomita and Funaishi (14), was a silver wire 40 μ in diameter, sharpened electrolytically in dilute nitric acid and sealed in a glass pipette by a microflame. The ommatidium selected for study was stimulated by a small (0.2 mm.) spot of light focussed on its corneal facet. Other ommatidia in its neighborhood could be stimulated independently of it by illuminating them by a large spot of light; the inhibitory effects of such activity of neighboring elements were measured

---

[1] The experimental work was done in the Thomas C. Jenkins Laboratory of Biophysics, Johns Hopkins University, Baltimore, Md., with the support of Contract ONR248 (11) (H. K. Hartline, Responsible Investigator) between the Johns Hopkins University and the Office of Naval Research. Reproduction in whole or in part is permitted for any purpose of the United States Government.

by the slowing produced in the rate of discharge of nerve impulses from the ommatidium under observation.

Antidromic nerve impulses were elicited by electrical stimulation of the stump of the optic nerve that had been removed with the eye. The whole nerve or a large bundle dissected from it was placed over a pair of electrodes and stimulated by repetitive monophasic electrical shocks (pulse duration 0.1–0.5 msec.), the strength and frequency of which could be varied. The nerve bundles could be chosen to include or exclude the fiber arising in the ommatidium whose responses were under observation.

The optical system, the timers for regulating the period of stimulation, and the recording system have been described by Hartline and McDonald (7). The experiments were carried out at 17.5°C.

RESULTS

Inhibition of impulse discharge of a single optic nerve fiber by antidromic volleys in rest of fibers. Volleys of antidromic impulses evoked in the optic nerve were found to reduce the frequency of the sensory discharge from an illuminated ommatidium, when the fibers stimulated antidromically did not include the one from that ommatidium. The slowing of the sensory discharge was very similar to the inhibition produced by illumination of other ommatidia in the neighborhood of the one whose sensory responses were under observation. An example is shown in Fig. 1. The top record shows the inhibition produced by illumination of neighboring ommatidia. The middle and bottom records show the slowing that resulted from supramaximal antidromic stimulation of all of the optic nerve fibers except a small bundle containing the fiber from the ommatidium whose responses to light were being recorded. This small bundle was on the recording electrodes; the eye

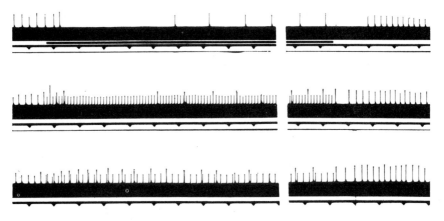

Fig. 1. Inhibition of sensory discharge in single optic nerve fiber by illumination of nearby ommatidia and by antidromic volleys in other optic nerve fibers. Top record: During steady state of impulse discharge in fiber, elicited by illumination of its ommatidium, nearby ommatidia were illuminated for period marked by black line. Middle record: Inhibition of activity of same fiber by antidromic volleys at 42/sec. in the other optic nerve fibers. Small spikes in record were due to physical spread of potentials of antidromic impulses in nerve trunk to lead-off electrodes; they indicate duration of antidromic stimulation. Bottom record: Antidromic volleys of 20/sec. Time marking: 0.2 sec.

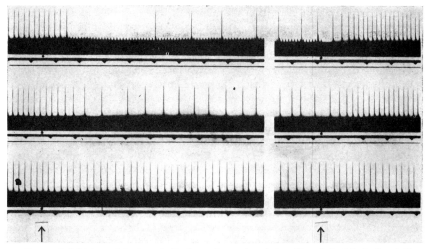

Fig. 2. Inhibition of single unit discharge by various intensities of electrical stimulation to optic nerve fibers with a fixed frequency (40/sec.). Onset and termination of stimulation are marked by dots in each record above arrows. Relative intensity of stimulation: For top record, 2.00 times threshold; for middle, 1.25 times threshold; for bottom, slightly above threshold. Time marking: 0.2 sec.

was intact. For the middle record the frequency of the antidromic stimulation was high and the slowing of the sensory discharge was pronounced. For the bottom record the frequency of the antidromic stimulation was lower, and the inhibition of the discharge was less marked. Thus the inhibitory effect produced by antidromic stimulation is graded: the higher the frequency of the antidromic volleys, the greater the degree of inhibition; however, no inhibition was seen at frequencies below 10/sec.

The records in Fig. 2 were obtained on the same preparation as in Fig. 1 with the rate of antidromic stimulation fixed but with different intensities of submaximal electrical pulses. For the top record of Fig. 2 the stimulus strength was high. For the middle record the intensity of the stimulus was somewhat lower and for the bottom record it was only slightly above threshold. As the number of fibers contributing to each volley was increased, the inhibitory effect increased. It is clear from the records in Figs. 1 and 2 that the inhibition of a given ommatidium was stronger the greater the total number of antidromic pulses per unit of time in the nerve fibers from the rest of the ommatidia in the eye.

The inhibitory effects of antidromic impulses set up in optic nerve fibers other than the one from the ommatidium whose sensory discharge is under observation thus resemble closely the inhibitory effects produced by illumination of ommatidia other than the one under observation. It has been shown (9) that the sensory discharge from an ommatidium is inhibited to a greater degree by increasing the intensity of illumination in neighboring ommatidia (thus increasing the frequency of discharge from each of them) and by increasing the number of neighboring ommatidia illuminated. Correspondingly, the present experiments have shown that the sensory discharge from an ommatidium is inhibited to a greater degree both by increased frequency of antidromic volleys and by increasing the number of optic nerve fibers participating in each volley. Thus it is thought reasonable to assume that the lateral inhibitory effect is caused by impulses in parallel fibers from other ommatidia no matter whether they are orthodromic or antidromic. A fact which may be worthy of noticing in this connection is that the inhibition produced by a steady train of antidromic volleys starts with a deep initial drop in frequency (cf. Figs. 1 and 2), and is similar to that produced by illuminating nearby receptors. There is no doubt that the inhibition by illumination reflects to some extent the pattern of discharge of illuminated receptors which are known to discharge more vigorously at the beginning of illumination. However, this is not the only cause of the strong initial inhibitory transient as evidenced by the fact that it is also produced by a steady train of antidromic volleys. Evidently, the inhibitory effect itself tends to "adapt."

It was stated by Hartline *et al.* (9), that the after-discharge of a strongly excited ommatidium is inhibited by illumination of nearby receptors. After-discharge is also inhibited by antidromic volleys in the nerve fibers other than the one from which the activity is being recorded. When an ommatidium was briefly exposed to strong light, yielding an after-discharge, antidromic stimulation of the nerve fibers from the other ommatidia caused marked slowing of this after-discharge.

It is important to know whether antidromic impulses evoked in the optic nerve penetrate the plexus all the way to the ommatidia. To determine this the eye was cut with a razor and the microelectrode was placed on a bundle of nerve fibers where it emerged from an ommatidium, as described in the section on Methods. Antidromic impulses were evoked by electrical stimulation of a bundle of optic nerve fibers that contained the one from the ommatidium under observation. These impulses were found to reach the origin of the nerve fiber where it emerged from the ommatidium with a correspondence of one shock to one impulse provided the fiber was undamaged throughout its course. (In the same experiment it was shown that orthodromic impulses, initiated by stimulation of the ommatidium by light, also had a one-to-one correspondence when recorded in the fiber both by the microelectrode close to the ommatidium and in the optic nerve proximal to the plexus.) These results, obtained in several experiments, show that the antidromic impulses set up in the optic nerve proximal to the plexus reach the ommatidia from which the nerve fibers take origin. Conduction through the plexus region of the eye can take place in either direction; there are no one-way synapses in the direct path of the optic nerve fibers.

With the same kind of preparation further observations were made on lateral inhibition. It was found that a discharge of impulses produced by illumination of an ommatidium was inhibited to an appreciable degree by antidromic stimulation of the entire optic nerve including the fiber from that ommatidium, even when the intensity of the shocks was adjusted to be just subliminal for the appearance of antidromic impulses in the fiber under the microelectrode. Obviously the inhibition was brought about by the activity of some other fibers that must have had lower thresholds than the one from the ommatidium under observation. The character of the inhibition was substantially the same, whether the impulses were recorded with a microelectrode on a fiber immediately behind an ommatidium, or with electrodes on the same fiber in the optic nerve at a point far behind the plexus. This finding suggests that the lateral inhibition is the result of suppression of the impulse generating mechanism near the origin of the fiber, a conclusion drawn by Hartline *et al.* (9) from similar experiments.

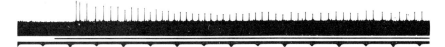

FIG. 3. Activity of single optic nerve fiber in response to illumination. Recording was made from point close to origin of fiber in its ommatidium by means of an extracellular microelectrode. Note decrease in spike height during course of illumination. Time marking: 0.2 sec.

Change in size of impulses in nerve fibers near their origin accompanying excitation and inhibition. When a nerve fiber response was recorded at a point close to an ommatidium with a microelectrode, a decrease in the spike height, similar to that observed by Katz (10) on the muscle spindle afferent fiber, occurred during illumination of the eye. As illustrated in Fig. 3, larger spikes at the beginning were followed by spikes gradually decreasing in height. The spike height at the steady state after a long illumination depended on the light intensity. With a very strong illumination, the impulses often dwindled into the noise level, and reappeared either when the light intensity was decreased or when the discharge was laterally inhibited. These changes in the spike height may be considered to be the result of depolarization and repolarization of the membrane of the optic nerve fiber at its origin in the ommatidium. An objection to this conclusion, however, is that the frequency of the impulses changed in the course of the excitation and the inhibition. This objection was overcome by pacing the impulses by antidromic stimulation of the bundle of fibers that included the one from the ommatidium under observation. The pace of the impulses remained unchanged at a rate determined by the antidromic shocks, whenever the illumination on the ommatidium produced a rate of discharge that was not higher than the rate of antidromic stimulation. Illumination of the ommatidium at such intensities, during steady antidromic stimulation, then elicited no extra impulses, but did produce a decrease in the height of the spikes recorded by the micro-

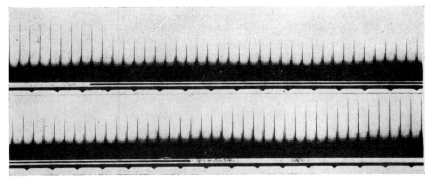

FIG. 4. Decrease in size of antidromic impulses following onset of illumination (black line in white band above time marks) and its recovery after cessation of illumination. Impulses recorded by an extracellular microelectrode on nerve fiber at point close to ommatidium of its origin. Time marking: 0.2 sec.

electrode. Figure 4 illustrates this effect. The rate of the antidromic stimulation was 15/sec. Decrease in the spike height by illumination and recovery to the initial height after cessation of the illumination are evident. Figure 5 is a plot of spike height against time obtained from similar records in two other experiments. The time course of the decrease in spike height during illumination and the time course of the recovery to the initial height after turning off the light were similar and nearly exponential, the time constant being 0.5–0.7 sec. It was noted that no overshoot was observed during excitation and recovery phases.

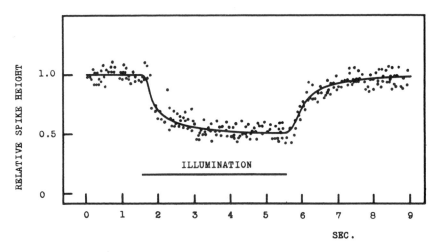

FIG. 5. Plot of spike heights of antidromic impulses (at 15/sec.) in nerve fiber at point close to its origin. From two series of records obtained from preparation different from that providing Fig. 4.

The above observation directed our interest to find out how the spike height at a steady state during steady illumination was influenced by lateral inhibition. By synchronizing the sweep of the oscilloscope beam with the stimulation, so that each of the antidromic impulses appeared at the same place on the screen, a slight increase in spike height was detected during illumination of nearby ommatidia, but the change seemed insignificant compared with the variability of the apparent spike heights due to noise. An attempt was made to substitute antidromic inhibitory volleys for the illumination of nearby ommatidia to avoid the effect of stray light, but the arrangement and the procedure were too complicated and the attempts failed. (However, cf. the next section.) Accordingly, the procedure was changed as follows. During steady illumination of an ommatidium the entire optic nerve including the fiber from that ommatidium was stimulated electrically at the same rate as that of the discharge elicited by illumination. The orthodromic impulses in the fiber were then replaced by antidromic ones without changing the rate of impulses. The effect of change in the rate of impulses upon their size was thus eliminated. In addition, the fiber received the inhibitory effect by the antidromic impulses simultaneously set up in the rest of fibers in the optic nerve. The height of the antidromic impulses in the fiber was then measured at a point close to its ommatidium, using a microelectrode as before. Although the results were not as clear as had been hoped, in some favorable cases a significant increase in spike height was observed during antidromic stimulation. Figure 6 was plotted from one such case.

From the above observations, it is inferred that, at the origin of the optic nerve fiber, a depolarization occurs in association with excitation and repolarization occurs with lateral inhibition. Further evidence supporting this view will be presented in the next section.

Effect of subliminal illumination and of antidromic inhibitory volleys upon electrical excitability of nerve fiber near its origin. It was thought that, if the optic nerve fiber was really depolarized at its origin by illumination and hyperpolarized by lateral inhibition, the threshold value of electrical stimulation of the fiber at a point close to its origin in the ommatidium would change accordingly. This idea was tested by the arrangement in the inset of Fig. 7. A single fiber originating in one of the superficial ommatidia along the cut edge of the eye was isolated from the rest of the fibers in the optic nerve. The lateral connections in the plexus were kept intact. A Ringer-filled capillary employed as a stimulating electrode was applied to this fiber at a point immediately behind the ommatidium. It was fixed at the position where the threshold to electrical stimulation was minimal. The threshold in darkness was determined, and this value was compared with that obtained during a subliminal illumination.

A distinct lowering of the threshold to single electrical shocks was observed at the onset of subliminal illumination, and the threshold remained low as long as the illumination continued. When a subliminal illumination was added to subliminal repetitive electrical shocks, summation occurred between them and repetitive impulses paced by the electrical shocks were seen

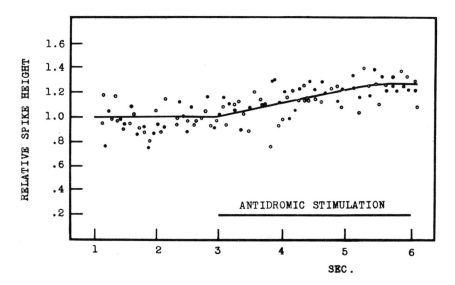

FIG. 6. Relative increase in impulse size as a result of antidromic inhibitory volleys in whole optic nerve (including nerve fiber from ommatidium under observation). Recording by means of an extracellular microelectrode on nerve fiber near its origin in ommatidium. Two series of records, differentiated from each other by dots and circles, were used for plot.

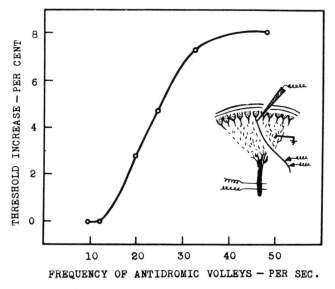

FIG. 7. Increase in threshold to electrical stimulation of nerve fiber at point close to its origin caused by various frequencies of antidromic inhibitory volleys in optic nerve. Threshold was measured with no light upon ommatidium.

on the oscilloscope screen. In the experiments in which the intensity of illumination was adjusted to be just subliminal by itself, the responses to the repetitive shocks did not disappear immediately after the light was turned off. An impulse continued to appear in response to each electrical shock for 1 or 2 sec. after the cessation of illumination. In such cases, a gradual increase in the latent period was observed until the final abrupt cessation of the response. The time course of the prolongation of the latency suggested a close relation to the time course of the change in the spike height after the cessation of illumination shown in Fig. 5.

To test the lateral inhibition, similar experiments were performed in the dark. The effect of antidromic inhibitory volleys upon the threshold to electrical stimulation applied to the fiber at a point just back of the ommatidium was measured. Figure 7 shows the elevation of the threshold by various frequencies of antidromic inhibitory volleys. The effect was almost nil when the frequency of the volleys was below 10/sec. and, as the frequency was raised, the threshold was elevated to a maximum at around 50/sec. The threshold shift was relatively small, but it was measured with a far greater accuracy compared with the change in the spike height.

DISCUSSION

From the experiments described above, it may be concluded that the lateral inhibition competes with excitation by repolarizing the membrane of the nerve fiber at its origin, where it has been depolarized by illumination. Even in darkness, a hyperpolarization may be considered to accompany lateral inhibition, since the threshold of the fiber to electrical stimulation is elevated by antidromic inhibitory volleys. In this regard, the lateral inhibition resembles inhibition in other structures. For example, Brock *et al.* (1) showed that the motoneuron is depolarized by excitatory volleys and hyperpolarized by inhibitory volleys, and, when excitatory and inhibitory volleys reach the motoneuron at the same time or after a short interval, there occurs interaction between the two opposite electrical events in the motoneuron membrane. The mechanism was further studied by Coombs *et al.* (2, 3, 4) from the ionic standpoint. Eyzaguirre and Kuffler (5, 6) and Kuffler and Eyzaguirre (11) revealed a similar mechanism of excitation and inhibition in crustacean stretch sensory cells.

In the eye of *Limulus*, however, the repolarizing effect of a single inhibitory volley appears to be very small. Appreciable effects are produced only by inhibitory volleys repeated at more than 10 times per sec. and then only after an appreciable latency. Even with the repetition of inhibitory volleys, the total effect appears not to be very strong. First, antidromic inhibitory volleys did not yield any detectable change in the ommatidial action potential that was produced by illumination and recorded with a pair of wick electrodes, one placed on the cornea, the other on the nerve bundle emerging from the ommatidium. Second, the change in spike height during lateral inhibition was small. As already mentioned, the curve in Fig. 6 showing a discernible spike height change during lateral inhibition represents one of the most favorable cases and in many other cases the increase in spike height was not clear.

In two preceding papers dealing with excitatory processes (12, 13), it was suggested that the site of impulse initiation is a little distance from the origin of the ommatidial action potential. The implication was that these two loci are electrically connected through relatively high resistance and so the site of impulse initiation receives only a fraction of the change of the ommatidial action potential at its origin. Therefore, if the inhibitory action opposes the ommatidial action potential not at its origin but at the region of the impulse initiation, the action, even if insufficient to change the ommatidial action potential as recorded in the above mentioned manner, might still be strong enough to suppress depolarization due to a function of the ommatidial action potential at the region of impulse initiation. With regard to the change in spike height it is important to notice that, in the motoneuron and also in the crustacean stretch sensory cell, the hyperpolarization due to inhibition has been found to be related to an increase of the membrane conductance to certain ions. If this is also the case in the eye of *Limulus*, the spike height that is actually recorded during lateral inhibition will be smaller than that predicted from a simple increase in the membrane potential level not accompanied by increase in the membrane conductance. Naturally, increase in membrane conductance means increase in the short-circuiting effect upon spike potentials. For more accurate estimation of the electrical events accompanying lateral inhibition, therefore, direct measurement of the membrane potential change with intracellular microelectrodes is considered to be indispensable.

SUMMARY

1. In the lateral eye of *Limulus*, the activity of a single optic nerve fiber elicited by a spot of light on its ommatidium was inhibited by antidromic impulses in the remaining optic nerve fibers (antidromic inhibitory volleys) in a manner similar to the lateral inhibition produced by illuminating nearby ommatidia. The after-discharge which was often observed in response to strong illumination was also inhibited by such antidromic inhibitory volleys.

2. With an extracellular microelectrode placed on a nerve fiber at a point close to its ommatidium, impulses were recorded when the ommatidium was illuminated. The size of the impulses showed a decrease in the course of steady illumination. When laterally inhibited while the illumination continued, the impulses increased again in height.

3. With the same placement of a microelectrode as above, antidromic impulses set up by repetitive stimulation of a proximal part of the optic nerve were found to reach the ommatidium with a correspondence of one shock to one impulse. The antidromic impulses thus recorded showed a decrease in size, when the ommatidium was illuminated with an intensity not strong enough to elicit any extra impulses, and they regained their full size after the light was turned off. The time courses of the changes in spike height

during and after illumination were similar and were exponential, the time constant being 0.5–0.7 sec. Antidromic inhibitory volleys appeared to augment the spike height of the antidromically paced impulses which had been made smaller by illumination.

4. The effects of subliminal illumination and of antidromic inhibitory volleys on the threshold to electrical stimulation of a nerve fiber at a point close to its origin were investigated. The threshold in the presence of subliminal illumination was lower than in darkness. The threshold in the dark was elevated by antidromic inhibitory volleys.

5. Resemblance of the mechanism of lateral inhibition in the eye of *Limulus* to inhibitory processes in other structures is discussed.

ACKNOWLEDGMENTS

I wish to express my most sincere appreciation to Dr. H. K. Hartline for making available the facilities of his laboratory, for his direction through the experiments and for his valuable criticisms of the results. I am also indebted to him and to Dr. W. H. Miller for assistance in preparing the manuscript. In addition I wish to thank Dr. E. F. MacNichol, Jr., for his assistance in some of the experiments.

REFERENCES

1. Brock, L. G., Coombs, J. S., and Eccles, J. C. The recording of potentials from motoneurones with an intracellular electrode. *J. Physiol.*, 1952, *117*: 431–460.
2. Coombs, J. S., Eccles, J. C., and Fatt, P. The specific ionic conductances and the ionic movements across the motoneuronal membrane that produce the inhibitory postsynaptic potential. *J. Physiol.*, 1955, *130*: 326–373.
3. Coombs, J. S., Eccles, J. C., and Fatt, P. Excitatory synaptic action in motoneurones. *J. Physiol.*, 1955, *130*: 374–395.
4. Coombs, J. S., Eccles, J. C., and Fatt, P. The inhibitory suppression of reflex discharges from motoneurones. *J. Physiol.*, 1955, *130*: 396–413.
5. Eyzaguirre, C. and Kuffler, S. W. Processes of excitation in the dendrites and in the soma of single isolated sensory nerve cells of the lobster and crayfish. *J. gen. Physiol.*, 1955, *39*: 87–119.
6. Eyzaguirre, C. and Kuffler, S. W. Further study of soma, dendrite, and axon excitation in single neurons. *J. gen. Physiol.*, 1955, *39*: 121–153.
7. Hartline, H. K. and McDonald, P. R. Light and dark adaptation of single photoreceptor elements in the eye of *Limulus*. *J. cell. comp. Physiol.*, 1947, *30*: 225–253.
8. Hartline, H. K., Wagner, H. G., and MacNichol, E. F. The peripheral origin of nervous activity in the visual system. *Cold Spr. Harb. Symp. quant. Biol.*, 1952, *17*: 125–141.
9. Hartline, H. K., Wagner, H. G., and Ratliff, F. Inhibition in the eye of *Limulus*. *J. gen. Physiol.*, 1956, *39*: 651–673.
10. Katz, B. Depolarization of sensory terminals and the initiation of impulses in the muscle spindle. *J. Physiol.*, 1950, *111*: 261–282.
11. Kuffler, S. W. and Eyzaguirre, C. Synaptic inhibition in an isolated nerve cell. *J. gen. Physiol.*, 1955, *39*: 155–184.
12. Tomita, T. The nature of action potentials in the lateral eye of the horseshoe crab as revealed by simultaneous intra- and extracellular recording. *Jap. J. Physiol.*, 1956, *6*: 327–340.
13. Tomita, T. Peripheral mechanism of nervous activity in lateral eye of horseshoe crab. *J. Neurophysiol.*, 1957, *20*: 245–254.
14. Tomita, T. and Funaishi, A. Studies on intraretinal action potential with low-resistance microelectrode. *J. Neurophysiol.*, 1952, *15*: 75–84.

Interaction of excitation and inhibition in the eccentric cell in the eye of *Limulus*

RICHARD L. PURPLE[1] AND FREDERICK A. DODGE[2]

Department of Physiology, University of Minnesota Medical School, Minneapolis, Minnesota,[1] *The Rockefeller Institute, New York, New York*[2]

Reprinted from COLD SPRING HARBOR SYMPOSIA ON QUANTITATIVE BIOLOGY, Vol. XXX, 1965

INTRODUCTION

To understand data processing by a nervous system, a neurophysiologist wants to know how the individual neurons work and how they are inter-connected. His ultimate goal is to obtain a quantitative specification of how information is utilized by the animal. To reduce a complex nervous system to manageable proportions the neurophysiologist often attempts to isolate quasi-independent subsystems. This approach gives some hope of being able to control the input and to obtain a quantitative measure of the output.

One of the simplest visual subsystems appears to be the excised lateral eye of the horseshoe crab, *Limulus*. This eye consists of a coarse, two-dimensional array of uniform photoreceptors, the ommatidia, and this arrangement permits a precise specification of the visual input. There is a one-to-one correspondence between the ommatidia and the fibers which conduct propagated impulses in the optic nerve, and thus the output directly represents the activity of the functional units. However, this simple system is not just a group of transducers and their data links. We know from the work of Hartline and his colleagues that significant processing of the visual data takes place via interaction among the units, and that this interaction is purely inhibitory.

Hartline and Ratliff (1957) have formulated quantitatively the steady-state input–output relations of the lateral eye. Their model consists of a set of linear, algebraic equations in which the output frequency of an ommatidium is given by the difference between two terms: excitation, which is dependent only upon illumination of this omma-tidium; and inhibition, which is dependent only upon the output frequency of other ommatidia.

The study which we are reporting was undertaken to elucidate the cellular mechanisms underlying the Hartline–Ratliff equations. This

345

was particularly simple in the *Limulus* eye because the integration of excitation and inhibition in each ommatidium takes place on one neuron, the eccentric cell. Our goal was to formulate an electrical equivalent circuit model of the eccentric cell, sufficiently detailed to provide a quantitative interpretation of electrical signals generated by that cell when it is integrating both excitatory and inhibitory effects.

In formulating this model, it has been necessary to take into account some of the anatomical information about the lateral nerve plexus which, at present, has received little emphasis. These details are more or less evident in the first figure (Fig. 1), which summarizes our current concepts of the eccentric cell anatomy. This is a composite sketch in which the dimensions for the dendrite, cell body, and axon-proper were scaled from histological cross-sections of a cell which we had impaled with a micropipette and electrophoretically stained after having taken our electrical measurements. The collateral branches and neuropile are schematic only, and are intended to portray the types of collaterals and the location of the neuropile with respect to the eccentric cell axon.

The first point that we would like to note is that many small axon collaterals branch from the axon of the eccentric cell along the axon-hillock region. From our own and from unpublished observations of Dr. Miller (personal com.), these collaterals are about one micron or less in diameter, and we estimate that at least fifty of them branch off before the first region of neuropile is encountered in the lateral plexus. Within the neuropile, the collateral branches are devoid of Schwann cell membranes and are filled with many presumed synaptic vesicles. The neuropile, then, is the most likely site across which inhibitory interaction occurs.

The second point, which has generally not been noted, is that all the areas of neuropile are closely apposed to an axon of an eccentric cell. In fact, electron micrographs typically show that at a neuropile a short collateral from the adjacent eccentric cell axon enters the neuropile and branches profusely where it interdigitates with the collaterals that are contributed by other ommatidia.

How the above points on structure correlate with the elements of our electrical model is illustrated in Fig. 2, which shows two abstractions of the eccentric cell. The upper diagram abstracts the essential structural elements of the cell, and the lower diagram shows the simplest equivalent circuit that has satisfied our goal in interpreting the simultaneous operation of both excitation and inhibition in the eccentric cell. Excitation occurs most probably at the dendrite, and the process of excitation is represented in the equivalent circuit as a fixed electromotive force in

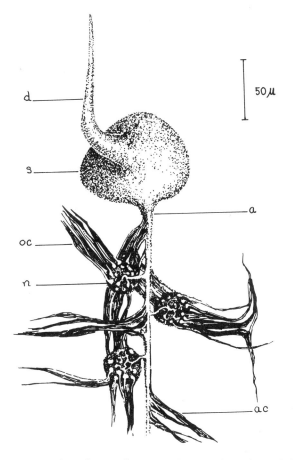

Fig. 1. Schematic illustration of a *Limulus* eccentric cell. Dimensions of the dendrite (d), soma (s), and main stem of the axon (a) are based on histological sections. The axon collaterals (ac) and neuropile (n) are diagramatic and based on electron micrographs by Miller (1957 and unpublished). Collateral branches (oc) are from other cells in the eye.

series with a variable conductance. The soma of the eccentric cell appears to be composed of passive membrane. It is, therefore, considered as a lumped resistance in the model. The initial portion of the axon and the numerous collateral branches which are spun from it before the neuropile is encountered, similarly are considered to have passive electrical properties, and we represent this portion of the cell as a cable structure interposed between the soma and the neuropile. Inhibition at the neuropile may be represented by the two-element circuit, a fixed electromotive force and a variable conductance. The inhibitory conductance is activated by lateral inhibition, which depends upon impulses in neighboring eccentric cells; and by a second pathway, which depends upon impulse activity within the axon of the cell itself, and is thus termed 'self-inhibition'. Completing the diagrams in Fig. 2, we have the rest of the axon and other collaterals below the area of neuropile which may be represented in the resting state as a cable-like structure, but which is also capable of producing regenerative propagated spike impulses. We have labeled this the spike transducing region of the axon.

To gain quantitative information about the elements of the model we employed a bridge technique (Purple, 1964), which enables simultaneous measurements of resistance and potential changes with a single intracellular pipette. In the operation of this bridge, we applied square steps of current of sufficient duration to charge the membrane capacitance to a steady value, thereby measuring the sum of the resistive components of the pipette and cell. The resistance of the pipette was then determined by employing high-frequency pulses for which the impedance of the cell was negligible, and the cell resistance was de-

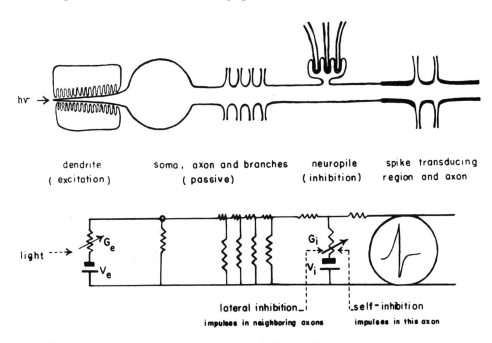

Fig. 2. Two abstractions of the eccentric cell. Upper diagram is a scheme of essential structural elements, lower diagram is the equivalent circuit based upon the structure.

termined by the difference in the two measurements. Furthermore, use of high-frequency pulses showed that the measurements of the slow conductance changes associated with activity were not perturbed by resistance changes of the pipette.

THE FUNCTIONAL ELEMENTS

In examining the main functional elements of the eccentric cell, we first directed our attention to the resting properties. With the micro-pipette in the cell soma, the resting resistance of a cell was typically 8 Mohms, with the values measured ranging from 5–10 Mohms. To interpret this effective cell resistance we cannot neglect the complex structure of the axon and its branches. We have assumed that in the resting state the membrane has essentially uniform characteristics, and we have applied the extended cable theory of Rall (1959, 1960, and 1962) to the anatomical structure of the cell. We use the measurement of the resting resistance and the surface area of the soma, which is typically about 3×10^{-4}cm^2, in conjunction with the geometry of the axon and its collaterals. Although the number and length of the collaterals are not precisely known, any reasonable set of branching models yields the estimate that the resistance of the axonal system to ground, as observed from the soma, is one-fourth to one-sixth that of the soma and dendrite. These values give an estimate for the specific transverse resistance of the membrane of 9000 ohm cm^2.

Two important implications can be drawn from a consideration of these cable properties. The first is that the distributed nature of the dendritic resistance can be neglected in the electrical analog model where we may treat the dendrite electrically as an integral part of the cell soma. Secondly, the distributed nature of the branches along the axon cannot be neglected. In this portion of the model, then, we include elements which represent the internal series resistance of the axon and the effective shunts to ground of the axon collaterals. This network is formally equivalent to a uniform cable.

An important parameter of the model will be the length of the euqivalent cable between the soma, where our pipettes were located, and the sites of inhibition and impulse initiation. The equivalent cable length (λ) must be expected to cause considerable attenuation of those signals which are generated in the axon and recorded at the soma.

Considering the excitatory elements, we have confirmed the measurements of Fuortes (1959) and of Rushton (1959), by measuring directly the conductance changes which are associated with depolarization of the cell induced by light. There is a linear relation between decrease in cell resistance and depolarization, and this gives a value for the excitatory equilibrium potential of approximately zero transmembrane potential – that is, about 50 mv depolarized from the resting potential.

The process of lateral inhibition can be studied in isolation by means of antidromic stimulation of axons from other ommatidia. As shown by Tomita (1958), antidromic stimulation produces lateral inhibition that is in most respects similar to lateral inhibition induced by light. In addition, antidromic stimulation provides us with a means of controlling the

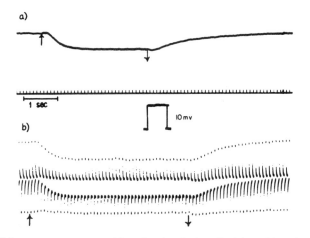

Fig. 3. Inhibitory responses to antidromic stimulation. In (a) antidromic stimulation of 30 impulse/sec was applied between the arrows. In (b) the same stimulus was applied with the bridge circuit operating. The steady-state portions of the lower pulses trace the potential change, and the separation of the traces chart the conductance increase. The pulse transients result from the charging and discharging of the cellular membrane capacitance. Calibration records are for both (a) and (b).

intensity of the inhibition, and of eliminating the effects of scattered light.

As examined with an intracellular pipette, there is a hyperpolarization of the membrane during lateral inhibition which is accompanied by an increase in membrane conductance. This is illustrated in Fig. 3. The upper record of Fig. 3 shows the hyperpolarization of the resting membrane when the optic nerve was stimulated at 30 impulse/sec. In the lower record, separation of the steady-state portions of the bridge measures the conductance increase associated with the hyperpolarization. That the measured decrease in resistance is strictly proportional to the inhibitory hyperpolarization is shown in curves (a) and (c) in Fig. 4. In the figure the ordinate gives the fractional decrease in

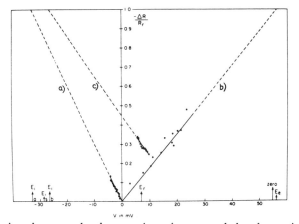

Fig. 4. Relations between the decrease in resistance and the change in membrane potential of an eccentric cell under different conditions of excitation and inhibition. The ordinate is the fractional decrease in cell resistance, and the abscissa is the change in membrane potential relative to the resting level. (The cell was hyperpolarized during measurements to allow for measurements of the excitatory conductance changes without the interference of excessive spiking. E_r is the true resting potential. Zero is the ground potential relative to the V scale and E_e is the extrapolated equilibrium potential for excitation. E_a is the apparent equilibrium potential from curve a and E_b is the apparent equilibrium potential from curve c.) E_s is the apparent equilibrium potential for 'self-inhibition' obtained from data which was not plotted in this figure.

resistance of the cell, and the abscissa is the potential change in mv, relative to the resting potential. The data for curve (a) were taken from a cell driven by antidromic stimulation alone. Curve (b) illustrates the linear relation between the decrease in resistance and depolarization during excitation by light, and curve (c) was from data in which the cell was first depolarized to a steady value using light, and antidromic stimulation was then applied.

Extrapolating the linear relations of either excitation or inhibition in Fig. 4 to where the fractional decrease in resistance is complete gives, in principle, the equilibrium potential for the process. This measure for the excitatory process was, as has been mentioned, about 50 mv deplorized relative to the resting level. In the case of excitation this is a valid measure because the excitatory process may be considered electrically to act directly on the soma. Extrapolation of the inhibitory relation gives an apparent equilibrium potential for that process. We qualify this as an apparent equilibrium potential because we must consider the effect of the electrical separation between the site of recording and the site of inhibition.

Figure 5 illustrates the relation predicted by the equivalent circuit model when inhibition is represented by a fixed electromotive force and a variable conductance applied at different distances along the axon. For curve (a) the inhibitory elements were applied directly to the soma of the model. If the inhibitory conductance is increased to infinity the fractional change in resistance is complete and the final potential is the true inhibitory equilibrium potential. However, if the inhibitory site is applied at 0.2λ from the soma, as in (b), then an infinite increase in

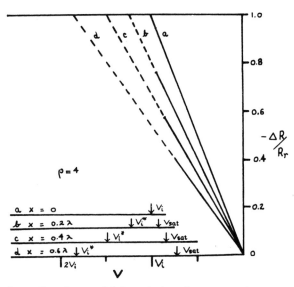

Fig. 5. Predictions of analog model for relations between resistance and potential changes. Ordinate is the fractional decrease in resistance measured from the soma, and the abscissa is the change in potential relative to the equilibrium potential for inhibition. ρ equals 4 is the ratio of the axon and somal input conductances used in constructing the model.

inhibitory conductance does not decrease the somal resistance completely, and the potential change saturates at a value less than the true equilibrium: this is given by the solid portion of (b). Extrapolation of the curve – the dashed line – yields an apparent equilibrium potential for inhibition which is greater than the true value. As we make the site of inhibition more remote from the soma, as in curves (c) and (d), the discrepancy between the saturation of inhibitory potential and the apparent equilibrium potential becomes greater.

In an experiment, of course, it is impossible to obtain an infinite inhibitory conductance, but we can estimate the saturation of the inhibitory potential indirectly. If we assume that the inhibitory conductance change is proportional to the frequency of antidromic impulses, then the expected relation between the potential change and frequency is hyperbolic, and the saturation potential is given by the asymptote of this hyperbola. The saturation potential estimated by this procedure and the apparent equilibrium potential are sufficient to determine the separation of the inhibitory site from the soma, and also the true equilibrium potential for inhibition. The results from four preparations which have been analyzed in this manner yielded an electrical separation which ranged from 0.4λ to 0.6λ, and a true equilibrium potential in the range of 10–17 mv negative to the resting potential.

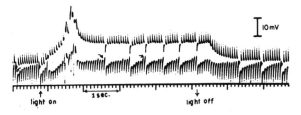

Fig. 6. Bridge records of 'self-inhibitory' conductance increase following spikes. The small arrows illustrate the time of occurrence of three of the spikes on the record. The steady-state portions of the lower pulses trace the depolarization induced by the stimulus, and the separation of the traces indicates the conductance increase.

While studying the conductance changes of light-induced excitation, we found, in addition to a general increase in conductance, a transient increase which occurred after each spike fired by the cell. This phenomenon is illustrated in Fig. 6. It should be noted that this transient increase in conductance is inhibitory, in the sense that there is a hyperpolarization of the membrane associated with it, which should act to decrease the frequency of firing of the cell.

If an eccentric cell is stimulated by a step of constant current, the instantaneous frequency response declines exponentially from an initial high value to a steady-state which is one-third to one-half of the initial frequency. This observation was first made by MacNichol (1956) and was later studied by Fuortes and Mantegazzini (1962), Fuortes and Poggio (1963), and Stevens (1963, 1964). Stevens' study showed that the decline in frequency was not due to the process of accommodation as we understand it in peripheral nerve, since the frequency changes were not dependent upon membrane potential (Hodgkin and Huxley, 1952). Stevens therefore proposed that the phenomenon responsible for this exponential frequency decline resulted from a temporal summation of synaptic inhibitory potentials which he termed 'self-inhibition'. He developed a formal model for this inhibitory action which adequately explained the temporal changes in frequency observed by stimulating the eccentric cell with various wave-forms of current.

We have extended the evidence for this 'self-inhibitory' mechanism by showing that both the conductance and potential changes following a spike sum in a manner expected of a synaptic mechanism, as illustrated in Fig. 7. In this experiment the cell was stimulated by brief

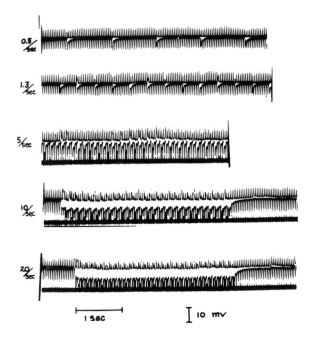

Fig. 7. Summation of 'self-inhibitory' potential and conductance changes as revealed by bridge records. Time and voltage calibration apply to all the responses illustrated. The depolarizing current pulse used to initiate each of the spikes was 1 msec in duration.

current pulses at various frequencies. From such data we determined that this process has the same linear relation between decrease in resistance and change in potential as does lateral inhibition and, hence, has the same equilibrium potential as lateral inhibition. Following each spike the unit 'self-inhibitory' conductance change has a peak value at the site of inhibition of 5×10^{-9} mho, and this declines exponentially with a time constant of typically 500 msec.

The final element in the model is the spike transducing region. Concerning the site of impulse initiation, many investigators have noted that the spikes recorded from the cell soma do not overshoot zero potential and that they undergo severe attenuation when the cell is depolarized by light. The postulate that the excitatory conductance change attenuates the spikes requires that they be generated at some site in the axon considerably remote from the cell-soma. With an analog model similar to the one we have presented, but which included the membrane capacitance, we have found the most likely site of spike initiation to lie between 0.5λ and 0.8λ from the soma; that is, at or beyond the site of inhibitory action on the model.

Furthermore, for considering interactions of excitation and inhibition we need a relation between depolarization and impulse frequency, once threshold has been reached. For this, we have used a single-valued linear relationship of 3.2 impulse/sec/mv depolarization at the site of impulse initiation. This is equivalent to roughly 2 impulse/sec/mv depolarization at the soma, which is about that found experimentally by Fuortes and Poggio (1963) between initial spike frequencies produced by steps of depolarizing current.

PREDICTIONS OF THE MODEL

Typical values for the parameters of the model have been determined experimentally, then, by studying each of the elements in isolation as far as this has been possible. We can now examine some of the predictions of the model.

According to Stevens' theoretical treatment, the interaction between self-inhibition and a constant depolarizing current should cause an exponential decline in frequency over a considerable range of stimulus intensities. By programming the model with a step of current at its soma we obtained the results illustrated in Fig. 8. In the left-hand column are records of depolarization at the soma. The vertical lines simply mark the time of occurrence of each spike. In the right-hand column are plotted the corresponding instantaneous frequencies. As predicted, the initial frequency declines exponentially to a steady-state which is little more than one-third the initial frequency. The time constant of the decline in frequency is 280 msec, which is half as long as the time constant of the unit of self-inhibitory conductance. This latter result and the predicted responses all agree well with experimental observations.

Many investigators have observed that inhibitory potential changes measured at the soma of the eccentric cell are disproportionately small compared to the effect on frequency of firing. The lower plot in Fig. 9

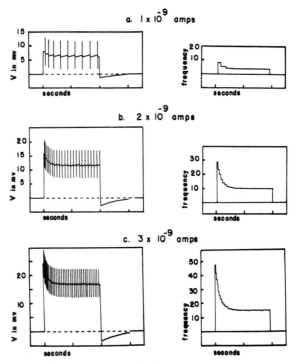

Fig. 8. Predictions of the analog model for responses induced by a depolarizing current injected at the soma. See text for explanation of the records.

illustrates this phenomenon. The solid line relates the steady-state frequencies obtained by illuminating a single facet at various intensities. At the highest steady-state frequency the cell was then progressively inhibited by increasing the frequency of antidromic stimulation, as shown by the open circles. It is immediately apparent that the reduction in frequency is disproportionately large compared to the membrane repolarization. Such an effect, it has been argued, can only be accounted for if the site of inhibitory action is remote from the cell soma, and close to the region of spike generation. Indeed, if both excitation and inhibition were applied at the soma, one would expect the two lines to superimpose. The upper graph is the prediction of our model. This predicted relation is quite sensitive to the value assigned to the electrical separation of the soma and neuropile. In this calculation, this was 0.5λ, and the agreement increased our confidence in this value which had been estimated from the conductance measurements.

Experiments show that a constant input of lateral inhibition depresses the spike frequency from a test ommatidium by an absolute number of

impulse/sec, no matter what the original firing rate of the test ommatidium. This 'constant decrement effect' is of fundamental importance
to the form of the Hartline–Ratliff equations (Hartline, Wagner, and

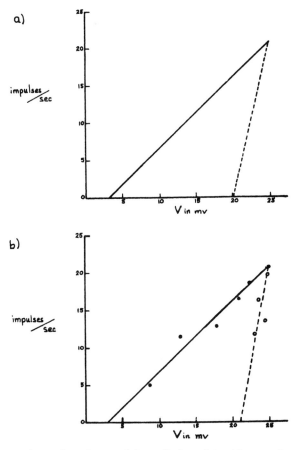

Fig. 9. Comparison of analog model predictions (a) with experimental measurements (b), for the relation between steady-state frequency and depolarization at the
soma. In (b) the dark circles were obtained by using only light stimuli of increasing
intensities, and the open circles then were obtained by inhibiting the cell with increasing frequencies of antidromic stimulation.

Ratliff, 1956), for it shows that lateral inhibition depends upon the
frequency of the inhibiting fibers, and not upon the firing frequency of
the fiber being inhibited.

Figure 10 illustrates both the experimental basis of the constant
decrement effect and the predictions of the model for this effect. The
lower graph is from Hartline, Wagner, and Ratliff (1956). The ordinate

is the decrease in steady-state frequency of the 'test' receptor, and the abscissa is the relative light intensities exciting the test receptor. The five solid lines chart the decrease in frequency produced by five different light intensities illuminating the inhibitory region. For each intensity of the inhibitory light an approximately constant number of impulse/sec are subtracted from the response of the test cell throughout the range of light intensities used to excite it.

The upper graph in Fig. 10 is the response of the model when the appropriate conductance changes were used to simulate excitation and inhibition. The conductance changes spanned the physiological ranges which we have measured in eccentric cells. Comparison of the model responses with the experimental data from actual cells shows that there is good qualitative agreement.

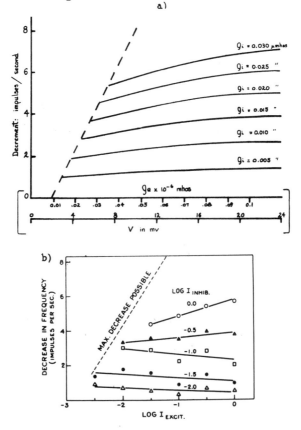

Fig. 10. Comparison of the predictions of the analog model (a) with experimental measurements (b) of the constant decrement effect. (b) is taken from Hartline, Wagner, and Ratliff (1956). See text for explanation of the figure.

As a final test of the model, we have examined the temporal interaction between an excitatory light stimulus and self-inhibition. If a small spot of light is directed upon a single ommatidium, the eccentric cell undergoes a rapid transient depolarization which usually decays rather smoothly to a maintained steady-state value. The frequency response of the cell, however, undergoes an initial transient which typically undershoots the final steady-state frequency in the manner illustrated by the records in the lower portion of Fig. 11. This under-

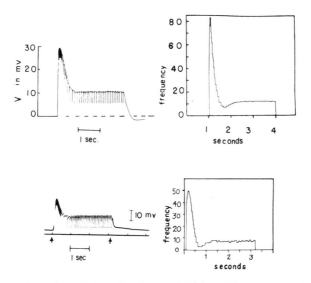

Fig. 11. Comparison of prediction of analog model (above) for a response to a constant light intensity with the response actually measured from an eccentric cell (below). The left-hand records are the potential changes, and the right-hand figures give the instantaneous frequencies of the respective responses.

shoot has commonly been referred to as the 'silent period'. The lower left record of Fig. 11 shows that the depolarization is actually greater during the silent period than in the steady-state. The upper response in Fig. 11 is the prediction of the model when the excitatory drive is a rapid increase of the excitatory conductance which subsequently declines exponentially to a steady-state. This conductance change has temporal characteristics that approximate those observed experimentally. The predicted response demonstrates qualitatively the essential features of the experimental record, in that the average potential at the soma declines monotonically, whereas the frequency shows pronounced undershoot.

CONCLUSION

These examples have demonstrated that the proposed model provides an adequate interpretation of the electrical signals recorded in an eccentric cell when both excitation and inhibition operate on it concurrently. We would wish to extend the model to predict the interaction of several ommatidia. However, at present we lack precise specifications for the kinetics of the excitatory conductance changes and for the spatial dependence of the inhibitory conductance changes. Nevertheless, we can offer this study of the special properties conferred on the eccentric cell by its particular structure as an illustration of a more general rule that the separation of synaptic sites on a neuron may play an important role in the integration of incoming signals and in the consequent output of the cell.

ACKNOWLEDGMENTS

This work was supported in part by United States Public Health Service grant number NB 00864 and in part by Public Health Service grant number NB 05756-01.

The authors wish to express their appreciation to Dr. H. K. Hartline, Dr. William H. Miller, and Dr. Floyd Ratliff for their help throughout the course of this work. The major portion of the research was carried out in Dr. Hartline's laboratory, and he and his colleagues did much to make the research possible.

REFERENCES

Fuortes, M. G. F. (1959), 'Initiation of impulses in visual cells of *Limulus*', *J. Physiol.*, **148**, 14–28.

Fuortes, M. G. F., and Mantegazzini, F. (1962), 'Interpretation of the repetitive firing of nerve cells', *J. Gen. Physiol.*, **45**, 1163–1179.

Fuortes, M. G. F., and Poggio, G. F. (1963), 'Transient responses to sudden illumination in cells of the eye in *Limulus*', *J. Gen. Physiol.*, **46**, 435–452.

Hartline, H. K., and Ratliff, F. (1957), 'Inhibitory interaction of receptor units in the eye of *Limulus*', *J. Gen. Physiol.*, **40**, 357–376.

Hartline, H. K., Wagner, H. G. and Ratliff, F. (1956), 'Inhibition in the eye of *Limulus*', *J. Gen. Physiol.*, **39**, 651–673.

Hodgkin, A. L., and Huxley, A. F. (1952), 'A quantitative description of membrane current and its application to conduction and excitation in nerve', *J. Physiol.*, **117**, 500–544.

MacNichol, E. F., Jr. (1956), 'Visual receptors as biological trans-
ducers', pp. 34–62, in R. G. Grenell and L. J. Mullins [ed.].
'Molecular structure and functional activity of nerve cells', *Amer.
Inst. Biol. Sci.*, Washington D.C.

Miller, W. H. (1957), 'Morphology of the ommatidia of the compound
eye of *Limulus*', *J. Biophys. and Biochem. Cytol.*, **3**, 421–428.

Purple, R. L. (1964), *The integration of excitatory and inhibitory influences
in the eccentric cell in the eye of* Limulus. Thesis, The Rockefeller
Institute.

Rall, W. (1959), 'Branching dendritic trees and motoneuron membrane
resistivity', *Exptl. Neurol.*, **1**, 491–527.

(1960), 'Membrane potential transients and membrane time constant
of motoneurons', *Exptl. Neurol.*, **2**, 503–532.

(1962), 'Theory of physiological properties of dendrites', *Ann. New
York Acad. Sci.*, **96**, 1071–1092.

Rushton, W. A. H. (1959), 'A thoretical treatment of Fuortes's
observations upon eccentric cell activity in *Limulus*', *J. Physiol.*,
148, 29–38.

Stevens, C. F. (1963), 'Input–output relation for *Limulus* receptor cells',
in Biophysical Society, *Abst.* 7th ann. meeting, New York City,
1963, item WF6.

(1964), *A quantitative theory of neural interactions: theoretical and experimental investigations.* Thesis, The Rockefeller Institute.

Tomita, T. (1958), 'Mechanism of lateral inhibition in eye of *Limulus*',
J. Neurophysiol., **21**, 419–429.

DISCUSSION

H. GRUNDFEST: I wonder what is the function of the branches which
lie close to the dendrite of the eccentric cell? They are located in a zone
which is electrically inexcitable and peripheral to the region where
spikes originate in the axon. Do these structures themselves perhaps
form the neuropile at which the inhibitory synapses are located?

R. L. PURPLE: We do not know the function of these branches. Some
of them do enter the neuropile, but they have not been traced completely. Whether they are electrically excitable beyond 0.5 of a characteristic cable length from the cell body also has not been determined.
However, since the numerous collateral branches in and below the
region of the neuropile are in a region of electrical excitability, it is
tempting to speculate that these collaterals mediate lateral inhibition
over relatively long distances, whereas the more distal, inexcitable

collaterals might possibly provide an electrotonic pathway for either lateral inhibition on neighboring units or for 'self-inhibition'.

R. W. MURRAY: Why do you suggest 'self-inhibition' by a collateral system of some kind, using chemical transmission, and not refractoriness with a long time course?

R. L. PURPLE: All our measurements of 'self-inhibition' have been consistent with the action of known synaptic mechanisms, whereas we have been able to satisfy ourselves that all the known mechanisms responsible for accommodation, refractoriness, and after-potentials in general cannot account for the measurements. Of course, we certainly cannot exclude the possibility that some as yet uncharacterized process in peripheral nerve can account for the 'self-inhibitory' component following an eccentric cell spike, but it would at least have to have very many properties in common with synaptic mechanisms.

Inhibitory interaction in the retina and its significance in vision *

H. KEFFER HARTLINE, FLOYD RATLIFF, AND
W. H. MILLER

The Rockefeller Institute, New York, N.Y.

Reprinted from *Nervous Inhibition*, Proceedings of an International
Symposium, 1961, Pergamon Press, London, pp. 241–284

THE importance of nervous inhibition in sensory processes has become increasingly evident in recent years. But it was nearly one hundred years ago that Ernst Mach (1865) first recognized the possible significance of reciprocal retinal inhibition in accentuating contours and borders in the visual field. More recently, Békésy (1928) pointed out a similar possible role of inhibition as a "sharpening" mechanism in the auditory system. These speculations, based primarily on indirect evidence from psychophysical experiments have since been borne out by the direct observation of neural activity made possible by the development of modern electrophysiological techniques, especially when applied to the study of the activity of single cellular units. As a few examples of the numerous modern studies that show the diverse roles that neural inhibition plays in the physiology of sensory systems we may cite Granit's work on the interplay of excitatory and inhibitory influences in the vertebrate retina (for reviews see Granit, 1947 and 1955); the observation of inhibition in the auditory pathways by Galambos and Davis (1944), and Mountcastle and Powell's (1960) studies of inhibition in the cutaneous system.

The interaction of nervous elements and the interplay of excitatory and inhibitory influences can mold particular patterns of neural activity in specific pathways. Less specific interactions also have an important integrative action in sensory systems. Thus in the visual system, inhibitory influences exerted quite indiscriminately on one another by neighboring receptors and neurons in the retina have the effect of enhancing contrast in the visual image. If each element in the retinal mosaic inhibits the activity of its neighbors, to a degree that is greater the more strongly it is excited, then brightly lighted elements will exert a stronger suppressing action on dimly lighted neighbors than the latter will exert on the former. As a consequence, the disparity in the activities in the pathways from the two regions will be exaggerated, and brightness contrast will be enhanced. If the inhibitory interaction is stronger for near

* This work was supported by a research grant (B864) from the National Institute of
Neurological Diseases and Blindness, Public Health Service, and by Contract Nonr 1442
(00) with the Office of Naval Research.

363

neighbors in the retinal mosaic than for more widely separated ones, such contrast effects will be greatest in the vicinity of sharp discontinuities in light intensity in the retinal image. That is, the outlines of objects imaged on the retina will tend to be emphasized. Thus patterns of neural activity generated by the receptor mosaic may be distorted in a useful way by inhibitory inter- action in the retina; such distortions constitute an early step in the integration of nervous activity in the visual pathway.

A simple inhibitory interaction has been found to exist in the lateral eye of the horse-shoe "crab", *Limulus*. This interaction was first noticed about twenty years ago when studies of the properties of single receptor units in the *Limulus* eye showed that these elements were not, as had previously been thought, independent of one another. The analysis of this interaction has been presented in several papers in recent years and has also been reviewed elsewhere (Hartline, 1959; Ratliff *et al.*, 1958; Ratliff, 1961). This paper will give a brief description of the histology of the *Limulus* eye, and a synopsis of the experimental studies will stress the principles on which the theory of this interaction has been developed.

The lateral eye of *Limulus* is a coarsely facetted compound eye containing approximately 1000 ommatidia, each with a corneal facet approximately 0·1 mm in diameter and a crystalline cone which is the dioptric system for the sensory structure of the ommatidium. This latter structure is composed of about a dozen retinular cells and a bipolar neuron ("eccentric cell") which sends a dendritic process up the axial canal in the center of the retinular cluster (see insert Fig. 2). The contiguous inner surfaces of the retinular cells near the axis of the ommatidium are elaborated into the rhabdom. This has been shown by electron microscopy to be a "honeycomb"-like structure composed of densely packed microvillous out-pouchings of the retinular cell surfaces (Miller, 1957, 1958): the rhabdom presumably contains the visual pigment. The visual pigment of *Limulus* has recently been isolated and studied by Hubbard and Wald (1960): it is a retinine$_1$ rhodopsin whose absorption spectrum adequately accounts for the action spectrum of the ommatidium as determined from measurements of single optic nerve fiber activity by Graham and Hartline (1935). Both the retinular cells and the eccentric cell give rise to axons which, emerging from the proximal tip of the ommatidium, travel in small bundles and collect with those from the other ommatidia of the eye to form the optic nerve.

Each ommatidium of the *Limulus* eye appears to function as a single "receptor unit". Bundles of nerve fibers can be dissected from the optic nerve and subdivided until the electrical record has the characteristics of the action of a single unit. By exploring the corneal facets one by one with a small spot of light, this unit can be identified with one and only one particular omma- tidium of the eye; in numerous experiments the nerve strand has been dissec- ted free all the way up to its ommatidium of origin. The eccentric cells in individual ommatidia can sometimes be seen in living preparations; a micro-pipette thrust into one of them yields electrical records consisting of a slow "generator potential" superimposed on which are large spikes which are synchronous with the nerve impulses recorded in the strand of fibers dissected from that ommatidium (Hartline *et al.*, 1952). The uniformity of the action potential spikes in the nerve bundle, and the regularity of their discharge, are evidence that they represent impulses in just one axon, presumably that of the impaled eccentric cell. It would appear then, that the trains of impulses that are recorded in "single" fibers dissected from the optic nerve originate in the eccentric cell of the particular ommatidium from which this fiber arises. Signs of activity of the retinular cells have not been identified. Perhaps they all fire impulses in exact synchrony with the eccentric cell; perhaps the action potentials in their axons are too small to have been recognized.

For the purposes of the present paper, each ommatidium may be con-sidered a single functional unit, excited only by light entering its own corneal facet; each ommatidium, when so excited, discharges trains of impulses in one and only one optic nerve fiber. These receptor units (ommatidia) as we have said, are not independent in their action: each one may be inhibited by its near neighbors and in turn may inhibit them. Thus, the activity of any given ommatidium, while principally determined by the light shining upon its facet, may be modified by the activity generated in the neighboring omma-tidia when they are stimulated by the light falling on their facets.

The anatomical basis for this interaction of the ommatidia of the *Limulus* compound eye is a plexus of fine nerve fibers—an extensive three-dimensional network of fiber bundles immediately proximal to the layer of ommatidia. In Fig. 1, a photograph of a silver-impregnated section of the eye, axons are seen emerging from the proximal ends of the ommatidia. Several inter-connecting bundles of fibers are labeled "*B*". At higher magnification (Fig. 2) the axons of the eccentric cells (*E. ax.*) may be distinguished from those of the retinular cells (*R. ax.*) by their greater thickness and density and by the presence of a juxtaposed substance that is lacey in appearance and continuous with the interconnecting bundles (*B*). In silver-stained sections such as this the interconnections appear to be composed of small branches of the axons of the retinular and eccentric cells. Electron micrographs of these structures have proved that this is the case (Ratliff *et al.*, 1958). This is illustrated by Fig. 3 and Fig. 4, electron micrographs of a retinular cell axon and an eccen-tric cell axon in cross-section. In Fig. 3 the arrow marks the point at which a small branch is seen emerging from a retinular cell axon (*R*) and joining a small bundle of similar branches (*B*). In Fig. 4 a well defined branch (*B*) emanates from an eccentric cell axon and joins a large bundle which cor-responds to the lacey substance seen in silver-impregnated sections. In silver-impregnated sections such as Fig. 2, areas of relatively greater density (*N*) are seen within the lacey substance. The electron microscope has shown that

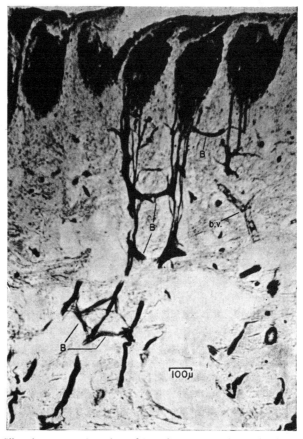

FIG. 1. Silver-impregnated section of *Limulus* compound eye. At the top of the figure are the heavily pigmented sensory portions of the ommatidia. Bundles containing about a dozen nerve fibers emerge from the proximal ends of the ommatidia. Interconnecting branches, (*B*); blood vessel (*b.v.*).

the fine axonal branches in such regions contain vesicular structures similar to those found in synaptic regions in a wide variety of animals. These knots of neuropile are therefore assumed to be synaptic regions. Figure 5 illustrates an eccentric cell axon (*E*) and a branch from the axon extending into a region of neuropile (*N*). A part of the branch and neuropile are also shown in Fig. 5 at high magnification. The synaptic vesicles are seen within the eccentric cell branch as well as other fibers comprising the neuropile. No nerve cell-bodies have been found in the plexus.

The inhibitory interaction of the ommatidia is dependent on the integrity of this plexus of interconnecting fibers. Cutting the plexus bundles around the strand of nerve fibers from an ommatidium abolishes all of the inhibitory

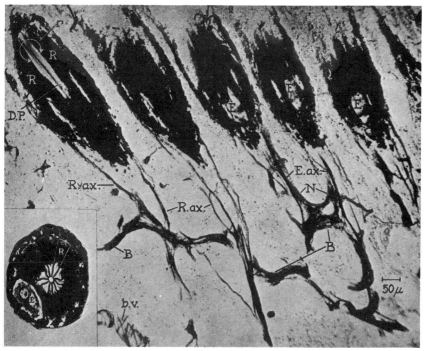

FIG. 2. Silver-impregnated section of *Limulus* compound eye. Unstained eccentric cells (*E*); pigment shrouded retinular cells (*R*); rhabdom (*r*); distal process (*D.P.*); retinular cell axons (*R. ax.*); eccentric cell axons (*E. ax.*); axonal branches (*B*); neuropile (*N*); blood vessel (*b.v.*).

(*Inset*)—Osmium-fixed ommatidium in cross-section. Eccentric cell (*E*). The border of a retinular cell (*R*) is indicated by a white line. (From Ratliff, 1961).

effects exerted on it by neighboring ommatidia. It is reasonable to suppose that the inhibitory interaction is mediated synaptically in the knots of neuropile that are located within the plexus.

Inhibition of a receptor unit by the activity of its neighbors is illustrated in Fig. 6. In the experiment from which this record was obtained a single fiber was dissected from the optic nerve and the ommatidium from which this fiber originated was located and illuminated by a small spot of light confined to its facet. After allowing a few seconds for the discharge to subside to its steady level, a region of the eye near this "test" receptor was illuminated as indicated by the signal above the time marks. This stimulation of the nearby ommatidia produced a marked slowing of the discharge of the test receptor, persisting as long as the neighboring elements were illuminated. When the illumination on them was turned off, the discharge of the test receptor rose again to its original value, with a very slight, but distinct, overshoot. There was a slight delay in the onset of the inhibitory action which can be attributed,

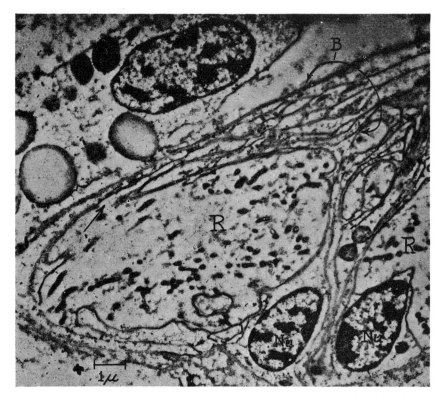

Fig. 3. Electron micrograph of retinular cell axon and branches. Retinular cell axons (*R*); axonal branch (arrow); bundle of axonal branches (*B*); nuclei of Schwann's cells (*Nu*).

in part, to the latent period of the action of light on the neighboring receptors. There was also a pronounced dip in frequency at the beginning of the period of inhibition, with partial recovery. This dip may be attributed, in part, to the strong transient outburst of impulses discharged initially when the neighboring receptors were illuminated after having been in darkness for some time.

The stronger the intensity of light on receptors that neighbor a given receptor, the greater is the depression of frequency of that receptor (Fig. 7). Similarly, the larger the area illuminated in the neighborhood of an ommatidium that is under observation, the greater is the depression of the frequency of its discharge, showing that there is spatial summation of the inhibitory influences exerted on a particular ommatidium by its neighbors. The nearer these neighbors are to a particular ommatidium, the stronger is their inhibitory effect on it; ommatidia that are widely separated in the eye interact little or not at all. A fixed degree of activity elicited in a given region of the eye

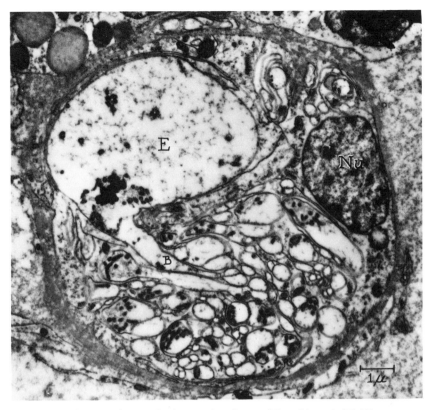

FIG. 4. Electron micrograph of eccentric cell axon (*E*) and branch (*B*). The axon and bundle of axonal branches are enclosed by a basement membrane and a thin layer of Schwann's cell cytoplasm. The nucleus of the Schwann's cell is labeled (*Nu*).

neighboring a particular ommatidium results in a fixed decrement in the frequency of discharge of that ommatidium, irrespective of its own level of excitation. These basic properties of the inhibition have been described in detail in an earlier paper (Hartline *et al.*, 1956).

Not only can inhibition be exerted by normally induced activity in the nervous pathways from regions neighboring an ommatidium, but antidromic stimulation of the optic nerve fibers from these regions also produces a slowing in the discharge rate from a test ommatidium (Tomita, 1958). The inhibition thus produced is similar in all of its aspects to that produced by the illumination of neighboring receptor units: the slowing is greater the higher the frequency of the antidromic volleys, and the larger the number of fibers recruited by submaximal shocks of increasing strength. Figure 8, showing the inhibition in response to trains of antidromic volleys, is noteworthy in showing

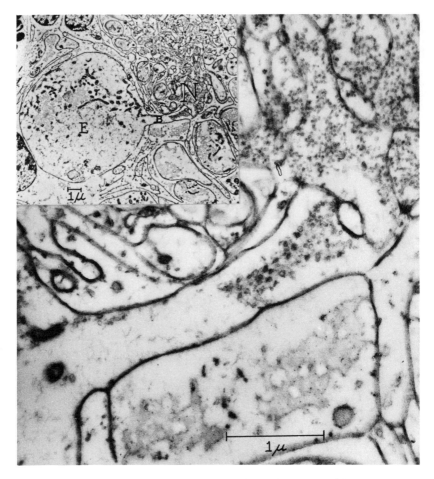

FIG. 5. Electron micrographs of eccentric cell axon (*E*), branch (*B*), and neuropile (*N*). The inset is low magnification; in the higher magnification micrograph of the same region (remainder of figure), showing part of the branch and neuropile, small dense circular outlines (synaptic vesicles) are seen. The significance of the difference in size of the vesicles is unknown.

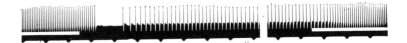

FIG. 6. Inhibition of the activity of an ommatidium in the eye of *Limulus* produced by illumination of a nearby retinal region. Oscillogram of action potentials in a single optic nerve fiber. See text for description. Time in $\frac{1}{5}$ sec. (From Hartline *et al.*, 1953).

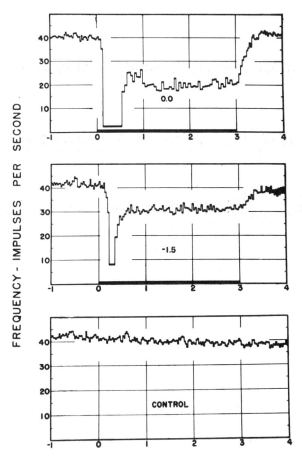

TIME - SECONDS

FIG. 7. Inhibition of the discharge of impulses from an ommatidium produced by illumination of a nearby retinal region for a period of 3 sec at a high intensity (top graph, log I inhib $= 0 \cdot 0$), and at a low intensity (middle graph, log I inhib $= - 1 \cdot 5$), with a control for comparison (bottom graph). Frequency of discharge (reciprocal of interval between successive impulses) is plotted as ordinate vs. time (sec) as abscissa. From oscillograms similar to that of Fig. 6. Throughout this paper the "magnitude of inhibition" is measured by the difference, over corresponding periods of time, between the frequency in the control and the frequency during the inhibiting illumination. (From Hartline *et al.*, 1956).

an appreciable delay in the onset of inhibitory effect. Also, a recognizable dip in frequency appears at the beginning of the period of antidromic stimulation, even though the antidromic impulses were uniformly spaced. Inhibition in the eye of *Limulus* has an appreciable lag, and shows something akin to adaptation.

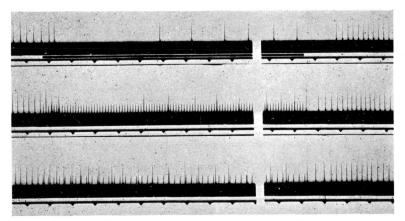

FIG. 8. Inhibition of impulse discharge in a single optic nerve fiber by illumination of nearby ommatidia and by antidromic volleys in other optic nerve fibers. (*Top record*)—During steady state of impulse discharge in fiber, elicited by illumination of its ommatidium, nearby ommatidia were illuminated for a period marked by black line. (*Middle record*)—Inhibition of activity of same fiber by antidromic volleys at 42/sec in the other optic nerve fibers. Small spikes in record were due to physical spread of action potentials of antidromic impulses in nerve trunk to lead-off electrodes; they indicate duration of antidromic stimulation. (*Bottom record*)—Antidromic volleys of 20/sec. Time in $\frac{1}{5}$ sec. (From Tomita, 1958.)

The observed slowing of the discharge of an ommatidium is not the result of interference with the access of light to its receptor mechanism, such as might result if, for example, there were some rapid migration of pigment, or other retino-motor response. This is proved by the fact that the after-discharge following intense illumination of a receptor can also be inhibited, and to the same degree as the discharge elicited during illumination (Fig. 9). Likewise the spontaneous activity that is sometimes observed in deteriorating preparations is usually inhibited in the same manner, and so is any dark discharge brought about by alteration in the ionic balance of the solutions bathing the eye. The frequency of discharge of impulses elicited by passing electric current into an eccentric cell impaled by a micropipette can also be slowed by illuminating neighboring regions of the eye.

The mechanism of the inhibition in the eye of *Limulus* is, of course, a subject of great interest. However, it has not yet been analyzed very thoroughly and we will not treat it in detail here. We have noted that the inhibitory action depends on the integrity of the nervous interconnections in the plexus and have speculated that the synaptic regions in the clumps of neuropile are sites of its mediation. It is evidently exerted at, or ahead of, the site of impulse generation within the receptor unit, for a microelectrode inserted in an ommatidium records the same slowing of the discharge as is observed more

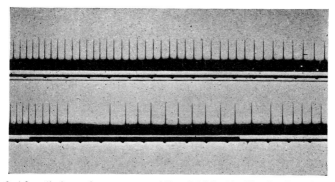

Fig. 9. After-discharge from an ommatidium inhibited by illumination of a nearby retinal region (*bottom record*); control (*top record*) for comparison. The after-discharges were elicited by intense illumination of the ommatidium for several seconds, ending just before the beginning of each record. Illumination of nearby region signalled by blackening of white band above time marks. Time in ⅕ sec.

proximally in the optic nerve; hence it is not the result of a dropping out of impulses as the fibers traverse the plexus.

We have some preliminary observations on a change in membrane potential of impaled eccentric cells inhibited by illumination of adjacent ommatidia. E. F. MacNichol found, in the case of an ommatidium that was spontaneously active and unresponsive to light, that on illumination of neighboring ommatidia, the spontaneous activity was slowed concomitantly with a small hyperpolarization of the eccentric cell membrane (personal communication). We have found that preparations showing no signs of injury (no spontaneous activity and unimpaired sensitivity to light) also show hyperpolarization concomitant with a slowing of the discharge of impulses. In the record shown in Fig. 10 (obtained in collaboration with F. A. Dodge) a constant frequency of spike discharge was maintained by passing a small depolarizing current through the recording pipette. An impulse occurred just before the start of the record. At the first arrow neighboring ommatidia were illuminated, taking care to prevent scattered light from stimulating the test ommatidium. After a short latency the baseline showed a negative deflection. The illumination was discontinued at the second arrow, whereupon the membrane potential returned to the firing level and the spike discharge was resumed. The fact that, during inhibition of slightly depolarized cells, the membrane potential tended towards the resting potential would seem to indicate a synaptic inhibitory mechanism similar to that of other preparations which have been analyzed more extensively (Fatt and Katz, 1953; Brock *et al.*, 1952; Kuffler and Eyzaguirre, 1955).

Even though we do not have a clear understanding of the cellular mechanisms of the inhibitory interaction, it is still possible to understand its consequences as a basis of an integrative mechanism in the eye. We begin our dis-

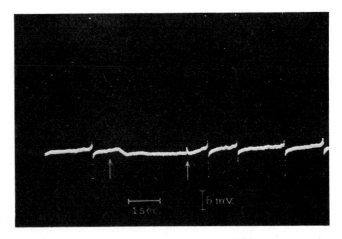

FIG. 10. Oscillograms of electric potential changes recorded by a micropipette electrode in an eccentric cell showing slight hyperpolarization (downward displacement of base-line) concomitant with inhibition of spike discharge, caused by illumination of nearby ommatidia during period between arrows (small switch artifact at second arrow). Tops of spikes marked by white dots. See text.

cussion with the consideration of the mutual action of the receptor units on one another.

A survey of single optic nerve fibers sampled successively from any one eye has shown that any ommatidium one picks can be inhibited at least to some degree by illumination of any retinal area within a few millimeters of it. More specifically, it has been shown by recording from two optic nerve fibers simultaneously that any two individual ommatidia, sufficiently close to one another in the retinal mosaic, inhibit one another by direct mutual action (Fig. 11). Often the inhibitory action is unequal in the two directions; occasionally it is quite one-sided, but it is safe to say that as a rule any ommatidium is inhibited by its neighbors and, being a neighbor of its neighbors, inhibits them in turn. This mutual interaction gives special interest to the phenomenon of inhibition in the eye of *Limulus*.

The first step in the quantitative analysis of this inhibitory interaction reveals a crucial point. The strength of the inhibitory influences exerted by a given ommatidium on other ommatidia in its neighborhood has been shown to depend not just on the stimulus to it, but rather on the net level of its activity. This level is the resultant of the excitation this ommatidium receives from light shining on its facet, diminished by whatever inhibitory influences are exerted on it by its neighbors. Now, the strength of those inhibitory influences from the neighbors depends in turn on the level of their activity, which is partially determined by the inhibition that the ommatidium in question exerts on them. Since these statements apply simultaneously to each

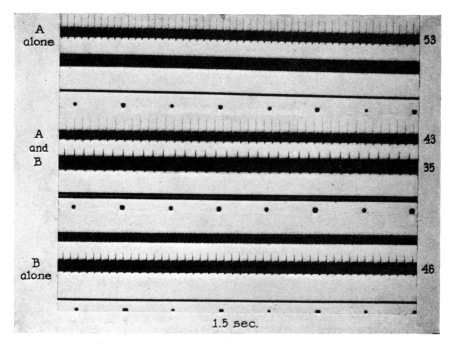

FIG. 11. Oscillograms of action potentials recorded simultaneously from two optic nerve fibers, showing the discharge of nerve impulses when the respective ommatidia in which these fibers arose were illuminated separately and together. The numbers on the right give the total number of impulses discharged in the period of 1·5 sec, for the respective cases. The inhibitory effect on A, 53–43, is to be associated with the concurrent frequency of B, 35; likewise the effect on B, 46–35, is to be associated with the concurrent frequency of A, 43 (see text). Time in $\frac{1}{5}$ sec. (From Hartline and Ratliff, 1957.)

ommatidium in the interacting set, it is evident that a closely-knit interdependence characterizes the activity of receptor units in this eye.

This crucial feature of the inhibitory interaction was unrecognized by us in the early years of our work. We were puzzled by confusing and seemingly contradictory results: spatial summation of inhibitory influences seemed to depend unpredictably on the location of the retinal regions with respect to one another and to the receptor on which the summating action was being tested; inhibitory effects could not be consistently related to intensities of retinal illumination. Only when we recognized that the inhibition exerted by a receptor depended on the level of its activity rather than on the level of its stimulation, could we make sense out of our results. When we recorded from two interacting ommatidia simultaneously, using different intensities on them, in various combinations, it became apparent that the decrement of

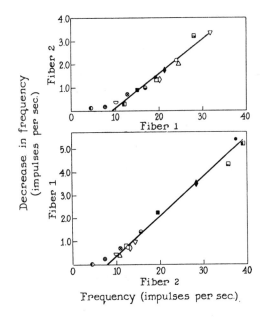

FIG. 12. Mutual inhibition of two receptor units. In each graph the magnitude of the inhibitory action (decrease in frequency of impulse discharge) exerted on one of the ommatidia is plotted (ordinate) as a function of the degree of concurrent activity (frequency) of the other (abscissa). See legend, Fig. 11. The different points were obtained by using various intensities of illumination on ommatidia 1 and 2, in various combinations. The data for points designated by the same symbol were obtained simultaneously. (From Hartline and Ratliff, 1957.)

frequency of each was an unambiguous function only of the *response* of the other (Fig. 12).

A more direct experimental proof that the inhibition exerted by receptors depends quantitatively on the level of their activity comes from experiments demonstrating "disinhibition". A region of the eye too far distant from a test receptor to affect it by direct action can nevertheless influence its response indirectly. If a nearer region of the eye, properly chosen in a position between the test receptor and the distant region, is illuminated at a fixed intensity, it will inhibit the discharge of the test receptor. If now the more distant region is illuminated, it will by its direct action on the receptors in the intermediate region inhibit their activity and as a consequence release the test receptor from the inhibition they exert on it (Fig. 13). Quantitatively, the degree of release is just that which could be produced by lowering the intensity on the intermediate receptors (in the absence of illumination on the distant region) by the amount necessary to reduce the frequency of their discharge to the level they had when illuminated at full intensity but inhibited by the distant region.

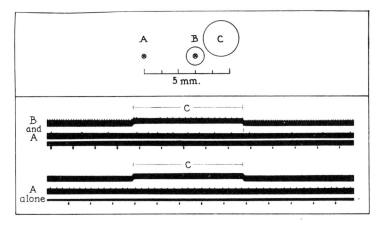

Fig. 13. Oscillograms of the electrical activity of two optic nerve fibers, showing disinhibition. In each record the lower oscillographic trace records the discharge of impulses from ommatidium A, stimulated by a spot of light confined to its facet. The upper trace records the activity of ommatidium B, stimulated by a spot of light centered on its facet, but which also illuminated approximately eight or ten ommatidia in addition to B. A third spot of light, C, was directed on to a region of the eye more distant from A than from B (the geometrical configuration of the pattern of illumination is sketched above). Exposure of C was signalled by the upward offset of the upper trace. (*Lower record*)—Activity of ommatidium A in the absence of illumination on B, showing that illumination of C had no perceptible effect under this condition. Upper record: activity of ommatidia A and B together, showing (i) lower frequency of discharge of A (as compared with lower record) resulting from activity of B, and (ii) effect of illumination of C, causing a drop in frequency of discharge of B and comitantly an increase in the frequency of discharge of A, as A was partially released from the inhibition exerted by B. Time in $\frac{1}{5}$ sec. The black band above the time marks is the signal of the illumination of A and B, thin when A was shining alone, thick when A and B were shining together. (From Hartline and Ratliff, 1957.)

These quantitative measurements compel us to accept the principle of mutual interdependence of receptor responses. Thus it appears that while the strength of the inhibitory influence generated by any receptor is determined by its output, the locus at which this influence is exerted on a neighboring receptor is at, or ahead of, the point at which the neighbor's output is determined. The inhibitory influences are transmitted reciprocally and in a sense recurrently over the plexus pathways. In this respect the inhibition in the *Limulus* eye is reminiscent of the recurrent (Renshaw) inhibition familiar in the physiology of spinal reflexes and discussed elsewhere in this symposium by Professor Granit. We note in this connection that it has been suggested that recurrent facilitation is a disinhibition which enhances reflex discharge by the removal of tonic inhibitory activity (Wilson *et al.*, 1960).

In the eye of *Limulus*, the quantitative expressions describing the essential properties of the inhibitory interaction have been found to be comparatively simple, once the principle of mutual interdependence of the receptor unit responses is recognized. This makes it possible to construct a useful formal theory describing the inhibitory interaction succinctly.

The value of such a theoretical formulation lies in the compactness with which a number of experimental observations are described, and the insight it gives into the understanding of relationships that, while inherently simple, sometimes yield phenomena of considerable complexity. It has predicted several experimental results. With the addition of simplifying assumptions, it furnishes a semiquantitative explanation of experimental phenomena associated with patterns of retinal illumination on the eye of *Limulus*. Applied with caution, it may be useful as a basis for hypothetical explanations of such phenomena as brightness contrast and sensitivity to moving patterns in human vision.

Perhaps the aspect of greatest interest for this symposium is the value this theory may have in furnishing a prototype for the construction of theories of more complex interacting systems. For highly organized nervous centers, basic principles may be difficult to establish by direct experiment, and patterns of interaction may be extremely complex. In such cases it may be of value to start with a simple model—one which possesses the merit that it describes fairly faithfully an interacting system that actually exists in at least one living organism.

We have based the theory of the inhibitory interaction in the eye of *Limulus* on postulates that have been derived inductively from certain empirical experimental observations. It would be much more desirable, of course, to have a complete knowledge of the underlying mechanism of the receptor unit and of the inhibitory process, and a complete description of the histological and functional interconnections of the interacting units. Undoubtedly, such knowledge would permit the derivation of fundamental postulates on which could be based an exact and rigorous theory of the interaction. In the absence of such basic knowledge, the postulates can only be worked out empirically, step by step, and of necessity still incompletely.

The construction of the theory must begin with a search for a parameter which, taken as the measure of the response of a receptor unit, yields a useful measure of the degree of its inhibition. It is no surprise to physiologists that the frequency of discharge, which seems a natural measure of a neuron's response, should turn out to be the required parameter. However, this should not necessarily be regarded as a consequence of any *a priori* considerations. Some other aspect of the discharge might have been more useful in the construction of an empirical theory of interaction: the magnitude of the time interval between successive impulses, for example, or the logarithm of the frequency. Less obvious is the experimental finding that it is the absolute decrease in frequency, independent of its absolute level, that is the most useful measure of the degree of inhibition exerted on a "test" receptor by a fixed inhibitory influence from neighboring receptors. This, too, is not the consequence of any *a priori* speculation. It could well be imagined that, for example, the relative decrease (percentage reduction in frequency) might have turned out to provide a more useful theoretical structure. For the *Limulus* eye, however, it is the fact that no matter what the level of activity of a parti-cular ommatidium whose nerve fiber is on the recording electrodes, the absolute decrease in frequency produced by a fixed inhibitory influence from neighboring elements is always the same.

We can express this experimental fact in the equation:

$$r = e - i \qquad (1)$$

In this equation the term r stands for the response of the ommatidium under observation, measured by the steady frequency of its discharge of nerve impulses while it is being subjected to inhibition from its steadily illuminated neighbors. The term e represents the magnitude of the external excitation supplied by the stimulating light of given intensity. It is to be measured by the frequency of discharge that the receptor would have in the absence of any inhibitory illumination, that is, when that ommatidium alone is illu-minated at the given intensity. The term i represents the inhibitory influence exerted on the ommatidium by its neighbors; it is some function, as yet to be specified, of the activity of those elements.

Implicit in our use of this notation is the understanding of several restric-tions: r and e, being frequencies cannot be negative; the quantity i likewise is to be restricted to positive values, since we are dealing with a purely in-hibitory interaction. In defining a notation for some other system, however, one might not wish to be bound by these particular restrictions. For example, the mechanoreceptors of lateral line organs and of vestibular ampullae dis-charge impulses "spontaneously" and one might wish to consider levels of activity both above and below the resting discharge. For the *Limulus* eye, however, these restrictions apply. For the present, moreover, we will restrict our consideration to the steady conditions of response, after all of the transi-ents have subsided that are associated with turning on the stimulating light and establishing the inhibitory interactions. Later in this paper we will de-scribe briefly some preliminary experiments on transient effects.

In the equation (1) the term i, representing the total inhibitory influence exerted by the combined action of all the neighboring elements that are activated by a given pattern of retinal illumination, is to be expressed as a set of "partial" terms, each representing the action of some one neighbor on the ommatidium under consideration, all combined in an appropriate manner as yet to be specified. Each partial inhibitory term is to be written as a function of the response r of the particular neighbor whose action it represents; this expresses the experimentally established principle of mutual interdependence of receptor responses, discussed above. As a consequence, the activity of each ommatidium in an interacting set will be described by an equation of the form of equation (1) expressing its response r in terms of its excitation e and an i which is a function of the r's of all the other ommatidia in the set. The resulting set of equations, one for each receptor, must be solved simultaneously to determine the values of any of the r's in terms of the e's (that is, in terms of a distribution of light over the retinal mosaic). It is the "recurrent" mutual interaction of the receptor units in the eye of *Limulus* that requires description by such sets of simultaneous equations.

Before we can give explicit form to the equations we have proposed, two pieces of information are required: we must know the form of the functions describing the partial inhibitory terms and we must know how these partial terms are to be combined to make up the function describing the total inhibition on a given receptor unit. Experiments provide the empirical answers to these two questions.

The form of the function that may be taken to describe the relation between the frequency of a given receptor and the amount of inhibitory influence it exerts on a particular neighbor is suggested by the graphs of Fig. 12. It is evident that, above a certain threshold, a linear relation describes the data satisfactorily. For example, the inhibitory action ($i_{1,\,2}$) exerted by ommatidium 2 on ommatidium 1 is proportional to the amount by which 2's frequency of discharge (r_2) exceeds the threshold $r^0_{1,\,2}$ for its action on 1:

$$i_{1,\,2} = K_{1,\,2}(r_2 - r^0_{1,\,2}). \tag{2}$$

A similar expression holds, of course, for 1's action on 2:

$$i_{2,\,1} = K_{2,\,1}(r_1 - r^0_{2,\,1}). \tag{2a}$$

These statements are true for any arbitrarily selected pair of ommatidia in a set of interacting receptor units—an inference from the fact that we have always observed this relationship in every experiment we have performed. Thus the partial inhibitory terms making up i in equation (1) are each of the form given by equation (2) with appropriate subscript labels to identify the pair of elements involved and the direction of the action that is being considered.

The law of combination of inhibitory influences also turns out to be a simple one; the partial inhibitory terms are merely *added* to express the total inhibition exerted on a given receptor. Thus for ommatidium 1 the total inhibition exerted by all of its neighbors (all of the *other* ommatidia in a group of n interacting units) is expressed by:

$$i_1 = i_{1,\,2} + i_{1,\,3} + \,\cdots\, i_{1,\,n} \tag{3}$$

This law of "spatial summation" of inhibitory influences is not an *a priori* assumption; it has been derived from experimental findings. Two patches of light were projected on to regions on either side of a test receptor, close enough to it to inhibit it but far enough from each other that they did not interact. The decrement in frequency of the test receptor's discharge when both regions were illuminated together was found to be equal to the sum of the frequency decrements produced by illumination of each separately (Fig. 14). This was true with considerable accuracy for a wide range of intensities on the two patches in various combinations. This is the basic fact on which the law of summation is based.

When, in an experiment similar to that just described, two patches of light

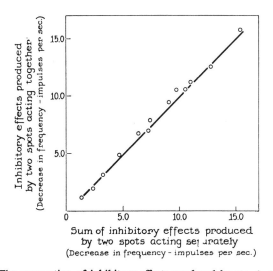

FIG. 14. The summation of inhibitory effects produced by steady illumination, at various intensities, of two widely separated groups of receptors. The sum of the inhibitory effects on a test receptor (steadily illuminated at a fixed intensity) produced by each group acting separately is plotted as abscissa; the effect produced by the two groups of receptors acting simultaneously is plotted as ordinate. (From Hartline and Ratliff, 1958.)

were put close together, their combined effect in inhibiting the test receptor became considerably less than the sum of their separate effects (Fig. 15). We attribute this to the interaction of the two groups of receptors illuminated, for we know that each group must have inhibited the activity of the other and that this must have reduced the net inhibition exerted on the test receptor. We now make the *assumption* that the law of spatial summation of inhibitory effects stated above can be extended to this case of interacting elements. According to this assumption, the reduction in intensity of inhibitory action is *quantitatively* accounted for solely by the reduction in activity of the two receptor groups (due to their mutual inhibition). In the formal description the partial inhibitory terms representing the influences exerted on the test receptor by the two regions will each be reduced by mutual action, but are

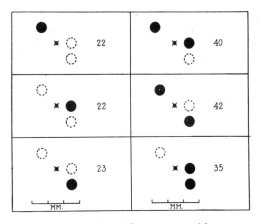

FIG. 15. The summation of inhibitory influences exerted by two widely separated groups of receptors and by two groups of receptors close together. Each panel in the figure is a map of the same small portion of the eye. The test receptor, location indicated by the symbol X, was illuminated steadily by a small spot of light confined to its facet. Larger spots of light were placed singly in one of three locations, as shown in the three panels on the left side of the figure, and in pairs, as shown in the three panels on the right. The filled circles indicate the spots illuminated in each case; the other locations (not illuminated) are indicated in dotted outline merely for purposes of orientation. The number of impulses discharged from the test receptor in a period of 8 sec was decreased upon illumination of the neighbouring spot or spots by the amount shown at the right in each panel. (From Hartline and Ratliff, 1958.)

still to be combined by simple addition to describe quantitatively the net inhibitory effect. An experiment served to establish the law of summation for a special case (no interaction); the assumption serves to extend it to the general case. The validity of this assumption will be demonstrated below, where we will present experimental evidence based on measurements of the simultaneous activity of three interacting ommatidia.

We can now write explicitly the set of n simultaneous linear equations describing the interaction of a set of n interacting receptor units:

$$r_p = e_p - \sum_{j}^{n} K_{pj}(r_j - r^0_{pj}) \qquad p = 1, 2, \ldots n \qquad (4)$$

(*n* equations)   Restrictions:

all $r, e, K \not< 0$

all $r_j \not< r^0_{pj}$

$j \neq p$

These equations can be solved by conventional methods, expressing all the r's as functions of the e's (distribution of light on the retinal mosaic), and of the K's and r^0's (parameters of the inhibitory interaction). All of these, in principle at least, can be measured by direct experiment.

The restrictions require comment. We have explained why only positive values of r, e and K are considered in this particular formalism. The second restriction, that no partial inhibitory term may be admitted for which the r is less than the r^0 with which it appears in that term, reflects experimental fact. Without exception, a receptor that affects a neighboring receptor has been found to do so only if its frequency of discharge exceeds a certain threshold value characteristic of the pair and of the direction of the action. No "subliminal" inhibitory effects have ever been observed: if an ommatidium is caused to discharge at a frequency below the threshold of its action on another ommatidium, it does not add anything to the inhibition exerted on that second one by other ommatidia in the neighborhood. (The absence of any subliminal effects that might sum to produce appreciable inhibition from large dimly lighted regions has an important practical bearing on this experimental work. It assures us that the halo of scattered light, so difficult to avoid entirely in any experiment, contributes nothing to the interaction, at least for moderate levels of "focal" illumination.) The restriction of equations (4) to r's that are suprathreshold for all partial inhibitory terms implies that the equations as written hold only for those values of the e's for which solutions meet this requirement. In any other case, the equations may be solved tentatively, the solutions inspected, and those partial terms for which $r < r^0$ set equal to zero. The resulting set of equations may then be solved, and the process repeated as often as necessary, until solutions have been found that meet the requirement for all terms.

The requirement $j \neq p$ in any of the summations is meant to express an unwillingness to consider the possibility of "self-inhibition" in this formal treatment (cf. equation 3). Now, there is no *a priori* reason to deny the existence of "self-inhibition"—it may well occur in the eye of *Limulus*, where the ommatidia are themselves complex cellular entities, or in other interacting systems that we might wish to consider. "Self-inhibition" might conceivably be demonstrated by the use of some pharmacological agent, for example, which could abolish all inhibition without otherwise affecting the neural elements. But "self-inhibition" really concerns the intimate mechanism of the ommatidium itself as a functional unit and therefore is properly excluded from a theory of *inter*action.

We choose to avoid the entire question of self-inhibition for the present by the following treatment. Suppose the receptor units did inhibit themselves by the same mechanism by which they inhibit each other; call the frequency with which a unit responds in the absence of *all* inhibitory influences e'; call its inhibitory coefficients K'. $K'_{p, j}$ will be the "actual" coefficient representing the inhibitory action of the jth receptor on the pth and, by admitting $j = p$, $K'_{p, p}$ appears as the "coefficient of self-inhibition" (with $r^0_{p, p}$ the threshold of the "self-inhibition"). Then in a set of equations (4') (not written here) where the primed letters replace the unprimed in (4), collect terms and divide by $1 + K'_{p, p}$ in each equation. This yields a set of equations of the same form as (4), in which the quantity $(e'_p + K'_{p, p}\, r^0{}_{p, p})/(1 + K'_{p, p})$ appears in place of e_p (unprimed) and $K'_{p, j}/(1 + K'_{p, p})$ appears in place of $K_{p, j}$, and in which the restriction $j \neq p$ must be restored in the summations. It is evident that these quantities are in fact the e's and K's (unprimed) of equation (4), according to the operational definition of these observable quantities (e_p is the frequency of discharge of ommatidium p, observed when it is illuminated by itself, $K_{p, q}$ is the coefficient of the inhibitory action of ommatidium q on ommatidium p, calculated from measurements of the responses of p and q when illuminated together at different intensities). It is also clear that "self-inhibition" cannot, indeed, be detected by the kind of experiments we have described in which optic nerve fiber activity is recorded under various conditions of retinal illumination. These considerations permit us to proceed without committing ourselves as to the presence or absence of "self-inhibition"; they indicate how the formal theory would have to be amended in case it became desirable to consider such self-action in an interacting system.

The theory so far developed has been subjected to test in a series of experiments in each of which three optic nerve fibers were isolated, coming from ommatidia close to one another in the eye. The ommatidia were illuminated independently, at various intensities in various combinations. The e's were determined, for the various intensities used, by illuminating the ommatidia separately and measuring the discharge frequency of each over a fixed interval of time, beginning at a fixed time after turning the light on (to permit the steady level of discharge to be attained). By pairwise illumination and measurement, the K's and r^0's were determined (from plots similar to Fig. 12). The responses (steady frequencies) in all three optic nerve fibers were then measured when all three ommatidia were illuminated together. The test of the theory was the comparison of these observed responses with values calculated from the solutions of a set of three simultaneous equations (equations (4), $n = 3$) using the measured values of the e's, K's and r^0's. The agreement has been satisfactory in all of the experiments done so far within the limits of the methods. An example is shown in Table 1. The different

TABLE 1. INHIBITORY EFFECTS (DEFICIT IN NUMBER OF IMPULSES OVER A 10 SEC PERIOD) OBSERVED IN THREE RECEPTOR UNITS ILLUMINATED SIMULTANEOUSLY, COMPARED WITH EFFECTS CALCULATED BY SOLUTION OF SIMULTANEOUS EQUATIONS (SEE TEXT)

Effect exerted on	Units illuminated pair-wise			Three units illuminated simultaneously	
	Separate effects produced by:			Observed effect	Calculated effect
	A	B	C		
A	—	27·1	14·8	36·2	35·0
B	6·8	—	11·1	14·0	13·5
C	6·0	18·9	—	20·4	22·0

experiments furnish a variety of combinations of interaction effects, all instructive but not all equally crucial as a test of the theory. The more interesting ones are those in which the interactions are strong between all three units in all directions but preferably unequal, to display instructive asymmetries in the actions. The satisfactory agreement between calculated values and observed measurements suggests that the theory has been properly constructed and the assumption extending the law of spatial summation to the general case of interacting receptors is valid under the conditions of our experiments.

It would be possible in principle to extend these experiments to larger numbers of interacting elements measured individually. However, this would be difficult in the *Limulus* preparation; the three fiber experiments are difficult enough and it is doubtful whether much more would be learned. It is instructive, however, to consider the interactions of groups of ommatidia.

By illuminating large enough regions of the eye (spots of light 1–2 mm in diameter) to include a moderate number of ommatidia (from 10 to 40) strong inhibitory effects can be elicited. A test receptor in the neighborhood of such groups can be used to analyze the properties of the inhibitory interaction as we have done in experiments on disinhibition and spatial summation. Effects of large groups on a test receptor are large; effects of a single test receptor, exerted back on to large groups are relatively small (though often recognizable) and the analysis is simplified. A more detailed analysis is provided by choosing one of the receptors within a group as a representative of the group. This is useful but not without its drawbacks, for individual receptor units differ appreciably in their individual properties and in their interactions with others.

The theoretical treatment of group interaction may be approached by considering idealized situations. We will assume that within small compact groups the receptor units have identical properties, that each receptor inhibits equally all others in the group and that each one of the group inhibits and is inhibited by any one receptor unit outside the group to the same degree. We know that actual receptor groups depart from these idealizations, often considerably, but the theory may be developed for the simpler ideal case and the results used to give understanding of the more complex actual ones.

Starting with the consideration of a single group of n receptor units, our assumptions state that all the e's, K's and r^0's are equal; the r's must then also be equal. Just one of the set of n equations suffices and the subscripts may be dropped:

$$r = e - (n-1) K(r - r^0) \tag{5}$$

or

$$r = \frac{e + (n-1) Kr^0}{1 + (n-1) K}$$

If the group is of a fixed size and is illuminated at various intensities, the frequency of any one of the units (r) will vary more slowly with the stimulus intensity than if it were illuminated alone (e), by the factor $1/\{1 + (n - 1)\,K\}$ (a slight displacement, due to the constant term, might be noticeable). Figure 16 shows that this expectation is borne out to a fair approximation. For large

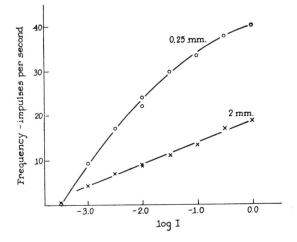

FIG. 16. Relations between intensity of light (log *I*, abscissae) and frequency of discharge (ordinates) of a single ommatidium when illuminated alone (upper curve, 0·25 mm spot of light centered on its facet), and when illuminated together with a large number (approx. 40) of neighboring ommatidia surrounding it (lower curve, 2·0 mm spot of light centered on its facet).

areas of retinal illumination, the activity of the individual receptors is reduced proportionately at each intensity. One of the consequences that this must have is that the range of intensities capable of being covered by the visual receptors is increased before a possible physiological limit to the frequency of the receptors is reached.

The relation between *r* and *n* for fixed *e* is hyperbolic, since (5) may be written

$$(r - r^0)\left(n + \frac{1}{K} - 1\right) = \frac{e - r^0}{K} \tag{5a}$$

If one of the receptors is considered a "test" receptor, the difference $(e - r)$ in the frequency of its response when illuminated alone and when illuminated with the rest of the n members of the group, measures the inhibition exerted by the group on each of its members. As a function of n this will increase along a hyperbolic curve from zero at $n = 1$ to $(e - r^0)$ at large values of n (in (5a) write $r - r^0$ as $(e - r^0) - (e - r)$). This is shown in the experiment reported in Fig. 6 of the paper by Hartline *et al.* (1956). The curve drawn in that figure is theoretical, based on equation (5a), but neglecting r^0. Too much weight must not be given to the exact form of the fitted curve, for the larger areas were great enough in linear extent that the falling off in inhibitory action between widely separated receptors undoubtedly contributed to the flattening of the upper part of the curve.

Experiments on the effect of area necessarily depart from the idealized situation, but the principle involved can usually be illustrated to a good approximation: as area is increased, receptors recruited in each new increment are subjected to increased inhibition from receptors in the rest of the area and so themselves add less and less to the total inhibition. We have shown this effect directly in the following experiment. A small fixed area was used as an "increment" to a contiguous area, the size of which was varied. The contribution of this fixed increment of area to the total inhibition exerted on a test receptor became less and less as the area of the contiguous region was increased (Fig. 17).

We now turn to the consideration of two groups of receptors, idealized by the assumption that all the receptors in any group have uniform properties, interact equally with one another in that group and also interact equally with

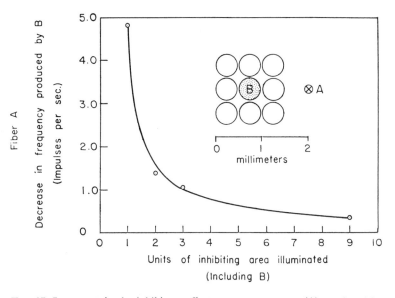

FIG. 17. Increment in the inhibitory effect on a test receptor (A) produced by adding a small retinal region (B, stippled) to various numbers of other small regions (arranged around B, as diagrammed). The decrease in A's frequency produced by the region B in combination with various other regions minus the decrease produced by those other regions alone is plotted (ordinate) as a function of the total number of regions illuminated (abscissa).

each receptor in the other group. In each group the r's of the receptors are equal and two simultaneous equations suffice:

$$r_A = e_A - [(n_A - 1) K_{AA}(r_A - r^0{}_{AA}) + n_B K_{AB}(r_B - r^0{}_{AB})] \qquad (6)$$

$$r_B = e_B - [n_A K_{BA}(r_A - r^0{}_{BA}) + (n_B - 1) K_{BB}(r_B - r^0{}_{BB})]$$

The validity of these equations is established by solving the entire set of $n_A + n_B$ equations (4), subject to the idealized assumptions. The notation used in these equations has the following meaning: the two groups are designated A and B, containing n_A and n_B receptor units, respectively. They are illuminated at intensities such that any single receptor in group A if illuminated by itself would have a frequency e_A; in group B, e_B. When the two groups are illuminated together, each receptor in group A responds at a frequency r_A; in group B, at r_B. K_{AA} is the coefficient of the inhibitory action between any two receptors in group A, and $r^0{}_{AA}$ is the threshold of that action. Likewise K_{BB} and $r^0{}_{BB}$ are the inhibitory parameters for the interaction within group B. K_{AB} is the coefficient of the inhibiting action ($r^0{}_{AB}$ its threshold) exerted by each unit in B on each unit in A; K_{BA} and $r^0{}_{BA}$ are the parameters of the action exerted by receptors in A on receptors in B. Collecting terms and dividing the first equation by $1 + (n_A - 1) K_{AA}$ and the second by $1 + (n_B - 1) K_{BB}$ we have

$$r_A = \bar{e}_A - \bar{K}_{AB}(r_B - r^0{}_{AB}) \qquad (6a)$$

$$r_B = \bar{e}_B - \bar{K}_{BA}(r_A - r^0{}_{BA})$$

where we define

$$\bar{e}_A \equiv \frac{e_A + (n_A - 1) K_{AA} r^0{}_{AA}}{1 + (n_A - 1) K_{AA}} \; ; \quad \bar{e}_B \text{ likewise} \qquad (6D)$$

$$\bar{K}_{AB} \equiv \frac{n_B K_{AB}}{1 + (n_A - 1) K_{AA}} \; ; \quad \bar{K}_{BA} \text{ likewise}$$

We note (cf. equation (5)) that $\bar{e}_A$ is the frequency we would obtain from each unit in A by illumination of the entire group A alone, at an intensity that would yield e_A if restricted to any one of the units in the group; likewise $\bar{e}_B$. The parameters $\bar{K}_{AB}$ and $\bar{K}_{BA}$ may be considered coefficients of group interactions (respectively, group B on group A, and group A on group B). Thus the two groups may be treated as units, each with a certain amount of self-inhibition, acting on each other with coefficients that depend on the numbers of ommatidia involved.

The variation of group inhibitory coefficients with group size has been examined experimentally. Figure 18 shows that enlarging a group increases

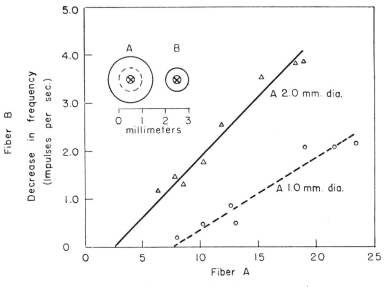

FIG. 18. Effect of size of group on the inhibition it exerts on a nearby ommatidium. Decrease in frequency of a receptor B (one of a small group of fixed size) produced by illumination of a nearby group, A, is plotted (ordinate) as a function of the frequency (abscissa) of one of the receptors in A. For the lower plot the diameter of the spot of light on A was 1·0 mm. For the upper plot the group A was enlarged by using a spot of light 2·0 mm in diameter, and the slope of the line (K_{BA}) was increased, as predicted by theory (the change in threshold is not expected according to the theory of *idealized* group action).

the coefficient of its inhibitory action on a nearby group of fixed size. It also decreases the coefficient of action of that fixed group on it (not shown). This is as predicted by the definitions (6D), for an idealized situation. Exact quantitative prediction cannot be made because of the departure of the actual groups from the ideal uniformity in receptor properties and interactions, required in the derivation of (6) and (6D).

Especially noteworthy is the case in which one of the groups is reduced to just one ommatidium (a "test receptor"). Then the coefficient of the other group (n receptors) on it is n times the coefficient of one of that group's receptors acting on the test receptor, while the action of the test receptor back on the receptors comprising the other group is diminished by the factor $1/\{1 + (n - 1) K'\}$. Here K' is used to designate the internal self-inhibition of the group—for a compact group perhaps of the order of 0·1 to 0·2. Hence for a large group, the test receptor's "back effect" might be substantially diminished compared with the effect it would have on any one of the receptors of the group by itself.

It is clear that this treatment may be extended to any number of groups. We will consider the case of three groups, but will have no occasion to go beyond this number. Our experiments have been confined to special cases concerning the separate and combined effects of two retinal regions on a third, from one of whose receptors we recorded optic nerve activity. Our results have been analyzed and published (Hartline and Ratliff, 1958). The coefficients required in the analysis are group coefficients, but only certain combinations are observable experimentally. The experimental results in all cases are interpretable in terms of the theory developed for three idealized groups of receptor units.

In most of these experiments, we illuminated independently two moderately large (1–2 mm in diameter) retinal regions, A and B together with a third small region X. One of the ommatidia in the region X served as a "test" receptor; its optic nerve fiber was isolated and the discharge of impulses in it recorded. Unless otherwise noted, we attempted to confine the spot of light to the ommatidium of the test receptor alone; when we wished to accentuate the effects of this third group in the interaction we then enlarged the spot of light to include the immediate neighbors of the test receptor. In some cases we also recorded from the optic nerve fiber of an ommatidium in one of the other regions. We will summarize our main results briefly.

When A and B were separated by 5 mm or more, and were on opposite sides of X, they interacted little if at all. As we have said earlier in this paper (cf. Fig. 14), their combined effect in lowering the frequency of X was then equal to the sum of the effects they produced separately

$$(\bar{K}_{XA}, \bar{K}_{XB} > 0; \ \bar{K}_{AB}, K_{BA} = 0).$$

However, if A and B were close together ($\bar{K}_{AB}, \bar{K}_{BA} > 0$), their combined effect was less than the sum of their separate effects, because of their mutual inhibition (cf. Fig. 15). To extend this latter experiment, we held constant the intensity on one, B, and varied the illumination on A; the combined effect on X of A and B together then increased as a linear function of the effect of A alone on X. This was true, of course, only in that range of intensities for which A was strongly enough excited to respond, in the presence of B, at a level that exceeded its threshold of action on X and on B. Examples of results obtained for various configurations of A, B and X are shown in Fig. 19. For A and B close together and at approximately the same distance from X, the slope of this linear function was always positive, but less than 1, being smaller the closer together we placed A and B. If A was placed farther from X than B, so as to inhibit X only slightly while still affecting B strongly, the action of the combination was principally determined by A's inhibition of B producing an indirect effect on X to release it from the inhibition exerted by B. The slope of the function was then negative. This is the case of disinhibition described earlier in this paper. If we placed B farther from X than A

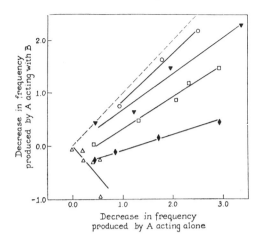

FIG. 19. Summation of inhibitory influences exerted on a test receptor (X) by two groups of receptors (A and B) at various distances from one another and from X. Each of the graphs was obtained from an experiment on a different preparation. In each case B refers to a group which was illuminated at a fixed intensity, A to a group illuminated at various intensities. (X was always illuminated at a fixed intensity.) As abscissa is plotted the magnitude of the inhibition (decreases in frequency of the discharge of X) resulting from illumination of A alone. As ordinate is plotted the change in frequency produced by A when it acted with B; that is, the decrease in frequency produced by A and B together less the decrease produced by B alone.

In the upper graph A and B were on opposite sides of X; in the others they were on the same side, in various configurations, the lowest being a case showing disinhibition. (From Hartline and Ratliff, 1958.)

(not shown in Fig. 19) then as the illumination on A was increased, it tended to release itself from B's inhibition (cf. Hartline and Ratliff, 1957, Fig. 7). Therefore the slope of the function was positive and in one experiment was as high as 1·0 (theoretically, the slope could be greater than 1). In all of these cases, the combined action of A and B was always less than the sum of their separate actions.

Returning to the case in which A and B were widely separated on either side of X, we note that a number of the individual observations in Fig. 14 showed the combined effect of A and B slightly to exceed the sum of their separate effects. This is a real phenomenon, greater than the scatter attributable to experimental error. It is readily understood, for in our first approximation we neglected the inhibition exerted by the test receptor itself back on A and B. When A and B were both illuminated they, of course, reduced the activity of X more than when only one of them was active, hence X inhibited each of them to a smaller degree when they were both active and in turn their individual contributions to the inhibition of X were greater when acting together than when acting separately. That this is indeed the correct interpretation was readily shown by enlarging the spot of light illuminating the test receptor so as to include several of its neighbors. Then the combined effect of A and B together was clearly greater than the sum of their separate effects (Fig. 4 in Hartline and Ratliff, 1958). Of course, the interaction of the group X, even when it consisted of the test ommatidium only, was of necessity present in all of the other experiments we have described. It is never possible in these simple experiments to provide an entirely unambiguous evaluation of the various inhibitory effects. The formulas for the combined and separate effects involve combinations of the inhibitory parameters of the several groups, and measurement of the activity in just one receptor does not provide enough information to calculate the parameters individually. Nevertheless, the theoretical formulas are useful in providing insight into the properties of the interacting system which can sometimes be unexpectedly complex even for relatively simple configurations of retinal illumination.

We need not reproduce here the analytic expressions derived theoretically to describe these experiments, but will show instead theoretical solutions plotted by an analog computer (Fig. 20). The examples chosen show all of the features found in actual experiments, and a few others not yet observed.

We will now turn to an aspect of the inhibitory interaction that has a special significance in visual physiology. In the foregoing analysis, we have treated the inhibitory interaction as determined by parameters r^0 and K whose numerical values were specified without inquiring how different values could arise. We will now discuss the principal factor that determines the values of these parameters. This is the distance separating any two ommatidia in the retinal mosaic (Ratliff and Hartline, 1959). Inhibitory influences are exerted more strongly, on the average, between near neighbors in the mosaic of retinal receptors than between widely separated ones. For example, Fig. 21 shows an instance in which the action of a group of receptors (A) on a nearby receptor (B) had a low threshold ($r^0_{BA} = 5$ impulses/sec) and a high coefficient of inhibition ($K_{BA} = 0.17$); on a more distant ommatidium (C) the threshold of A's inhibitory action was higher ($r^0_{CA} = 18$ impulses/sec) and its coefficient lower ($K_{CA} = 0.07$). C was approximately 3 mm from A; ommatidia separated by more than 5 mm rarely exert any observable influence on one another. The explanation of this dependence of inhibitory interaction on retinal separation is unknown. Perhaps inhibitory influences are conducted decrementally over the fine nerve branches of the plexus; perhaps there are merely less profuse connections between ommatidia that are widely separated than there are between near neighbors. More complete knowledge of the inhibitory mechanism and of the histology of the plexus is required.

The rule we stated above for the diminution of the inhibitory influence with distance, while true on the average, often fails in specific instances when applied to the interaction of individual ommatidia. The interaction of pairs of ommatidia of equal separation may vary considerably even in the same

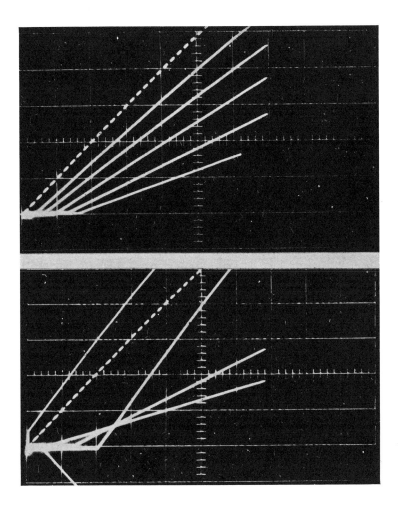

Fig. 20. Solutions generated by an analog computer (constructed by C. C. Yang) imitating the responses of three interacting receptor groups. The traces are analogous to the experimental plots of Fig. 19. The decrease in response of a test element (X) inhibited by two interacting elements, A and B, in combination minus the decrease produced by B alone is traced (ordinate) as a function of the decrease in response of X when inhibited by A alone (abscissa). In the upper figure, A and B were caused to inhibit one another to varying degrees (increasing from top to bottom). In the lower figure, various degrees of interaction between A and B are portrayed. The lowest trace (negative slope) illustrates disinhibition. The topmost trace is the only one for which X was caused to inhibit A and B. In this latter case A and B did not interact: this illustrates how their combined effect can sometimes exceed the sum of their separate effects, as in the points above the line in Fig. 14. In both figures the dotted line represents the case for equality of the combined and separate effects of A and B (solid line of Fig. 14).

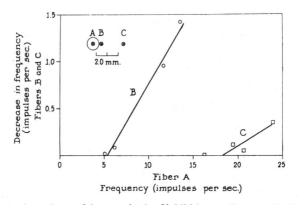

FIG. 21. The dependence of the magnitude of inhibition on distance. The inhibition exerted by a small group of receptors (A) on two other receptors (B and C) is plotted as ordinate. As abscissa is plotted the concurrent frequency of the discharge of impulses of one of the receptors in the group A. The geometrical configuration of the pattern of illumination on the eye is shown in the insert. The locations of the facets of the receptors whose discharges were recorded are indicated by the symbol ⊗. The receptor A was at the center of a group of six or seven receptors illuminated by a spot of light 1 mm in diameter. The illumination on B and C was provided by spots of light 0·2 mm in diameter and of fixed intensity. The effects of the group A on B and C were determined separately. (From Ratliff and Hartline, 1959).

region of the eye. Sometimes a near neighbor of an ommatidium will exert a much weaker influence on it than will its more distant neighbors. Furthermore, the correlation between the threshold and the coefficients of the inhibitory action is not perfect. We have even seen a few cases in which it is the reverse of that shown in Fig. 21. We have already noted that the strength of the inhibitory influences between two receptor units is not necessarily equal for the two directions of action, as it was, approximately, for the pair represented in Fig. 12. Sometimes, but rarely, the inequality is considerable: an ommatidium may effect a particular neighbor quite strongly but be only slightly affected by it. However, when we measure the interactions of moderately sized, compact groups of receptors we find greater regularity and the rule we have stated is followed in the manner illustrated in Fig. 21.

It is evident that any law relating the strength of the mutual inhibitory interaction of any two individual ommatidia in the retinal mosaic to the distance by which they are separated must take a statistical form. At the present we do not have enough data to formulate such a law quantitatively. Nevertheless, the broad rule we have stated is significant. The fact that the inhibitory parameters are strongly dependent, albeit statistically, on retinal separation, introduces a topographic factor into the inhibitory interaction which gives it special significance in pattern vision.

We have alluded to the possible role of retinal inhibition in explaining the enhancement of visual contrast at borders or steep intensity gradients in the retinal image. Consider two contiguous regions of different retinal illumination with a sharp transition between them. A receptor that is within the region of high illumination but close to the transition will receive less inhibition than a receptor that is well inside that region, where all of the closely neighboring receptors are brightly lighted. Consequently, the receptors near the transition will respond more vigorously than those well inside the region and the bright area will appear a little brighter near its border. Conversely, the dimly lighted region will appear a little dimmer near the border where it adjoins the bright region. These bands of greater and lesser brightness, flanking and accentuating a transition between two areas of unequal illumination, are Mach's bands. They are specially noticeable if the transition is not perfectly sharp but is an extended though fairly steep gradation in intensity. The penumbra of a shadow formed by a small extended source usually shows Mach's bands clearly. A double shadow cast by an object illuminated by two point sources of light usually shows striking variations in apparent brightness across its double edge—variations that have no counterpart in the actual distribution of light but are entirely the result of "border contrast" in the eye.

We have demonstrated the physiological counterpart of Mach's bands in the eye of *Limulus*, recording from a single receptor unit as the eye was caused to scan, slowly, a pattern consisting of two regions of different brightness separated by a transitional gradient (Ratliff and Hartline, 1959). When the eye was masked so that only the one receptor from which we were recording viewed the pattern, then the frequency of optic nerve impulse discharge mapped faithfully the distribution of physical brightness in the pattern. But when the mask was removed, so that the entire eye viewed the pattern, then as the pattern was scanned the receptor from which activity was being recorded showed maxima and minima of discharge rates correlated with those regions of the pattern where a human observer saw Mach's bands (Fig. 22, upper graph). Even more pronounced border contrast effects were recorded when the intensity step was abrupt (Fig. 22, lower graph). In the *Limulus* eye, this phenomenon is the inevitable consequence of mutual inhibitory interaction; for the human observer, a similar inhibitory interaction in the visual system may be postulated to explain this and related subjective phenomena of simultaneous "brightness contrast". Indeed, an inhibitory *Wechselwirkung* of adjacent retinal regions is precisely what Mach postulated to explain his now well known bands.

An exact theoretical treatment of "border contrast" cannot be given as yet for the eye of *Limulus* or for any other visual system because the exact law relating the magnitude of the inhibitory parameters to retinal distance between receptors is not known. We have, however, considered theoretically an idealized system—a uniform, fine-grained mosaic of large extent with respect to the range of inhibitory interaction. We postulated convenient plausible

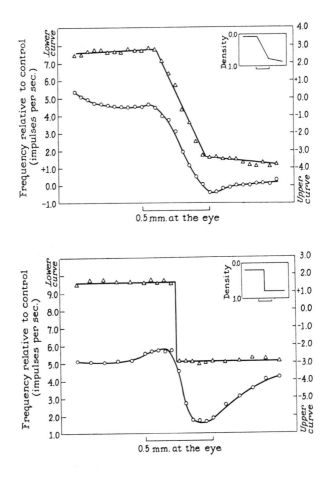

Fig. 22. The discharge of impulses from a single receptor unit in response to simple patterns of illumination in various positions on the retinal mosaic. Upper figure: the so-called "Mach pattern" (a simple gradient of intensity). The demagnified image of a photographic plate was projected on the surface of the eye. The insert shows the relative density of the plate along its length as measured, prior to the experiment, by means of a photomultiplier tube in the image plane where the eye was to be placed. The density of the plate was uniform across its entire width at every point. The upper (rectilinear) graph shows the frequency of discharge of the test receptor, when the illumination was occluded from the rest of the eye by a mask with a small aperture, minus the frequency of discharge elicited by a small control spot of light of constant intensity also confined to the facet of the test receptor. Scale of ordinate on the right. The lower (curvilinear) graph is the frequency of discharge from the same test receptor when the mask was removed and the entire pattern of illumination was projected on the eye in various positions, minus the frequency of discharge elicited by a small control spot of constant intensity confined to the facet of the receptor. Scale of ordinate on the left. Lower figure: a simple "step pattern" of illumination. Same procedure as in upper figure. (From Ratliff and Hartline, 1959).

guesses as to the quantitative form of the spatial function of interaction (we have considered only K, neglecting, for the present, the thresholds). This function should be symmetric, falling off equally in opposite directions from any given receptor. For simplicity, it should be isotropic in the retinal mosaic although this may not be the case in actuality (in *Limulus*, the inhibitory influences fall off more rapidly in the dorsoventral direction from any given receptor than in the anteroposterior direction). We have explored several forms of functional relation: one in which the inhibition had a constant non-zero value up to a given distance and was zero beyond; one in which it decayed exponentially in all directions with a given space constant. For one numerical solution, we chose a function which had the form of a Gaussian error curve (used by Fry (1948) in a similar treatment of "border contrast"). We have considered only patterns in which the intensity varied along one co-ordinate, and have dealt mostly with a simple step in intensity from a low value on one side of the step to a higher one on the other. Numerical solutions of equations (4) were obtained by an iterative method of successive approximations, as is sometimes done when dealing with integral equations. Indeed, a Fredholm integral equation of the second type may be considered an approximation to the present set of simultaneous equations representing the interaction of discrete elements. The first step in the computation is to substitute the e's in place of the r's under the summation (integration) sign; this yields an approximate solution which is next substituted, and the process is repeated as often as necessary. If the total inhibition on any element, $\sum_j K_{pj}$, is less than unity, as it must be in any actual retina, the successive approximations converge to a solution in which maxima and minima of r flank the intensity step on the high and low sides, respectively. We may note that Fry (1948) has made a somewhat similar calculation to explain Mach's bands in human vision. His treatment, however, does not involve a mutual interaction of the "recurrent" type demonstrated in the *Limulus* eye; the inhibition was assumed to depend only on the intensity of the stimulating light rather than on the activity of the receptors. This assumption is equivalent to using the e's in place of the r's under the summation sign in our equation (4) and is, indeed, the first step in our approximation procedure. Fry's model generates "Mach bands"; computation with it is much easier than with ours, of course, and for many purposes it may be useful in explaining contrast effects in human vision even though some evidence has been presented favoring "recurrent" inhibition in the human visual system (Alpern and David, 1959).

The form of the curves we obtained by our numerical solution differs very little from that obtained by Fry; there are, however, very weak minima and maxima flanking the main maxima and minima of the Mach bands—second-order Mach bands, so to speak. They could not be present, of course, in Fry's curves but are so weak in the particular case we have computed, that there would be little chance of detecting them in an effort to decide between the two models for human vision. In *Limulus*, they must be present and perhaps could be demonstrated.

These exercises with idealized models are perhaps instructive but they are so speculative at present that we will not give any numerical results here.

Up to this point our analysis of the inhibitory interaction in the eye of *Limulus* has been confined to the "steady state", in which light was allowed to shine steadily on the eye for a long enough time to permit sensory adaptation of the receptors to take place and to permit the inhibiting influences to take effect and come to a mutual equilibrium. Whenever the pattern of illumination on the eye is changed, transient changes in receptor activity take place and readjustments of the inhibitory influences follow. These transient changes are no less interesting than the steady-state interaction, and are of equal or greater significance in visual physiology.

Transient inhibitory effects are demonstrated in an experiment in which the responses of two ommatidia were observed (Fig. 23). To begin with, the receptors were steadily illuminated; then the light intensity on one of them was increased for a period of several seconds. An isolated receptor similarly stimulated responds to the increment of intensity, after brief latency, with a sharp peak in frequency; as the receptor adapts the frequency soon subsides to a steady level, higher than the value it had before the increment was applied. When the increment is turned off, there is again a short delay and then a sharp dip in the frequency of discharge which reaches a minimum and then returns to a value close to the initial level (MacNichol and Hartline, 1948). The upper curve of Fig. 23 illustrates these phenomena in the experiment under consideration; these frequency changes were determined primarily by the response of the first receptor to the stimulus increment that was applied to it. The second receptor, whose responses are plotted in the lower curve, was steadily illuminated throughout the entire period. Its frequency changes mirrored those of the first, with maxima and minima inverted with respect to those of the first fiber. Evidently the inhibition exerted by the first receptor varied with its discharge rate and these variations were followed with some fidelity by the frequency of the second. It must now be recognized that the variations in the frequency of the second receptor must also have produced changes in the inhibition it exerted back on the first so that the responses of the two receptors, being mutually interdependent, must have affected one another so as to modify each other's transient responses reciprocally. Since there are time delays in the exertion of inhibitory actions, and since the inhibitory process may itself exhibit transient changes in magnitude, it is evident that the temporal interactions of a group of receptors may become quite complex.

We have begun the analysis of the temporal aspects of the inhibitory inter-

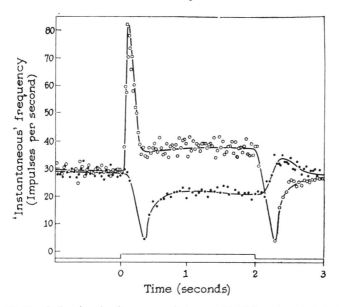

FIG. 23. Graph showing simultaneous excitatory and inhibitory transients in two adjacent receptor units. One ommatidium, black filled circles, was illuminated steadily throughout the period shown in the graph. The other unit, open circles, was illuminated steadily until time 0 when the illumination on it was increased abruptly to a new steady level at which it remained for 2 sec, then was decreased abruptly to the original level. The added illumination produced a large transient increase in frequency of that receptor which subsided quickly to a steady rate of responding ; the subsequent decrease in illumination to the original level produced a large transient decrement in the frequency of response after which the frequency returned to approximately the level it had prior to these changes. Accompanying these marked excitatory transients are large transient inhibitory effects in the adjacent, steadily illuminated receptor unit. A large decrease in frequency is produced by the inhibitory effect resulting from the large excitatory transient; during the steady illumination the inhibitory effect is still present but less marked; and finally, accompanying the decrement in the frequency of response of the ommatidium on which the level of excitation was decreased, there is a marked release from inhibition. (From Ratliff, 1961.)

action by studying the effects of short flashes of light applied to one receptor while a second receptor was illuminated steadily. Figure 24 shows the brief burst of impulses elicited by a short flash applied to one receptor and the brief transient dip in frequency elicited by this burst of impulses in the response of the second. The delay in the action is noteworthy: the dip in frequency did not begin until about 0·13 sec after the onset of the burst of impulses in the first receptor's fiber (0·20 sec after the flash of light). Indeed, we chose this record to show that if the burst of impulses is short, the inhibitory effect may not begin until the burst is nearly all over.

We can measure the total inhibitory effect produced by a burst of impulses in one fiber by counting the number of impulses discharged in the second fiber over a period containing the entire transient dip in frequency, and comparing this with the number discharged in a comparable control period of equal length. The deficit measures the integrated inhibition; it may be correlated with the integrated activity of the inhibiting receptor, that is, with the total number of impulses discharged in the first fiber in response to the flash. When this was done in an experiment in which various flash intensities were used, the relation was found to be a linear one similar to that shown for the steady state (Fig. 12). The slope of the plot may be taken as an inhibitory coefficient and the intercept with the axis of abscissae suggests a threshold for the action of the flash. We are therefore led to hope that the linearity found to hold for the steady-state interaction may also find a useful extension in the analysis of the transient phenomena. Our work on this phase of the problem, however, is still at its beginning.

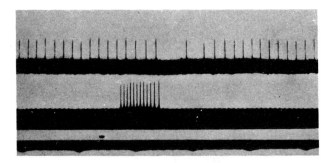

FIG. 24. Transient inhibition of the discharge from a steadily illuminated ommatidium (upper trace) by a burst of impulses discharged by a second ommatidium nearby (bottom trace) in response to a 0·01 sec flash of light (signalled by the black dot in the white band above the time marks). Time in $\frac{1}{5}$ sec.

The spatial summation of transient inhibitory effects exerted on a test receptor when brief flashes were applied to two regions of the eye in its neighborhood has been examined briefly. The experiments reveal a point of some interest. Since the bursts of impulses from such regions in response to short flashes of moderate intensity may be completed before the beginning of inhibitory effects they produce (as in Fig. 24), two regions that can be shown to interact under conditions of steady illumination may give no evidence of affecting one another when their inhibitory actions on a test receptor are produced by sufficiently short flashes. This is illustrated in Table 2, where the inhibitory effects of two regions, A and B, on a test receptor X are shown for these two conditions. When the frequencies of X were measured during steady illumination of A and B separately and in combination, the combined effect of A and B illuminated together (measured by the decrement produced in X's steady frequency), was less than the sum of their separate effects—the consequence of their mutual inhibition, as we have explained in the earlier

TABLE 2. SUMMATION OF INHIBITORY EFFECTS IN A TEST RECEPTOR (DEFICIT IN NUMBER OF IMPULSES OVER A 1 SEC PERIOD) PRODUCED BY TWO CLOSELY SPACED RETINAL REGIONS (A AND B) WHEN ILLUMINATED STEADILY, COMPARED WITH THE SUMMATION OF THEIR EFFECTS WHEN ILLUMINATED BY BRIEF FLASHES

Illumination	Separate inhibitory effects produced by		Sum of separate effects	Combined effect produced by A and B together
	A	B		
Steady	4·5	4·7	9·2	6·0
Flash	4·7	2·2	6·9	7·0

part of this paper. But when short flashes were used, the deficits in X's discharges showed no evidence of interaction between A and B: the combined effect equalled the sum of the separate effects. This we interpret to mean that the mutually exerted inhibitory interaction of A and B on each other did not have time to act before the bursts of impulses from them had been completed. Evidently, the process of combining the effects from the two receptor groups is able to operate linearly for short flashes as well as for steady illumination. Our assumption is strengthened, that the combination of inhibitory influences always takes place by simple addition and one need only take into account mutual interaction to explain all the effects observed under both the steady and the transient conditions.

Complex transient effects are to be expected when a receptor's activity lasts for a long enough time to be affected in turn by the modifications it produces in the activity of its neighbors. The principles, however, can be demonstrated in a rather simple experiment. The response of an ommatidium to turning on a small spot of light confined to its facet was compared with that obtained when the stimulus spot was enlarged to include a number of near neighbors. Figure 25 illustrates the difference. When the receptor was illuminated alone, the initial peak in its discharge was followed, as the receptor adapted, by a monotonic decrease in frequency to a lower level which was then maintained steadily. When a larger area was illuminated, surrounding and including this same ommatidium, the initial part of the discharge was the same, but just after the peak there was a sudden drop in frequency—a "silent period"—after which the discharge was resumed, but at a lower level than when the light was confined to a single receptor. We are familiar with the lowering of the steady level of a receptor's response when it is one of a large group of interacting units. The "silent period" in this experiment we interpret as the result of the transient in the inhibitory influences from the neighboring elements, reflecting the initial peak in their responses, acting, after a delay, on the receptor unit whose activity we were observing. It is no different from

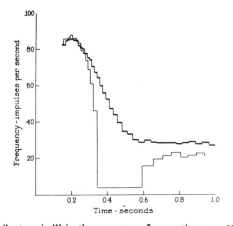

FIG. 25. The "silent period" in the response of an optic nerve fiber. The upper heavy line shows the frequency of discharge of impulses from an ommatidium illuminated alone. The lower curve shows the frequency of discharge in the same fiber when the area of illumination (same intensity as before) was enlarged so that neighboring ommatidia were also stimulated. The time delay of their inhibitory action on the test receptor was long enough that the initial peak of the discharge was unaffected; it was complete before the inhibitory influences affected the test receptor. Soon after, however, the inhibitory influences affected the test receptor and its response dropped abruptly. Since the inhibition is mutual, similar effects were produced on the neighboring receptors themselves, the inhibition they exerted became smaller, and the response of the test receptor increased somewhat.

the deep minimum observed in the response of a steadily illuminated test receptor when a neighboring group of units is suddenly illuminated (Fig. 7).

One can readily understand how several groups of receptors, under suitable conditions, might respond to sudden changes of intensity with rather complex transient oscillations, as the groups interact with time delays. An actual experimental example is given in Fig. 26. It is easy to simulate such oscillations in the output of a pair of interacting amplifiers, connected through an electrical delay network (Fig. 27). However, the detailed quantitative analysis of these complex transient effects in the eye of *Limulus* must wait for a more thorough experimental study of the temporal features of the inhibitory interaction.

Vigorous and complex transient responses to sudden changes in light intensity are familiar to students of visual physiology. "Charpentier's bands", for example, are oscillations in brightness perceived by a human subject under suitable stimulus configurations. Of much greater importance is the pronounced sensitivity of animals to movements in their visual fields. A physiological basis for this sensitivity is found in the "on" and "off" bursts of impulses characteristic of the responses of certain ganglion cells of the vertebrate retina, and in the visual pathways of many invertebrates as well. Such elements are often extremely sensitive to slight changes in intensity of

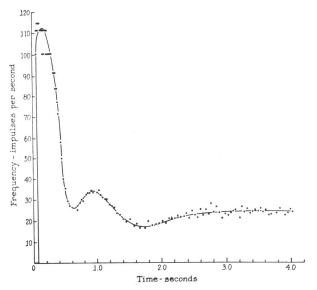
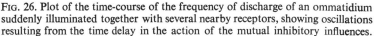

FIG. 26. Plot of the time-course of the frequency of discharge of an ommatidium suddenly illuminated together with several nearby receptors, showing oscillations resulting from the time delay in the action of the mutual inhibitory influences.

retinal illumination, and also respond to minute movements of a spot of light or a shadow across their receptive fields (Hartline, 1940). Similarly, as the eye itself moves—even minutely—neural responses occur. That minute motions

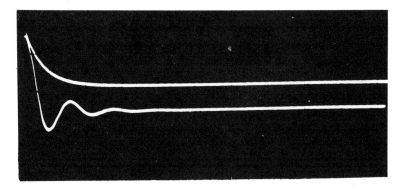

FIG. 27. Oscillations in the output of one of a pair of interacting amplifiers connected to "inhibit" one another through electrical delay circuits, to imitate the receptor responses shown in Figs. 25 and 26. The amplifiers were "excited" by a wave form imitating approximately the response (frequency of discharge) of an ommatidium when suddenly illuminated and showing the usual sensory adaptation. Upper trace shows the response of just one amplifier excited alone; lower trace the output of the same amplifier when interconnected through the delay circuits with the second amplifier (similarly excited).

of the eye actually play an important role in human vision has been shown in experiments in which an optical device is used to cancel all the effects of eye movements. When a retinal image is formed that is stationary with respect to the retinal mosaic, all contours and discontinuities gradually fade out, and within a few seconds the visual field appears uniform, although the image is physically unchanged on the retina (Riggs, Ratliff, Cornsweet and Cornsweet, 1953; for a review of work by Ditchburn and his associates see Ditchburn, 1955).

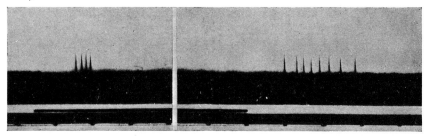

Fig. 28. Oscillogram of a "synthetic" on–off discharge in a single fiber of *Limulus* optic nerve. The typical response to steady illumination of a single receptor is a sustained discharge. In the record shown, the receptor was illuminated simultaneously with other nearby receptors which exerted inhibition on it. By properly balancing the excitatory and inhibitory influences against one another transient burst of impulses at the onset and cessation of illumination were obtained. A section 0·8 sec long (no impulses) was cut from the center of the record (cf. Ratliff and Mueller, 1957).

Responses to movement are but one instance of a retinal action that serves as a step in the integration of sensory information; the wide diversity of response characteristics of the ganglion cells of the vertebrate retina undoubtedly subserve other integrative processes that have their beginnings in the sense organ itself. Receptive fields of retinal ganglion cells have an elaborate functional organization (Kuffler, 1953; Barlow, 1953). The full significance of this organization is one of the important problems of visual physiology; in some animals, antagonistic actions within the receptive fields of single ganglion cells are "color-coded" (Wagner *et al.*, 1960). The neural mechanisms involved in these various phenomena are not fully understood, but it is clear that they are based on an interplay of excitatory and inhibitory influences, and on the interactions of retinal receptors and neurons (Granit, 1955). In the simpler eye of *Limulus*, these mechanisms are not elaborated, but a simple integrative process is nevertheless present in the form of the inhibitory interaction.

Although "on–off" and "off" responses are never observed in the optic nerve fibers of *Limulus* under ordinary conditions of stimulation, such response patterns can be "synthesized" by careful balancing of the excitation furnished directly by illumination on an ommatidium and the inhibition from its neighbors (Ratliff and Mueller, 1957). An example is shown in Fig. 28, where the strengths of the excitatory and inhibitory influences, their transients and their relative time delays were favorable to the development of an "on–off" response. This shows that an interplay of excitatory and inhibitory influences can indeed generate complex response patterns, that may resemble those produced in the vertebrate retina where neural interactions are more elaborate.

The eye of *Limulus* has provided a useful object for the study of neural interaction in a form that is complex enough to have general interest, and yet simple enough to permit quantitative analysis and the development of a formal theory for its concise representation. This analysis has been successful for the steady-state condition, and offers promise of useful extension to the transients. Its significance to visual physiology has been indicated, and its extension to other sensory systems should be useful. It is hoped that it may have general value in the analysis of the complex interactions that characterize the action of all nervous centers.

REFERENCES

ALPERN, M. and DAVID, H. (1959) The additivity of contrast in the human eye. *J. Gen. Physiol.* **43** : 109–127.

BARLOW, H. B. (1953) Summation and inhibition in the frog's retina. *J. Physiol. (London)* **119** : 69–88.

BÉKÉSY, G. VON (1928) Zur Theorie des Hörens; Die Schwingungsform der Basilarmembran. *Physik. Z.* **29** : 793–810.

BROCK, L. G., COOMBS, J. S. and ECCLES, J. C. (1952) The recording of potentials from motoneurones with an intracellular electrode. *J. Physiol. (London)* **117** : 431–460.

DITCHBURN, R. W. (1955) Eye movements in relation to retinal action. *Optica Acta (Paris)* **4** : 171–176.

FATT, P. and KATZ, B. (1953) The effect of inhibitory nerve impulses on a crustacean muscle fiber. *J. Physiol. (London)* **121** : 374–389.

FRY, G. A. (1948) Mechanisms subserving simultaneous brightness contrast. *Am. J. Optom. and Arch. Am. Acad. Optom.* **25** : 162–178.

GALAMBOS, R. and DAVIS, H. (1944) Inhibition of activity in single auditory nerve fibers by acoustic stimulation. *J. Neurophysiol.* **7** : 287–304.

GRAHAM, C. H. and HARTLINE, H. K. (1935) The response of single visual sense cells to lights of different wave-lengths. *J. Gen. Physiol.* **18** : 917–931.

GRANIT, R. (1947) *Sensory Mechanisms of the Retina.* Oxford University Press, London.

GRANIT, R. (1955) *Receptors and Sensory Perception.* Yale University Press, New Haven.

HARTLINE, H. K. (1940) The receptive fields of optic nerve fibers. *Am. J. Physiol.* **130** : 690–699.

HARTLINE, H. K. (1959) Receptor mechanisms and the integration of sensory information in the eye. *Rev. Mod. Phys.* **31** : 515–523.

HARTLINE, H. K. and RATLIFF, F. (1957) Inhibitory interaction of receptor units in the eye of *Limulus. J. Gen. Physiol.* **40** : 357–376.

HARTLINE, H. K. and RATLIFF, F. (1958) Spatial summation of inhibitory influences in the eye of *Limulus,* and the mutual interaction of receptor units. *J. Gen. Physiol.* **41** : 1049–1066.

HARTLINE, H. K., WAGNER, H. G. and MACNICHOL, E. F., JR. (1952) The peripheral origin of nervous activity in the visual system. *Cold Spring Harbor Symposia Quant. Biol.* **17** : 125–141.

HARTLINE, H. K., WAGNER, H. G. and RATLIFF, F. (1956) Inhibition in the eye of *Limulus. J. Gen. Physiol.* **39** : 651–673.

HUBBARD, R. and WALD, G. (1960) Visual pigment of the horseshoe crab, *Limulus polyphemus. Nature* **186** : 212–215.

KUFFLER, S. W. (1953) Discharge patterns and functional organization of mammalian retina. *J. Neurophysiol.* **16** : 37–68.

KUFFLER, S. W. and EYZAGUIRRE, C. (1955) Synaptic inhibition in an isolated nerve cell. *J. Gen. Physiol.* **39** : 155–184.

MACH, E. (1865) Über die Wirkung der räumlichen Vertheilung des Lichtreizes auf die Netzhaut—I. *Sitzber. Akad. Wiss. Wien Math. naturw. Kl.* II, **52** : 303–322.

MACNICHOL, E. F. and HARTLINE, H. K. (1948) Responses to small changes of light intensity by the light-adapted photoreceptor. *Federation Proc.* **7** : 76.

MILLER, W. H. (1957) Morphology of the ommitidia of the compound eye of *Limulus. J. Biophys. Biochem. Cytol.* **3** : 421–428.

MILLER, W. H. (1958) Fine structure of some invertebrate photoreceptors. *Ann. N.Y. Acad. Sci.* **74** : 204–209.

MOUNTCASTLE, V. B. and POWELL, P. S. (1960) Neural mechanisms subserving cutaneous sensibility, with special reference to the role of afferent inhibition in sensory perception and discrimination. *Bull. Johns Hopkins Hosp.* **105** : 201–232.

RATLIFF, F. (1961) Inhibitory interaction and the detection and enhancement of contours. *Sensory Communication* (ed. by ROSENBLITH, W. A.) Chap. 11. Technology Press, Cambridge, and John Wiley, New York.

RATLIFF, F. and HARTLINE, H. K. (1959) The responses of *Limulus* optic nerve fibers to patterns of illumination on the receptor mosaic. *J. Gen. Physiol.* **42** : 1241–1255.

RATLIFF, F., MILLER, W. H. and HARTLINE, H. K. (1958) Neural interaction in the eye and the integration of receptor activity. *Ann. N.Y. Acad. Sci.* **74** : 210–222.

RATLIFF, F. and MUELLER, C. G. (1957) Synthesis of "on-off" and "off" responses in a visual-neural system. *Science* **126** : 840–841.

RIGGS, L. A., RATLIFF, F., CORNSWEET, J. C. and CORNSWEET, T. N. (1953) The disappearance of steadily fixated test objects. *J. Opt. Soc. Am.* **43** : 491–501.

TOMITA, T. (1958) Mechanism of lateral inhibition in the eye of *Limulus. J. Neurophysiol.* **21** : 419–429.

WAGNER, H. G., MACNICHOL, E. F., JR. and WOLBARSHT, M. L. (1960) The response properties of single ganglion cells in the goldfish retina. *J. Gen. Physiol.* **43**, pt. 2 : 45–62.

WILSON, V. J., DIECKE, F. P. J. and TALBOT, W. H. (1960) Action of tetanus toxin on conditioning of spinal motoneurons. *J. Neurophysiol.* **23** : 659–666.

Part Five

Inhibitory Interaction in the Lateral Eye of *Limulus*: Dynamics

INTRODUCTION by F. Ratliff

> '*The sun also ariseth, and the sun goeth down, and hasteth to his place where he arose.*
> *The wind goeth toward the south, and turneth about unto the north; it whirleth about continually, and the wind returneth again according to his circuits.*
> *All the rivers run into the sea; yet the sea is not full; unto the place from whence the rivers come, thither they return again.*'
>
> Ecclesiastes, 1:5–7.

If anything is 'constant' in nature, it is the unceasing change and turmoil. Even the progression of time – which in the abstract we regard as uniform, although we do not perceive it as such – is marked out by grand cycles of change: night follows day, the moon waxes and wanes, and the seasons come and go. Everywhere there is change: from the atom to the cosmos, all things are restless. At the molecular, cellular, and organic levels, in living organisms, change – and reaction to change – is the norm. Only by careful control of many variables can a steady state even be approximated for any length of time. And under such unusual conditions many sense organs respond little or not at all. Indeed, most have evidently been designed, by evolution, to respond to changes in the environment; to survive in a continually changing world an organism must be able to detect and respond to the changes that affect it. The eye is especially well adapted to aid in achieving this purpose.

To show how highly specialized our own eyes are in this regard let us consider what happens when all change is prevented – when a near steady state in the conditions of illumination is achieved. Then, by way of introduction to the work on dynamics in the lateral eye of *Limulus*, we will survey the recent application of Fourier methods and linear systems analysis to the study of various visual systems, and review briefly some of the current developments.

The Purkinje Tree. Because of the peculiar inversion of the vertebrate retina, light that reaches the rods and cones must pass through not only the cornea, lens, and aqueous and vitreous humors, but also through the entire retina itself and the blood vessels that supply it. Why, then, do we not see the shadows of all these intervening structures? For one reason, most are quite transparent. But the blood vessels are not, and they do cast shadows on the photoreceptors. But a beam of light focused on any point of the retina always reaches that point along essentially the same path – that defined by the pupil. Under ordinary circumstances, therefore, the shadows of the blood vessels, like the blood vessels themselves, are fixed on the retina. And only because these shadows are unchanging are they not visible.

Jan Purkinje, the famous Czech physiologist, noticed 150 years ago that if the retina is illuminated from an unusual direction (as by strong light through the sclera, rather than through the pupil – a small pen light held next to the lower lid will do) the shadows of the branched blood vessels appear distinctly. (The phenomenon is now known as the Purkinje Tree.) If both the eye and the light are held still, this 'vascular tree' soon becomes invisible as before, and remains so, until its shadows are moved again by moving either the eye or the light. It then reappears for a while, and gradually fades out once more. The shadows remain visible continuously only if they are moved from time to time. Why, then, does not any object upon which we fix our gaze also disappear? The answer is that it does – if fixation is truly steady.

Fixation Blindness. So-called fixation blindness is a well-known effect. It, too, is easy to demonstrate. Stare fixedly at an already indistinct object, such as a blurred 'soft' shadow on a uniform surface, or the lectern in a dimly lit auditorium. What is seen at first, although indistinctly, gradually disappears from view altogether. Any sudden movement of the eyes, however, restores the image to view. As in the case of the Purkinje Tree, movement of the retinal image across the retinal mosaic is all that is required to maintain visibility. But the demonstration of 'fixation blindness' succeeds only under the special conditions mentioned: dim illumination, or – in brighter light – already blurred contours of the object viewed. The reason that these conditions must exist is that the eyes are continually in motion – even during steady fixation. To demonstrate these small involuntary movements, observe the relative positions of a small afterimage and some reference mark viewed normally. The two cannot be kept in perfect register; fixation on the mark, therefore, is not steady.

Physiological Nystagmus. The very small involuntary motions of the eye (physiological nystagmus) can be measured by means of an optical lever provided by a beam of light reflected from a mirror mounted directly on the eye (Adler and Fliegelman, 1934), or – more accurately and more comfortably for the subject – on a contact lens tightly fitted to the eye (Ratliff and Riggs, 1950). The small high-frequency components (up to 100 cycles per second or more) move the retinal image only across a few receptors – at most – and are probably insignificant. Gradual drifts of the eye and miniature saccadic movements, which occur from time to time, are larger, and move the image across some 10–15 receptors. When the image of an object is already blurred or indistinct, these movements are insufficient to bring about a substantial change in illumination on a receptor. With careful steady fixation under these conditions, 'fixation blindness' then occurs.

Stabilized Retinal Images. The same optical lever used to record eye movements can be used to produce images that are stationary on the eye (Ditchburn and Ginsborg, 1952; Riggs and Ratliff, 1952; Riggs, Ratliff, Cornsweet and Cornsweet, 1953). The mirror on the contact lens is used as part of a projection system, and the image to be viewed is projected by way of it to a screen. The image on the screen thus moves as the eye moves, but, unfortunately, a reflected image turns through twice the angle that a moving mirror does. To compensate for this, all that is required is to view the image along an optical path that is twice the distance from the mirror to the screen, thus halving the effective angle of motion. Under these conditions, the image seen moves as the eye moves, and the stationary image on the retina gradually disappears from view. For a detailed review of the work on this subject, see Yarbus (1967).

There have been reports that some parts of a stabilized image may reappear, and that those parts that do reappear are determined by their perceptual content or significance. Others claim that any reappearance of a stabilized image occurs only because of some inadvertent motion of that image, such as might be caused by slight slippage of the contact lens. The work of Yarbus (1967), who used very tightly fitting suction devices to hold attachments to the eye strongly supports this latter view. Under these very best conditions of stabilization the image disappears quickly and does not reappear. It does reappear, however, when flickered in place (Cornsweet, 1956) or caused to move on the retina (Krauskopf, 1957).

These movements do not appear to aid acuity significantly (Ratliff, 1952; Riggs, Ratliff, Cornsweet and Cornsweet, 1953; and Gilbert and Fender, 1969). They serve only to counter the 'adaptation' effects that lead to the disappearance of the image. It is evident that the ability of the eye to respond to temporal changes is not only of significance in the detection of those changes themselves, such responses are also essential for the maintenance of continuous vision.

Temporal Contrast. Some basic features of the dynamics of visual systems can be regarded as a form of 'temporal contrast' and interpreted in somewhat the same way as are the better known spatial contrast effects. The distribution of excitatory and inhibitory influences in both time and space account for these temporal effects. The delay between the excitation of an element in a network and the inhibition that the element ultimately exerts on its neighbors, or upon itself, and the time course of that inhibition are especially significant in accentuating responses to temporal changes. In particular, the response to an abrupt step increase in illumination will be maximal immediately following the step. The inhibition (either self or lateral) will reach its maximum effect on the response only some time later. Similarly, the response to a step decrease will be minimal immediately following the decrement because the inhibition from the preceding higher response will be greatest then. The exact course of these transients will depend upon the various excitatory and inhibitory time constants involved, just as the spatial contrast effects depend upon the space constants of the fields of excitation and inhibition. For example, if the time constant of the self-inhibition of a unit is longer than that of the lateral inhibition exerted on it, then a post inhibitory rebound will occur (Lange, Hartline, and Ratliff, 1966).

Mechanisms of this sort have been proposed to account quantitatively for the dynamic responses – the 'on', 'on-off', and 'off' transients – of the vertebrate retina (see Bicking, 1965; Bishop and Rodieck, 1965; Rodieck, 1965; and Rodiek and Stone, 1965). Since color appears to be coded in terms of these 'on' and 'off' transients, one might expect to find some strong dependence of perceived color on the temporal variations in a stimulus. The color phenomena seen in Benham's Top is one such example: when the top is rapidly rotated, a black and white pattern painted on it appears colored; the particular color seen depends upon the particular pattern used. The movement itself is not essential, it is the temporal and spatial distribution of the black and white pattern that is significant. According to Campenhausen (1968) these and other similar color phenomena can be accounted for in terms of the phase relations between the modulation of excitation and inhibition produced by the periodic variations in the black and white stimulus.

Flicker Fusion. If a wheel, top, or other rotatable device is turned at a sufficiently high frequency it will appear to be of uniform color and brightness at all points equidistant from the center of rotation. These basic principles of flicker fusion have been known since ancient times, and have always been of great interest to students of vision. Indeed flicker fusion is one of the most studied of all visual phenomena; a bibliography on the subject covering the period 1740–1952 which was compiled by Landis (1953) contains over a thousand references. Until

liography on the subject covering the period 1740–1952 which was compiled by Landis (1953) contains over a thousand references. Until relatively recent times, however, the work in this area was more voluminous than informative. Every new investigation that was carried out under somewhat different conditions than the preceding ones seemed to show some new, different, and interesting effect. But, except for the Talbot-Plateau law (apparent luminance above flicker fusion equals the mean varying luminance) and the Ferry-Porter law (relating flicker fusion frequency and log luminance), there were few unifying principles to tie the whole together.

A major advance, upon which much of the modern work on flicker is based, came in 1922 when Ives applied Fourier methods to the problem, and attempted to formulate a general mathematical theory of intermittent vision. He also expressed his theory in the form of an electrical analog of the dynamic characteristics of the eye that consisted mainly of a series of RC circuits forming a 'cable' between the photo-sensitive element and the final detector (the analog proposed for the *Limulus* photoreceptor by Fuortes and Hodgkin, 1964, has a similar form). Ives's investigations did not attract much attention at the time, however, and only during the past decade or so has the use of Fourier methods had a significant impact on psychophysical and electro-physiological research in this area.

Psychophysical Experiments. The theoretical work of Ives (1922) was based almost entirely on experiments by other investigators. New experimental work, specifically designed to exploit Fourier methods and techniques of linear systems analysis, was first carried out by de Lange (1952, 1957, 1958) and, later, by Levinson (1959, 1960) and Kelly (1960, 1961, 1962, 1964). These experiments immediately clarified many of the existing theoretical difficulties. The effects of many apparently unrelated variables became subsumed at once under a few characteristics of the visual system: namely, those characteristics that could be described as the effects of attenuation by a system of filters (cf. Sperling, 1964, and Sperling and Sondhi, 1968). For a review, see Levinson (1968).

The typical form of a so-called de Lange curve (sensitivity to sinu-soidal flicker as a function of the frequency of that flicker) is a gradual rise to maximum sensitivity at about 10 cycles per second followed by a rapid decline to no significant sensitivity at about 50 cycles per second. This 'typical' curve is for a moderate mean level of illumination. At higher adaptation levels the overall sensitivity is greater, the peak is more pronounced, and the upper frequency cut-off is higher. At low

declines still further as the frequency is increased), and the upper frequency cut-off is lower. These results with sinusoidal modulation of the stimulus in time are similar to the analogous results obtained with sinusoidal spatial stimuli, and have been interpreted similarly: the low-frequency cut-off is believed to result from inhibitory processes, the high-frequency cut-off is attributed to the limitations of the excitatory mechanisms.

Under ordinary conditions of viewing, the normal involuntary eye movements contribute an uncontrolled component to the temporal variation of the flickering stimulus. The effects produced appear to be small, however. For a flickering stimulus they are significant only with small fields (about 1.5°) in the fovea (West, 1968). For the analogous spatial frequencies, the stabilized image contrast thresholds are slightly but not very significantly higher than those measured with normal eye movements (Gilbert and Fender, 1969), and the forms of the function are essentially the same under both conditions.

In order to determine some of the perceptual correlates of inhibitory and excitatory spatial interactions in the visual system, Fiorentini and Maffei (1968) have measured responses of the human visual system to a modulated disc of illumination surrounded by an annulus of steady light. A small annulus was found to facilitate the perception of the disc when illuminated steadily, but to inhibit the detection of the time-varying component of the modulated signal. The converse effect was found with an annulus of much larger diameter. These results are similar, in some respects, to those obtained in similar electrophysiological experiments on retinal ganglion cells of the cat, and can be interpreted in terms of the properties of retinal receptive fields.

Electrophysiological Experiments. Responses to intermittent stimuli were used early in the study of the electroretinogram (Creed and Granit, 1933) to measure effects of adaptation (Granit and Riddell, 1934) and effects of alcohol (Bernhard and Skoglund, 1941). In these experiments, an intermittent stimulus, continuously varying in frequency, yielded – in a single record of responses – an approximation to what we would now regard as the 'transfer function' of the system. The first systematic study on flicker fusion by recording responses of single optic nerve fibers was by Enroth (1952). See, also, Dodt (1964) for similar investigations. Fourier methods and linear systems analysis were first explicitly applied to electrophysiological work in a study on mechano-receptors (Pringle and Wilson, 1952), and only some years later on visual systems (Stark and Sherman, 1957; Stark, 1959; and De Voe, 1962). Because of their wide generality and great power, these methods are now used in many diverse branches of electrophysiology. Following are a few examples of recent applications of these methods in electrophysiological experiments on vision (for general review see Graham and Ratliff, 1974; for a review of experiments on *Limulus* see: Hartline, 1972, and Hartline and Ratliff, 1972).

Most of the studies have been carried out on the retinas of *Limulus*, the goldfish, and the cat. Pinter (1966) measured the transfer function from light to generator potential in the eye of *Limulus*, subsequently Dodge, Knight, and Toyoda (1968) and Knight, Toyoda, and Dodge (1970) extended the investigation to include transfer functions for light to nerve impulses, and generator potential to impulses, as well as effects of adaptation level analogous to those seen in the family of de Lange curves for human vision. For a study of responses to very slow frequencies see Biederman-Thorson, M. and Thorson, J. (1971). The effect of increasing the area of illumination has been investigated by Ratliff, Knight, Toyoda, and Hartline (1967). As expected, increasing the area increased the amount of lateral inhibition, and thus diminished the response to low frequencies. Unexpectedly, however, responses to intermediate frequencies, with periods about twice the time to the peak of the inhibitory potential, were enhanced by the lateral inhibition; the maximum inhibitory effect coincides with the minimum excitatory effect, and vice versa. For a theoretical treatment of this 'tuning' and 'amplification' by lateral inhibition, see Ratliff, Knight, and Graham (1969).

The characteristics of cat retinal ganglion cell receptive fields have been mapped with sinusoidal stimuli (Maffei, 1968) and the distributions of the inhibitory and excitatory components and their interactions determined. In much the same way Maffei and Cervetto (1968) measured the dynamic interactions within a receptive field. For a study of the dynamics of retinal ganglion cell responses in goldfish, see Schellart and Spekreijse (1972). They found that by adjusting the phase relations between a stimulus on the center of the field and one on the surrounds, the resulting response may be either attenuated or amplified. The maximum response occurs when the stimuli producing the antagonistic influences are nearly in antiphase, the minimum when they are nearly in phase. These effects appear to be attributable, as in the *Limulus* retina, to the various delays and time constants of the excitatory and inhibitory influences. The results cannot be accounted for exactly in terms of a linear system. Indeed, earlier experiments by Cleland and Enroth-Cugell (1966) and by Hughes and Maffei (1966) had already shown that the cat retina is definitely non-linear. This comes as no surprise, of course, for no real physical system can be strictly linear. Why, then, the wide application of linear methods to non-linear systems?

The Problem of Linearity. Real non-linear systems can be treated in such a way that their behavior is linear – for all practical purposes. In the linear analysis of a visual system this is commonly done by using small signals so that the departures from linearity are insignificant. Such a procedure is not physiologically unrealistic. Although the range of light intensities in nature is enormous (about 10^{14} from the faintest visible star to a direct view of the midday sun!), the variations in ordinary indoor surroundings are often of the same small order of magnitude as the variations of stimuli required in a typical psycho-physical or electrophysiological experiment on vision. Nevertheless, some of the most interesting features of any visual system are in those parts of the range of operation where the departures from linearity are so great that even small signal linear techniques cannot be applied. This is especially true at or near thresholds in the system. But the problem is not altogether insoluble. As Spekreijse (1969) has shown, noise added to a sinusoidal stimulus can act as a carrier signal, the effect of which can be to shift the amplitude domain of a signal away from a non-linear region and into a linear portion. By means of ingenious techniques of this sort, and by proper and careful choice of amplitude and range of stimuli being used, techniques of linear systems analysis can be, and are being, widely and fruitfully applied to the analysis of visual systems. But however useful the results may be, they are none the less first approximations. Sooner or later, the non-linearities have to be dealt with directly. A number of investigators are now doing so – for example: Cleland and Enroth-Cugell (1968, 1970), Stone and Fabian (1968), Enroth-Cugell and Pinto (1972), Levine (1972), and Shapley, Enroth-Cugell, Bonds, and Kirby (1972). In the application of linear methods to the mathematical analysis of the electrophysiology of vision one must always keep in mind that it is the system of equations which is strictly linear, not the visual system itself.

REFERENCES

Adler, F. H., and Fliegelman, F. (1934), 'Influence of Fixation on the Visual Acuity', *Arch. Ophthal.*, **12**, 475–483.

Bernhard, C. G., and Skoglund, C. R. (1941), 'Selective Suppression with Ethylalcohol of Inhibition in the Optic Nerve and of the Negative Component PIII of the Electroretinogram', *Acta Physiol. Scand.*, **2**, 10–21.

Bicking, L. A. (1965), 'Some Quantitative Studies on Retinal Ganglion Cells', Thesis, The Johns Hopkins University.

Bishop, P. O., and Rodieck, R. W. (1965), 'Discharge Patterns of Cat Retinal Ganglion Cells', in *Proceedings of the Symposium on Information Processing in Sight Sensory Systems*, P. W. Nye, ed., California Institute of Technology, Pasadena, pp. 116–127.

Biederman-Thorson, M., and Thorson, J. (1971), 'Dynamics of excitation and inhibition in the light-adapted *Limulus* eye *in situ*', *J. Gen. Physiol.*, **58**, 1–19.

Campenhausen, C. von (1968), 'Über die Farben der Benhamschen Scheibe', *Zeit. vergl. Physiol.*, **60**, 351–374.

Cleland, B., and Enroth-Cugell, C. (1966), 'Cat Retinal Ganglion Cell Responses to Changing Light Intensities: Sinusoidal Modulation in the Time Domain', *Acta Physiol. Scand.*, **68**, 365–381.

Cleland, B. G., and Enroth-Cugell, C. (1968), 'Quantitative aspects of sensitivity and summation in the cat retina', *J. Physiol* (Lond.), **198**, 17–38.

Cleland, B. G., and Enroth-Cugell, C. (1970), 'Quantitative aspects of gain and latency in the cat retina', *J. Physiol.* (Lond.), **206**, 73–82.

Cornsweet, T. N. (1956), 'The Determination of the Stimuli for Involuntary Drifts and Saccadic Eye Movements', *J. Opt. Soc. Amer.*, **46**, 987–993.

Creed, R. S., and Granit, R. (1933), 'Observations on the Retinal Action Potential with Especial Reference to the Response to Intermittent Stimulation', *J. Physiol.*, **78**, 419–441.

De Lange, H. (1952), 'Relationship between Critical Flicker-Frequency and a Set of Low Frequency Characteristics of the Eye', *J. Opt. Soc. Amer.*, **44**, 380–389.

De Lange, H. (1957), *Attenuation Characteristics and Phase-Shift Characteristics of the Human Fovea-Cortex Systems in Relation to Flicker-Fusion Phenomena*, Thesis, Technical University, Delft, Holland.

De Lange, H. (1958), 'Research into the Dynamic Nature of the Human Fovea – Cortex Systems with Intermittent and Modulated Light. I. Attenuation Characteristics with White and Coloured Light. II. Phase Shift in Brightness and Delay in Color Perception', *J. Opt. Soc. Amer.*, **48**, 777–789.

De Voe, R. D. (1962), 'Linear Superposition of Retinal Action Potentials to Predict Electrical Flicker Responses from the Eye of the Wolf Spider, *Lycosa baltimoriana* (Keyserling)', *J. Gen. Physiol.*, **46**, 75–96.

Ditchburn, R. W., and Ginsborg, B. L. (1952), 'Vision with a Stabilized Retinal Image', *Nature*, **170**, 36.

Dodge, F. A., Knight, B. W., and Toyoda, J. (1968), 'Voltage Noise in *Limulus* Visual Cells', *Science*, **160**, 88–90.

Dodt, E. (1964), 'Erregung und Hemmung Retinaler Neurone bei Intermittierender Belichtung', *Doc. Ophthal.*, **18**, 259–274.

Enroth-Cugell, C. (1952), 'The Mechanism of Flicker and Fusion Studied on Single Retinal Elements in the Dark-Adapted Eye of the Cat', *Acta Physiol*. Scand., **27**, 5–67.

Enroth-Cugell, C., and Pinto, L. (1972a), 'Properties of the surround response mechanism of cat retinal ganglion cells and center-surround interaction', *J. Physiol*. (Lond.), **220**, 403–441.

Fiorentini, A., and Maffei, L. (1968), 'Perceptual Correlates on Inhibitory and Facilitatory Spatial Interactions in the Visual System', *Vision Res.*, **8**, 1195–1203.

Fuortes, M. G. F., and Hodgkin, A. L. (1964), 'Changes in Time Scale and Sensitivity in the Ommatidia of *Limulus*', *J. Physiol.*, **172**, 239–263.

Hartline, H. K. (1972), 'Introduction', *Handbook of Sensory Physiology*, V.VII/2, *Physiology of Photoreceptor Organs*, M. G. F. Fuortes, ed., Springer Verlag, Berlin, pp. 1–3.

Hartline, H. K., and Ratliff, F. (1972), 'Inhibitory Interaction in the Eye of Limulus', *Handbook of Sensory Physiology*, V.VII/2, *Physiology of Photoreceptor Organs*, M. G. F. Fuortxs, ed., Springer Verlag, Berlin, pp. 381–447.

Gilbert, D. S., and Fender, D. H. (1969), 'Contrast Thresholds Measured with Stabilized and Non-Stabilized Sine-Wave Gratings', *Optica Acta*, **16**, 191–204.

Graham, N., and Ratliff, F., 'Quantitative theories of the integrative action of the retina', in *Contemporary Developments in Mathematical Psychology*, Editors: R. C. Atkinson, D. H. Krantz, R. D. Luce, and P. Suppes, W. H. Freeman Co. 1974.

Granit, R., and Riddell, H. A. (1934), 'The Electrical Responses of Light- and Dark-Adapted Frog's Eyes to Rhythmic and Continuous Stimuli', *J. Physiol.*, **81**, 1–28.

Hughes, G. W., and Maffei, L. (1966), 'Retinal Ganglion Cell Response to Sinusoidal Light Stimulation', *J. Neurophysiol.*, **29**, 333–352.

Ives, H. E. (1922), 'A Theory of Intermittent Vision', *J. Opt. Soc. Amer.*, **6**, 343–361.

Kelly, D. H. (1960), 'Stimulus Patterns for Visual Research', *J. Opt. Soc. Amer.*, **50**, 1115–1116.

Kelly, D. H. (1961), 'Visual Responses to Time-Dependent Stimuli.

I. Amplitude Sensitivity Measurements', *J. Opt. Soc. Amer.*, **51**, 422–429.

Kelly, D. H. (1961), 'Visual Responses to Time-Dependent Stimuli. II. Single Channel Model of the Photopic Visual System', *J. Opt. Soc. Amer.*, **51**, 747–754.

Kelly, D. H. (1961), 'Flicker Fusion and Harmonic Analysis', *J. Opt. Soc. Amer.*, **51**, 917–918.

Kelly, D. H. (1962), 'Visual Responses to Time-Dependent Stimuli. III. Individual Variations', *J. Opt. Soc. Amer.*, **52**, 89–95.

Kelly, D. H. (1962), 'Visual Responses to Time-Dependent Stimuli. IV. Effects of Chromatic Adaptation', *J. Opt. Soc. Amer.*, **52**, 940–947.

Kelly, D. H. (1964), 'Sine Waves and Flicker Fusion', *Doc. Ophthal.*, **18**, 16–35.

Knight, B. W., Toyoda, J.–I., and Dodge, F. A. (1970), 'A quantitative description of excitation and inhibition in the eye of *Limulus*', *J. Gen. Physiol.*, **56**, 421–437.

Krauskopf, J. (1957), 'Effect of Retinal Motion on Contrast Thresholds for Maintained Vision', *J. Opt. Soc. Amer.*, **47**, 740–744.

Landis, C. (1953), *An Annotated Bibliography of Flicker Fusion Phenomena Covering the Period 1740–1952*, Armed Forces National Research Council, Michigan.

Lange, D., Hartline, H. K., and Ratliff, F. (1966), 'The Dynamics of Lateral Inhibition in the Compound Eye of *Limulus*. II', *Proc. of Internat. Symp. on the Functional Organization of the Compound Eye*, Pergamon Press, Oxford, 425–449.

Levine, M. (1972), *An analysis of spatial summation in the receptive fields of goldfish ganglion cells*, Thesis, The Rockefeller University, New York.

Levinson, J. (1959), 'Fusion of Complex Flicker', *Science*, **130**, 919–921.

Levinson, J. (1960), 'Fusion of Complex Flicker. II', *Science*, **131**, 1438–1440.

Levinson, J. (1968), 'Flicker Fusion Phenomena', *Science*, **160**, 21–28.

Maffei, L. (1968), 'Inhibitory and Facilitatory Spatial Interactions in Retinal Receptive Fields', *Vision Res.*, **8**, 1187–1195.

Maffei, L., and Cervetto, L. (1968), 'Dynamic Interactions in Retinal Receptive Fields', *Vision Res.*, **8**, 1299–1303.

Pinter, R. B. (1966), 'Sinusoidal and Delta Function Responses of Visual Cells of the *Limulus* Eye', *J. Gen. Physiol.*, **49**, 565.

Pringle, J. W. S., and Wilson, V. J. (1952), 'The Response of a Sense Organ to a Harmonic Stimulus', *J. Exp. Biol.*, **29**, 220–234.

Ratliff, F., and Riggs, L. A. (1950), 'Involuntary Motions of the Eye During Monocular Fixation', *J. Exp. Psychol.*, **40**, 687–701.

Ratliff, F. (1952), 'The Role of Physiological Nystagmus in Monocular Acuity', *J. Exp. Psychol.*, **43**, 163–172.

Ratliff, F., Knight, B. W., Toyoda, J., and Hartline, H. K. (1967), 'Enhancement of Flicker by Lateral Inhibition', *Science*, **158**, 392–393.

Ratliff, F. Knight, B. W., and Graham, N. (1969), 'On Tuning and Amplification by Lateral Inhibition', *Proc. Nat. Acad. Sci.*, **62**, 733–740.

Riggs, L. A., and Ratliff, F. (1952), 'Effects of Counteracting the Normal Movements of the Eye', *J. Opt. Soc. Amer.*, **42**, 872–873.

Riggs, L. A., Ratliff, F., Cornsweet, J. C., and Cornsweet, T. N. (1953), 'The Disappearance of Steadily Fixated Visual Test Objects', *J. Opt. Soc. Amer.*, **43**, 495–501.

Rodieck, R. W. (1965), 'Quantitative Analysis of the Cat Retinal Ganglion Cell Responses to Visual Stimuli', *Vision Res.*, **5**, 583–601.

Rodieck, R. W., and Stone, J. (1965), 'Response of Cat Retinal Ganglion Cells to Moving Visual Patterns', *J. Neurophysiol.*, **28**, 819–832.

Rodieck, R. W., and Stone, J. (1965), 'Analysis of Receptive Fields of Cat Retinal Ganglion Cells', *J. Neurophysiol.*, **28**, 833–849.

Schellart, N., and Spekreijse, H. (1972), 'Dynamic characteristics of retinal ganglion cell responses in goldfish', *J. Gen. Physiol.*, **59**, 1, 1–21.

Shapley, R. M., Enroth-Cugell, C., Bonds, A. B., and Kirby, A. (1972), 'The automatic gain control of the retina and retinal dynamics', *Nature*, **236**, 352–353.

Spekreijse, H. (1969), 'Rectification in the goldfish retina: Analysis by Sinusoidal and Auxiliary stimulation', *Vision Res.*, **9**, 1461–1472.

Sperling, G. (1964), 'Linear Theory and the Psychophysics of Flicker', *Doc. Ophthal*, **18**, 3–15.

Sperling, G., and Sondhi, M. M. (1968), 'Model for Visual Luminance Discrimination and Flicker Detection', *J. Opt. Soc. Amer.*, **58**, 1133–1145.

Stark, L., and Sherman, P. M. (1957), 'A Servoanalytic Study of the Consensual Pupil Reflex to Light', *J. Neurophysiol.*, **20**, 17–26.

Stark, L. (1959), *Transfer Function of a Biological Photoreceptor*, Aerospace Medical Laboratory, Ohio.

Stone, J., and Fabian, M. (1968), 'Summing Properties of the Cat's Retinal Ganglion Cell', *Vision Research*, **8**, 1023–1040.

West, D. C. (1968), 'Effect of Retinal Image Motion on Critical Flicker-Fusion Measurement', *Optica Acta*, **15**, 317–328.

Yarbus, A. L. (1967), *Eye Movements and Vision*, Plenum Press, New York.

Spatial and temporal aspects of retinal inhibitory interaction[1,2]

FLOYD RATLIFF, H. KEFFER HARTLINE, AND
W. H. MILLER

The Rockefeller University, New York, N.Y.

Reprinted from JOURNAL OF THE OPTICAL SOCIETY OF
AMERICA, Vol. 53, no. 1, 110–120, January 1963

ABSTRACT

The inhibitory interaction among neural elements in the compound eye
of *Limulus* was investigated by recording impulses from two or more
optic nerve fibers simultaneously. The inhibitory influences are exerted
mutually and recurrently, with an appreciable time delay, over a network of interconnections among the interacting elements.

Under steady conditions of retinal illumination the activity of any
group of interacting elements may be described by a set of simultaneous
equations, one equation for each element. In each equation the activity
of the particular element represented is expressed as the resultant of the
excitatory stimulus to it and the opposing inhibitory influences exerted
on it by all the others. By also taking account of the time required for
an inhibitory effect exerted by one element to act upon another, this
quantitative description may be extended to include transient phenomena associated with changes in the pattern of retinal illumination.

The influences exerted over the inhibitory network give rise to,
maxima and minima in the optic nerve responses to spatial patterns of
illumination, and to fluctuations in the responses to temporal patterns.
The spatial and temporal properties of the responses of the population
of interacting elements are analogous to a number of familiar phenomena in human vision and may offer an explanation for them. These
properties also lend support to the view that inhibition may play a role
in the generation of the transient 'on' and 'off' responses observed in a
wide variety of visual systems.

[1] Invited paper presented at the Symposium on Physiological Optics, Joint Session
of the Armed Forces–NRC Committee on Vision, the Inter-Society Color Council,
and the Optical Society of America, 14–15 March 1962, Washington, D.C.

[2] This work was supported by a research grant (B864) from the National Institute
of Neurological Diseases and Blindness, Public Health Service, and by Contract
Nonr 1442(00) with the Office of Naval Research.

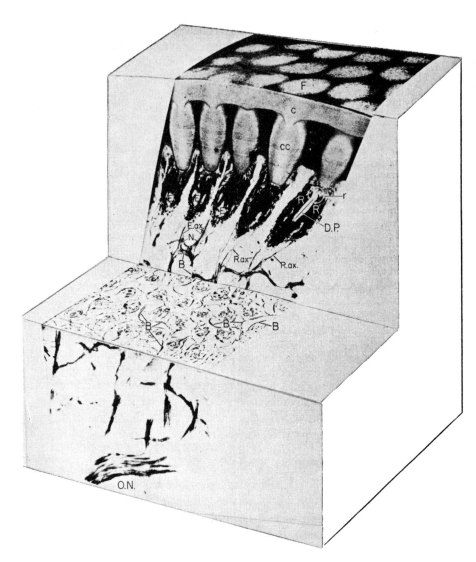

Fig. 1. Composite three-dimensional micrograph of the compound lateral eye of *Limulus*. In the Upper horizontal plane, the facets F of the individual ommatidia may be seen on the outer surface of the cornea C. (The facets would appear dark in the living eye). The upper vertical plane is a section perpendicular to the outer surface of the cornea. The crystalline cones CC are lens-like structures formed in the inner portion of the chitinous cornea. The rhabdom r is the sensory portion of the ommatidia. It is formed by the inner portions of a dozen or more wedge-shaped retinular cells R which are arranged radially around the distal process D.P. of the eccentric cell E. Axons arise from the eccentric cell E.ax. and from the retinular cells R.ax. and course downward. Both types of axons give off fine branches which run laterally in small bundles B and terminate in clumps of neuropile N near the eccentric cell axons

I. INTRODUCTION

A retina, as its name implies, is a network. The functional units in it are interconnected and interact with one another; the neural activity generated by illumination of any one receptor may influence, or be influenced by, the activity generated by many others. Consequently, many visual phenomena may depend as much upon the properties of the network of interconnected receptors and retinal neurons, acting as a whole, as they do upon the properties of the individual components, acting alone.

In the eyes of higher animals, both excitatory and inhibitory influences interplay to generate complex patterns of neural response. This paper surveys some recent electrophysiological studies on temporal and spatial properties of a purely inhibitory interaction in the less complicated retina of the lateral eye of the horseshoe crab *Limulus*.

II. STEADY-STATE INHIBITION IN THE LATERAL EYE OF 'LIMULUS'

The compound eye of *Limulus* (Figs. 1–4) is a favorable preparation for the study of inhibitory interaction. The eye has a relatively small population of fairly large receptor units (ommatidia) on which the pattern of illumination can be controlled with considerable precision; it contains a three-dimensional network, or plexus, of neural interconnections which form a true retina, and the interactions mediated over this network appear to be purely inhibitory (Hartline, 1949; Hartline, Wagner, and Ratliff, 1956).

The interaction of a pair of receptor units in the steady state can be described by a pair of simultaneous linear equations (Hartline and Ratliff, 1957):

$$r_1 = e_1 - K_{1,2}(r_2 - r^0_{1,2}),$$
$$r_2 = e_2 - K_{2,1}(r_1 - r^0_{2,1}). \tag{1}$$

The activity of each receptor unit (its response r) is measured by the frequency of discharge of impulses in its eccentric-cell axon. Each

E.ax. The numerous bundles B form a network, or plexus, interconnecting the axons immediately below the receptor layer (lower horizontal plane). After passing through the plexus the eccentric-cell axons and retinular-cell axons come together to form the optic nerve O.N., lower vertical plane. Diameter of a single ommatidium approximately 150 μ. In the experiments described in this paper, impulses conducted in the eccentric-cell axons E.ax. were recorded. No propagated impulses have been observed, as yet, in the axons of the retinular cells R.ax. or in the interconnecting bundles B of fine fibers that form the plexus.

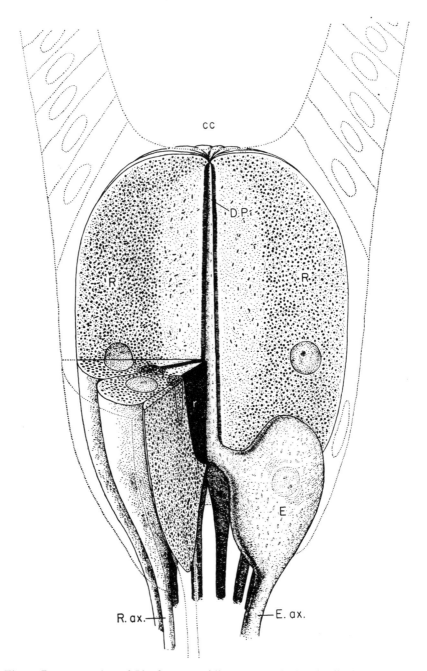

Fig. 2. Representation of *Limulus* ommatidium as seen in longitudinal section. CC, crystalline cone; r, rhabdom; R, retinular cell; D.P., distal process; E.ax., eccentric-cell axon; R.ax., retinular-cell axon. Based on a drawing by B. Tagawa, *Scientific American*.

response is determined by the excitation e supplied by the external stimulus diminished by the inhibitory influence exerted by the other member of the pair. The subscripts label the individual receptor units. In each of these equations, the magnitude of the inhibitory influence is given by the last term. The 'threshold' frequency that must be exceeded before a receptor can exert any inhibition is represented by r^0. It and the 'inhibitory coefficient' K are labeled to indicate the direction of the action: $r^0_{1,2}$ is the frequency of Receptor 2 at which it begins to inhibit

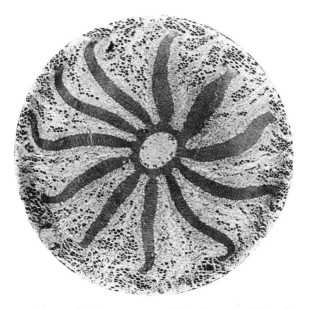

Fig. 3. Electron micrograph of sensory part of *Limulus* ommatidium in cross-section. In the center is the distal process of the eccentric cell. The rhabdom appears to be shaped like the hub and spokes of a wheel in this two-dimensional micrograph. For further details see Miller (1957, 1958). Magnification approximately 2500 ×.

Receptor 1; $r^0_{2,1}$ is the reverse. In the same way, $K_{1,2}$ is the coefficient of the inhibitory action of Receptor 2 on Receptor 1; $K_{2,1}$ the reverse. In general, K decreases with increasing separation of interacting elements and r^0 increases (Ratliff and Hartline, 1959). Negative frequencies, of course, cannot occur; when the inhibitory term $K(r-r^0)$ is greater than the excitation e, the corresponding response r must be set equal to zero. Furthermore, when $(r-r^0)$ is negative, the inhibitory term must be dropped.

Equations (1) above describe a network in which the strength of the inhibitory influence exerted by each receptor unit on the other is

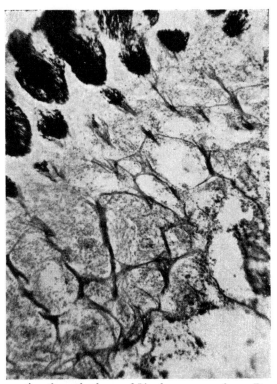

Fig. 4. Oblique section through plexus of *Limulus* compound eye. Densely pigmented proximal portions of ommatidia at top. Silver impregnated axons and axonal branches interconnecting bundles from ommatidia are seen. Paraffin section, Samuel's silver stain.

determined by its level of activity, which, in turn, is the resultant of the excitatory stimulus to that receptor unit and the inhibitory influences exerted back upon it from the other [Fig. 5(a)]. In this respect, the system is reminiscent of the so-called recurrent (Renshaw) inhibition in the spinal cord (cf. Granit, Pascoe, and Steg, 1957; Brooks and Wilson, 1959), and we shall refer to it hereafter as a 'recurrent' system.

In an alternative 'non-recurrent' system, a type which has often been postulated for various inhibitory networks, the strength of the inhibitory influence exerted by each unit on the other depends upon its level of activity *ahead* of the site at which inhibitory influences from the others are exerted upon it [Fig. 5(b)].

The differences between these two types of inhibitory networks are important. In the recurrent system influences are not only exerted directly on neighbors but also indirectly on others by way of those affected directly. For example, when additional receptors are illuminated in the vicinity of an interacting pair too far from one receptor unit to affect it directly, but near enough to the second to inhibit it, the frequency of discharge of the first increases as it is partially released from the inhibition exerted on it by the second (Hartline and Ratliff, 1957). Such 'disinhibition' can occur in a single stage of a recurrent system; in a single stage of a non-recurrent system it cannot. [Alpern and David (1959) and Mackavey, Bartley, and Casella (1962) have obtained evidence of a similar disinhibition in the human visual system, suggesting that the inhibitory influences there may also be recurrent.

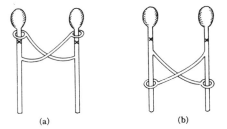

(a)   (b)

Fig. 5. Schematic diagram of (a) 'recurrent' and (b) 'non-recurrent' inhibitory systems. In both systems the magnitude of the inhibitory influence exerted by each unit on the other depends upon the level of activity generated at the site X ahead of the interconnecting branches. In the recurrent system (a) each unit exerts inhibitory influences back upon the other at or ahead of the site X at which impulses are generated and which is also ahead of the lateral branches. In the non-recurrent system (b) each unit exerts influences on the other at some point below the lateral branches.

The same results could be obtained, however, with a multiple-stage non-recurrent system.] In addition to the above differences, Reichardt and MacGinitie (1962) have pointed out that single-stage non-recurrent inhibitory systems are stable, while single-stage recurrent systems may or may not be stable depending upon the magnitudes of the inhibitory coefficients (see also Melzak 1962).

There is much indirect proof that the inhibition in the eye of *Limulus* is recurrent. For one thing, the anatomy of the interconnections suggests this; also, the disinhibition and other results of combined inhibitory influences that we have observed in a number of experiments using a variety of configurations of illumination and numbers of interacting elements all seem to require description in terms of the recurrent types of equations (Hartline and Ratliff, 1957, 1958; Ratliff and Hartline, 1959). In addition, more direct evidence has been obtained by recording from a micropipette inserted into the ommatidium at or ahead of the site at which impulses are generated. The discharge of impulses observed there is slowed by inhibition in the same manner as in the axon of the eccentric cell (Hartline, Wagner, and Ratliff, 1956). More recently, by recording impulses simultaneously with a pipette in the ommatidium and with wick electrodes on the axon which arises from the eccentric cell we have shown that there is a one-to-one correspondence – even during inhibition – between the impulses which are observed in the ommatidium and in the eccentric-cell axon (Fig. 6). It is evident that impulses are not first generated by the light and then sometime later abolished by the inhibition.

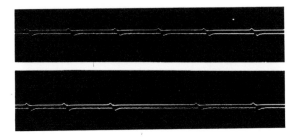

Fig. 6. Impulses recorded simultaneously with a micropipette electrode (upper trace) inserted in the ommatidium and wick electrodes (lower trace) placed on the axon of the eccentric cell of the same ommatidium. Upper record: no inhibition. Lower record: response during inhibition produced by illumination of neighboring ommatidia. Inhibitory influence begins following third pair of impulses. Note one-to-one correspondence between impulses recorded simultaneously from the two different sites. (Amplifier inputs capacitatively coupled.)

Studies of the mechanism of the inhibition reveal the basis of the recurrent effects. Stimulation by light produces a 'generator potential' – a decrease in the membrane potential of the eccentric cell (Hartline, Wagner, and MacNichol, 1952). During steady illumination the discharge of impulses in the eccentric-cell axon increases linearly with increasing magnitudes of the depolarization of the eccentric cell (Mac-Nichol, 1956; Fuortes, 1959). Conversely, an increase in the membrane potential of the eccentric cell, produced either by decreasing the level of illumination or by passing current through the recording micro-electrode, slows the discharge of impulses. Similarly, inhibitory influences exerted on a discharging eccentric cell produce a slight increase in the membrane potential of the cell (Fig. 7) with a concomitant slowing of the discharge of impulses (Tomita, Kikuchi, and Tanaka, 1960; see also Hartline, Ratliff, and Miller, 1961). Presumably, these are post-synaptic influences exerted upon the eccentric-cell axon where branches of the interconnecting fibers terminate in clumps of neuropile in the plexus. [These influences are comparable to inhibitory post-synaptic potentials observed in other preparations. See Eccles (1961).] Thus, the photoexcitatory mechanism and the inhibitory mechanism appear to exert their opposite influences simultaneously at or near a common point: the site of impulse generation. The net level of the membrane potential at this site determines the frequency of impulses (Tomita, 1958; Fuortes, 1960).

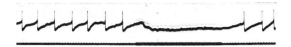

Fig. 7. Decrease in magnitude of 'generator potential' and concomitant cessation of impulse discharge resulting from inhibitory influences. The inhibition was produced by antidromic stimulation of the axons of neighboring ommatidia (cf. Tomita, 1958; Tomita, Kikuchi, and Tanaka, 1960). Antidromic stimuli (66 per sec. for 1·5 sec.) signaled by thickening of lower trace and shock artifacts on upper trace. Downward movement of the trace indicates increasing negativity of the recording microelectrode in the interior of the cell. Amplitude of spikes approximately 10 mV.

The inhibitory influences from two regions of the eye combine when they affect a third region. This combination is by a simple addition of the separate influences (Hartline and Ratliff, 1958). Therefore, Eqs. (1) above can be extended to a system of n interacting elements simply by summing, in each of the n equations, all of the $(n-1)$ influences exerted on a particular element p by each of the others j:

$$r_p = e_p - \sum_{j=1}^{n} K_{p,j} \ (r_j - r^0_{p,j}). \qquad (2)$$

Terms for which $j=p$ are omitted. This excludes consideration of possible 'self-inhibition' in this formal treatment (see Hartline, Ratliff, and Miller, 1961). The restrictions on Eqs. (1), mentioned above, apply here also.

This more general formulation was first tested indirectly by observing the effects – on single elements – of two neighboring inhibiting areas of various sizes, locations, and intensities of illumination (Hartline and Ratliff, 1958; Ratliff and Hartline, 1959). More recently, it has been possible to test the validity of the formulation directly by recording from three fibers simultaneously, as shown schematically in Fig. 8. In these experiments the six sets of inhibitory coefficients and thresholds of inhibitory action were determined directly by illuminating the three elements in pairs. Once the inhibitory coefficients and thresholds were obtained in this manner then a number of values of e were determined

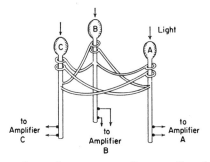

Fig. 8. Diagram of experimental arrangement for recording simultaneously from the eccentric cell axons of three interacting receptor units. Highly schematic.

by illuminating the three elements singly at several different levels of intensity. By using the values of e obtained when the elements were illuminated singly and the values of K and r^0 obtained by illuminating the elements in pairs, the responses expected when all three were illuminated simultaneously were calculated from the general Eqs. (2) above for this special case of $n = 3$. (No arbitrary adjustment of constants was permitted.) In Fig. 9 the results of these calculations are compared with the observed simultaneous responses of the three elements. The theoretical prediction agrees reasonably well with the observed data. If the same data are used in solving equations written to express non-recurrent inhibition (that is, letting the inhibition depend on e_j rather than r_j) then the magnitude of the predicted inhibition is generally too great. The equations for recurrent inhibition that we have adopted give the best fit.

The responses of such an interacting population of photoreceptors suggest an explanation for some familiar phenomena in human vision. It is evident, for example, that border contrast, Mach bands, and other forms of brightness contrast could all conceivably result from inhibitory interaction at some level or other in the visual pathways. Indeed, we have used the eye of *Limulus* as a model of such phenomena, and have generated patterns of optic nerve responses in which border contrast and the Mach effect appear (Ratliff and Hartline, 1959). Any extension to problems of color and color contrast would require, of course, a number of additional assumptions about the spectral sensitivity of the individual photoreceptors, and the manner in which fibers arising from them are interconnected with one another at various levels in the visual system. A theory of color vision advanced by Hurvich and Jameson (1957) is an example of one which utilizes principles of opposing influences exerted among various receptor elements.

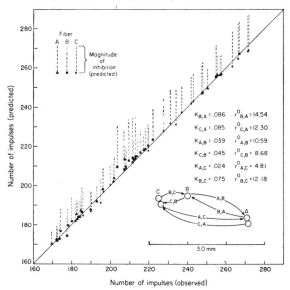

Fig. 9. Comparison of observed and predicted responses of three interacting receptor units (number of impulses generated in a steady-state period of 10 sec.). The values of K and r^0 obtained by illuminating the elements in pairs are shown in the table. The configuration of the illuminated ommatidia is shown in the inset. The spots of light A and C each illuminated two ommatidia; the response of only one member of each pair was observed, however, and this response was taken as a measure of the activity of both members of the pair. The spot of light B illuminated only one ommatidium. The uninhibited responses of the three receptor units are indicated – on the ordinate – by the upper end of the dashed lines (A, B, and C illuminated alone). The filled symbols plot the responses of A, B, and C illuminated together; predicted responses as ordinates, observed responses as abscissas.

III. TEMPORAL PROPERTIES OF THE INHIBITORY INTERACTION IN THE EYE OF 'LIMULUS'

In the experiment illustrated in Fig. 10, one element in the eye of *Limulus* was illuminated steadily to give a steady discharge of nerve impulses. A group of nearby elements was illuminated with a short flash to give a compact burst of impulses of nearly uniform frequency (monitored by recording the response of one element in the center of the group.) The familiar latent period of about 100 msec between the onset of the flash and the appearance of the first impulse in the burst is evident. Following this, a comparable time elapsed before there was an appreciable slowing of the activity in the neighboring steadily illuminated element. Following the end of the burst, it took approximately 300 msec for the steadily illuminated element to resume its original frequency of discharge. These time delays can be seen more clearly if the

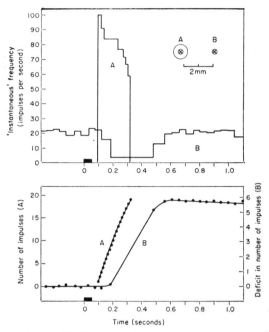

Fig. 10. Inhibition of a steadily illuminated receptor unit B produced by a short flash of illumination on neighboring ommatidia A. Configuration of the pattern of illumination shown in the inset. Spot A illuminated a small group of approximately 6 ommatidia. The activity of only the one in the center of the group was recorded. In the upper graph the 'instantaneous' frequencies (reciprocals of intervals between successive impulses) of A and B are plotted. In the lower graph the same data are plotted in terms of the cumulative number of impulses in the burst of activity produced by illumination of A (left-hand ordinate) and the corresponding cumulative deficit in number of impulses in B (right-hand ordinate). The ordinates were adjusted to match the total number of impulses in A and the total deficit in B. Illumination of A for 0.05 sec. at $t = 0$ indicated by black rectangle.

impulses in the burst, and – similarly – the loss of impulses by the inhibited element, are integrated (Fig. 10, lower graph).

Data obtained from just two interacting elements (Fig. 11) show similar, but smaller, mutual inhibitory effects resulting from the influence of transient bursts in each exerted on the other. The relative sizes of the effects are comparable to the relative magnitudes of the steady-state inhibitory coefficients determined for these two elements. The time delays in the two directions are approximately (but not exactly) equal.

In the steady state the time delays involved in the inhibitory interaction are of no significance, but they are important in the dynamic

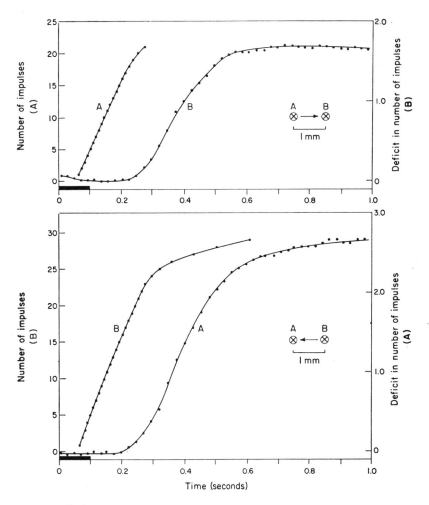

Fig. 11. Inhibition of one steadily responding receptor unit by a burst of activity in another. Upper graph, B steadily illuminated, A illuminated by 0.1 sec. flash at $t = 0.0$. Lower graph, A steadily illuminated, B illuminated by 0.1 sec. flash. Separation of the two ommatidia and the direction of the transient influence shown in the insets. Ordinates adjusted as in Fig. 10, lower graph.

response of the inhibitory network. For one thing, the dynamic system may be thought of as non-recurrent in time. That is, the successive states of a pair of interacting elements may be regarded as linked in time, as shown in the schematic diagram of Fig. 12. Neither element affects the other immediately; each affects the response of the other at some later time. The modified response of each then affects the response of the other at a still later time, and so on. The process, of course, is probably more or less continuous, not stepwise as the diagram might suggest.

As a first approximation, we can include the temporal properties of this system in Eqs. (2) above with the following modification:

$$r_p(t) = e_p(t) - \sum_{j=1}^{n} K_{p,j}[r_j(t - T_{p,j}) - r^0{}_{p,j}].$$
(3)

In these equations the response, r_p of a particular element at any time t is determined by the level of excitation e_p of the element at that same time, diminished by the summated inhibitory influences exerted on it by the other elements j. These influences are the ones initiated by the elements j at some earlier time $t - T_{p,j}$, where $T_{p,j}$ is the time-lag of the action of any particular element j on the element p, as defined above. The restrictions on Eqs. (1) and (2) above also apply here.

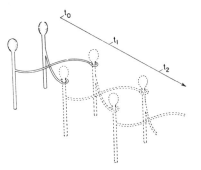

Fig. 12. Diagram of the temporal sequence of the mutual inhibitory influences exerted between a pair of interacting elements. Highly schematic.

We wish to emphasize that this quantitative formulation of the temporal properties of the inhibition is only a first approximation in which a number of important details are omitted. In the first place, we have assumed, for the sake of simplicity, that the inhibitory influence has no appreciable duration. That is, the inhibitory influence produced by r_j at the time $t - T_{p,j}$ is treated as if it were exerted on r_p only at the one instant of time t. Undoubtedly, the influence takes some time to build up and to decay. Second, there may be a natural transient in the initial phases of any prolonged inhibitory influence in addition to that which might be attributed to the initial high-frequency burst of impulses (Tomita, 1958; Hartline, Ratliff, and Miller, 1961). Third, some experiments indicate that the inhibitory coefficients may not be constant in time, as we have assumed here. We have found, for example, that the second of two short bursts of impulses, spaced 1.0 sec. apart, may produce a greater inhibitory effect than the first. Fourth, the time delay of the action may not be the same at all levels of frequency. Furthermore, there is a small overshoot, or 'post-inhibitory rebound', following inhibition, which is neglected in our present treatment. Further experimental study is needed to elucidate these points.

Despite its shortcomings, this formal description is a useful approximation. It is intuitively clear that a time-lag in the action of such a system is likely to lead to oscillations if there is a sudden increment in the stimulation on one or several members of an interacting group. Indeed, we have observed oscillations in the frequency of the optic nerve discharge in the eye of *Limulus* (Fig. 13). The inhibitory co-

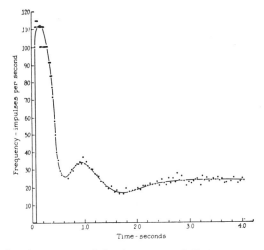

Fig. 13. Plot of the time course of the frequency of discharge of an ommatidium illuminated together with several nearby ommatidia, showing oscillations resulting from the time delay in the action of the mutual inhibitory influences.

efficients in the *Limulus* eye are usually not very large, even for near neighbors $(K \cong 0.2)$, and as might be expected, the oscillations are strongly damped. We have calculated the expected time course of these oscillations and the relative amplitudes of their maxima and minima, using the above Eqs. (3). The calculated values agree reasonably well with those observed. [In these calculations we used time delays $(T_{p,j})$ estimated from graphs such as those in Fig. 10; the inhibitory co-efficients $K_{p,j}$ were determined from steady-state experiments.]

The various transients in the responses of steadily illuminated receptor units are not all the result of inhibitory interaction. The initial maximum is a property of the receptor, and the first minimum following it may also be, in part, an expression of a receptor mechanism (Hartline and Graham, 1932). This 'silent period' is usually absent in the response of the light-adapted receptor, however. Furthermore, this first minimum may be greatly enhanced by enlarging the area of illumination and thus increasing the strength of the inhibition exerted on the particular receptor unit under observation. The subsequent oscillations appear to be entirely the result of the mutual inhibitory influences in the group of receptors.

These damped oscillations, which result from time delays in the interacting network, resemble some well-known human visual phenomena. Oscillations in the Broca Sulzer effect at high intensities, Charpentier's bands – and similar 'ghosts' – have often been attributed to the effects of delayed inhibition in the visual pathways. Indeed, the formal similarities between the temporal properties of the inhibitory network we have described and the temporal properties of these visual phenomena

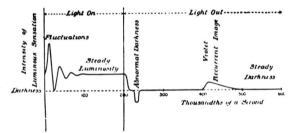

Fig. 14. Diagrammatic representation of visual sensations in the human in response to a short flash of light (from Bidwell, 1899).

are striking. For example, Bidwell's measurements (1899) of the changes in apparent brightness of a flash of light (based on observations of Charpentier's bands) show a damped oscillation (Fig. 14) very much like the system we have described. Our direct observations that an inhibitory network can produce such phenomena offer support for the view that similar inhibitory mechanisms are operating in our own visual systems.

In Eqs. (1)–(3) above, the response of a receptor unit illuminated alone is defined as an immediate and direct measure of the level of excitation e of that unit. In these formulations it is not necessary to take into account the latent period between the onset of the external stimulus and the production of the excitatory influence in the receptor. Indeed, this latent period is of no significance in our treatment of the steady-state inhibitory interaction [Eq. (2)]. Also, in some of the examples of the temporal properties of inhibitory interaction given above, the latent periods need not be considered; they are nearly identical for all elements. In all such cases, responses determined by solutions of the Eqs. (3) may be related to the external stimulus simply by a constant displacement in time equal to the latent period. In other situations, however, differences in the latent periods of the various elements may be enormous. They may range from 40 to 1000 msec or more, depending upon the intensity of illumination, state of adaptation, inhibitory influences exerted by neighbors, etc. The effects of these differences are of considerable interest.

One of the effects of different latent periods in neighboring receptor units is illustrated in the following experiment. A test receptor A and a neighbouring group of receptors B were illuminated by short flashes so as to produce short compact bursts of impulses in their axons. (The response of one receptor in the center of the group B was taken as a measure of the activity of the whole group.) The latencies of the responses to these short flashes were adjusted by setting the level of

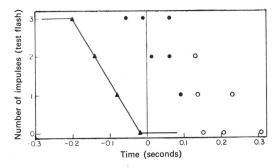

Fig. 15. Apparent 'backward' inhibition in the lateral eye of *Limulus*. A single ommatidium A was illuminated with 0.05-sec. flashes of low-intensity illumination, and the impulses discharged in response to these test flashes were recorded. A neighboring group of five ommatidia B were illuminated with 0.05-sec. flashes of high-intensity illumination and the discharge of impulses from the ommatidium in the center of the group was recorded. The times of presentation of the two stimuli were varied so that the weak test flash on the single ommatidium either preceded, coincided with, or followed the strong flash on the neighboring group. The number of impulses discharged from the single ommatidium A in response to the test flash is plotted (filled triangles and solid line) as a function of the time of the test *flash* relative to the time of the *flash* of illumination on the neighboring group B. When plotted in this manner the inhibitory effect appears to occur before the flash of light on the group exerting the effect. The actual time of occurrence of each *impulse* discharged by A is plotted (filled circles) relative to the time of occurrence of the first *impulse* in the response of the neighboring group B. Times at which the missing impulses (open circles) would have occurred, had there been no inhibition, were estimated from control observations of the discharge of impulses in response to the test flash alone. When plotted in this manner it is evident that approximately 0.1 sec. elapses between the first impulse in the response of the group and the first impulse lost in the response of the test receptor.

adaptation and intensity of illumination such that the test receptor A had an extremely long latent period and the group B an extremely short latent period. When the stimuli were presented asynchronously it was possible to find time relations such that there appeared to be an inhibitory influence exerted 'backwards' in time. That is, a stimulus to receptor unit A came on some time ahead of the stimulus to the neighbouring receptor units B, but since the latent period of A was very long, the response of the group B had time to appear and exert its inhibitory effects before the appearance of the response of A, which was illuminated first. If the data are plotted in terms of the times of *stimulus* onsets, then the effect of B on A seemed to appear before B was illuminated (Fig. 15). The inhibition is truly forward in time, of course, as can be seen if the data are plotted in terms of the times of occurrence of the *responses* rather than the times of the stimuli.

A similar interpretation of the effects of latent periods or other time delays is often advanced as an explanation of various 'backward masking' effects observed in the eye of the human (e.g. Crawford, 1947). In this experiment, however, we have the advantage that the neural response can actually be observed, and it can therefore be demonstrated directly that an inhibitory network with certain temporal properties can produce an apparent 'backward' inhibition.

IV. ROLE OF INHIBITORY INTERACTION IN THE GENERATION .OF SPECIALIZED TRANSIENT RESPONSES

The specialized 'on-off' and 'off' responses to changes in the level of illumination are familiar properties of the retinal ganglion cells of the vertebrate eye (Hartline, 1938). (Such responses are not unique to the vertebrate, however; they also appear – at some level or another – in the visual systems of many invertebrates.) The nature of these transient responses depends upon both the spatial and temporal configuration of the pattern of illumination (Hartline, 1941; Barlow, 1953; Kuffler, 1953; Wagner and Wolbarsht, 1958; Maturana, Lettvin, McCulloch, and Pitts, 1960). Furthermore, in some animals the transient responses are 'color-coded' (Wagner, MacNichol, and Wolbarsht, 1960). All are responses to *change*, and thus they carry information of great significance to the organism about its environment. Furthermore – in the human eye, at least – change is essential for the maintenance of vision; stationary images on the retina gradually fade from view (Ditchburn and Ginsborg, 1952; Riggs, Ratliff, Cornsweet, and Cornsweet, 1953).

The transient responses are generally believed to result from the complex interplay of excitatory and inhibitory influences (see Granit, 1947). The manner in which the inhibitory interaction may contribute to the generation of transient responses is less obvious than the role it may play in contrast phenomena. Nevertheless, it is easy to show a number of possibilities inherent in an interacting system such as the one we have just described.

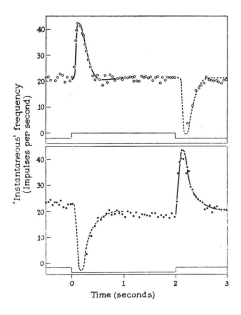

Fig. 16. Changes in optic-nerve discharge frequency for incremental and decremental stimuli. Light-adapted, steadily discharging *Limulus* single optic-nerve preparation stimulated by an incremental 2-sec. flash (top) or 2-sec. decrement (bottom). Open and closed circles represent experimental determinations of 'instantaneous' frequency of response. Bottommost lines in each half of the figure indicate onset and termination of the stimulus. Solid lines fitted by inspection to changes in frequency of response during upward-step stimuli; dashed lines are mirror images of the solid lines (for each half of the figure, respectively). Log adapting $I = -0.26$; log I during increment $= 0.0$; log I during decrement $= -0.50$.

Both the excitatory and inhibitory components of activity in the optic nerve of the lateral eye of *Limulus* exhibit marked transient responses to stimulus changes. MacNichol and Hartline (1948) found that the steady discharge of a single receptor unit in response to constant illumination is modulated in a characteristic way by step increments or decrements in the intensity of the illumination. A relatively small increase in intensity produces a large transient increase in frequency of discharge which quickly subsides to a steady level only slightly greater than that preceding the change in illumination. Similarly, a small decrease in intensity produces a large decrease in frequency which quickly returns to a level slightly below that preceding the change in illumination (Fig. 16). Because of the inhibition, these excitatory transients produce similar but opposite effects in the frequency of response of steadily illuminated neighboring receptor units (Fig. 17).

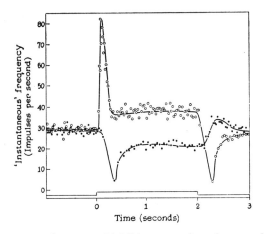

Fig. 17. Simultaneous excitatory and inhibitory transients in two adjacent receptor units in the lateral eye of *Limulus*. One receptor unit, black dots, was illuminated steadily throughout the period shown in the graph. The other unit, open circles, was illuminated steadily until time 0, when the illumination on it was increased abruptly to a new steady level where it remained for 2 sec. and then was decreased abruptly to the original level. The added illumination produced a large transient increase in frequency of the second receptor, which subsided quickly to a steady rate of responding; the subsequent decrease in illumination to the original level produced a large transient decrement in the frequency of response, after which the frequency returned to approximately the level it had prior to these changes (cf. Fig. 16). Accompanying these marked excitatory transients are large transient inhibitory effects in the adjacent, steadily illuminated receptor unit. A large decrease in frequency is produced by the inhibitory effect resulting from the large excitatory transient; during the steady illumination the inhibitory effect is still present but less marked; and finally, accompanying the decrement in the frequency of response of the element on which the level of excitation was decreased, there is a marked release from inhibition (from Ratliff, 1961).

It is evident that with proper adjustment of latencies of response, as in the masking experiment described above, it should be possible to obtain the response of some elements far in advance of the response of others even though all are stimulated simultaneously. This is indeed the case. Under proper conditions one group of elements can completely

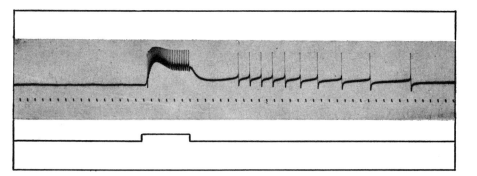

Fig. 18. Intracellular record showing afterdischarge following direct response to intense illumination of *Limulus* compound eye. Spikes in afterdischarge approximately 60 mV. Time 1/10 sec.

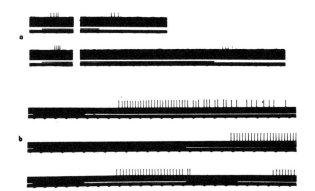

Fig. 19. Oscillograms of diverse 'types' of impulse discharge patterns in single fibers of *Limulus* optic nerve. The typical response to steady illumination of a single ommatidium is a sustained discharge. In the records shown the receptor was illuminated simultaneously with other nearby receptors, which exerted inhibition upon it. Depending on the conditions of illumination, various kinds of responses can be 'synthesized'. (a) Records of synthetic 'on-off' responses produced by two different durations of illumination; approximately 1 sec. was cut from the middle of each record. (b) Records of synthetic 'off' responses for various durations of illumination. In the lower record of (b) the 'off' response, comparable to that in the upper record, was inhibited by reillumination. Time is marked in fifths of a second. Signal of exposure to light blackens the white line above the time marks. (From Ratliff, Hartline, and Miller, 1958. See also Ratliff and Mueller, 1957.)

inhibit the other. That is, the inhibitory influences from the one group can reach the other group before it has time to respond at all, and thus suppress its response throughout an entire period of maintained illumination. Or, by suitably adjusting the latent period, it is possible for the response of the stronger member of the two groups to come in just late enough so that a few impulses escape from the weaker before it is completely inhibited. In this manner a simple 'on' burst of responses can be generated. Similarly, a combination of factors such as after-discharge (Fig. 18) and the overshoot following inhibition can lead to an 'off' discharge of impulses from one of the elements.

By a suitable combination of the principles just described and by careful adjustment of the stimulus conditions, it has been possible to generate 'on-off' and 'off' responses in some members of an interacting group of receptors in the eye of *Limulus* (Fig. 19), each of which – when illuminated singly – would ordinarily give a maintained discharge in response to illumination. These 'synthesized' transient responses resemble those which normally occur in the vertebrate retina and in optic ganglia of a number of species, both vertebrates and invertebrates. In these cases complex ganglionic structures provide ample opportunity for the interplay of excitatory and inhibitory influences.

Mutual inhibitory interaction in the retina not only serves to enhance spatial contrast in the retinal image, but also appears to play a role in generating complex responses to temporal changes in illumination. Those produced by movements of the eye, or by movements of objects in the visual field, are of special significance, for – as Ulysses remarked when upbraiding Achilles for his inaction – 'Things in motion sooner catch the eye than what stirs not' (*Troilus and Cressida*, Act III, Scene III).

REFERENCES

Alpern, M., and David, H., 'The Additivity of Contrast in the Human Eye', *J. Gen. Physiol.*, **43,** 109 (1959).

Barlow, H. B., 'Summation and Inhibition in the Frog's Retina', *J. Physiol.*, **119,** 69 (1953).

Bidwell, S., *Curiosities of Light and Sight* (Swann Sonnenschein and Company, London, 1899).

Brooks, V. B., and Wilson, V. J., 'Recurrent Inhibition in the Cat's Spinal Cord', *J. Physiol.* **146,** 380 (1959).

Crawford, B. H., 'Visual Adaptation in Relation to Brief Conditioning Stimuli', *Proc. Roy. Soc.* (London) **B134,** 283 (1947).

Ditchburn, R. W., and Ginsborg, B. L., 'Vision with a Stabilized Retinal Image', *Nature* **170,** 36 (1952).

Eccles, J. C., 'The Mechanism of Synaptic Transmission', Ergeb. *Physiol. biol. Chem. u. exp. Pharmakol.* **51,** 300 (1961).

Fuortes, M. G. F., 'Initiation of Impulses in Visual Cells of *Limulus*', *J. Physiol.* **148,** 14 (1959).

Fuortes, M. G. F., 'Inhibition in *Limulus* Eye', *Inhibitions of the Nervous System and γ-Aminobutyric Acid* (Pergamon Press, New York, 1960).

Granit, R., *Sensory Mechanisms of the Retina* (Oxford University Press, London, 1947).

Granit, R., Pascoe, J. E., and Steg, G., 'The Behavior of Tonic *a* and γ Motoneurones during Stimulation of Recurrent Collaterals', *J. Physiol.* **138,** 381 (1957).

Hartline, H. K. 'The Response of Single Optic Nerve Fibers of the Vertebrate Eye to Illumination of the Retina', *Am. J. Physiol.* **121,** 400 (1938).

—, 'The Neural Mechanisms of Vision', The Harvey Lectures, Ser. XXXVII, 39 (1941–1942).

—, 'Inhibition of Activity of Visual Receptors by Illuminating nearby Retinal Elements in the *Limulus* Eye', Federation Proc. **8,** 69 (1949).

Hartline, H. K., and Graham, C. H., 'Nerve Impulses from Single Receptors in the Eye', *J. Cell. Comp. Physiol.* **1,** 277 (1932).

Hartline, H. K., and Ratliff, F., 'Inhibitory Interaction of Receptor Units in the Eye of *Limulus*', *J. Gen. Physiol.* **40,** 357 (1957).

—, 'Spatial Summation of Inhibitory Influences in the Eye of *Limulus*, and the Mutual Interaction of Receptor Units', *J. Gen. Physiol.* **41,** 1049 (1958).

Hartline, H. K., Ratliff, F., and Miller, W. H., 'Inhibitory Interaction in the Retina and its Significance in Vision', *Nervous Inhibition* edited by E. Florey (Pergamon Press, New York, 1961).

Hartline, H. K., Wagner, H. G., and MacNichol, E. F., Jr., 'The Peripheral Origin of Nervous Activity in the Visual System', Cold Spring Harbor *Symposia Quant. Biol.* **17,** 125 (1952).

Hartline, H. K., Wagner, H. G., and Ratliff, F., 'Inhibition in the Eye of *Limulus*', *J. Gen. Physiol.* **39,** 651 (1956).

Hurvich, L. M. and Jameson, D., 'An Opponent-Process Theory of Color Vision', *Psychol. Rev.* **64,** 384 (1957).

Kuffler, S. W., 'Discharge Patterns and Functional Organization of Mammalian Retina', *J. Neurophysiol.* **16,** 37 (1953).

Mackavey, W. R., Bartley, S. H., and Casella, C., 'Disinhibition in the Human Visual System', *J. Opt. Soc. Am.* **52,** 85 (1962).

MacNichol, E. F., Jr., 'Visual Receptors as Biological Transducers', in 'Molecular Structure and Functional Activity of Nerve Cells', American Institute of Biological Sciences Publ. No. 1 (1956), p. 34.

MacNichol, E. F., and Hartline, H. K., 'Responses to Small Changes of Light Intensity by the Light-Adapted Photoreceptor', *Federation Proc.* **7,** 76 (1948).

Maturana, H. R., Lettvin, J. Y., McCulloch, W. S., and Pitts, W. H., 'Anatomy and Physiology of Vision in the Frog (*Rana pipiens*)', *J. Gen. Physiol.* **43,** No. 6, Pt. 2, 129 (1960).

Melzak, Z. A., 'On a Uniqueness Theorem and its Application to a Neurophysiological Control Mechanism', Information and Control **5,** 163 (1962).

Miller, W. H., 'Morphology of the Ommatidia of the Compound Eye of *Limulus*', *J. Biophys. Biochem. Cytol.* **3,** 421 (1957).

—, 'Fine Structure of Some Invertebrate Photoreceptors', *Ann. N.Y. Acad. Sci.* **74,** 204 (1958).

Ratliff, F., 'Inhibitory Interaction and the Detection and Enhancement of Contours', *Sensory Communication* edited by W. A. Rosenblith (MIT Press, Cambridge, Mass., 1961).

Ratliff, F., and Hartline, H. K., 'The Responses of *Limulus* Optic Nerve Fibers to Patterns of Illumination on the Receptor Mosaic', *J. Gen. Physiol.* **42,** 1241 (1959).

Ratliff, F., Miller, W. H., and Hartline, H. K., 'Neural Interaction in the Eye and the Integration of Receptor Activity', *Ann. N.Y. Acad. Sci.* **74,** 210 (1958).

Ratliff, F. and Mueller, C. G., 'Synthesis of "on-off" and "off" Responses in a Visual-Neural System', *Science* **126,** 840 (1957).

Reichart, W., and MacGinitie, G., 'Zur Theorie der lateralen Inhibition', Kybernetik (to be published). **1/7,** 155–165 (1962).

Riggs, L. A., Ratliff, F., Cornsweet, J. C., and Cornsweet, T. N., 'The Disappearance of Steadily Fixated Test Objects', *J. Opt. Soc. Am.* **43,** 495 (1953).

Tomita, T., 'Mechanism of Lateral Inhibition in the Eye of *Limulus*', *J. Neurophysiol.* **21,** 419 (1958).

Tomita, T., Kikuchi, R., and Tanaka, I., 'Excitation and Inhibition in Lateral Eye of Horsehoe Crab', *Electrical Activity of Single Cells* edited by Y. Katsuki (Igaku Shoin Ltd., Tokyo, 1960).

Wagner, H. G., MacNichol, E. F., Jr., and Wolbarsht, M. L., 'The

Response Properties of Single Ganglion Cells in the Goldfish Retina', *J. Gen. Physiol.* **43,** No. 6, Pt. 2, 45 (1960).

Wagner, H. G., and Wolbarsht, M. L., 'Studies on the Functional Organization of the Vertebrate Retina', *Am. J. Ophthal.* **46,** No. 3, Pt. 2, 46 (1958).

Inhibitory interaction in the retina: techniques of experimental and theoretical analysis*

DAVID LANGE, H. KEFFER HARTLINE, AND
FLOYD RATLIFF

The Rockefeller University, New York, N.Y.

Reprinted from ANNALS OF THE NEW YORK ACADEMY OF
SCIENCES, 31 January 1966, Vol. 128, Art. 3, pp. 955-971

This paper describes the use of a small general purpose digital computer (Control Data Corporation 160-A) as an aid to experimental and theoretical studies of nervous interactions in visual systems. The experimental work has been primarily concerned with the inhibitory interaction in the lateral eye of the horseshoe crab, *Limulus polyphemus*. The theoretical work has been concerned with developing models of the spatial and dynamical properties of the interactions in this eye, and with the application of these models to the study of the vertebrate retina and to the explanation of more complex visual phenomena encountered in human psychophysics.

The earlier experimental work on steady state properties of the eye of *Limulus* was amenable to relatively simple techniques of data collection such as gated counters and photography. For reviews of this work see Hartline, Ratliff, and Miller (1961) and Ratliff (1961). The work is now being extended to the dynamical properties of the eye. For a review of some of the preliminary observations on dynamics see Ratliff, Hartline, and Miller (1963). In the case of dynamics, the continuous, impulse-by-impulse, collection of very large volumes of data is required. It is also necessary to have immediate information on the course of the experiment so that adjustments can be made in procedures. The computer is therefore employed at all levels of the study; namely, data collection, data storage, data processing, model simulation, and comparison of experimental and theoretical results.

Complete descriptions of the experimental procedure and results of previous studies are readily available in the references cited above, and therefore we will limit ourselves to a short summary as a background to the discussion of the computer techniques.

The anatomy of the *Limulus* lateral eye has been extensively studied by Miller (1957, 1958). FIGURE 1 is a composite three-dimensional light micrograph of a portion of the eye. The upper horizontal plane contains the facets (*F*) of the corneal surface (*c*). Light enters more or less perpendicularly to this plane. The upper vertical plane is a view of the longitudinal aspect of the functional units or ommatidia. Each unit has a crystalline cone lens (*cc*) which focuses an image onto the rhabdom (*r*). The rhabdom is formed from the convergence of the microvillous borders of a dozen or more retinular cells (*R*). These retinular cells are radially arranged around the distal process (D. P.)

*This investigation was supported by a research grant (NB864) from the National Institute of Neurological Diseases and Blindness, Public Health Service.

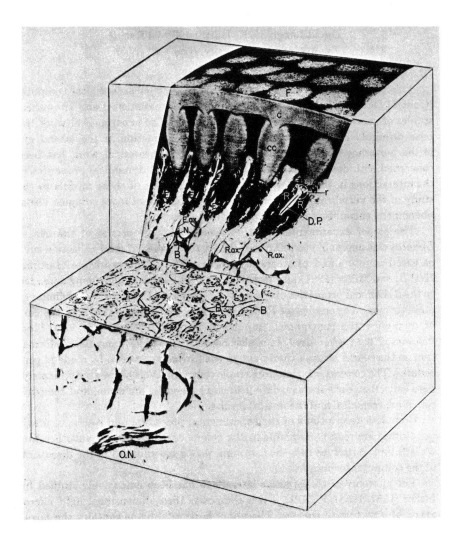

FIGURE 1. Composite, three dimensional light micrograph of a portion of the lateral eye of *Limulus*. See text for explanation. Reproduced from Ratliff, Hartline, and Miller (1963).

of a biopolar neuron, the eccentric cell (E). The rhabdom is in close contact with this dendrite. The eccentric cell and the many retinular cells have axons (E. ax and R. ax) which pass through a three-dimensional network of fibers and finally come together to form the optic nerve (O.N.). Each ommatidium seems to function as a unit as far as its output via the eccentric cell axon is concerned. For this reason we will refer to ommatidia as receptor units. We will refer to specific receptor units, the outputs of which we are using as a measure of inhibition, as test units.

Within the network, or lateral plexus, the axons of eccentric and retinular cells give off fine branches that course laterally in bundles (B in FIGURE 1). Clumps of neuropile (N) may be seen in the plexus and are usually found near eccentric cell axons. Under the electron microscope, this neuropile shows characteristic morphology usually associated with synapses. There are no nerve cell bodies within the neuropile. Because of the synaptic character of these regions it is believed that the inhibitory interactions within the eye are mediated through the neuropile.

The primary data in this work are spike-like electrical signs of nerve impulses recorded from single optic nerve fibers at points well beyond the lateral plexus. (The terms nerve spike and impulse will be used interchangeably.) When one confines a small spot of light to a single ommatidium and records the nerve spikes from the associated optic nerve fiber, one observes a spike frequency roughly proportional to the logarithm of the light intensity. If, however, one also illuminates the neighboring units, the spike frequency is reduced. This is the phenomenon of lateral inhibition. The brighter the light on the neighbors, the greater is the reduction in frequency. The smaller the distance between the test unit and illuminated neighbors, the greater is the inhibition. The larger the number of neighbors illuminated, the greater is the inhibition. The laws governing this phenomenon can be formulated in terms of a set of equations relating the steady state nerve spike frequencies in each optic nerve fiber to those in all its neighbors. The equations may be written as follows:

$$r_p = e_p - \sum_{\substack{j=1 \\ j \neq p}}^{n} k_{p,j}\,(r_j - r_{p,j}^0)$$

In words, the frequency, r_p, of the pth optic nerve fiber is the result of an excitatory frequency, e_p, related to the light intensity on it, diminished by a summation of frequencies from the n other ommatidia of the eye, r_j, reduced by values, $r_{p,j}^0$, and weighted by constants, $k_{p,j}$. Some further rules for the summation are necessary. Negative frequencies are not allowed, and $r_{p,j}^0$ is to be interpreted as a threshold frequency. Therefore $r_j - r_{p,j}^0$ must be taken as either positive (if $r_j > r_{p,j}^0$) or zero (if $r_j < r_{p,j}^0$). FIGURE 2 shows the results of an experiment where $n = 2$ and the solid lines are solutions of the resulting pairs of equations where $e_A - r_A$ is plotted against r_B and vice versa. This formulation adequately describes the steady state frequencies obtained after the lights have been on for some time. Our more recent interests have centered on the behavior of this lateral inhibitory system as a function of time with varying inhibitory input. Detailed accounts of the results will be published elsewhere, and we will confine the following discussion primarily to techniques.

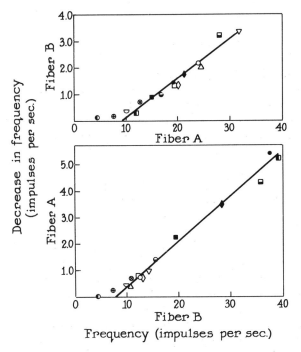

FIGURE 2. Graphs showing mutual inhibition of two receptor units. In each graph the inhibition (measured as a decrease in frequency relative to a control) exerted on one unit was plotted as a function of the concurrent activity (measured as a frequency) in the other. In order to obtain one point on each graph, three patterns of illumination were required: (1) light on A alone (A control), (2) B alone (B control), (3) light on both simultaneously (A and B experimental). Corresponding symbols on the two plots are from corresponding sets of illumination. The slopes of the lines are the inhibitory constants, K_{BA} and K_{AB}. The intercepts on the abscissa are the inhibitory thresholds r_{BA}^0 and r_{AB}^0. Reproduced from Hartline and Ratliff (1957).

Two methods of introducing time varying inhibition into the eye are used. One which follows immediately from the discussion above is to vary the light intensity as a function of time and record the changes in nerve impulse frequencies thus induced. The other is based on a technique developed by Tomita (1958). He found that one can induce inhibition by antidromically stimulating the optic nerve fibers of the neighboring ommatidia. That is, nerve spikes are propagated backward up the optic nerve and through the lateral plexus, thus causing inhibition. Although spikes enter the plexus from the "wrong" direction, inhibitory influences apparently propagate through it normally, and indeed the same laws hold for the steady state dependence of inhibition on spike frequency as in the case of light induced inhibition (Lange, 1965). This technique has the advantage of allowing very precise control over the inhibitory input.

The primary instrumental problems in these studies arise from the need to control precisely the temporal and spatial patterns of light flashes and electrical stimulations while simultaneously collecting large amounts of nerve spike data. The control aspects have been solved by using the solid state programmed timer described by Milkman and Schoenfeld (1965) in this monograph, while the data collection problem has been solved by using the digital computer and its associated input interfaces. A preliminary description of the system has been presented by Schoenfeld (1964).

FIGURE 3 diagrammatically outlines both the control and data collection aspects of the laboratory. We will confine the following discussion to the latter. The set-up as shown in the figure utilizes electrical stimulation of the optic nerve as the means of introducing inhibition, while light is used to provide the excitatory input. The techniques are not basically different if light is used to excite the neighbors.

The eccentric cell axon from the test unit is placed on a wick electrode in air. The electrode is connected to the input of a high input impedence pre-amplifier. The preamplifier output is AC-coupled to the oscilloscope input. The oscilloscope output from the vertical deflection circuit is then fed to an audio amplifier-speaker system and to the input of a discriminator and pulse former. The discriminator produces a pulse with each nerve spike recorded. An adjustable threshold on the discriminator allows for the removal of baseline noise.

The standard pulses from the discriminator provide an input to a special digital conversion device attached in turn to the input of the digital com-

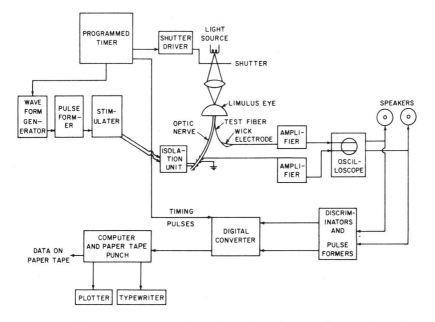

FIGURE 3. Diagramatic representation of experimental set-up. See text for explanation. Reproduced from Lange (1965).

puter (Control Data Corporation 160-A). The converter was designed and constructed by the Rockefeller Institute electronics laboratory and has been described by Schoenfeld (1964) and Schoenfeld and Milkman (1964). The function of this device is to feed a seven bit (digit) binary number to the computer in synchrony with the ten kilocycle oscillator of the programmed timer. Each of the seven bits represents one of seven possible input channels. A binary *one* in a particular bit indicates an event occurring since the last clock pulse; a *zero* indicates quiescence. Ordinarily only three or four of these channels are used. An event on the channel corresponding to the test unit is the presence of a nerve spike. Another channel signals antidromic stimulus pulses, while one or two others may signal the opening or closing of shutters. One line is used to control the computer itself and to designate the onset and end of an experiment. The computer is programmed to count the number of clock pulses between events on each channel and to store numbers representing these times. Therefore a list representing interspike or inter-stimulus intervals is made in the memory. These numbers are punched out on paper tape as a permanent record of the experiment and are considered the primary data at later stages in data processing. The oscilloscope tracings, which are more conventionally considered primary data, are not preserved.

Some preliminary data processing is done immediately by the computer, and the results are displayed between experimental runs. The most useful of these monitoring facilities is a plot of reciprocal interspike interval versus time. Such a display is commonly called an instantaneous frequency plot. A sample plot is seen in FIGURE 4a. The plot provides not only a good quantitative estimate of responses in a run but also a very sensitive indication of the discriminator adjustment. (See FIGURE 4, b and c.) In the lower figures the sudden drops of apparent frequency to half value signal a loss of one impulse, while the very high apparent frequencies result from added noise pulses. A type-out of an interval count over coarse time marks is also a useful measure of average frequency of impulses. In general these two monitors are the only data processing required at the time of the experiment. They provide adequate immediate feedback to the experimenter for control of the significant variables and for evaluation of the state of the preparation.

At a later date the paper tape output from the computer can be re-entered and used for more sophisticated processing. In general the most useful processing consists of averaging many experimental runs together to eliminate random variations and comparing them to similarly averaged control runs.

The averaging of data in the form of interspike intervals leads to a basic problem. One cannot merely add the nth interspike intervals from several experiments and divide. This is because the nth intervals from two experiments do not necessarily occur at the same time with respect to the onset of the experiments. Therefore, if one wishes to preserve absolute time information, some scheme must be used to assign an appropriate interval length, or a pulse frequency, to each point in time. The nearest approximation one can

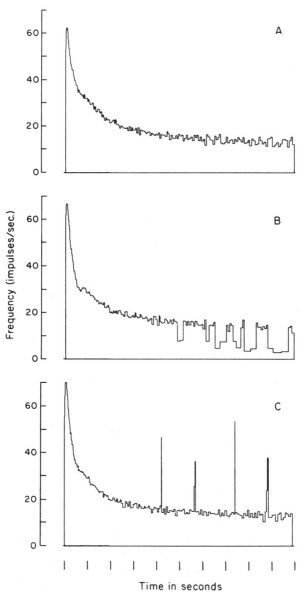

Time in seconds

FIGURE 4. "Instantaneous" frequency plots showing error detection. FIGURE A is a typical "instantaneous" frequency plot of the reciprocals of interspike intervals as a function of time. Frequency is calculated as the reciprocal of the interspike intervals. FIGURE B demonstrates the use of this display to detect failures in the electronic discriminators. At the points where the indicated frequency suddenly drops to one-half its value one nerve impulse was lost. Where it drops to one-third two were lost, etc. This indicates that the threshold should be lowered on the discriminator. In FIGURE C added pulses due to noisy signals have been recorded. Because of the random phasing of the noise it may cause a discrepancy ranging from double the frequency up to 10,000 cps (the reciprocal of the basic clock pulse). This type of plot indicates that the discriminator threshold should be raised. Reproduced from Lange (1965).

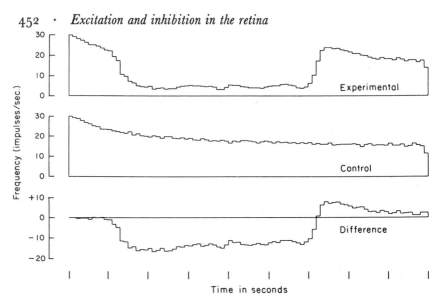

FIGURE 5. Comparison of experimental runs with control runs by subtraction. The figure demonstrates the method by which the response curves of FIGURE 11 were calculated. The second experiment from 11 A is illustrated. The upper trace is an average of four experimental runs. The middle trace is a similar average of four control runs where no inhibitory stimuli were delivered. The lowest trace is the algebraic difference between the first and second. Notice that this procedure eliminates the downward drift of frequencies. Reproduced from Lange (1965).

make to the pulse frequency at any time is to use the reciprocal of the interval occurring at that time. The program was therefore arranged to do the following: Time is divided into short periods. The lengths of these periods are varied depending on the use to which the data is put, but they are most often 0.1 second. The reciprocal of the interspike interval occurring during that time is associated with that period. If spikes occur during the period, the relevant reciprocals are weighted according to the fraction of the period they occupy. Another way of putting this would be to say that the number of interspike intervals in each period is counted with fractions of intervals included.

Once frequencies have been assigned to particular times, the results of several experimental runs can then be averaged. Such an averaging is done for both experimental and control runs, and these are compared. It is in fact most useful to subtract the averaged controls from the averaged experimental runs (see FIGURE 5). Inhibition appears then as a negative frequency difference. This frequency difference can then be plotted on the incremental plotter attached to the computer. The curves in FIGURE 5 were plotted in this way. The scales and lettering were then added by an artist. Differences in average frequencies over longer periods can also be typed out for use in computing inhibitory constants and thresholds with the help of curve fitting programs.

The averaging technique should be compared to the more commonly used technique of constructing post-stimulus-time histograms, which also measure an empirical probability of firing. The latter methods are sensitive to small changes in probability of firing and to patterning of firing with respect to the onset of the stimulus. Our technique is insensitive to correlations in absolute time of arrival of pulses but allows for a smooth estimate of frequency with a relatively small number of experimental repetitions. Time resolution below the width of an interspike interval is lost, however. The methods must be suited to the desired results. If one wishes to preserve the absolute times of arrival of individual impulses the post-stimulus-time histogram is more appropriate. If on the other hand one wishes to assign as smooth a frequency as possible to all times, our averaging methods are more appropriate.

Another useful averaging technique has been to reproduce the behavior of computers of average transients. These have been useful in studying the results of experiments with flickering light. In these experiments, the light on the test unit remains constant while that on its neighbors is switched between two intensity values. The switching pulses which are fed to the electromagnetic shutters of the optical system are also available to the computer input. These pulses are then used to cut the data into segments of constant phase with respect to the flicker. These segments are then averaged. The result is that only those changes in nerve impulse frequency, either excitatory or inhibitory, which are locked to the flickering input, survive the averaging. FIGURE 6 shows the raw data, and FIGURE 7 the results of averaging in such an experiment.

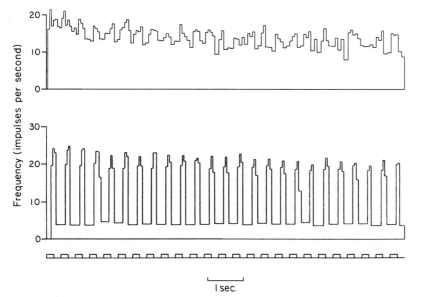

1 sec.

FIGURE 6. Plots of raw data from flicker experiment. The upper trace is the response of the test unit. The lower trace is the response of the inhibiting unit which is receiving flickering light. The boxes at the bottom represent the opening and closing of the shutters. See also the legend of FIGURE 7.

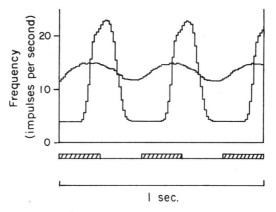

FIGURE 7. Plots of processed data from flicker experiment. See text for description of averaging technique. The low amplitude trace was extracted from the data represented in the top trace of FIGURE 6. The high amplitude trace was extracted from the data in the bottom trace of FIGURE 6. Notice changes of scale.

Let us now turn to some of the ways we are applying the computer to the theoretical problems related to our experiments. The first of these applications concerns problems in spatial contrast phenomena.

Lateral inhibitory mechanisms have long been hypothesized to explain contrast or edge effects, which occur at the boundaries between light and dark regions in the visual field. In particular, the phenomenon discovered by the well-known Austrian physicist, philosopher and psychologist, Ernst Mach, in 1865, which is now known as Mach bands, has been explained in these terms. [For a complete review of this and related phenomena and for translations of Mach's original papers in this field the reader should refer to Ratliff (1965).] Given a graded distribution of illumination, as in the penumbra of a shadow cast by an object in the light of an extended source, the apparent brightness differs from the measured luminance. Wherever there is a flection in the luminance there is seen either a dark band or a light band, depending on the sign of the second derivative of the luminance curve (see FIGURE 8).

One can observe the Mach bands at the edges of almost any shadow cast on a fairly uniform surface by an object in sunlight. The transition from the full shadow to the graded half-shadow provides the necessary convex flection; the transition from the half-shadow to the fully illuminated space provides the concave flection. At these points respectively, dark and light bands are seen. Indoors the Mach bands can easily be seen at the edge of a shadow cast on a piece of white paper by a card held under a fluorescent desk lamp, which provides the necessary extended source of light. (Covering the ends of the lamp, which usually are not uniformly bright, enhances the effect somewhat.) For best results, the card should be held about one or two inches above the white

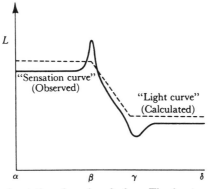

FIGURE 8. Mach bands at the edge of a shadow. The luminance or "light curve" (dashed line) is an ideal curve based on physical calculations. The point α is in the fully illuminated space, β is at the outer edge of the half-shadow, γ at the inner edge, and δ is in the full shadow. The solid line represents the apparent luminance or "sensation curve" actually observed. The maximum and minimum in the curve correspond to the bright and dark Mach bands. Reproduced from Ratliff (1965).

paper. Slight lateral movements of the card may enhance the visibility of the bands.

Neural nets having the properties of lateral inhibition described above will demonstrate spatial distributions of activity related to stimulus patterns in this same way. Simulation of such neural nets on a computer enables one to explore quickly the effects of many variables.

These simulations, unlike the collection and monitoring of real data, do not have to be carried out in real time, and therefore it is possible to use interpretive languages for programming. The simulations below were programmed in SICOM, a floating point decimal interpreter written especially for the CDC 160-A computer.

Although many models of lateral inhibition are linear, some contain inhibitory thresholds and the requirement for positive pulse frequencies. These restrictions make analytic solutions difficult. Furthermore, the equations for *Limulus* lateral inhibition are recurrent, that is, they are simultaneous equations. Since they are only piecewise linear this necessitates an iterative solution procedure which is nearly impossible by hand. The computer is, of course, well suited for such calculations.

A typical iterative solution is as follows. Let p represent any particular one of the n elements in the network and j all the others. Assume $e = kI$. The first step in the iteration is

$$r_p^{|1|} = e_p,$$

which gives the uninhibited response of any particular element in the network. The first approximation to the inhibited response—the second step in the iteration—uses these uninhibited responses to determine the inhibition on any particular element

$$r_p^{[2]} = e_p - \sum_{j=1}^{n} k_{p,j}(r_j^{[1]} - r_{p,j}^0).$$

Similarly, the third step in the iteration uses the inhibited responses determined in the second step in the iteration

$$r_p^{[3]} = e_p - \sum_{j=1}^{n} k_{p,j}(r_j^{[2]} - r_{p,j}^0)$$

and so on to the *s*th step in the iteration

$$r_p^{[s]} = e_p - \sum_{j=1}^{n} k_{p,j}(r_j^{[s-1]} - r_{p,j}^0).$$

The response r_p at all (or representative) points along the stimulus distribution $I(x)$ yields the corresponding response distributions $R(x)$ for each of the successive stages (FIGURE 9). The successive steps in a converging iterative solution are, of course, alternately over-estimates and underestimates which gradually approach the final solution that is shown in FIGURE 9. Inset in the figure is a geometrical representation of the dependence of $k_{p,j}$ on distance. (To simplify the figure, the thresholds have been omitted and negative frequencies allowed to occur.)

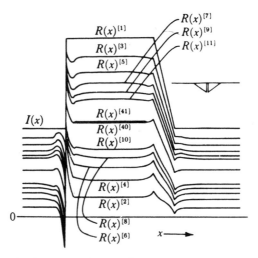

FIGURE 9. A graphical representation of the successive steps in the iterative solution of the response of a recurrent network to a rectilinear stimulus distribution. Only the results of the first 10 and the 40th and 41st steps are shown. In the computation the two ends of the stimulus distribution were extended a great distance to the right and left so that no edge effects would appear in the figure. Note that $r(x)^{[1]}$ equals $I(x)$, the top line in the graph. The maxima and minima in the calculated responses to the abrupt step are analogous to "border contrast" effects, and the maxima and minima in the responses to the gradient are analogous to the Mach bands. Reproduced from Ratliff (1965).

For linear cases, one can avoid repeated iterations by using a delta function input. The $R(x)^{[\infty]}$ resulting from a delta function input can be used as a single pass weighting function (Green's function) for other stimulus patterns thus obviating the need to iterate every solution.

The calculations done so far have been for one dimensional models in the steady state. In the future, we plan to make similar calculations for two dimensional nets as a function of time. The results of such calculations should have relevance to questions of form and motion perception.

All the discussion to this point has centered on steady state interactions among receptor units. It is well known, however, that changes in light intensity are most important to the behavior of an animal. In particular there are cells in some retinas which are sensitive to the onset, or cessation (or both) of a light stimulus but are not sensitive to steady illumination. Likewise there are cells which are sensitive to movement of patterns in the visual field. It is very likely that lateral interactions of the type described in this paper are of importance in (if not responsible for) these specialized responses (see, for example, Ratliff and Mueller, 1957). We have therefore been studying the dynamics of the lateral inhibitory system in *Limulus* and have been using the computer in creating models of these dynamics.

The specific physiological considerations which lead to the current models we are using have been discussed elsewhere (Lange, 1965). The basic assumptions in these models are as follows. It is assumed that impulse propagation occurs in the lateral plexus of axonal branches as well as in the main optic nerve fibers and that inhibitory information is transmitted along these plexus fibers. Associated with the arrival of each nerve impulse is an inhibitory event. These inhibitory events can be described as having a sharp onset and an exponential decay and as summing linearly with one another.

Physiologically, a potential, termed the generator potential, precedes and is responsible for the generation of spikes. The nerve spike frequency is proportional, at least in the steady state, to the magnitude of this potential (MacNichol, 1956). For our purposes we can consider the generator potential as a mathematical entity which describes the state of the test unit.

A generator potential is formed for the unit which is a linear sum of all excitatory input and the current value of the sum of all inhibitory influences where the latter have an opposite sign to the former, of course. The programs are primarily concerned with the generation of the time dependent inhibitory level. This is made up of two parts: (1) a summation of all lateral inhibitory events resulting from pulses in the lateral plexus and (2) a summation of inhibitory events associated with the firing of the cell itself. This latter phenomenon of self-inhibition is fully discussed by Stevens (1964), and in fact his model forms the basis for ours.

Once the current generator is formed from the summation of excitatory and inhibitory influences, a spike frequency proportional to this generator is produced.

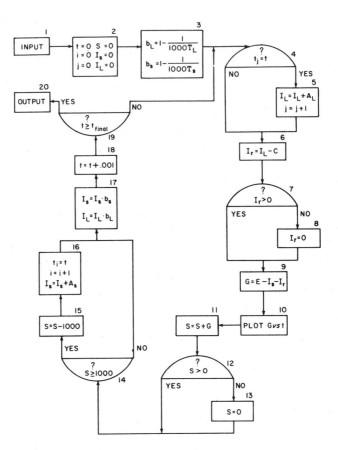

FIGURE 10. Flow diagram of model of dynamics. A table defining the terms and a description of each step follow. The numbers refer to the box numbers in the diagram.

E:	excitatory input	τ_s:	self-inhibitory time constant
t:	time of cycle	A_L:	lateral inhibitory quantum
i:	index of generated impulses	A_s:	self-inhibitory quantum
j:	index of inhibitory pulses	G:	generator
t_i:	times of impulses generated	I_s:	self-inhibitory pool
t_j:	times of inhibitory pulses	I_L:	lateral inhibitory pool
b_L:	lateral inhibitory decay factor	I_r:	reduced lateral inhibition
b_s:	self-inhibitory decay factor	S:	running sum (integral) of G
τ_L:	lateral inhibitory time constant	C:	threshold of lateral inhibition

1. Reads in paper tape data of inhibitory pulses $(t_j, j = 1$ to $n)$. Allows for setting of parameters and of the initial values of E on the typewriter.

2. Initialization of impulse list variables (i and j) of time (t) of the spike generating integral (S) and of the inhibition (I_s and I_L).

3. Formation of multiplicative decay constants (b_L and b_s) from each of the time constants (τ_L and τ_s).

4. Check for an inhibitory pulse at this time. If there is one go to 5, if not to 6.

5. Add quantum (A_L) to lateral inhibitory pool (I_L) and increase the inhibitory pulse index (j) to the next inhibitory pulse.

6. Form I_r by subtracting C from I_L.

The algorithm for spike generation is based on empirical observations and is formally similar to one proposed by Hodgkin (1948) for the repetitive firing in crab nerve. The generator is integrated with respect to time, and when this integral reaches a critical value a spike is produced. For steady generators, this produces a steady spike frequency proportional to the generator.

Let us now look in more detail at the actual programming of such a model. The original data consists first of a list of times of inhibitory pulses. This list is in fact usually constructed from the input, as recorded by the computer, of the real experiment to be simulated. The rest of the data are time constants for self and lateral inhibition, the amplitude of inhibitory events, the size of the inhibitory threshold, and a number describing the excitatory generator before inhibition.

At each point in time, the program must construct the generator (excitation diminished by inhibition), integrate the generator by one more time division, and decide whether to produce a spike. FIGURE 10 shows a flow diagram of the program, which is described in detail in the figure legend.

At each time (usually each millisecond), the lateral inhibitory pulse list is consulted. If there is an inhibitory pulse a constant quantity, representing the amplitude of the inhibitory event, is added to a lateral inhibitory pool. This pool and the self inhibitory pool are each allowed to decay to some fraction of their values determined by the two inhibitory time constants. The lateral inhibitory pool is then diminished by a threshold amount (which makes the program nonlinear) and the two inhibitory pools are subtracted from the excitatory level to form the generator. The generator is integrated one more time mark and if it produces an impulse, a quantity is added to the self-inhibitory pool. At the end of the simulation a plot of the "instantaneous"

---

7. Is I_r positive, if yes go to 9, if no to 8.

8. Make negative I_r equal to 0.

9. Form generator (G) by subtracting self-inhibitory pool (I_s) and reduced lateral inhibition (I_r) from the excitation (E).

10. Plot G as a function of t.

11. Add G to the running sum (integral) S.

12. Is the sum (S) positive, if yes go to 14, if no go to 13.

13. Make negative S equal to 0.

14. Has S reached 1000 (is $\int_{t_i-1}^{t_i} G(t)dt \geq 1$), if yes go to 15, if no to 17.

15. Subtract 1000 from S. (Begin integration again saving remainder to avoid truncation error.)

16. Record a spike at time t. ($t_i = t$). Increase the spike index i by one. Add self-inhibitory quantum (A_s) to self-inhibitory pool (I_s).

17. Decay self and lateral inhibitory pools.

18. Add one millisecond to the clock (t).

19. Has the program reached the end, if yes go to 20, if no recycle at 4.

20. Output instantaneous frequency plot (reciprocals of intervals between spikes) of model test unit response and of inhibitory input. Punch on paper tape the results of the calculation so that they may be replotted at a later date. (Reproduced from Lange, 1965.)

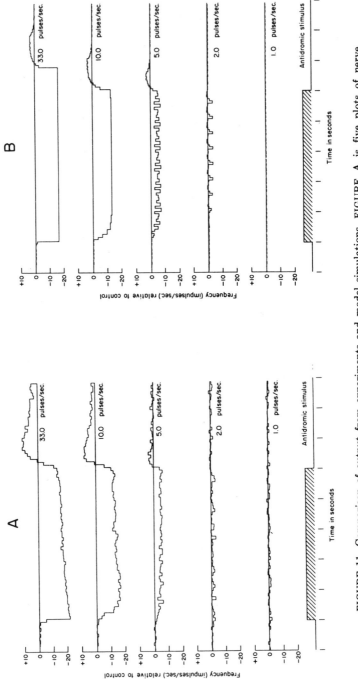

FIGURE 11. Comparison of output from experiments and model simulations. FIGURE A is five plots of nerve spike frequency relative to a control. Inhibition was delivered to the eye by antidromic stimulation during the time represented by the hatched bar. Curves were calculated as described in the legend of FIGURE 5. FIGURE B is five plots of the output of the dynamical model using the same input as the real experiment. The parameters used in the model were $\tau_s = \tau_L = 0.67$. $A_s = 4.125$. $A_L = 9.0$. $C = 12.0$. For definitions of these symbols see legend of FIGURE 10. (Modified from Lange, 1965.)

frequency of the spikes produced by the model is made so that it can be compared with the output of the real cell. FIGURE 11 shows output from five model cases (B) and the five corresponding real experiments (A). Again, all the plots were made by the computer, and the scales were added by the artist.

In summary, it is clear that the computer has been found nearly indispensable for multichannel, impulse-by-impulse, recording and processing of data. Its use in model simulation not only provides a succinct description of the properties of the systems but also allows for manipulation of parameters and prediction of the outcome of complicated experiments. In this sense the computer programs fulfill the same function as more conventional mathematical theories.

References

HARTLINE, H. K. & F. RATLIFF. 1957. Inhibitory interaction of receptor units in the eye of *Limulus*. J. Gen. Physiol. **40**: 357–376.

HARTLINE, H. K., F. RATLIFF & W. H. MILLER. 1961. Inhibitory interaction in the retina and its significance in vision. *In* Nervous Inhibition, E. Florey, ed. : 241–284. Pergamon Press, New York, N. Y.

HODGKIN, A. L. 1948. The local electric changes associated with repetitive action in a nonmedulated axon. J. Physiol. (London) **107**: 165–181.

LANGE, D. 1965. Dynamics of Inhibitory Interactions in the Eye of *Limulus:* Experimental and Theoretical Studies. Thesis. Rockefeller Institute, New York, N. Y.

MACNICHOL, E. F., JR. 1956. Visual receptors as biological transducers. *In* Molecular Structure and Functional Activity of Nerve Cells. Publ. No. 1 Am. Inst. Biol. Sci. 34–53.

MILKMAN, N. & R. L. SCHOENFELD. 1965. A digital programmer for stimuli and computer control in neurophysiological experiments. Ann. N. Y. Acad. Sci. (This monograph.)

MILLER, W. H. 1957. Morphology of the ommatidia of the compound eye of *Limulus*. J. Biophys. and Biochem. Cyt. **3**: 421–428.

MILLER, W. H. 1958. Fine structure of some invertebrate photoreceptors. Ann. N. Y. Acad. Sci. **74**: 204–209.

RATLIFF, F. 1961. Inhibitory interaction and the detection and enhancement of contours. *In* Sensory Communication, W. A. Rosenblith, ed. M. I. T. Press, Cambridge, Mass. and John Wiley & Sons, New York, N. Y.

RATLIFF, F. 1965. Mach Bands: Quantitative Studies on Neural Networks in the Retina. Holden-Day, Inc., San Francisco, Calif.

RATLIFF, F., H. K. HARTLINE & W. H. MILLER. 1963. Spatial and temporal aspects of retinal inhibitory interaction. J. Opt. Soc. Amer. **53**: 110–120.

RATLIFF, F. & C. G. MUELLER. 1957. Synthesis of "on-off" and "off" responses in a visual-neural system. Science. **126**: 840–841.

SCHOENFELD, R. L. 1964. The role of a digital computer as a biological instrument. Ann. N. Y. Acad. Sci. **115**: 915–942.

SCHOENFELD, R. L. & N. MILKMAN. 1964. Digital computers in the biological laboratory. Science **146**: 190–198.

STEVENS, C. F. 1964. A Quantitative Theory of Neural Interactions: Theoretical and Experimental Investigations. Thesis. Rockefeller Institute, New York, N. Y.

The dynamics of lateral inhibition in the compound eye of *Limulus*. I*

FLOYD RATLIFF, H. KEFFER HARTLINE, AND D. LANGE

The Rockefeller University, New York, N.Y.

Reprinted from Proceedings of the International Symposium on THE FUNCTIONAL ORGANIZATION OF THE COMPOUND EYE, 1966, Pergamon Press, Oxford, pp. 399-424

PRONOUNCED transient responses to changes in the spatial, temporal, and spectral distribution of illumination on the retina are characteristic features of the activity of the optic nerve in all well-developed visual systems, both vertebrate and invertebrate. These transient responses may result from the separate or combined effects of many and diverse processes, including the photochemical processes in the receptor itself, the electrochemical processes underlying the generation of nerve impulses, and the interplay of excitatory and inhibitory influences among neighboring elements in the retina.

The purpose of this paper is to examine a few major aspects of the dynamics of inhibition in the retina of the compound eye of *Limulus*. Our aim is to provide an empirical basis for the extension of our mathematical account of inhibitory interaction in the steady state to include the dynamic behavior of the lateral and self-inhibition in the neural network in this retina. This study is confined to the influences that are revealed by the discharge of impulses in the fibers of the optic nerve in response to various spatial and temporal patterns of illumination on the receptor mosaic. In a subsequent paper in this symposium we consider the dynamics of the inhibitory influences that result from various temporal patterns of antidromic impulses produced by electrical stimulation of the optic nerve, and develop a mathematical formulation of the dynamics. To provide a background for both studies let us first consider a few salient features of the anatomy and function of the compound eye of *Limulus* and briefly review our earlier quantitative account of the steady-state inhibitory interactions.

GROSS AND MICRO ANATOMY
OF THE COMPOUND EYE OF LIMULUS

The corneal surface of the compound eye of *Limulus* forms an ellipsoidal bulge on the carapace of the prosoma just below a spine-like projection of the ophthalmic ridge. In very young animals the projecting spine is quite

* This investigation was supported by a research grant (NB–00864) from the National Institute of Neurological Diseases and Blindness, U.S. Public Health Service, and by an Equipment Loan Contract Nonr. [1442(00)] with the U.S. Office of Naval Research.

prominent and the surface of the cornea is nearly spherical. The older the animal, the more oblate is the corneal bulge and the less prominent is the ophthalmic ridge and spine. When full maturity is reached (at about 10 years of age) the cornea is usually very much flattened and the protective spine on the ophthalmic ridge is almost completely absent.

Photographs of several aspects of the corneal surface of the right lateral eye of an adult male *Limulus* (width of carapace 22·5 cm) are shown in Fig. 1.

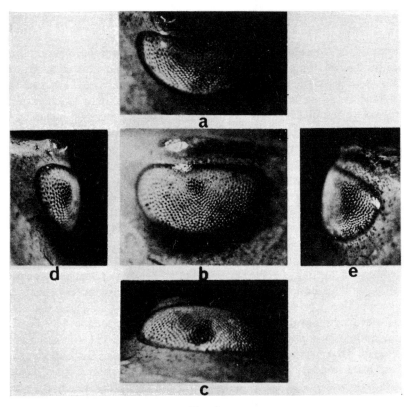

FIG. 1

Various aspects of the corneal surface of the compound eye of *Limulus*. a, dorsal; b, high lateral; c, low lateral; d, posterior; e, anterior. Length of eye: approximately 1·5 cm.

The optical axes of the approximately 1000 ommatidia diverge so that the visual field of the eye as a whole covers approximately a hemisphere. The divergence of the optical axes is greater than the divergence of the morphological axes because of the slant of the corneal surface, especially near the anterior and posterior margins of the eye. The acceptance angle of each ommatidium is quite large, the half-width being about 8° (Waterman, 1954; Kirschfeld and Reichardt, 1964), and the visual fields of closely neighboring ommatidia overlap one another to a considerable extent. The pseudopupil resulting from the low reflectance of the ommatidia oriented in the direction of the camera is not the same from all angles of view, for the divergence of the optical axes of neighboring ommatidia is not the same everywhere.

The optical axes of the ommatidia near the anterior portion of the eye, for example, are nearly all oriented in the anterior direction. Therefore, when viewed from the front, the pseudopupil appears very large—filling almost the entire anterior portion of the eye. Viewed from the side, the pseudopupil appears small and nearly circular. From the rear, it appears somewhat larger, but not as large as in the frontal view. Viewed from above, the pseudopupil generally appears somewhat elongated and flattened against the margin of the eye. From a low side view it appears large and circular. Occasionally, two distinct pseudopupils can be seen from some directions of view. In addition to these normal variations, deep scars on the cornea and malformations of the arrangement of the ommatidia resulting from injury or disease are common, particularly in the eyes of older animals obtained from the northern part of their range along the east coast of America (Nova Scotia to Yucatan). We mention these points because it is easy to fall into the error of thinking of the compound eye of *Limulus* as a more or less homogeneous structure. The normal variations in the size and shape of the pseudopupil, seen from different points of view, suggest that there may be some corresponding differences in the functional organization of the interconnections among the ommatidia in the retina or among the ganglion cells in the optic lobe. Excepting a few crude maps of iso-inhibitory contours (Hartline, Wagner, and Ratliff, 1956), however, these possibilities remain to be investigated.

A photomicrograph of a section of the compound eye of *Limulus* is shown in Fig. 2. It was cut more or less perpendicularly to the plane of Fig. 1b. At the top of the micrograph are the lower ends of the densely stained pigmented sheaths of the ommatidia, *O*. A portion of the photosensitive rhabdom, *Rh*, is visible in one ommatidium. (See Fig. 5 for a detailed drawing.) Axons, labeled *Rax* and *Eax*, arise from the several retinular cells and the one eccentric cell* in each ommatidium. These axons form small bundles which eventually come together to form the optic nerve, *ON*, a portion of which is shown at the bottom of the micrograph.

At various short distances below the layer of ommatidia, both the retinular cell axons and the eccentric cell axons give rise to numerous fine lateral

---

* Occasionally one finds an ommatidium with two eccentric cells, and—less frequently— one with no eccentric cell. The double eccentric cells probably generate the nearly synchronous double spikes sometimes observed in small strands of the optic nerve (see Tomita, 1957).

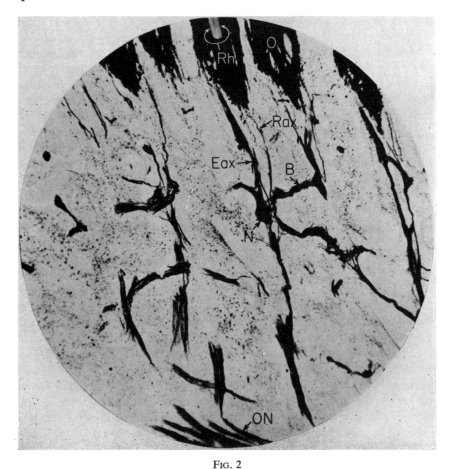

FIG. 2

Photomicrograph of a horizontal section through the compound eye of *Limulus*
(cornea and crystalline cones removed). Samuel's silver stain. Micrograph prepared
by W. H. Miller.

branches. Bundles of these branches, *B*, form a complex three-dimensional
plexus of interconnections among the axons of the retinular and eccentric
cells. The fibers in these bundles appear to terminate and form clumps of
neuropile, *N*, mainly around the axons of the eccentric cells. The inhibitory
interaction, discussed in this and in our succeeding paper, is mediated by this
plexus of interconnections: cutting the lateral branches abolishes the inhibition (Hartline, Wagner, and Ratliff, 1956).

Sections through the plexus in planes perpendicular to the plane of Fig. 2
are shown in Figs. 3 and 4. The section in Fig. 3 gives a rough idea of the
nature of the interconnections among the bundles of axons from about 30

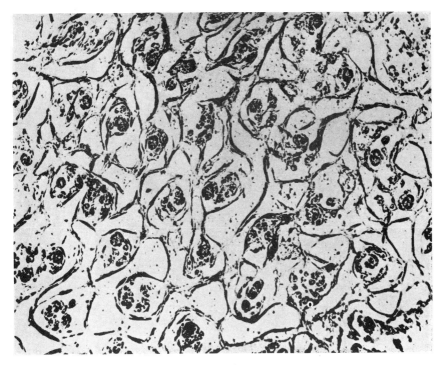

FIG. 3

Photomicrograph of section through the plexus, cut perpendicular to the bundles of retinular cell and eccentric cell axons. Hematoxylin and eosin stain. Micrograph prepared by W. H. Miller.

ommatidia. The section was fixed in osmium and stained with hematoxylin and eosin and, since this stain is not specific for neural tissue, shows many non-neural structures in addition to the lateral plexus and the axons of the retinular and eccentric cells.

Samuel's silver stain was used to prepare the section shown in Fig. 4 and the dark linear structures in it are all branches of the plexus. Note that in some cases (one of which is indicated by the arrow) the branches do not seem to go directly from one bundle of axons to the next nearest bundle, but instead loop around neighboring bundles and go to more distant ones. A section through a higher or lower plane, however, may show direct connections between next nearest neighbors where none exist in this section.

It has not yet been possible to determine the origin, course, and termination of individual fibers in the plexus. This much is known, however: both the retinular cell axons and the eccentric cell axons give rise to the small fibers that form, and run laterally in, the bundles of the plexus. These fibers end in clumps of neuropile which appear to be located mainly around the axons of the eccentric cells. In addition to the relatively long lateral fibers, the eccentric cell axons give rise to short branches which extend some distance into the immediately surrounding neuropile where they appear to make intimate synaptic contact with the terminations of the plexus fibers. For a detailed study of the microanatomy of the plexus see Miller (1966).

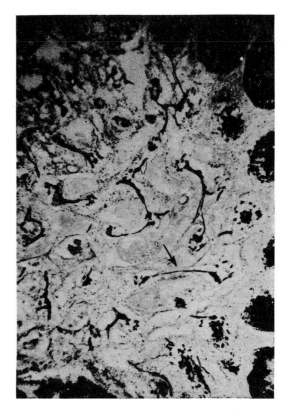

FIG. 4

Photomicrograph of section through the plexus at a somewhat higher magnification than Fig. 3. Samuel's silver stain. Micrograph prepared by W. H. Miller.

THE FUNCTIONAL PROPERTIES OF SINGLE OMMATIDIA

The photochemical and electrophysiological properties of an ommatidium in the compound eye of *Limulus* are summarized in a much oversimplified and highly schematic way in the drawing shown in Fig. 5.

Light enters the ommatidium through the cornea (not shown), passes through the crystalline cone, *CC*, and is at least partly absorbed by photo-pigment located in the rhabdomeres, *Rh*, of the retinular cells, *R*. The photo-pigment has been isolated and identified by Hubbard and Wald (1960): it is a retinene$_1$ rhodopsin, the absorption spectrum of which adequately accounts for the action spectrum of the ommatidium that was determined by measurements of the activity of single optic nerve fibers by Graham and Hartline

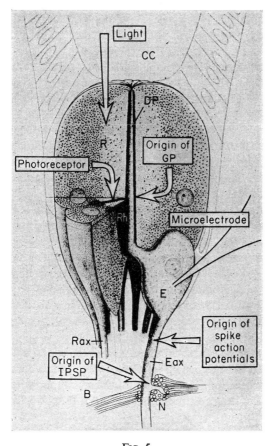

FIG. 5

Schema of structure and function of an ommatidium in the compound eye of *Limulus*.

(1935). The photochemical action leads to conductance changes and an accompanying depolarization of the eccentric cell, commonly referred to as the "generator potential", *GP*. For studies on these conductance changes see Tomita (1958), Fuortes (1959), Rushton (1959), and Purple (1964). The mechanism and exact locus of the conductance changes have not yet been determined; the label in Fig. 5, "Origin of *GP*", merely indicates a *possible* locus. For recent studies on the electrical connections between cells in the ommatidium see Tomita, Kikuchi, and Tanaka (1960); Purple (1964); Behrens and Wulff (1965); and Smith, Baumann, and Fuortes (1965).

The magnitude of the generator potential increases approximately linearly with the logarithm of the intensity of illumination (Hartline, Wagner, and MacNichol, 1952; MacNichol, 1956; Fuortes, 1959). (See Pinter, 1966, for a study on the dynamics of the generator potential.) Nerve impulses originate in the axon of the eccentric cell just below the cell body, and are conducted along the axon to the optic ganglion in the brain.* In the steady state, the frequency of discharge of nerve impulses is proportional to the amplitude of the generator potential.

Illumination of neighboring ommatidia—or antidromic electrical stimulation of the axons that arise from them—produces an inhibitory postsynaptic potential, *IPSP*, by way of influences transmitted across the lateral branches of the plexus to the neuropile (see Tomita, Kikuchi, and Tanaka, 1960; Hartline, Ratliff, and Miller, 1961; Ratliff, Hartline, and Miller, 1963; Purple, 1964). This inhibitory potential is in the hyperpolarizing direction and decreases the frequency of firing in the axon of the eccentric cell by an amount which, in the steady state, is proportional to the increase in frequency of discharge of impulses (or antidromic volleys) in the neighboring units. (The magnitude of the inhibitory post-synaptic potential also depends upon the number of neighboring elements activated and upon their distance from the ommatidium under observation.) In addition, each nerve impulse discharged by an eccentric cell is followed by an inhibitory potential in the discharging cell itself (see Stevens, 1964; Purple, 1964). Because of its similarity to the above-mentioned lateral inhibition, this phenomenon has been called "self-inhibition".

In brief, the photoexcitatory mechanism and the lateral and self-inhibitory mechanisms exert their opposing influences at or near a common point: the site of impulse generation. The net level of the membrane potential at this site determines the frequency of impulses (Tomita, 1958; Fuortes, 1960; Purple, 1964).

* Evidence has been obtained from time to time which suggests that the retinular cell axons may also conduct impulses. For example, some unpublished experiments by Gasser and Miller (personal communication, 1955) revealed two discrete components in the compound action potential elicited by electrical stimulation of the optic nerve. The latency of the large initial component indicated a conduction velocity (measured over 11·5 cm of nerve trunk) of 2·3 m/sec. The smaller later component indicated a conduction velocity of about 1·3 m/sec. Similar experiments by Stevens and Lange (personal communication, 1963) indicated conduction velocities of 1·9 m/sec for the large initial component and 0·7 m/sec for the small component (measured over 2·2 cm of nerve at 15°C). Presumably, the large component results from the activity of the eccentric cell axons and the small component from the activity of the retinular cell axons, but this is by no means firmly established. Furthermore, clear-cut evidence of unitary spike action potentials in the retinular cell axons, as obvious and unmistakable as in the eccentric cell, has not yet been obtained.

REVIEW OF THE QUANTITATIVE ACCOUNT
OF INHIBITORY INTERACTION

The interaction of two ommatidia may be expressed (to a first approximation) by a pair of simultaneous linear equations (Hartline and Ratliff, 1957):

$$r_1 = e_1 - K_{1,2}(r_2 - r^0_{1,2}),$$
$$r_2 = e_2 - K_{2,1}(r_1 - r^0_{2,1}). \tag{1}$$

The activity of each ommatidium is to be measured by the frequency of discharge of impulses in its eccentric cell axon. This response r is determined by the excitation e supplied by the external stimulus to the receptor, diminished by whatever inhibitory influence may be acting upon the receptor as a result of the activity of neighboring receptors. (The excitation of a particular receptor is to be measured by its response when it is illuminated by itself, thus lumping together in e the physical parameters of the stimulus and the characteristics of the photoexcitatory mechanism of the receptor.) The "threshold" frequency that must be exceeded before a receptor can exert any inhibition is represented by r^0. This and the inhibitory coefficient K are labelled in each equation to identify the direction of the action: $r^0_{1,2}$ is the frequency of receptor 2 at which it begins to inhibit receptor 1; $r^0_{2,1}$ is the reverse. In the same way $K_{1,2}$ is the coefficient of the inhibitory action of receptor 2 on receptor 1; $K_{2,1}$, the reverse.*

The inhibitory coefficients and thresholds must be labelled because they are not necessarily symmetrical. In one experiment on the eye of a large adult *Limulus*, for example, we found: $K_{1,2} = 0.15$ and $K_{2,1} = 0.06$; and $r^0_{1,2} = 10.9$ and $r^0_{2,1} = 9.9$. The two optic nerve fibers were not isolated by dissection; instead, rather large bundles containing several active fibers were placed on each of the two electrodes. An opaque wax (Cenco Tackiwax, loaded with lampblack) was melted and distributed evenly over the surface of the cornea. Small holes were then drilled through the wax so that illumination could reach just one ommatidium through each hole. The two ommatidia thus exposed were about 0.75 mm apart (center to center) and were separated by the width of at least one ommatidium. The fibers from the neighboring ommatidia on the electrodes served to monitor for possible scattered light. No impulses were recorded from them during the experiment and we were therefore fairly confident that there was little or no scatter to neighbors.

---

* Negative frequencies, of course, are not allowed; when the inhibitory term $K(r - r^0)$ is greater than the excitation e, the corresponding response r must be set equal to zero; when $(r - r^0)$ is negative, the inhibitory term must be dropped. Thus, the equations are not strictly linear; they are only piece-wise or segmentally linear. For discussions of the limitations of these linear approximations, see Hartline, Wagner, and Ratliff (1956), Purple (1964), and Lange (1965).

The inhibitory coefficient of 0·15, found in the above experiment, was unusually large and so was the degree of asymmetry. Although we cannot exclude with certainty the possibility that the much larger effect in one direction may have resulted from some light scattered to neighboring ommatidia that were not monitored, it seems likely—in view of the precautions taken—that the asymmetry was real. Indeed, only the degree of asymmetry was unusual—some asymmetry is the rule rather than the exception.

With more refined techniques of stimulation that make use of fiber optics (developed in our laboratory in collaboration with Robert B. Barlow, Jr.), we have frequently noticed that there are "holes" in the inhibitory field of a particular ommatidium. That is, an ommatidium may produce little or no effect on one of its near neighbors and yet a fairly strong effect on another neighbor at the same or even greater distance from it. When a compact group of several neighboring ommatidia are illuminated, however, the inhibitory effects that they produce do not seem to be so spotty. On the average, the effects of such a group clearly diminish with distance in a systematic way and seldom does one find, when using several ommatidia to produce the inhibition, that a nearby element is not affected by the group as a whole.*

When several ommatidia act simultaneously, the total inhibition they exert on a particular neighbor appears to be determined quantitatively by the separate inhibitory influences exerted by each, combined by simple addition. As a consequence, the responses of n ommatidia interacting with one another may be described (to a first approximation) by a set of n simultaneous equations, linear in the frequencies of the interacting units:

$$r_p = e_p - \sum_{j=1}^{n} K_{p,j}(r_j - r_{p,j}^0), \qquad (2)$$

where $p = 1, 2, \ldots, n$. (The restrictions on the equations mentioned above apply here also.) Self-inhibition is not considered here; that is, $j \neq p$.

---

* These kinds of effects may account, in part, for the quantitative discrepancies between the directly observed inhibitory coefficients reported by us and those calculated indirectly by Kirschfeld and Reichardt (1964), although their results and ours are qualitatively similar. In general, we select for our most extensive experiments those pairs that show a strong interaction and usually do not report results of numerous experiments in which little or no interaction is observed. The averages of our results, calculated by Kirschfeld and Reichardt, could not take this selection into account. Moreover, calculations of the inhibitory coefficients by Kirschfeld and Reichardt are based on the assumption that all of the ommatidia are interacting and that the influences are more or less homogeneous. If some ommatidia should fail to respond, or to inhibit near neighbors, this would tend to bias their estimates of the inhibitory coefficients in the opposite direction from the bias inherent in the averages of our selected results. In any event, the inhibitory coefficients between two ommatidia are small (we have never observed an inhibitory coefficient as large as 0·2; generally they are smaller than 0·1, even for near neighbors), and frequently no inhibition by one element on a near neighbor can be observed at all.

The strength of the inhibitory influence exerted by any one ommatidium on its neighbors diminishes markedly with distance; in terms of the above equations, the inhibitory coefficients $K_{p,j}$ decrease and the thresholds of inhibition $r^0_{p,j}$ increase. The distance effects are therefore implicit in the present form of the equations and no additional terms for distance appear to be required, at least not in the steady state.

Some preliminary experiments on the transient, dynamic phases of the inhibitory interaction have been described elsewhere (Hartline, Ratliff, and Miller, 1961; Ratliff, Hartline, and Miller, 1963; Ratliff, Hartline, and Lange, 1964). On the basis of these experiments, one of which is illustrated in Fig. 6, the steady-state equations (2) above were modified to include the temporal properties of the system as follows:

$$r_p(t) = e_p(t) - \sum_{j=1}^{n} K_{p,j} \left[r_j(t - T_{p,j}) - r^0_{p,j} \right]. \tag{3}$$

In these equations the response r_p of a particular ommatidium at any time t is determined by the level of excitation e_p of the ommatidium at that same time, diminished by the summated inhibitory influences exerted on it by the other ommatidia j. These influences are the ones initiated by the elements j at some earlier time $t - T_{p,j}$, where $T_{p,j}$ is the time lag of the action of any ommatidium j on the ommatidium p. This simple modification gives qualitatively correct results in most cases but is obviously only a rough first approximation.

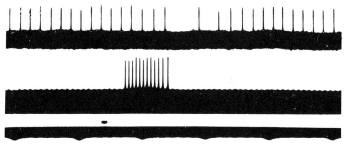

FIG. 6

Transient inhibition of the discharge from a steadily illuminated ommatidium (upper trace) by a burst of impulses discharged from a neighboring ommatidium (bottom trace) in response to a 0·01 sec flash of light (signaled by the black dot in the white band above the 1/5 sec time marks). From Hartline. Ratliff, and Miller, 1961.

AN ILLUSTRATIVE EXPERIMENT ON THE DYNAMICS
OF EXCITATION AND INHIBITION

In the experiment summarized in Fig. 7, records of responses to step increments and decrements in illumination were obtained from two optic nerve fibers. These fibers arose from two ommatidia which were separated by the width of just one ommatidium. The test ommatidium, which we will call *B*, was illuminated by a very small spot (about 0·075 mm in diameter) confined to the facet of that ommatidium. The other ommatidium, which we will call *A*, was illuminated—along with at least two of its neighbors—by a larger spot of light, approximately 0·25 mm in diameter. The eye was partially covered with opaque wax and a razor blade was inserted a fraction of a millimeter into the cornea between the small group of ommatidia including *A* and the test ommatidium *B* so that light from one beam could not scatter into the region that was supposed to be illuminated by the other.

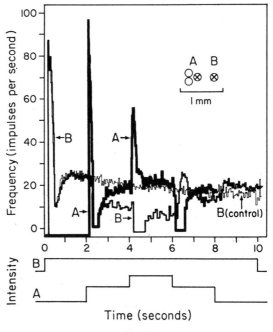

FIG. 7

Concurrent excitatory and inhibitory transients in the responses of neighboring ommatidia. Note that the intensity scale for *B* is displaced upward (both *A* and *B* begin and end at zero intensity).

The test ommatidium *B* was illuminated for 10 sec. Its response to this illumination alone is shown by the light line marked "*B* (control)" in Fig. 7. The one response of *A* shown in the figure resulted from illumination of it (and two of its adjacent neighbors) beginning 2 sec after the onset of another 10 sec period of illumination of *B*. The intensity of illumination on *A* remained at a steady level until the fourth second, at which time it was abruptly increased. The intensity then remained at this higher level until the sixth second, at which time it stepped down to the original level. The intensity of illumination then continued at this level until the eighth second, when the light was turned off.

Several expected excitatory transients appear in the record of the response of the fiber *A*, which served as the monitor of the response of the whole group of three adjacent ommatidia. First, there is an initial high frequency transient appearing about 75 msec after the onset of illumination. A pronounced silent period then follows, after which the frequency of response gradually climbs up and nearly reaches a steady level by the fourth second. The increment in illumination added at the fourth second yields a second excitatory transient (much smaller than the first, even though the intensity of illumination is greater), following which the response subsides to a steady frequency just slightly greater than that prior to the increment.

The response continues at this higher steady level until the intensity of the illumination is decreased to the original level at the sixth second. Following this decrease there is an abrupt and marked undershoot in the frequency of the response of *A* after which it returns to approximately the same steady level that it had during the initial period of illumination of the same intensity. When the illumination is turned off at the eighth second the discharge of impulses stops abruptly.

The frequency of response of the steadily illuminated test ommatidium *B* undergoes multiple changes concomitant with the changes observed in the activity of the small neighboring group monitored by *A*. First, corresponding to the initial transient in *A* following the onset of illumination on it and two of its adjacent neighbors at $t = 2 \cdot 0$ sec, there is a marked decrease in frequency of the response of the test ommatidium *B*. (Compare with "*B* control".) Following this large transient inhibitory effect, the frequency of *B* increases somewhat but still remains substantially below the corresponding control frequency.

With the second transient in *A*, produced by the increment in illumination at $t = 4 \cdot 0$ sec, there is an even larger transient inhibitory effect on the test ommatidium *B*. But it has a much shorter latency than the initial inhibitory transient, even though the excitatory transient is less pronounced than the first one. Following this second large inhibitory transient, the frequency of discharge of *B* increases as before, but still remains not only below the control level but also below its frequency during the first period of more or less steady inhibition because of the now higher frequency of response of *A*.

Following the sixth second, when the intensity of illumination on *A* and its two adjacent neighbors is abruptly decreased, producing a marked undershoot in the frequency of response of *A*, there is a marked increase in the frequency of discharge of the test ommatidium *B*, and it overshoots the control frequency by a substantial amount. As the frequency of *A* increases, returning to a high steady level, the frequency of *B* once again falls to a steady level considerably below the control frequency. Finally, when the light on *A* and its two adjacent neighbors is turned off, the frequency of *B* once again overshoots the control frequency and remains substantially above it until near the end of the tenth second, at which time the two no longer differ significantly.

The above experiment illustrates most of the major features of the dynamics of the inhibitory interaction. But the experiment is much too complex, and the effects of too many variables confounded, to permit the precise analyses required for a further more exact development of our quantitative formulation. Nevertheless, one can see in this illustrative experiment the direction that a more analytic approach must take and the nature of the modifications of the theory that will be required.

In general, the inhibitory effects are a slightly delayed and much reduced "mirror image" of the excitatory effects that produce them—as predicted by the simple modification of our steady-state equations (to include a constant time delay) that is represented in equations (3) above. In detail, however, these equations are not in accord with the observed phenomena.

First of all, the time delays are not constant. Indeed, the inhibitory effect produced by the large initial excitatory transient (at $t = 2 \cdot 0$) takes longer to develop than does the effect produced by the smaller excitatory transient resulting from the increment in illumination (at $t = 4 \cdot 0$). Second, the inhibitory transients are not simple mirror images of the excitatory transients. There is a marked overshoot, well above the control frequency, in the responses of the test ommatidium—not only following a similar undershoot in the response of the neighboring ommatidia exerting the inhibition (at $t = 6 \cdot 0$), but also following cessation of their response (at $t = 8 \cdot 0$). In addition, the magnitude of the inhibitory effect produced by the second smaller transient (at $t = 4 \cdot 0$) is larger than that produced by the initial large transient (at $t = 2 \cdot 0$). Let us now consider these problems in some detail.

FACILITATION OF THE INHIBITION

We have shown, in experiments not to be reported in detail here, that the time at which a single transient inhibitory influence is exerted on a test ommatidium—once the response of that ommatidium has reached a steady state—has no significant effect on the latency and magnitude of the inhibition.*
For example, a burst of impulses discharged by neighboring ommatidia two sec after the beginning of the discharge of impulses from the test ommatidium

* This differs from the recurrent inhibition of motoneurones in the spinal cord of the cat. Granit and Rutledge (1960) found that the effects of antidromic volleys of constant frequency and duration are stronger the later they occur with respect to the maintained stretch reflex discharge.

produces essentially the same inhibitory effect on the test ommatidium as does an identical burst at the fourth second (each effect measured independently during a different period of illumination). Therefore, the difference between the latent periods and between the magnitudes of the transient inhibitory effects produced by the excitatory transients at $t = 2 \cdot 0$ and $t = 4 \cdot 0$ in the experiment illustrated in Fig. 7 cannot be attributed to the times at which the transients occur with respect to the onset of illumination on, or discharge of impulses from, the test ommatidium. Instead, such differences appear to result from *facilitation* of the second inhibitory transient—either by the concurrent steady suprathreshold inhibition produced by the ongoing steady discharge on which the second excitatory transient is superimposed, or by concurrent subthreshold inhibitory influences that are produced by, and persist for a time after, the initial excitatory transient, or both.

The difference between the inhibitory transients in the experiment illustrated in Fig. 7 can be seen more clearly in the actual film records of the oscilloscope traces obtained in a later part of this same experiment (Fig. 8). The numbers on the records are the times of occurrence of the impulses, to the nearest millisecond, which were flashed on the film by an automatic counting and gating device as the record was taken. (For details of the method of recording see Eisenberg and Ratliff, 1960.) The upper record shows the inhibitory effects produced by the initial excitatory transient at $t = 2 \cdot 0$. The lower record shows the inhibitory effects produced by the excitatory transient at $t = 4 \cdot 0$. (The numbers printed on the records show only fractions of seconds; the millisecond counters were reset to zero at the end of each second.)

Note that the first inhibitory transient (upper trace in upper record), when there was no ongoing inhibition, took longer to appear than did the second inhibitory transient (upper trace in lower record), when the test ommatidium was already subjected to some inhibition. Also, the first inhibitory transient appears to be smaller than the second. The experiment is not definitive, however: the two excitatory transients that produce the two different inhibitory transients are themselves dissimilar, and the steady frequencies of discharge from the test ommatidium preceding the two transients are not comparable.

The following experiment, some results of which are illustrated in Fig. 9, was designed to remedy these defects. The inhibitory transient was produced by a single compact burst of impulses from a group of about 6 neighboring ommatidia located approximately 0·75 mm from the test ommatidium. (The discharge of only one ommatidium in the center of the group was recorded.) First, the transient inhibitory effect exerted on the steady discharge of the test ommatidium by this burst of activity alone was determined (left half of the figure). The plot of the burst and the plot of the concomitant transient inhibitory effect are each the average of 5 experimental runs. The nearly straight line across the graph is a smoothed average of 11 control runs (no inhibition). For details of our method of computation of average frequencies see Schoenfeld (1964). Except during the inhibitory transient and the short post-inhibitory rebound, the control and experimental frequencies of the test ommatidium coincide. The lower graph shows the accumulating deficit of

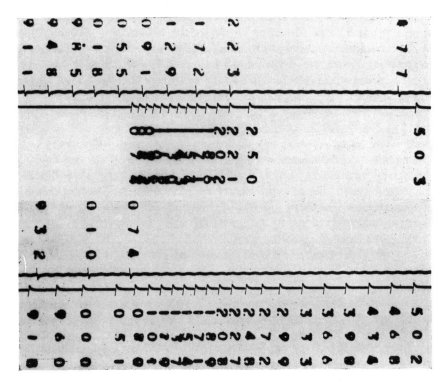

Fig. 8

Initial inhibitory transients (upper record) and subsequent inhibitory transient superimposed on steady inhibition (lower record). Millisecond counters reset to zero at $t = 2 \cdot 0$ sec in upper record and at $t = 4 \cdot 0$ sec in lower record. Compare with Fig. 7.

impulses over the same period of time, in the discharge of the test ommatidium, relative to the discharge immediately preceding the inhibition.

In the second part of the experiment (right half of the figure) the conditions were the same except that a low level of ongoing "background" inhibition was provided by steady low intensity illumination of another nearby group of about a half-dozen ommatidia. This group was also located about 0·75 mm from the test ommatidium, but on the side opposite the group that exerted the transient inhibition and therefore about 1·5 mm from it.

The steady inhibition was weak; the average frequency of the 5 experimental runs prior to and following the inhibitory transient and post-inhibitory rebound was only slightly less than the smoothed average of the 11 control runs. Nevertheless, this low level of background inhibition significantly increased the inhibitory transient and post-inhibitory rebound resulting from the short high frequency burst of impulses. The increase in magnitude of the effect is shown more clearly in the lower right hand graph where the deficit in number of impulses discharged in the test ommatidium (relative to the discharge just prior to the onset of inhibition) is plotted. Note, however, that the greater post-inhibitory rebound almost exactly compensates for the greater inhibitory effect, and thus there is no significant difference in the total deficit of impulses under the two different conditions from about $t = 6·8$ sec onwards. Differences in latency—if any—are slight. Unfortunately, such differences have to be rather large in order not to be obscured by "noise" on the baseline. Also, the accuracy of detection of the time of changes in average frequency is limited by the size of the intervals between impulses—about 40 msec at the critical point in this experiment.

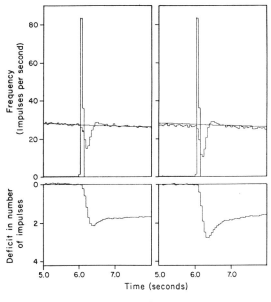

FIG. 9

Comparison of the transient inhibitory influences produced by a compact burst of impulses acting alone (left half of figure) and superimposed on a steady background of weak inhibition (right half of figure).

Facilitation of inhibition resulting from previous inhibition is illustrated in Figs. 10 and 11. The test ommatidium was illuminated, throughout the period shown, with a small spot of light of constant intensity confined to the facet of that ommatidium. To produce the inhibitory effects a neighboring ommatidium, at a distance of about 0·5 mm from the test ommatidium, was illuminated with short flashes of light. Presumably only one neighbor was

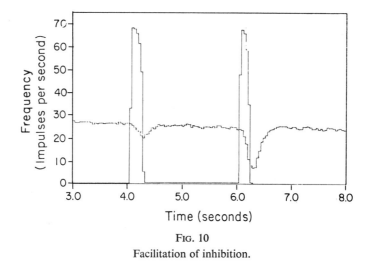

FIG. 10

Facilitation of inhibition.

illuminated, but no special precautions (such as masking with opaque wax) were taken to ensure that there was no light scatter from the focused spot. Prior to each experimental run this ommatidium was partially light-adapted so that the short flashes would generate short compact bursts of impulses with little or no after discharge. The intensities of the two flashes were the same. In order to generate nearly equal bursts of impulses it was therefore necessary to make the second flash longer than the first. In the experiment illustrated, the duration of the first flash was 0·01 sec, the duration of the second flash was 0·1 sec. (The curves plotted are the averages of 5 experimental runs.)

When the second burst of impulses followed soon after the first, the inhibitory effect that it produced was very much enhanced. The effect was greater the closer the second burst was to the first. With separations of about 4 or 5 sec between the two bursts (not illustrated here), there was no facilitation of the second inhibitory effect by the first. Evidently, some residual subthreshold inhibitory influence follows the first burst, takes several seconds to decay, and—while it still persists—adds to the inhibitory influence generated by the second burst. Even though these residual influences alone produce no observable effect on the discharge of impulses from the test ommatidium, they are, nevertheless, still present as is evidenced by the facilitation of the inhibition produced by the second burst.

It might be objected that the greater effect of the second burst is simply the result of the greater amount of light in the longer second flash that is required to produce a discharge approximately equal to that in the first burst.

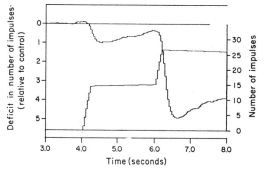

FIG. 11

Facilitation of inhibition. Same experiment as illustrated in Fig. 10. Deficit in number of impulses discharged from test ommatidium, relative to control, shown on left-hand ordinate. Number of impulses discharged from the neighboring ommatidium that produced the inhibitory effect is shown on the right-hand ordinate.

This is not the case, however. Indeed, we have observed that a weaker response, generated by the second of two flashes of *equal* duration and intensity, often produces an effect as great as or greater than that produced by the first flash. Furthermore, as we shall show in the subsequent paper, a similar facilitation of inhibition occurs when two identical bursts of antidromic activity are generated by electrical stimulation of the optic nerve.*

THE EFFECTS OF DISTANCE ON THE INHIBITORY TRANSIENT

The frequencies of impulses discharged from three widely separated ommatidia are illustrated in Fig. 12. The relative locations of the corneal facets of the three ommatidia, each indicated by a circle and cross, are shown at the right of the graph. The steady illumination on the two test ommatidia B and C was confined to their facets, and the intensities of the two spots were adjusted

* One preliminary experiment that we have carried out indicates that the facilitation of inhibition by residual subthreshold influences may not occur if the two inhibitory influences are produced by illuminating two separate groups of ommatidia. Further experiments are required, however, to elucidate this point.

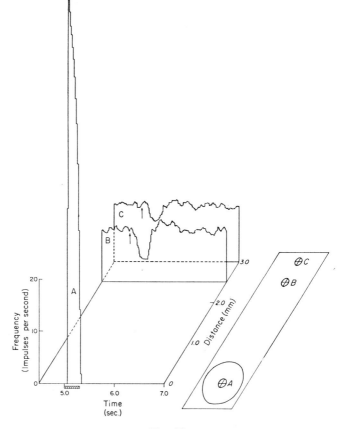

FIG. 12

The dependence of a transient inhibitory effect on distance.

so that the frequency of discharge of impulses from both was approximately the same. Ommatidium *A*, along with a group of its immediate neighbors, was illuminated by a short (0·3 sec) flash of light. The approximate dimensions of the spot of light are indicated by the large circle enclosing the ommatidium *A*.

To avoid possible complications due to interaction between *B* and *C*, the transient inhibitory effect of *A* on each was measured separately. The burst of impulses from *A* itself was so short that there was little or no possibility that the transients produced in the responses of *B* and *C* had any effect back on it.

The results of this experiment are more or less as would be expected from our previous experiments on the effects of distance on the steady-state inhibition. That is, the greater the distance the smaller are the inhibitory transient and the post-inhibitory rebound. Also, the greater the distance the longer the latency of the inhibitory transient. To make this latter point clearer in this three-dimensional figure, the time of occurrence of the first impulse in *A* is indicated by the small arrows in the planes of the graphs of the frequency of discharge of impulses from the test ommatidia *B* and *C*. The graphs shown are averages of 6 experimental runs.

Results of a similar experiment, on a different preparation, are illustrated

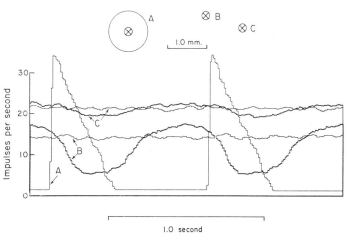

FIG. 13

The dependence of periodic transient inhibitory effects on distance.

in Fig. 13. In this experiment, however, the excitatory transients were produced by a succession of 0·2 sec flashes on *A*, repeated at 1·0 sec intervals within the 10 sec periods of steady illumination on *B* and *C*. The two full cycles shown are the average of 15 similar periods (the last six cycles in each of five experimental runs). The controls for *B* and *C* (no inhibition) are represented by the thin nearly straight lines across the graph. In general, the results are the same as those obtained in the single flash experiment illustrated in Fig. 12. The nearer the ommatidium inhibited, the greater is the amplitude of the effect and the shorter the latency. The results of this experiment appear simple, but in fact are difficult to interpret. The falling phase of the overshoot and the onset of the inhibition overlap in such a way that the inhibitory effect on *B* appears to begin before the occurrence of the impulses in *A* that cause it.

Ideally, if one could measure the spatial and temporal properties of the inhibitory effects produced by a single impulse and determine how these effects combine with those produced by a second impulse, then one could predict the effects produced by any temporal pattern of impulses. To achieve this ideal would require far more sensitive techniques than those we now have. The best we can do—at the moment—is to approximate this ideal by generating short compact bursts of impulses which produce easily measurable effects.

Using this technique we have performed a number of three-fiber experiments, similar to the one illustrated in Fig. 12, but as yet have insufficient data on which to base a general law relating the dynamics of the inhibition and distance on the retina. The amplitude and extent of the inhibitory influence varies somewhat from place to place in the same eye (see our remarks above on the pseudopupil) and from one preparation to another. For these reasons it is not permissible to combine the data obtained from these several experiments. Unfortunately, the technique outlined above does not permit one to map out the amplitude and extent of the inhibitory influence that a particular ommatidium exerts on all, or on a representative large sample, of its neighbors. The small sample that is obtained is selected more or less by chance in the process of dissection, and the necessary large number of control and experimental measurements do not allow sufficient time to vary the frequency of discharge of the ommatidia in question over a large range, or to dissect out additional fibers coming from other locations. The new technique using fiber optics, that we mentioned above, promises to solve some of these problems and to enable us to map more accurately and in more detail the inhibitory fields around single ommatidia.

VARIATIONS IN THE LATENT PERIOD OF THE INHIBITION

Early in the course of these three-fiber experiments we thought that it might be possible to measure the velocity of the conduction of the lateral inhibitory influences even though no propagated activity can be observed, as yet, in the fibers of the plexus. The plan was to measure the differences between the times of onset of inhibition exerted on two test ommatidia by a third ommatidium—or group of ommatidia. There was some hope that this adaptation of Helmholtz's classic technique for measuring the velocity of conduction in a nerve-muscle preparation might yield an estimate of the conduction time over the plexus between the two test ommatidia.

The hopes we had were slight, for the accuracy of pin-pointing changes in the frequency of discharge of discrete impulses is limited by the size of the intervals between impulses. Furthermore, the slight hopes we did have were short-lived. The *apparent* conduction times indicated by this method were of the order of a *millimeter* per second and seemed to depend more strongly on the frequency of discharge of impulses from the ommatidium (or group of ommatidia) exerting the inhibition than on the distance to, or between, the test receptors inhibited.

Details of one such experiment are illustrated in Fig. 14. The discharge of impulses was recorded from three ommatidia located on a nearly straight line, as indicated in the diagram inset in the figure. Ommatidia B and C—the test ommatidia—were steadily illuminated for 10 sec by small spots of light of constant intensity. Ommatidium A, along with a group of its neighbors, was illuminated by a large spot of light, centered on A, as indicated in the inset. This large spot of light was turned on for 0·05 sec at $t = 6·0$ (indicated by the small black rectangle on the abscissa) to produce a short compact burst of activity. As in the three-fiber experiment described above, the transient inhibitory effects on the two test ommatidia B and C were determined separately in order to avoid possible complications resulting from interaction between them.

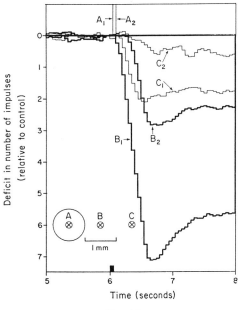

FIG. 14

Variations in the latent periods of transient inhibitory effects.

Each curve in the figure (an average of four comparable runs) is the integral of the difference between the frequencies of impulses in control and experimental runs following $t = 6·0$, the time at which A and its near neighbors were illuminated by a short flash of the large spot of light. The integral in each case is relative to the discharge of impulses in the one second period preceding the flash. Only small portions of the integrals of the bursts of impulses

486 · *Excitation and inhibition in the retina*

discharged from *A*—sufficient to indicate the time of the first impulse in the burst—are shown. (There was a low frequency after-discharge of impulses from *A* which began at about $t = 6 \cdot 7$ sec—too late to affect either the magnitude or latent period of the initial transient in the inhibitory effect.)

Consider first the curves A_1, B_1, and C_1. They were obtained when the intensity of illumination of the flash was high, producing a burst of impulses in *A* with a short latency and high frequency. The expected inhibitory effects on *B* and *C* were observed: a large effect with a short latent period on *B* (curve B_1) and a much smaller effect with a longer latent period on the more distant ommatidium *C* (curve C_1).

On the basis of these observations alone one might be tempted to attribute the time delay between the appearance of the first impulse in *A* and the onset of the inhibitory effect on *B* (and the difference between this latent period and the latent period of the effect on *C*) to the distance that the inhibitory influence has to traverse in the lateral plexus. Undoubtedly, a finite amount of time *is* required for the inhibitory influence to be conducted from one ommatidium to another, but it should be very small and nearly constant, according to all generally accepted notions about nervous conduction. The second half of this experiment shows that this apparent conduction time is *not* constant, but instead varies with the frequency of discharge of impulses from the group *A* that is exerting the inhibition on *B* and *C*.

Consider now the curves A_2, B_2, and C_2. These data were obtained in the same way as in the first half of the experiment. The only change was that the intensity of the flash on *A* was reduced. The result of this lower intensity was to produce a burst of impulses in *A* with a longer latency and a lower frequency than before.

As expected, the less vigorous discharge from *A* yielded a smaller inhibitory effect on the test ommatidia *B* and *C*. Also, because of the longer latent period in the response of *A*, one would expect to find all three curves A_2, B_2, and C_2 shifted to the right—which they are. But the shift of B_2 and C_2 is much greater than can be accounted for on the basis of the increased latency of response of *A*. Indeed, the difference between the times of the onset of inhibition on ommatidium *B* (curves B_1 and B_2) is about three times larger than the difference between the times of appearance of the first impulse in *A* (curves A_1 and A_2). Unfortunately, the weaker effect on *C* is so small (curve C_2) that no definite conclusions can be drawn from it. The increased delay, however, does appear to be much larger than could be accounted for on the basis of the longer latent period in the response of *A*.

The increases in the apparent conduction time of the inhibitory effect from *A* to *B* and *C* are not merely the result of the smaller inhibitory effect produced by the less vigorous burst of activity from *A*. In fact, there is a shorter delay to the weak effect on *C* (curves A_1 and C_1) than to the slightly stronger effect on *B* (curves A_2 and B_2). Judging by these latter two cases alone, it would appear that the longer the distance the shorter is the time delay. Evidently such anomalous results cannot be explained in terms of a constant velocity of conduction over the distance traversed by the inhibitory influence. Instead, the apparent transmission time *seems* to depend as much or more on the activity of the ommatidia exerting the inhibition. Further experiments with more flexible and more precise control over the excitatory transients than that afforded by short flashes of light are required, however, to determine whether this tentative interpretation is correct.

SUMMARY

Some of the gross features of the dynamics of the inhibitory interaction in the compound eye of *Limulus* are implicit in our earlier analysis of the steady-state interaction: the inhibitory effects are "mirror images"—more or less—of the excitatory effects that produce them and they diminish with distance. Furthermore, as expected, some time elapses between any excitatory transient and the inhibitory transients that result from it; in general, the greater the distance between the interacting ommatidia, the greater are the time delays.

Three major phenomena that appear in the dynamics of the inhibitory interaction, however, are not adequately accounted for by the mere addition of simple constant time delays to the steady-state equations. These include: (1) the facilitation of the inhibition by ongoing inhibition or by recent prior inhibition; (2) the overshoot or post-inhibitory rebound following a reduction in or cessation of inhibition; and (3) the apparent greater dependence of the latent period of the inhibition on the frequency of discharge of the ommatidia exerting the inhibition than upon the distance traversed by the inhibitory influence.

The problem we now face is to develop a comprehensive quantitative description of the inhibitory interaction which will not only account fully for these and other features of the dynamics but which will also reduce to the steady-state equations. In our subsequent paper we attempt such a formulation and subject it to a variety of tests.

REFERENCES

BEHRENS, M. E. and WULFF, V. J. 1965. Light-initiated responses of retinula and eccentric cells in the *Limulus* lateral eye. *J. Gen. Physiol.* **48**, 1081–93.

EISENBERG, L. and RATLIFF, F. 1960. Gating system for photographic printout of counts in neurophysiological research. *Review of Scientific Instruments*, **31**, 630–3.

FUORTES, M. G. F. 1959. Initiation of impulses in visual cells of *Limulus*. *J. Physiol.* **148**, 14–28.

FUORTES, M. G. F. 1960. Inhibition in *Limulus* eye, in *Inhibition of the Nervous System and γ-Aminobutyric Acid*. Pergamon Press, New York, 418–23.

GRAHAM, C. H. and HARTLINE, H. K. 1935. The response of single visual sense cells to lights of different wave length. *J. Gen. Physiol.* **18**, 917–31.

GRANIT, R. and RUTLEDGE, L. T. 1960. Surplus excitation in reflex action of motoneurones as measured by recurrent inhibition. *J. Physiol.* **154**, 288–307.

HARTLINE, H. K. and RATLIFF, F. 1957. Inhibitory interaction of receptor units in the eye of *Limulus. J. Gen. Physiol.* **40**, 357–76.

HARTLINE, H. K., RATLIFF, F. and MILLER, W. H. 1961. Inhibitory interaction in the retina and its significance in vision, in *Nervous Inhibition*, E. Florey, ed. Pergamon Press, New York, 241–84.

HARTLINE, H. K., WAGNER, H. G. and MACNICHOL, E. F., Jr. 1952. The peripheral origin of nervous activity in the visual system. *Cold Spring Harbor Symposia on Quantitative Biology*, **17**, 125–41.

HARTLINE, H. K., WAGNER, H. G. and RATLIFF, F. 1956. Inhibition in the eye of *Limulus. J. Gen. Physiol.* **39**, 651–73.

HUBBARD, R. and WALD, G. 1960. Visual pigment of the horseshoe crab, *Limulus polyphemus. Nature* **186**, 212–5.

KIRSCHFELD, K. and REICHARDT, W. 1964. *Die Verarbeitung stationärer optischer Nachrichten im Komplexauge von* Limulus **2**, 43–61.

LANGE, D. 1965. Dynamics of inhibitory interaction in the eye of *Limulus*. Experimental and theoretical studies, Thesis, Rockefeller Institute.

MACNICHOL, E. F., Jr. 1956. Visual receptors as biological transducers. *Molecular Structure and Functional Activity of Nerve Cells*, Publication No. 1 of American Institute of Biological Sciences, 34–53.

MILLER, W. H. 1966. The anatomy of the neuropile in the compound eye of *Limulus*, in *Proceedings of the Second International Symposium on the Structure of the Eye* (held in Wiesbaden, August 1965) Pergamon Press 1966—in press.

PINTER, R. B. 1966. Sinusoidal and delta function responses of visual cells of the *Limulus* eye. *J. Gen. Physiol.* **49**, 565–93.

PURPLE, R. L. 1964. The integration of excitatory and inhibitory influences in the eccentric cell in the eye of *Limulus*. Thesis, Rockefeller Institute.

RATLIFF, F., HARTLINE, H. K. and LANGE, D. 1964. Studies on the dynamics of inhibitory interaction in the retina, in *Physiological Basis for Form Discrimination*, Symposium, Brown University, Providence, R.I.

RATLIFF, F., HARTLINE, H. K. and MILLER, W. H. 1963. Spatial and temporal aspects of retinal inhibitory interaction. *J. Opt. Soc. Amer.* **53**, 110–20.

RUSHTON, W. A. H. 1959. A theoretical treatment of Fuortes' observations upon eccentric cell activity in *Limulus. J. Physiol.* **148**, 29–38.

SCHOENFELD, R. L. 1964. The role of a digital computer as a biological instrument. *Ann. N.Y. Acad. Sci.* **115**, 915–42.

SMITH, T. G., BAUMANN, F. and FUORTES, M. G. F. 1965. Electrical connections between visual cells in the ommatidium of *Limulus. Science* **147**, 1446–7.

STEVENS, C. F. 1964. A quantitative theory of neural interactions: theoretical and experimental investigations, Thesis, Rockefeller Institute.

TOMITA, T. 1957. Peripheral mechanisms of nervous activity in lateral eye of horseshoe crab. *J. Neurophysiol.* **20**, 245–54.

TOMITA, T. 1958. Mechanism of lateral inhibition in the eye of *Limulus. J. Neurophysiol.* **21**, 419–29.

TOMITA, T., KIKUCHI, R. and TANAKA, I. 1960. Excitation and inhibition in lateral eye of horseshoe crab. *Electrical Activity of Single Cells*, Igakushion, Hongo, Tokyo, 11–23.

WATERMAN, T. H. 1954. Directional sensitivity of single ommatidia in the compound eye of *Limulus. Proc. Nat. Acad. Sci.* **40**, 252–7.

The dynamics of lateral inhibition in the compound eye of *Limulus*. II*

D. LANGE, H. KEFFER HARTLINE, AND FLOYD RATLIFF

The Rockefeller University, New York, N.Y.

Reprinted from Proceedings of the International Symposium on THE
FUNCTIONAL ORGANIZATION OF THE COMPOUND EYE,
1966, Pergamon Press, Oxford, pp. 425–449

THE inhibitory effects produced by illumination of the lateral eye of *Limulus* have a very complex form as a function of time. Part of this complexity is inherent in the inhibitory process, but much of it stems from the complex excitatory transients in the responses of the photoreceptors themselves—as was evidenced by the results of the several experiments reported by Ratliff, Hartline and Lange (1966). To achieve better control over the activity of the optic nerve and the resulting inhibitory effects we have resorted to an electrical technique for stimulating the optic nerve proximal to the eye to provide trains of antidromic volleys. In this paper we will discuss the results of some experiments in which this technique is utilized, and then propose a quantitative mathematical model that accounts for many features of the experimental results.

ANTIDROMIC INHIBITION

Tomita (1958) showed that inhibition in the *Limulus* eye can be produced by antidromic volleys in the optic nerve. In our experiments, as in his, a single eccentric cell fiber was isolated by dissection and stimulated by light confined to the facet of the ommatidium from which it arose (the test ommatidium or test unit). Inhibition was produced by stimulating the rest of the optic nerve with brief electric shocks to generate volleys of antidromic impulses (see Fig. 1). The advantage of the antidromic technique is that it allows very precise control of the excitation of the optic nerve and enables one to avoid effects of the complex excitatory transients associated with light stimulation of the receptors. This element of control provided by the antidromic stimulation is valuable for a quantitative study of input–output relations.

* Substantial portions of this paper are based on a dissertation submitted by D. Lange to the faculty of the Rockefeller University in partial fulfilment of the requirements for the degree of Doctor of Philosophy.

This investigation was supported by a research grant (NB–00864) from the National Institute of Neurological Diseases and Blindness, U.S. Public Health Service, and by an Equipment Loan Contract Nonr. [1442(00)] with the U.S. Office of Naval Research.

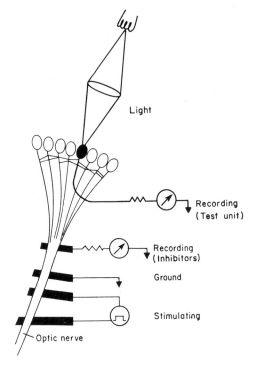

FIG. 1

Diagrammatic representation of the experimental set-up for producing antidromic inhibition. The eccentric cell fiber from the test unit (black) is isolated from the rest of the optic nerve. The remaining portion of the nerve is stimulated to produce the inhibition. Inhibition is measured by measuring changes in impulse frequency in the test fiber. (Figure modified from Purple, 1964.)

The inhibition produced by antidromic stimulation, although admittedly unphysiological, had many properties similar to that produced normally by light. Thus, steady-state inhibition increased with the pulse frequency of the antidromic stimulus, following a piecewise linear relationship as in light-induced inhibition. Antidromic inhibition also exhibited many of the same temporal properties as that produced by light: there was a substantial latent period before the inhibition appeared, an initial transient—or undershoot—preceding the steady state, and an overshoot above the control frequency, for a time, upon cessation of the antidromic impulses. It is important to note that some of these transients—so very prominent in the mirroring of excitatory transients—appear at the onset and cessation of *steady* antidromic stimulation. These transients (undershoots and overshoots) must therefore, in part at least, be ascribed to the inhibitory system itself.

The experimental methods employed in this work are similar to those used by Tomita (1958) and have been described fully elsewhere (Lange, 1965). The electronic equipment has also been described (Schoenfeld, 1964; Milkman and Schoenfeld, 1966) as has our use of computer techniques (Lange, Hartline and Ratliff, 1966).

In a typical experiment the light focused on the test ommatidium (test unit in Fig. 1) was allowed to shine steadily for 10–15 sec. Within 3 or 4 sec after the onset of this illumination the frequency of impulses generated by the receptor reached a more or less steady value. At this time stimulus pulses were delivered to a large bundle of optic nerve fibers that did not include the fiber from the test ommatidium. The changes in impulse frequency in the test unit fiber constituted the measure of inhibition. "Experimental" runs of this sort interspersed with "controls" (no antidromic stimulation) were repeated at intervals of 2–4 min.

There is some difficulty, of course, in assigning a significant pulse frequency to a non-uniform train of pulses. We have defined the "instantaneous frequency" at any time as the reciprocal of the interspike interval coincident with that time. We have used this measure of frequency throughout this paper.

STEADY-STATE EXPERIMENTS

Although the main reason for using antidromic inhibition was the ease of control of its temporal properties, it was necessary to collect some steady-state data as well. There were two reasons for this. First, we had to determine whether the steady-state equations were applicable in this artificial situation. Second, steady-state data were required to calculate the parameters of the mathematical model.

We have taken as our measure of activity the difference in instantaneous frequency between an experimental and a control run. Inhibition is thus indicated by a negative ordinate in plots of frequency difference versus time (see Fig. 2).

As seen in Fig. 3A the firing frequency of the test ommatidium tends to reach a steady inhibited level in the second or third second of the antidromic stimulus. Once this steady state has been reached it is appropriate to apply the same analysis as previously applied to the steady-state light-induced inhibition. Figure 4 is a typical plot of inhibition as a function of antidromic pulse frequency. The deviations from linearity are discussed later in the section entitled "Comparison of experimental results and model calculations". In the linear approximation drawn, the slope of the line gives the inhibitory constant, K. The inhibitory constants in antidromic inhibition are characteristically much larger than those published previously ($0 \cdot 5$–1 as opposed to $0 \cdot 1$). This is reasonable, considering the probable linear summation of effects from all inputs to a cell.

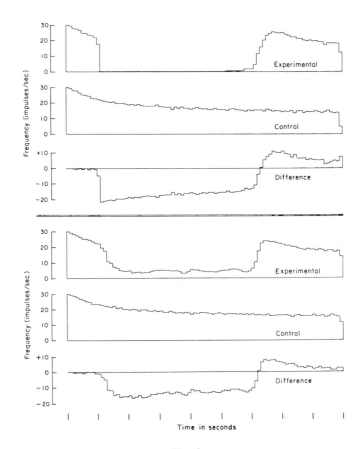

FIG. 2

Comparison of experimental runs with control runs by subtraction. The figure demonstrates the method by which the response curves of Fig. 3A were calculated. The first two experiments from that series are illustrated. The upper trace of each group is an average of four experimental runs. The middle trace is a similar average of four control runs in which no inhibitory stimuli were delivered. The lowest trace is the algebraic difference between the first and second traces. Notice that this procedure eliminates the downward drift of frequencies. In the upper experiment, however, where the experimental frequency reaches zero impulses per second, the drift cannot appear. The subtraction of the downward drifting control then leads to the misleading upward drift of the difference.

(Figure from Lange, Hartline and Ratliff, 1966.)

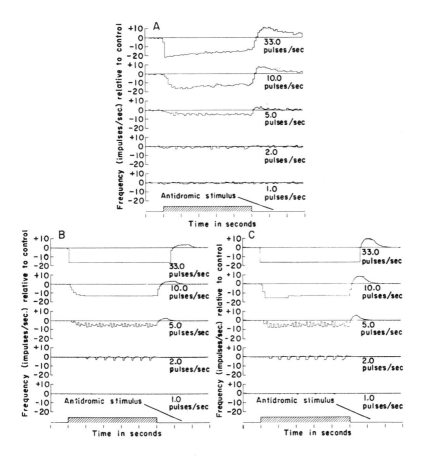

FIG. 3

Step function responses. Fig. 3A shows the' response of an ommatidium in an
actual experiment. The curves were obtained as described in the legend of Fig. 2.
The numbers to the right of each trace are the pulse frequencies of the antidromic
stimuli, the duration of which is designated by the hatched bar. The average control frequency was 18 impulses/sec. See text for detailed description of the dynamics. Figure 3B and C displays the results of calculations based on the theoretical
"model" described later in the text. Figure 3B was produced by the model when a
single time constant ($\tau_s = \tau_L = 0 \cdot 67$) was used. Other constants were: $A_s =$
$4 \cdot 125$; $A_L = 9 \cdot 0$; and $C = 12$. Compare asymmetry of response, approach to
steady state, apparent effects of single volleys at 2 impulses/sec and post-inhibitory rebound. Figure 3C was produced by the model when the time constants
were allowed to differ ($\tau_s = 1 \cdot 0$; $\tau_L = 0 \cdot 5$). A_s and A_L were adjusted to keep
steady-state inhibition constant ($A_s = 2 \cdot 75$; $A_L = 12 \cdot 0$). Notice better simulation
of transients at onset of inhibition and during post-inhibitory rebound. (Figure
modified from Lange, Hartline and Ratliff, 1966.)

493

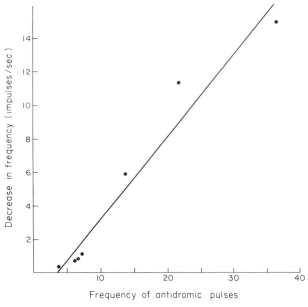

FIG. 4

Inhibition versus antidromic frequency. The ordinate values were calculated by subtracting the steady-state inhibited frequency from a control uninhibited frequency. The slope of the line (antidromic inhibitory constant) is 0·48 and was fit by a least squares method. The intercept (threshold frequency) is 3·5 impulses/sec.

The steady-state equations (see preceding paper) are:

$$r_p = e_p - \sum_j K_{p,j}(r_j - r^0_{p,j}). \tag{1}$$

As in our previous formulations, the response r_p of a particular ommatidium p is measured in terms of the frequency of discharge of impulses from that ommatidium. It is equal to the uninhibited response e_p of that same ommatidium, diminished by the summation of whatever inhibitory influences may be exerted on it by the other ommatidia j. Each of the separate inhibitory influences is the product of that part of the response r_j that exceeds the threshold of inhibitory action $r^0_{p,j}$, multiplied by the corresponding inhibitory coefficient $K_{p,j}$.

In the case where all pertinent thresholds have been exceeded the equations reduce to a special form in antidromic inhibition. Since an antidromic pulse frequency r_a is being imposed on the entire optic nerve (exclusive of the test bundle), eqn. (1) becomes:

$$r_p = e_p - r_a \sum_j K_{p,j} + \sum_j K_{p,j} r^0_{p,j}, \tag{2a}$$

$$r_p = e_p - \left(\sum_j K_{p,j} \right) \left(r_a - \frac{\sum_j K_{p,j} r_{p,j}^0}{\sum_j K_{p,j}} \right), \tag{2b}$$

or

$$I_p = e_p - r_p = \left(\sum_j K_{p,j} \right) \left(r_a - \frac{\sum_j K_{p,j} r_{p,j}^0}{\sum_j K_{p,j}} \right). \tag{2c}$$

The plot in Fig. 4 is of I_p (the total inhibition on the test unit p) versus r_a. The slope of the line is therefore the sum of the inhibitory constants

$$\left(\sum_j K_{p,j} \right)$$

and the intercept on the antidromic frequency axis is a mean of individual thresholds weighted according to their corresponding inhibitory constants. The line in the figure was plotted by the digital computer using a least squares fit.

DYNAMICS

The primary goal of this work is to describe in some detail, and perhaps to explain, the dynamical properties of the lateral inhibitory system. Since the steady-state equations are at least piecewise linear, some of the principles of linear systems analysis are applicable. Therefore, we have applied step function and delta function inputs to the lateral inhibitory system. As is well known, the responses of a linear system to such inputs are sufficient to characterize completely that system. In other words, if one knows the response of a linear system to either a step function or a delta function input, one can predict its response to all other inputs.

The definition of a step function or a delta function in a system where the input is a train of nerve spikes leads to some difficulty. Assuming that it is the spike frequency that is important, however, the step function input may be defined as an abrupt change from one pulse frequency to another.

Similarly, a delta function input may be most naturally defined as the input of one nerve impulse. This idealized definition can be achieved in the antidromic case to the extent that one impulse per optic nerve fiber (i.e. one volley) can be generated. (Such an experiment is discussed later in the paper, and the results are illustrated in Fig. 6.) In such experiments, however, the inhibition is often small. One may consider the inhibition from a short burst of volleys of inhibitory input as a delta function response in these cases. Such a generalization will hold as long as the burst is shorter than the important characteristic times of the system, and as long as the number of pulses in the burst is used to normalize the results. Of course, non-linearities in the system, which most assuredly exist, can completely invalidate the assertion that the response to *n* impulses is merely *n* times the response to one.

STEP FUNCTION RESPONSE

Figure 3A illustrates a typical set of step function responses. The number to the right of each plot represents the frequency of antidromic pulses occurring during the time represented by the hatched bar. Outside of this time there were no antidromic pulses.

At high input frequencies, production of impulses by the test unit stops; then, of course, no details of the inhibitory time course can be seen. (The technique of subtracting the control from the experimental frequency in this case leads to a misleading result, explained in the legend of Fig. 2.) On cessation of the antidromic input the unit began to respond at a low frequency, rapidly recovered to the control level (0·0) and finally transiently exceeded the control level and slowly reapproached it. In this plot the frequency never returned to the control frequency. This long-lasting post-inhibitory rebound at high input frequencies was observed in some but not all experiments. The shorter rebounds seen in the lower plots were always present and are seen with light-induced inhibition as well.

At lower input frequencies the activity of the test fiber is not completely suppressed but rather approaches a uniform inhibited level. As is seen in the second plot, the approach to this steady state is not necessarily monotonic; rather the frequency falls below the steady-state level and then returns. This behavior, which we will call the undershoot, was seen in some but not all the preparations. On cessation of inhibitory input the frequency quickly rises, overshoots and finally settles to the control level.

At still lower input frequencies (5 impulses/sec, here) the onset of inhibition seems decidedly sluggish with none of the undershoot seen above, while the release from inhibition is quick with a decided overshoot. This asymmetry between onset and release of inhibition will be of foremost importance in the discussions to follow.

At the lowest frequency showing inhibition (2 impulses/sec) we see what seem to be small inhibitory responses with a virtual return to the control level between them. These are very likely responses to individual inhibitory volleys which occur at each of the time marks and halfway between them. At these low frequencies it is perhaps unwise to continue to think in terms of a "step response" and of pulse frequency at all. The apparent response times of the system are such that responses to individual inputs are evident and hence the input is not seen as an integrated single step of frequency. These individual responses will be discussed further in the sections on delta function responses and in terms of the experimental model.

Returning to the description of Fig. 3A, it can be seen that at the very lowest input frequency (1 impulse/sec) there is no apparent inhibition. This is a manifestation of the inhibitory threshold in the steady-state analysis.

The theoretical model we will propose is based on the principles of linear analysis. It will therefore be useful to discuss the main features of the responses in terms of the expectations from a linear system.

First, were the system linear, we should expect the general shape of the responses to be unchanged as the magnitude of the input is changed. This is more or less the case for the release from inhibition but does not seem to hold well at the onset. Second, were the system linear, we should expect the onset of inhibition and the release from inhibition to be mirror images of one another. That this is not the case with very high inhibition is a trivial result of the fact that the fiber stops responding altogether and hence the frequency can have no undershoot. The response at 20 impulses/sec is most nearly symmetrical, having transient undershoots and overshoots at both onset and release. The responses at lower frequencies are again asymmetric with a sharper release than onset. At the frequencies where individual responses are seen the apparently non-linear effects are quite obviously due to the pulsatile character of the input.

In conclusion, then, it is apparent that although the steady-state levels of inhibition in the *Limulus* eye can be nicely predicted by a piecewise linear formulation, the time-dependent step responses show signs of asymmetries which are certainly the result of non-linear behavior. It will be seen, however, that the non-linearities necessary to explain the data again have the character of piecewise linearity.

TIME DELAYS

Delays in the onset of light-induced inhibition have been extensively discussed in the preceding paper. Delays also appear in the antidromic experiments. They can be as long as several hundred milliseconds. Figure 5 illustrates an experiment designed to study the properties of the time delay and, in particular, its dependence on the level of inhibition and past history of inhibition. The figure illustrates two experimental situations.

In the experimental run designated by the dashed arrow an antidromic frequency of 20 impulses/sec was begun at 1·0 sec and was then stepped to 33 impulses/sec at 3·0 sec (as indicated by the dashed lines). A delay of about 400 msec is observed before the first noticeable inhibition at the first step. The delay is very short at the second step.

In the run identified by a solid arrow a just suprathreshold antidromic frequency of 10 impulses/sec was begun 2 sec prior to the beginning of the record, and stepped to 33 impulses/sec at 3·0 sec (indicated by the solid lines). In this case the delay was greatly reduced (to about 100 msec), the same steady state was reached, and when the next step was imposed the response was identical to that in the first experiment. We see, therefore, that the time delay to the onset of inhibition is not constant but depends on the previous history of inhibition. In another part of this experiment (not illustrated) the last step was imposed without any previous inhibition. In this case, with this rather high frequency, the delay was not much affected by the history. We see, therefore, that the time delay is shortened both by a previous background of

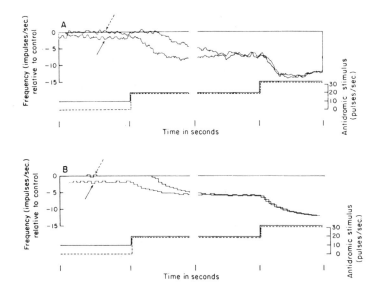

FIG. 5

Responses of an ommatidium (A) and of the model (B) to steps of antidromic frequency, showing changes in delay. The average frequency of controls in this experiment was 20 impulses/sec. See the text for further details. In Fig. 5B the same inhibitory input was introduced into the model as described later in the paper. The difference in the time delay due to previous inhibition is evident. The constants used in the calculations were: $A_L = 1\cdot3$; $A_s = 2\cdot0$; $\tau_s = \tau_L = 1\cdot0$; and $C = 7\cdot2$.

inhibition and by a large step in frequency. Similar results have been obtained using the light-induced inhibition. We have previously proposed (Ratliff, Hartline and Lange, 1964) that these delays may be partly explained in terms of the times necessary to overcome the steady-state inhibitory threshold. In this paper we hope to make this conjecture both plausible and quantitative. A similar explanation in terms of hypothetical interneurons was proposed by Stevens (1964) for both the threshold and the delays.

With antidromic stimulation of the whole nerve or a bundle of many fibers coming from different parts of the eye, we cannot say anything about the dependence of the time delays on distance. In fact these experiments are subject to a dispersion error to the extent that delays are distance-dependent. These distance effects are discussed in the preceding paper.

DELTA FUNCTION RESPONSES

As stated above, either single volleys of antidromic stimulation or short groups of volleys can be considered delta function inputs to the lateral inhibitory system.

Figure 6 illustrates the response to a single antidromic volley. This experiment was performed in a slightly different manner from those previously described. In this case the recording is from a bundle of fibers rather than a single test fiber. The upper trace in each photograph is the recording of the

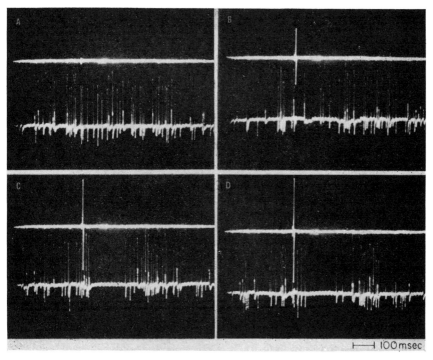

FIG. 6

Responses to single antidromic volleys. The upper trace in each oscillogram records the compound action potential from the electrically stimulated optic nerve. The lower traces are recordings from a bundle of fibers whose ommatidia were stimulated by light. The stimulus voltages are 2·5 (A), 2·8 (B), 5·0 (C) and 50·0 (D). See text for discussion.

compound action potential from the optic nerve, associated with the anti-dromic volleys. The lower trace of each photograph records the nerve action potentials from the test bundle.

In Fig. 6A the shock to the optic nerve was subthreshold (2·5 V) as is indicated by the lack of a compound action potential. There was no effect on the test bundle. In B there was submaximal stimulation (2·8 V) and a detectable deficit of impulses in the test bundle just after the antidromic volley. In C the stimulation (5·0 V) produced a maximal compound action potential and a larger inhibitory effect. In D the stimulation was increased 10 times over C (50 V). Both the compound action potential and the inhibitory effect remained sensibly the same in D as in C. This maneuver served as a control against the remote possibility that the electrical shock to the optic nerve was producing its inhibitory effect directly on the eye rather than through the response of the nerve fibers. Both this control and the sharp onset of inhibition closely following the compound action potential (compare A and B) argue against the possibility of a direct artifactual effect.

Although it is not possible to say much quantitatively about this composite response, it can be seen that the inhibition lasts for only about 200 msec and is followed by a post-inhibitory rebound of about the same duration.

GROUPS OF VOLLEYS

The use of short groups of antidromic volleys produces inhibitory inputs similar to those produced by short flashes of light to neighboring ommatidia that were described in the preceding paper. One of the most striking findings has been that if one separates two short flashes of light on a neighboring ommatidium by one to a few seconds there is an enhancement of the inhibition produced by the second burst which depends on the presence of the first burst. The enhancement is so strong that it often appears even when the second burst contains fewer impulses. The antidromic technique is an ideal one to use in studying this facilitation because it is possible to make the inhibitory inputs highly reproducible.

Figure 7A and C illustrates such an experiment. It is evident that the inhibitory response to the second burst is greater than that to the first. This is true even though there is no directly observable effect remaining from the first burst at the time the second occurs. Again, discussing these results in terms of a linear system we would expect the response to two bursts to be the sum of the responses to each burst taken separately. This is clearly not the case. This phenomenon can be explained using the same reasoning as that used to explain the variable time delay. That is, the presence of a threshold masks persisting subthreshold—and hence, by definition, nonobservable—events which contribute to the inhibition produced by the second burst of antidromic impulses.

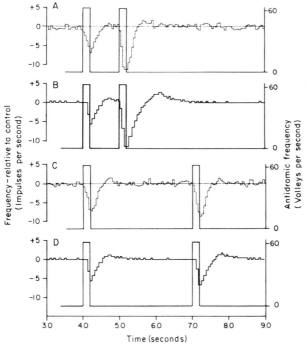

Facilitation. Figure 7A and C illustrates the facilitation of inhibition when a burst of inhibitory pulses (at 4 sec) is followed by another (at 5 sec in A and 7 sec in C). It is evident that the facilitation decreases with increasing time between bursts. Figure 7B and D illustrates the model simulation of this experiment, as described later in the text.

This explanation of facilitation is strengthened by the following experiment. Bursts of antidromic volleys were produced at a constant pulse frequency but with different numbers of pulses in the burst. A plot was then made of the number of impulses lost by the test fiber in a given period versus the number of pulses in the inhibitory input (Fig. 8). Such a plot is analogous to the inhibitory plot in Fig. 4 except that Fig. 8 displays changes in number versus number rather than changes in frequency versus frequency. (Analogous results have been obtained using two flashes of light.)

As one might expect if the bursts of pulses in the inhibitory input are short enough to be essentially delta functions, these plots produce straight lines just as do the steady-state plots. The line through the open circles is for the first of two bursts while the line through the closed circles is for the second. Notice that the plots demonstrate an apparent threshold. That is, for this preparation no effect is seen when fewer than three volleys of antidromic pulses appear together. Once this threshold is exceeded the number of impulses lost is linearly related to the number of pulses in the burst. It can be seen that the slopes of the two lines are the same, but the threshold is lower in the case of the second burst. Evidently some subthreshold inhibitory influences persist for a time after the first burst and, in effect, lower the threshold for the inhibitory influences produced by the second burst.

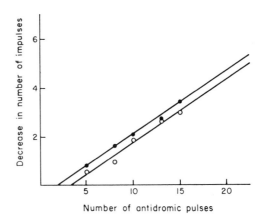

FIG. 8

Inhibition as a function of the number of antidromic volleys in a burst. The ordinates were calculated as the difference in the number of impulses from the test ommatidium in one second, in a control and in an experimental run. The abscissa is the number of pulses in the antidromic burst causing the inhibition. The open circles are for the first burst in a series similar to Fig. 7A, while the closed circles are for the second burst. The slopes of the lines (fit by least squares) are identical (0·25) but the intercept (threshold) has been decreased by the presence of a previous burst.

SUMMARY OF EXPERIMENTAL FINDINGS

We can now summarize the main features of the responses of the lateral inhibitory system in the *Limulus* eye. We may list these features in order of their appearance in the response:

(1) The onset of inhibition is delayed by an amount dependent on the previous inhibitory level and on the amplitude of the change in input.

(2) The onset of inhibition is sluggish at low levels of inhibitory input.

(3) The frequency undershoots at high levels of inhibitory input (not seen in all experiments).

(4) The level of inhibition in the steady state is linearly related to the inhibitory input.

(5) There is a steady-state threshold.

(6) There is a post-inhibitory rebound.

(7) Inhibitory deficits resulting from short bursts of antidromic volleys are linearly related to the number of volleys in the bursts; there is a threshold for the inhibitory responses.

(8) The inhibitory responses to short bursts of antidromic volleys are facilitated by previous inhibition.

Points 2 and 3 taken together with 6 are evidence of an asymmetry between the onset and release of inhibition.

Any theoretical treatment of this system should account for all of these phenomena if it is to be complete. It is clear, however, that a purely linear model will not account for the asymmetries, delays, or facilitations mentioned above. At this point we can anticipate, therefore, that any adequate model of the activity of this system will probably be non-linear.

THEORETICAL MODEL

We have developed a quantitative theoretical formulation which accounts for many of the features seen in the inhibitory response (cf. Lange, 1965). This formulation, or model, has been expressed in two ways. One, in the form of an integral equation, is a generalization of the steady-state formulation. This form will not be discussed in this paper. A complete treatment will be published in the future.

The second form of the model is expressed as a computer program. It is based on the impulse-by-impulse calculation of input and output and is equivalent to the integral form where individual nerve spikes are expressed as delta functions. It is this form of the model which is used to compute the responses of the system.

Both forms are based on the concept of nervous integration by summation. That is, it is asserted that the output of each cell of a nervous system is largely determined by, and is more or less proportional to, the sum of all excitatory and inhibitory influences on it. The extent to which this principle holds in various nervous systems varies widely. It is evident from the steady-state formulation, however, that the addition (or subtraction) principle holds well in the *Limulus* eye.

GENERAL PROGRAMMING CONSIDERATIONS

The model program was written in Control Data 160 Fortran A, a language nearly identical to the widely used forms of IBM Fortran. The calculations were performed on the Control Data Corporation 160-A computer in our laboratory.

A program is a set of rules for transforming one set of numbers into another. This transformation or mapping property of programs is really no different from the transformation or mapping property of mathematical operators and functions. The program can therefore perform the same function as that of a mathematical theory of a physical system. That is, it can predict the outcome of new experiments and thereby put the theory in a quantitatively testable form. In the present application, use of a digital computer program was particularly convenient because input data generated during experiments could be used directly as input data for the model.

The program was divided into three parts: input, model and output. There was provision for input of either real or idealized stimulus data and for input of the parameters of the model. Output consisted of typed and plotted displays of exactly the same form as that produced by the data processing program, thus facilitating the comparison of experimental and theoretical results.

The model itself was written in cyclic form. The basic cycle, called a clock cycle, represented one millisecond of time. The operations performed during each clock cycle will be described with the appropriate sections of the model.

SPIKE GENERATION

On the basis of empirical observations, a model for spike generation has been formulated over the past few years. This model asserts that the spike generating mechanism of the *Limulus* eccentric cell integrates the generator potential until a critical value of this integral is reached, at which time a spike is generated and the integration begins again. Stevens (1964) put this model into a formal statement in his discussion of slow potential theory as applied to the eccentric cell. The model is formally identical with one hypothesized by Hodgkin (1948) which was based on the classical notion of strength-duration reciprocity. At the time of production of each impulse the reciprocal of the interval since the last impulse is proportional to the average value of the generator potential during that interval. For constant generator potentials, such a model produces a frequency of impulses linearly related to the generator potential (cf. MacNichol, 1956).

In more symbolic terms we may say that a generator (g) was formed from the excitatory term (e) minus all inhibitory terms to be defined later. At each clock cycle of the program, the generator (g) was added to a running sum (s). When this sum reached a critical value a spike was recorded for the eccentric cell and the summation was begun again. The operation amounted to an integration of the generator and produced an impulse frequency proportional to it.

SELF-INHIBITION

In conformity with the work of Stevens (1964), Purple (1964) and Purple and Dodge (1966) the model was provided with self-inhibition in the following manner. A self-inhibitory pool (I_s) was set to zero at the beginning of the program. When the spike generator produced a spike, a quantity of inhibition (A_s) (in the same units as the generator) was added to this pool. At each cycle of the program a portion of this pool proportional to its current values and to the reciprocal of the self-inhibitory time constant (τ_s) was subtracted from it.

The total effect of the steps outlined above was to produce an exponentially decaying inhibitory potential following each impulse generated, leading to an exponential approach to the steady state of the spike frequency. This is consistent with Stevens' formulation and reproduces curves very similar to those calculated by a self-inhibitory simulation program written by F. A. Dodge (see Purple, 1964).

A neuron model of this type, with a summable inhibition following each impulse, should be carefully distinguished from models which set the membrane potential to a particular value following each impulse (Perkel *et al.*, 1964). The latter type of model destroys all information concerning the size of the generator previous to the last spike produced. Transients in the firing rate of such models cannot be any longer than the time between impulses. This is clearly not the case in the *Limulus* eccentric cell where transients to a step change in generator potential can persist over many tens of interspike intervals.

So far we have discussed three variables in the model: the initial size of the generator (e), the time constant of decay of self-inhibition (τ_s) and the magnitude of the inhibitory quantum (A_s), added to the self-inhibitory pool following each spike.

LATERAL INHIBITION

The success of the self-inhibitory model in predicting the dynamical behavior of the eccentric cell naturally leads one to attempt to extend the same ideas to the case of lateral inhibition. This was done by Schoenfeld (1964) with some qualitative success.

The straightforward way to apply these concepts to antidromic inhibition in the model is as follows:

A list of times of occurrence of antidromic pulses is entered into the computer memory. At each cycle of the program (each millisecond) this list is consulted. If an antidromic pulse is encountered, a quantity of inhibition (A_L) is added to a lateral inhibitory pool (I_L). At each cycle the lateral inhibitory pool is diminished as in the self-inhibitory case, the decay being governed by the lateral inhibitory time constant (τ_L). Thus, two more parameters have been added to the model: the lateral inhibitory quantum of inhibition (A_L) and the lateral inhibitory time constant (τ_L).

THE LINEAR MODEL

At this point we can construct the total model in a linear form. In the case of the computer program this amounts to adding a step at each cycle which calculates the generator (g) by subtracting the two inhibitory terms from the excitatory term

$$g = e - I_s - I_L. \tag{3}$$

This generator (g) is the one we then apply to the sum (s) in the spike generating program.

The linear model has some of the necessary properties of lateral inhibition (see Fig. 9 and legend). It may be recalled, however, that many of the pro-

No Threshold

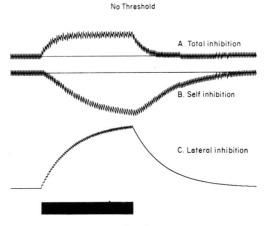

A. Total inhibition

B. Self inhibition

C. Lateral inhibition

FIG. 9

Model inhibitory pools with no threshold. Trace C shows the lateral inhibitory pool as it builds up during a train of inhibitory pulses designated by the black bar. The sawtooth build-up is essentially exponential. Trace B shows the self-inhibitory pool changing during the inhibition. The rate of increase and decrease of self-inhibition is such that it matches the lateral inhibition so that their sum (Trace A) has no overshoot. (Increase in total inhibition corresponds to decrease in the firing frequency of the test unit.)

perties of lateral inhibition discussed above were inconsistent with a linear model. Foremost among these were the lack of symmetry between onset and release of inhibition and the steady-state threshold. It should be noted that it is possible to produce inhibitory transients with an entirely linear model. If one makes the self-inhibitory time constant (τ_s) larger than the lateral inhibitory time constant (τ_L) an initial undershoot in the frequency and a post-inhibitory rebound will be present. The response will be symmetric, however.

INTRODUCTION OF A NON-LINEARITY

The responses displayed earlier were on the whole non-linear in their time-dependent properties. Recall that there were strong asymmetries in the step function response, there was facilitation and there were apparently non-linear time delays. We (Ratliff, Hartline and Lange, 1964) have previously suggested that there may be a connection between the delay phenomenon and the steady-state threshold. Ratliff (1965) has pointed out that there is an apparent relationship between threshold and inhibitory constant in a given eye. This relationship seems to be one of reciprocity, that is

$$r_{p,j}^0 = \frac{C_p}{K_{p,j}} \tag{4}$$

where C_p is a constant depending on the test unit only. This relationship demands that all plots of the inhibition exerted on a unit p from its neighbors j will have a common intercept on the inhibition ordinate. This simplification substantially reduces the number of empirical constants required. With these approximate relations in mind, we have introduced a threshold into the model.

NON-LINEAR MODEL

The imposition of a critical level on the lateral inhibitory pool makes the model non-linear. As before, at the time corresponding to each inhibitory impulse a quantity (A_L) of inhibition was added to the pool (I_L). The full value of the pool was not used, however, in the calculation of the generator (g). Instead, a reduced inhibition (I) was used, calculated by subtracting a constant (C) from I_L (see Fig. 10C). If this subtraction produced a negative number, zero was substituted for I_r. Therefore, the expression for the generator becomes $g = e - I_s - I_r$.

A flow diagram of the complete model program has been published elsewhere (Lange, Hartline and Ratliff, 1966).

CONSISTENCY WITH THE STEADY-STATE EQUATIONS

The model is consistent with the steady-state equations. It provides an inhibition which is linear above threshold. In fact, one can calculate most of the parameters of the model from steady-state data. One can rigorously derive the steady-state equations from the integral equation formulation of the model. This has been done (see Lange, 1965), but its details are outside the scope of this paper.

When the integral equations are reduced to the steady state, relationships between the steady-state parameters and those of the dynamic model are established.

These are:
$$\frac{A_L \tau_L}{1 + A_s \tau_s} = \sum_j K_{p,j} \qquad \frac{C}{A_L \tau_L} = \frac{\sum_j K_{p,j} r_{p,j}^0}{\sum_j K_{p,j}} \tag{5}$$

With Threshold

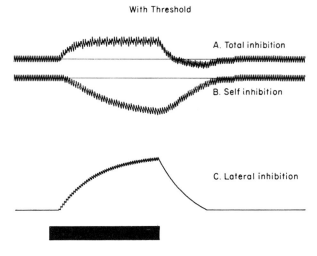

A. Total inhibition

B. Self inhibition

C. Lateral inhibition

FIG. 10

Model inhibitory pools with a threshold. Trace C shows the lateral inhibitory pool. Notice the delay due to the time to achieve threshold; notice also the shortened decay. Because of this shortened decay the self-inhibition (Trace B) cannot compensate exactly for the lateral inhibition (Trace C), and therefore their sum (Trace A) exhibits an undershoot which leads to a post-inhibitory overshoot in the frequency of the test unit. The apparent noise in the total inhibition is a consequence of beats between the sawteeth of the lateral and self-inhibitory pools.

where the terms on the right of the identities are from eqn. (2c). If we plot inhibition as a function of antidromic frequency, as was done in Fig. 6, then $\dfrac{A_L \tau_L}{1 + A_s \tau_s}$ is the slope of the line while $\dfrac{C}{A_L \tau_L}$ is the intercept on the abscissa or the apparent threshold frequency. These quantities are therefore measurable. In order to evaluate the individual parameters we must make some assumptions. In the light-adapted state the initial transient to the onset of light in the test ommatidium follows a nearly exponential time course. In this case $(1 + A_s \tau_s)$ is the ratio of the initial frequency to the steady-state frequency. This allows $A_s \tau_s$ to be calculated from the experimental data. It only remains to estimate the time constants. This can be done by fitting the model to a typical inhibition curve or by assuming, as above, that the approach to steady state exhibited in the light-adapted state is primarily the result of self-inhibition. A third alternative is to choose an arbitrary time constant in the range found by Stevens.

PHYSIOLOGICAL SIGNIFICANCE OF PARAMETERS

The question now arises as to the physiological meaning of the parameters. The terms A_L and A_s can be conceptually associated with the release of unitary quantities of some inhibitory substance. Adolph has reported in this symposium that gamma amino butyric acid seems to mimic the effects of lateral inhibition when applied to the eye. Perhaps the assumption of a chemical transmitter substance is, therefore, not without some basis. If it is assumed that each synaptic ending produces some constant amount of inhibitory substance, then the magnitudes of A_L and A_s should be proportional to the number of active synaptic endings impinging on the test unit.

It would also be reasonable to assume that the dependence of the inhibitory constant on distance may be through a dependence of A_L on the distance to the inhibitors; perhaps widely separated receptors have fewer inhibitory endings on one another; perhaps conduction in the plexus is with decrement. Without specifying the actual mechanism, the assumption that A_L depends on distance will be made in future attempts to tie together spatial and temporal phenomena. Once we have made these assumptions concerning A_s and A_L, the time constants τ_s and τ_L might be associated with inactivation or diffusion of the transmitter substance.

The physiological interpretation of the thresholds is difficult. Their introduction into the model is most easily justified by pointing to the formal importance they have in properly predicting the data. There does, however, appear to be some real barrier in the lateral inhibitory system which affects the appearance of the hyperpolarizing inhibito.y potential in intracellular recordings. Purple (1964) found that the inhibitory potential did not appear until the antidromic frequency had reached about 3 impulses/sec. The seat of the threshold must lie, then, either in the synaptic cleft or in the presynaptic ending. The dynamics, which require that the threshold be applied both as the inhibition is rising and as it is falling, would seem to place the barrier or inactivation in the synaptic cleft or at the site where the inhibitory substance first affects the post-synaptic membrane. At this time we can only make these speculations and hope that future experiments may shed more light on the mechanism.

COMPARISON OF EXPERIMENTAL RESULTS AND MODEL CALCULATIONS

Having set numerical values of the constants needed in the model, we can calculate with the computer the time course of "responses" the model generates, and display outputs which are of the same form as those produced by the data processing of the actual experiment, Comparisons of experimental results with the "responses" generated by the model are shown in Figs. 3, 5 and 7. Referring to these figures, we will now discuss in detail the successes and failures of the model.

Figures 3B and C represent simulations of the experiment in Fig. 3A. In Fig. 3B the time constants of self- and lateral inhibition were equal, while in Fig. 3C they were allowed to differ. Both simulations reproduce the gross features of the response reasonably well. We expect the steady-state levels of inhibition to fit well because these were used to calculate the parameters of the model. We see, however, that the model has reproduced other features of the response as well, including asymmetries and post-inhibitory rebound.

The undershoot seen in the second run of Fig. 3A and the post-inhibitory overshoots are best fit by the second simulation (C). The sluggish onset of the inhibition in the third run is best fit by the first simulation (B). These discrepancies in detail suggest that the exponential time course for inhibitory events is probably too simple.

The recovery from inhibition in the first run of each simulation is too slow. This could result from either of two faults. Either the time constant for lateral inhibition is too long or the absence of a saturation of inhibition in the model is allowing it to be driven too far out of range. In the eye the level to which the generator can be driven in a hyperpolarizing direction is determined by the inhibitory equilibrium potential. The model has no such limit and hence at high frequency input the inhibition can continue to grow without bound, thus leading to an overly long recovery time.

Examination of Fig. 4 reveals a saturation phenomenon in the steady state. It can be seen that the experimental points are better fit by an *S*-shaped curve than by a straight line, and indeed this is a feature commonly observed. The upper curvature at high inhibitory levels is consistent with saturation. The curvature near threshold can be explained by assuming that there is a distribution of thresholds in the antidromic experiment due to the dependence of threshold on inhibitory constants and distance.

Some other successful results which were not, so to speak, built into the model are the individual inhibitory responses in the experimental curves corresponding to an antidromic frequency of 2 pulses/sec. These are represented in the model's response, and seem to be of about the right magnitude. This detail can only be reproduced by a model which calculates the response impulse-by-impulse.

Another phenomenon in the model's response which depends on the impulse-by-impulse calculations is the apparent "noise" during the inhibition in the curves corresponding to 5 pulses/sec in Fig. 3B and C. This phenomenon results from the beats generated between the antidromic input frequency and the average frequency of the simulated unit during inhibition (see also Fig. 10A). There is some indication of a similar phenomenon in the real experiment as well.

The time delays associated with the inhibitory interaction are the subject of the experiment illustrated in Fig. 5A. For the model, parameters were estimated from the steady-state results of the experiment and from the transients ascribed to self-inhibition. The reader will recall that in this experiment the difference between the two runs is the presence of a previous inhibitory input. As can be seen, the model accounts well for the *difference* between the two time delays (Fig. 5B). There is a residual delay in the real experiment which has no parallel in the model. The results do seem to confirm the earlier speculation that a substantial part of the delay is related to the threshold phenomenon. The delay in the model is clearly due to the time necessary for the inhibitory pool to exceed the threshold, the details of these events being illustrated in Fig. 10C, which shows the rise and fall of the inhibitory pools in the model.

Figure 7 compares the performance of the model with the experiments on facilitation of inhibition. Plots A and C show the experimental results while plots B and D show the results of the simulation. The simulation is good, except that the recovery from inhibition seems to be somewhat slower in the model than it is in the experiment on the eye. Facilitation is explained by a residuum of subthreshold inhibition from the first burst of antidromic volleys which is added to the effects of the second burst.

CONCLUSION

We have described some of the dynamic properties of the inhibitory interaction in the eye of *Limulus,* and proposed a theoretical model which describes quite well the results of a variety of experiments involving antidromic inhibition.

The parallels between the results of antidromic experiments and those with light-induced inhibition make it very likely that the model will also describe that body of data as well. The model is written in such a way that it is accessible to the use of data actually recorded from single fibers and, therefore, these data will be tried. The computed model has the advantage that it automatically considers the sampling problem and can reproduce the microstructure (that is, the detailed responses to each impulse) of the inhibitory response. Adding to these the simplicity of the theory and the fact that the parameters are few in number and have meaningful physiological interpretation leads us to hope that this may be a significant contribution.

The question arises as to the possible applications of a theory of this type to systems other than lateral inhibition in *Limulus.* One of the goals would seem to be to try to explain the behavior of more complex systems in terms of cells or subsystems having the same dynamical characteristics seen in this eye. It is quite clear that changes play a very impoitant role in the veitebrate visual system. Hartline (1938) found that the large majority of optic nerve fibers in the frog retina showed little or no activity in response to steady illumination, and in recent years there has been a profusion of excellent studies of the visual systems of vertebrates, emphasizing the strongly phasic nature of much of the activity of retinal and central neurons. The importance of such responses in human vision is exemplified by the studies of Ditchburn and Ginsborg (1952) and by Riggs *et al.* (1953), who demonstrated the disappearance of objects whose image is stabilized on the retina. Therefore, it is quite clear that dynamical theories will be needed to explain the characteristics of these visual systems. Indeed, even in *Limulus*, where the optic nerve certainly does carry steady-state information, nervous activity in the optic lobes has elements of a phasic nature (Wilska and Hartline, 1941). Another type of study seeks to characterize the input to complex sensory motor systems by analyzing their transfer properties. With the *Limulus* photoreceptors this has recently been done by Pinter (1966) and by Purple and Dodge (1966). There have also been studies of the overall characteristics of arthropod sensory motor systems: the optomotor responses of the beetle (Reichardt, 1962), of the locust (Thorson, 1964, 1965), and of the fly (McCann and MacGinitie, 1965).

We believe that the area of application of our model probably lies between these extremes. Attempts have already been made to explain some aspects of motion perception in terms of lateral inhibition. Barlow and Levick (1965) have hypothesized lateral inhibition with time delays to explain the selective sensitivity of ganglion cells in the rabbit retina to direction of motion of the retinal image. In this case, the lateral inhibitory system is presumed to be at the bipolar cell or receptor level. Thorson (1965) has discussed the possibility that a non-linear lateral inhibitory system might provide the mechanism for motion perception necessary to explain the optomotor response in insects. Bicking (1965) has proposed an inhibitory model similar to ours, which seems to explain on and off responses in the goldfish retina. A model of the type discussed in the present paper can, hopefully, provide the necessary basis for putting some of these explanations in a quantitative and hence more precise and more testable form.

REFERENCES

ADOLPH, A. R. 1966. Excitation and inhibition of electrical activity in the *Limulus* eye by neuropharmacological agents. This volume.

BARLOW, H. B. and LEVICK, W. R. 1965. The mechanism of directionally selective units in the rabbit's retina, *J. Physiol.* **178**, 477–504.

BICKLING, L. A. 1965. Some quantitative studies on retinal ganglion cells, Thesis, the Johns Hopkins University.

DITCHBURN, R. W. and GINSBORG, B. L. 1952. Vision with a stabilized retinal image, *Nature* **170**, 36.

HARTLINE, H. K. 1938. The response of single optic nerve fibers of the vertebrate eye to illumination of the retina, *Amer. J. Physiol.* **121**, 400–15.

HODGKIN, A. L. 1948. The local electric changes associated with repetitive action in a non-medullated axon, *J. Physiol. (London)* **107**, 165–81.

LANGE, D. 1965. Dynamics of inhibitory interactions in the eye of *Limulus*: Experimental and theoretical studies, Thesis, the Rockefeller University.

LANGE, D., HARTLINE, H. K. and RATLIFF, F. 1966. Inhibitory interactions in the retina: techniques of experimental and theoretical analysis. *Ann. N.Y. Acad. Sci.* **128**, 955–71.

MACNICHOL, E. F., Jr. 1956. Visual receptors as biological transducers, in *Molecular Structure and Functional Activity of Nerve Cells*, Publ. No. 1, Am. Inst. Biol. Sci., 34–53.

MCCANN, G. and MACGINITIE, G. 1965. Optomotor response studies of insect vision, *Proc. Roy. Soc. B*, **163**, 369–401.

MILKMAN, N. and SCHOENFELD, R. L. 1966. A digital programmer for stimuli and computer control in neurophysiological experiments, *Ann. N.Y. Acad. Sci.* **128**, 861–75.

PERKEL, D. H., SCHULMAN, J. H., BULLOCK, T. H., MOORE, G. P. and SEGUNDO, J. P. 1964. Pacemaker neurons: effects of regularly spaced synaptic input, *Science* **145**, 61–3.

PINTER, R. B. 1966. Sinusoidal and delta function responses of visual cells of the *Limulus* eye, *J. Gen. Physiol.* **49**, 565–93.

PURPLE, R. L. 1964. The integration of excitatory and inhibitory influences in the eccentric cell in the eye of *Limulus*, Thesis, the Rockefeller Institute.

PURPLE, R. L. and DODGE, F. 1966. Self-inhibition in the eye of *Limulus*. This volume.

RATLIFF, F. 1965. *Mach Bands: Quantitative Studies on Neural Networks in the Retina*, Holden Day, San Francisco.

RATLIFF, F., HARTLINE, H. K. and LANGE, D. 1964. Studies on the dynamics of inhibitory interaction in the retina, in *Physiological Basis for Form Discrimination*, Symposium, Brown University, Providence, R. I.

RATLIFF, F., HARTLINE, H. K., and LANGE, D. 1966. The dynamics of lateral inhibition in the compound eye of *Limulus*. I. This volume.

REICHARDT, W. 1962. Nervous integration in the facet eye, *Biophys. J.* **2**, 121–44.

RIGGS, L. A., RATLIFF, F., CORNSWEET, J. C. and CORNSWEET, T. N. 1953. The disappearance of steadily fixated test objects, *J. Opt. Soc. Amer.* **43**, 495–501.

SCHOENFELD, R. L. 1964. The role of a digital computer as a biological instrument, *Ann. N.Y. Acad. Sci.* **115**, 915–42.

STEVENS, C. F. 1964. A quantitative theory of neural interactions: theoretical and experimental investigations, Thesis, the Rockefeller Institute.

THORSON, J. W. 1964. Dynamics of motion perception in the desert locust, *Science* **145**, 69–71.

THORSON, J. W. 1965. Small signal analysis of a visual reflex in the desert locust, Thesis, University of California, Los Angeles.

TOMITA, T. 1958. Mechanism of lateral inhibition in the eye of *Limulus*, *J. Neurophysiol.* **21**, 419–29.

WILSKA, A. and HARTLINE, H. K. 1941. The origin of "off-responses" in the optic pathway, *Amer. J. Physiol.* **133**, 491.

Synthesis of "on-off" and "off" responses in a visual-neural system

FLOYD RATLIFF AND CONRAD G. MUELLER[1]

The Rockefeller Institute for Medical Research, New York, N.Y.

Reprinted from SCIENCE, 25 October 1957, Vol. 126, no. 3278, pp. 840–841.

The most distinctive feature of the discharge of impulses in the vertebrate optic nerve in response to a light stimulus is the marked activity elicited by changes in the level of illumination. The early records of Adrian and Matthews from the whole optic nerve (1) demonstrate a strong burst of activity when the light is turned on, a continuing discharge at a lower rate as long as the light remains on, and, upon the cessation of light, a renewed burst which gradually subsides.

Hartline (2) has shown that this composite response results from individual fibers whose activity differs markedly: some fibers discharge regularly as long as the light shines; others discharge only briefly when the light is turned on and again when it is turned off, with no activity during steady illumination; still others respond only when the light is turned off. These complex responses, observed in third-order neurones, have been ascribed by Hartline (2) and Granit (3) to the excitatory and inhibitory interactions of retinal structures interposed between these neurones and the photoreceptors rather than to special properties of the photoreceptors themselves.

The reasons for this interpretation are many. One reason derives from the nature of these 'transient' responses. Hartline (4) found that, in the eye of the frog, an 'off' response elicited in a single fiber by illuminating one group of receptors may be suppressed by illuminating another group of receptors in the same receptive field, and Barlow (5) has obtained a similar suppression using stimuli outside the receptive field. Also, Kuffler (6) has shown that, in the cat, these diverse response 'types' are labile and that, depending on the locus of illumination and the level of background illumination, a particular fiber may exhibit a variety of responses. Furthermore, the fibers arising directly from the ommatidia in the lateral eye of the invertebrate, *Limulus*, do not exhibit the diversity of response found in the vertebrate nerve. Although 'off' responses have been found in the *Limulus* optic ganglion (Wilska and

---

[1] National Academy of Sciences–National Research Council senior postdoctoral fellow in physiological psychology.

Hartline, 7), the typical response of *Limulus* optic nerve fibers to stimuli of long duration is a sustained discharge while the light is on and an immediate cessation of impulses when the light is turned off (Fig. 1*A*).

The relatively simple discharge pattern typically observed in fibers of the optic nerve of *Limulus* may be greatly modified by various means.

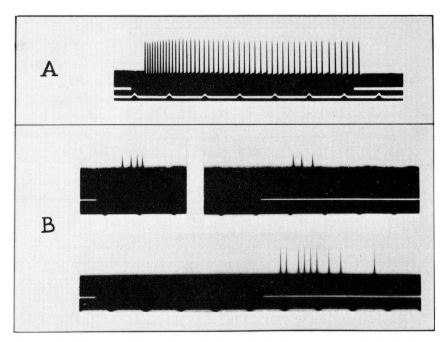

Fig. 1. Oscillograms of diverse 'types' of impulse discharge patterns in single fibers of *Limulus* optic nerve. *A*, Typical sustained discharge in response to steady illumination. *B*, Upper record; a synthetic 'on-off' response (approximately 1 sec. was cut from the middle of this record). Lower record; a synthetic 'off' response. Time is marked in 1/5-sec. periods. Signal of exposure of eye to light blackens the white line above the time marker. Fibers whose activity is shown in the two *B* records gave a sustained discharge like that shown in *A* when the ommatidia from which they arose were illuminated alone.

First, a pronounced afterdischarge may be obtained by proper control of exposure time, intensity of the stimulus, and state of adaptation. Second, the frequency of the discharge of impulses may be decreased by illuminating neighboring ommatidia; this inhibition seems to be mediated by a plexus of lateral interconnections immediately behind the ommatidia (Hartline, Wagner, and Ratliff, and Hartline and Ratliff, 8).

By combining these various influences on the discharge of impulses, 'on-off' and 'off' responses have been 'synthesized' in individual fibers of the *Limulus* optic nerve (9). Examples are shown in Fig. 1*B*. These responses possess the properties of the analogous responses in the vertebrate eye. The 'on-off' responses are characterized by a burst of activity when the light is turned on, no further activity as the light stays on, and a final burst of activity after the light is turned off. The pure 'off' responses also have the properties of the vertebrate response: no discharge appears until after the light goes off, and the discharge may be inhibited by reillumination. Both types of response have been obtained over a considerable range of stimulus durations.

A very delicate balance of excitatory and inhibitory influences is required to obtain these 'on-off' and 'off' responses in the optic nerve fibers of *Limulus*. The responses are not obtained under ordinary conditions of stimulation and have never been obtained when only one ommatidium is stimulated. From what we know of the properties of the inhibitory effect and of the temporal characteristics of the after-discharge, we view the 'on-off' response as occurring in the following manner: the onset of light stimulates several ommatidia, one of which gives rise to the fiber whose activity is being recorded. A few impulses are discharged in this fiber before the inhibitory influences from the neighboring elements completely suppress its activity. This suppression continues until the light is turned off. If the duration of the stimulus and the relative states of adaptation of the various receptors are adjusted so as to enhance the after discharge of the inhibited fiber and to minimize the afterdischarge of the neighboring elements, an 'off' response is obtained. To obtain a pure 'off' response the latency of excitation of the element whose activity is being recorded must be longer than the latency of the inhibition exerted upon it. This can be achieved by adjusting the angle of incidence of the light so that the element whose activity is being recorded is stimulated less effectively than are the neighboring elements which inhibit it.

The consequences of these experiments are twofold. (i) They lend support to the view that 'on-off' and 'off' responses are the result of the complex interplay of excitatory and inhibitory influences by showing that the experimental manipulation of these influences can, indeed, yield such transient responses; and (ii) they show the feasibility of using the *Limulus* preparation in the further study of these transient responses. This preparation offers distinct experimental advantages over the vertebrate preparation because the excitation and inhibition of individual receptor units may be easily and independently controlled and measured.

REFERENCES

1. Adrian, E. D., and Matthews, R., *J. Physiol. (London)* **63,** 378 (1927).
2. Hartline, H. K., *Amer. J. Physiol.,* **121,** 400 (1938).
3. Granit, R., *J. Physiol. (London),* **77,** 207 (1933).
4. Hartline, H. K., *Amer. J. Physiol.,* **126,** P527 (1939).
5. Barlow, H. B., *J. Physiol. (London),* **119,** 69 (1953).
6. Kuffler, S. W., *J. Neurophysiol.* **16,** 37 (1953).
7. Wilska, A., and Hartline, H. K., *Amer. J. Physiol.* **133,** P491 (1941).
8. Hartline, H. K., Wagner, H. G., Ratliff, F., *J. Gen. Physiol.* **39,** 651 (1956); Hartline, H. K., and Ratliff, F., ibid. **40,** 357 (1957).
9. This investigation was supported by a research grant (B864) from the National Institute of Neurological Diseases and Blindness, U.S. Public Health Service, and by contract Nonr 1442(00) with the Office of Naval Research (H. K. Hartline, principal investigator).

Enhancement of flicker by lateral inhibition

FLOYD RATLIFF, B. W. KNIGHT, JUN-ICHI TOYODA,
AND H. K. HARTLINE

Rockefeller University, New York 10021

Reprinted from SCIENCE, 20 October 1967, Vol. 158, no. 3799, pp. 392–393

Abstract. *Sinusoidal modulation of illumination on the compound eye of the horseshoe crab,* Limulus, *produces a corresponding variation in the rate of discharge of optic nerve impulses. Increasing the area of illumination decreases the variation at low frequencies of modulation, but unexpectedly enhances – or 'amplifies' – the variation at the intermediate frequencies to which the eye is most sensitive. Both effects must result from inhibition since it is the only significant lateral influence in this eye.*

The appearance of flicker in a light that varies periodically depends upon several variables (1). For example, whether a flicker will be observed in a light with sinusoidally varying luminance depends on both the amplitude and frequency of the variation. Results typical of those obtained by De Lange in 1957 from a human observer viewing a small sinusoidally modulated 2-deg field of white light are represented by the solid curve in Fig. 1A. Increase in frequency, up to about 10 cycle/sec, decreases the percentage of modulation about the mean luminance required for the observer to see flicker. At this point the modulation to reach threshold is minimal; that is, flicker sensitivity is maximal. With additional increases in frequency, the percentage of modulation required to reach threshold increases rapidly, and at some point between 50 to 75 cycle/sec even a light modulated 100 per cent does not appear to flicker.

The size of the retinal area stimulated has a marked effect on the threshold of flicker. Measurements made by Kelly in 1960, using a large, 85-deg field, are represented by the dashed curve in Fig. 1A. The dash-dot curve, extending from 1 to 10 cycle/sec, represents some results obtained by Thomas and Kendall in 1962 in an experiment in which a sinusoidal modulation was applied to the illumination of the entire room in which the subject was seated.

The increase, at low frequencies, in the percentage of modulation required to reach threshold that results from an increase in the area of the stimulus has been attributed to the effects of lateral inhibition (1).

In order to test this hypothesis by direct electrophysiological observations we have carried out some comparable experiments with sinusoidal stimuli (2) on the compound eye of the horseshoe crab, *Limulus*, in which lateral influences are predominantly inhibitory (3).

Modulation of the intensity of light shining on an ommatidium of the *Limulus* eye causes a modulation in the rate of discharge of impulses in

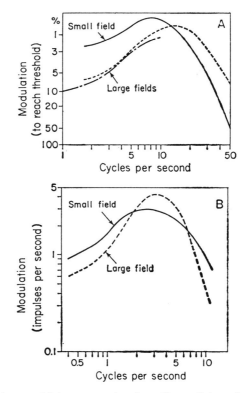

Fig. 1. Modulation sensitivity curves showing effects of size of retinal area stimulated. (A) Psychophysical measurements on human subjects [redrawn after Kelly (1)]. (B) Electrophysiological measurements on the compound eye of the horseshoe crab, *Limulus*.

the optic nerve fiber from that ommatidium. The amplitude of this modulation of the discharge may be taken as a measure of the 'flicker response' of the receptor. Figure 1B shows that this response varies in a characteristic manner with frequency of modulation, and that it is affected by varying the area of the eye illuminated by the modulated light.

In order to obtain the results illustrated in Fig. 1B, a *Limulus* eye was excised and mounted in a moist chamber. A single active optic nerve fiber, arising from an ommatidium near the center of the eye, was dissected from the optic nerve and placed on wick electrodes in the input circuit of an amplifier. A spot of light was centered on the ommatidium from which the nerve fiber arose. The mean intensity of this spot was set by neutral density wedges inserted in the beam. The intensity was then varied sinusoidally, with a constant modulation about this mean, by a rotating polarizer and a fixed analyzer. (Other experiments showed that the polarization itself played no role in the effects reported here.)

The modulated light was turned on for 20 seconds every 3 minutes. The discharge of impulses by the single optic nerve fiber was recorded on line by a small digital computer (4). In order to avoid the transient response at the onset of the illumination, only the final 15 seconds of each record were processed. The sum of a constant plus a sine was fitted, by the method of least squares, to the reciprocals of the intervals between successive impulses. In this way average discharge rate (impulses per second) and amplitude and phase of the response modulation were determined (5).

The results for a small field (a spot of light about 0.25 mm in diameter which is slightly larger than the facet of one ommatidium) are represented by the solid curve in Fig. 1B. The results that were obtained with a large field (a spot about 1.5 mm in diameter that covered about 20 ommatidia) are represented by the dashed curve. In Fig. 1B *modulation* refers to the various peak-to-peak amplitudes of the neural flicker responses to stimuli of constant amplitude; in Fig. 1A *modulation* refers to the various amplitudes of the stimuli required to produce a constant response – that is, to reach the observer's threshold of flicker. Note that the scale of frequency in Fig. 1A is three times that in Fig. 1B.

Increasing the area of illumination produced two major effects. (i) There was the expected decrease in the amplitude of the flicker response to low-frequency modulation of the light. (ii) At its maximum, the dashed curve in Fig. 1B actually exceeds the maximum of the solid curve. This enhancement or 'amplification' of the amplitude of the flicker response to intermediate modulation frequencies was unexpected. Both effects are the result of lateral inhibition.

Previous experiments on single ommatidia have shown that the transfer functions relating intensity of illumination to generator potential (6) and intensity of illumination or of generator potential to frequency of discharge of impulses (5, 7) have characteristic shapes. In brief, there is some frequency of modulation of the light to which the ommatidium is most sensitive. Typically, there is a span of lower frequencies over which the visual sensitivity is somewhat reduced, and when the optimal frequency is exceeded, there is a very pronounced high-frequency cut-off. In general, the crest of the flicker response leads the crest of the modulation of the stimulus at frequencies below the optimum. As the frequency of the modulation of the stimulus increases, the phase lead turns into a phase lag, generally reversing somewhere near the optimum. Thus, the photoreceptor and its axon are a 'tuned' system which responds maximally to frequencies of modulation of the illumination of about 3 cycle/sec.

In this experiment, a further depression of the low-frequency portion of the transfer function resulted from increasing the area of illumination. Lateral inhibition must account for this effect, because the only significant neural effect of increasing the area of illumination is to increase the amount of inhibition exerted on the ommatidium under observation. Lateral inhibition must therefore also account for the unexpected amplification.

This amplification appears to result mainly from a substantial delay between the generation of an impulse in one ommatidium and the production of its inhibitory effect in a neighboring ommatidium. Because this delay is about 150 msec (8), the opposed excitatory and inhibitory influences are about half cycle out of phase at stimulus frequencies of about 3 cycle/sec (period of 333 msec). The transfer function for the large field passes through its maximum at the frequency at which the opposed excitatory and inhibitory influences are most out of phase, because that is the frequency at which the greatest inhibitory influence coincides with the smallest excitatory influence. This general conclusion is borne out by extensive theoretical calculations which will be reported elsewhere (9). Whether a similar amplification of the maximal flicker sensitivity occurs in the human visual system has yet to be determined.

'Amplification' by lateral inhibition is not necessarily restricted to the responses to stimuli that vary in time. Responses to variations in the spatial distribution of stimuli may be similarly affected. It has been known, since Mach's work in 1865 (10), that inhibitory interaction can produce maxima and minima in the neural response where there are no corresponding maxima and minima in the spatial distribution of illumination – only steps or flections. Thus inhibition accentuates the neural responses to certain features of the stimulus pattern. It has been generally assumed, however, that the peak-to-peak distance between the maxima and minima, such as those produced by a step, cannot exceed the step that would appear in the response without inhibition.

But, according to theory, lateral inhibition can amplify the peak-to-peak distance above that found in the uninhibited response. These spatial amplification effects, resulting from particular spatial distributions of the inhibitory influence, have been demonstrated in calculations by von Békésy (11) for a sinusoidal distribution of illumination and by Barlow and Quarles (12) for a step pattern of illumination. A more general theoretical treatment by Ratliff, Knight, and Graham is in preparation (9). None of these spatial ampification effects have been demonstrated experimentally as yet.

In the experiment reported here, the amplification of the variations in the response by lateral inhibition is accomplished at the expense of a reduction in the mean level of response. The same is also true in all the theoretical calculations mentioned earlier for either temporal or spatial modulation. Lateral inhibition provides a mechanism for enhancing significant variations in both spatial and temporal patterns of illumination.

REFERENCES

1. The use of sinusoidal stimuli in the study of human flicker thresholds, beginning with Ives's work in 1922, is reviewed by D. H. Kelly, in *Information Processing in Sight Sensory Systems*, P. W. Nye, ed. (California Inst. of Technology, Pasadena, 1965), pp. 162–176.
2. The use of sinusoidal stimuli in neurophysiological experiments on various invertebrate and vertebrate eyes is reviewed by B. Cleland and C. Enroth-Cugell, *Acta Physiol. Scand.* **68,** 365 (1966).
3. Hartline, H. K., Wagner, H. G., Ratliff, F., *J. Gen. Physiol.* **39,** 651 (1956). However, we have since confirmed an observation, by R. L. Purple ['The interpretation of excitatory and inhibitory influences in the eccentric cell in the eye of *Limulus*', thesis, Rockefeller University (1964)] that the lateral inhibitory hyperpolarization is preceded by a brief, small depolarization. This complication has slight effects upon the *Limulus* flicker response.
4. Lange, D., Hartline, H. K., Ratliff, F., *Ann. N.Y. Acad. Sci.* **128,** 955 (1966); Schoenfeld, R. L., and Milkman, N., *Science* **146,** 190 (1964).
5. Dodge, F. A., Jr., Knight, B. W., Toyoda, J., *Science,* **160,** 88–90 (1968).
6. Pinter, R. B., *J. Gen. Physiol.* **49,** 565 (1966).
7. Purple, R. L. and Dodge, F. A., Jr., in *The Functional Organization of the Compound Eye*, Bernhard, C. G., ed. (Pergamon, Oxford, 1966), pp. 451–464.

8. Hartline, H. K., Ratliff, F., Miller, W. H., in *Nervous Inhibition*, Florey, E., ed. (Pergamon Press, New York, 1961), pp. 241–284; Ratliff, F., Hartline, H. K., Miller, W. H., *J. Opt. Soc. Amer.* **53,** 110 (1963).

9. Ratliff, F., Knight, B. W., Graham, N., *Proc. Natl. Acad. Sci.*, **67,** 1558–1569 (1970).

10. Ratliff, F., *Mach Bands: Quantitative Studies on Neural Networks in the Retina* (Holden-Day, San Francisco, 1965).

11. von Békésy, G., *Sensory Inhibition* (Princeton Univ. Press, Princeton, N.J., 1967).

12. Barlow, R. B., Jr., 'Inhibitory fields in the *Limulus* lateral eye', thesis, Rockefeller University, New York (1967).

13. Supported by research grant B864 from the National Institute of Neurological Diseases and Blindness and grant GB-6540X from the National Science Foundation.

On tuning and amplification by lateral inhibition *

FLOYD RATLIFF, B. W. KNIGHT, AND NORMA GRAHAM†

The Rockefeller University, New York, N.Y.

Reprinted from the PROCEEDINGS OF THE NATIONAL ACADEMY
OF SCIENCES, Vol. 62, no. 3, pp. 733-740, March 1969

Abstract.—Lateral inhibition in a neural network generally attenuates the amplitudes of the responses to sinusoidal stimuli—both spatial and temporal. For an inhibitory influence with an abrupt onset and an exponential decay in time, and with a Gaussian distribution in space (the forms often assumed in theoretical calculations), the attenuation is greatest at low temporal and spatial frequencies. The attenuation diminishes with increasing frequencies until ultimately the amplitudes of inhibited responses become equal to, but never exceed, the amplitudes of the uninhibited.

For an inhibitory influence with a delay to the maximum in time or with eccentric maxima in space, however, the amplitudes of inhibited responses to certain intermediate frequencies may be greater than those of the uninhibited responses. This "amplification" results because the delay and the spatial separation "tune" the network to particular temporal and spatial frequencies; the inhibition is turned on at the trough of the response and off at the crest, thus tending to produce the greatest possible amplitude. The amplification has been observed in one neural network, the retina of the lateral eye of *Limulus*. The basic principles are general, and the effects may be expected in any system with negative feedback.

The theory developed here illustrates some effects of spatial and temporal distributions of inhibitory influences. It is based on earlier experimental analyses of interactions among receptor units (ommatidia) in the retina of the compound lateral eye of the horseshoe crab, *Limulus*. In the steady state [1,2] the mth ommatidium, when illuminated alone, discharges optic nerve impulses at a rate e_m. Because of the lateral inhibition, illuminating the rest of the eye will produce a generally lower rate r_m, which is given by the linear equation

$$r_m = e_m - \sum_{n \neq m} k_{mn}(r_n - r^0{}_{mn}), \tag{1}$$

where the r_n are the rates of discharge of the elements other than r_m; k_{mn} are constants specifying the inhibition for particular spatial separations of m and n, independent of rate of discharge; and the summation extends over all elements for which the rate of discharge is above the threshold of effectiveness $r^0{}_{mn}$. Further analyses have extended the theory to include the dynamics of lateral inhibition.[3,4] Such a translationally invariant linear system may be characterized by its response to sine-wave input. The response is a sine wave of the same frequency, generally differing in amplitude and phase. The relationship of the amplitude and phase of the output to that of the input is commonly called the "transfer function" of the system.

The diagonal lines in Figure 1 illustrate the steady-state operation of a linear

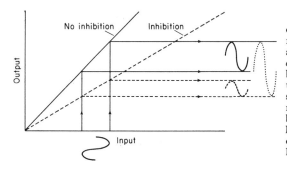

FIG. 1.—Steady-state input-output curves for a network with no inhibition (*solid diagonal line*) and with inhibition (*dashed diagonal line*). Calculated on the basis of these steady-state curves, the two outputs for a sinusoidally modulated input would not exceed the limits indicated by the pair of horizontal solid lines (no inhibition) and the pair of horizontal dashed lines (inhibition).

neural network, such as that represented by equation (1), in which the lateral influence is inhibition (to simplify the illustration, effects of thresholds of inhibition are omitted). Also shown are the responses to a sinusoidal modulation of the input. (For a retinal network, an example of an input sinusoidally modulated in time is a flickering light where the intensity is a sinusoidal function of time t; an example of an input sinusoidally modulated in space, in one dimension, is a pattern of striations where intensity changes sinusoidally along the spatial axis x, perpendicular to the stria.) If the modulation is very slow in time or very much spread out in space (long wavelength in t or x), the temporal characteristics of the inhibitory influences or the spatial characteristics of the inhibitory field may be neglected. Under these conditions any output, inhibited or uninhibited, would be given simply by drawing a reflection of the input from the appropriate steady-state input-output curve, as illustrated.

Thus, for very low frequency inputs, the difference between maxima and minima in the response is less with inhibition than without inhibition. Accordingly, the expectation has been that the amplitude of the response of an inhibited system cannot exceed the comparable response without inhibition. Indeed, as the frequency increases, the amplitude of the inhibited response to a sine wave increases and must eventually become the same as the uninhibited. This happens because the wavelength of the stimulus at the higher frequencies is short compared to the extent of the inhibitory field or the duration of the influence.

As a result of the attenuation of the amplitudes of the responses to low frequencies, inhibition will produce a low-frequency cutoff in the transfer function. In general, there is also a high-frequency cutoff resulting from other mechanisms (Fig. 5), and so the network is "tuned" to the intermediate frequencies. Note, however, that the limit on this best transmission is fixed by the difference between the maximum *uninhibited* response and the minimum *inhibited* response. If the inhibition could be turned completely off at the crests of the modulation of the input and completely on at the troughs, the output would be amplified as indicated by the dotted curve in Figure 1. A tuning of the system to particular intermediate wavelengths in either space or time can actually lead to such an amplification.

In order to make a comparison of various functions easier, the following modification of equation (1) is used:

$$r(x,t) = e(x,t) - \int_{-\infty}^{\infty} dx' \int_{-\infty}^{t} dt' k(x - x', t - t') r(x',t'). \tag{2}$$

Here $r(x,t)$ is the response at spatial position x and time t, $e(x,t)$ is the stimulus, and $k(x - x',t - t')$ is the amount of inhibition exerted by the ommatidium at x' at time t' on the ommatidium at x at time t.

In this model the amount of inhibition exerted by one point on another depends on the response at the first point. A reasonable alternative is a system where the inhibition depends on the stimulus at a point, rather than on the response.[5] This is expressed by integration over e rather than r:

$$r(x,t) = e(x,t) - \int_{-\infty}^{\infty}dx' \int_{-\infty}^{t}dt'k(x - x',t - t')e(x',t'). \qquad (3)$$

In line with earlier terminology,[6] we will call equations (2) and (3) "recurrent" and "nonrecurrent" systems, respectively.

A recent investigation[7] of the spatial distribution of inhibition in the *Limulus* eye showed that inhibition is greatest, not at points immediately adjacent to the inhibiting ommatidium,[8,9] but at some distance from it. This observed distribution of the inhibition k as a function of distance x from the inhibited ommatidium is closely approximated by the difference between a broad Gaussian distribution and a narrow one.

For this and for a simple Gaussian inhibitory field, the transfer functions for responses to spatial sinusoids by both recurrent and nonrecurrent networks were calculated by the usual techniques of linear systems analysis. As expected (Fig. 2), the responses to low spatial frequencies are always depressed by inhibition, and for high frequencies the inhibited response approaches that of the uninhibited. For intermediate frequencies, however, there is a difference in the behavior of the two networks. One amplifies the response (i.e., the ratio goes above unity) and the other does not. Note that there is little difference between the recurrent and nonrecurrent networks.

Mathematically there is a straightforward answer to the question of what

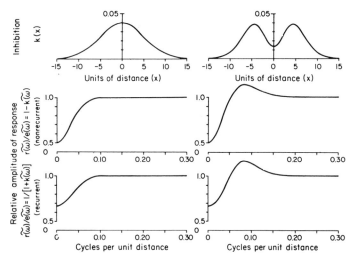

FIG. 2.—Normalized transfer functions for examples of symmetrical unimodal (*left graph*) and symmetrical bimodal (*right graph*) inhibitory fields $k(x)$ in a nonrecurrent network (*upper graph*) and a recurrent network (*lower graph*).

produces amplification in the spatial case. Since the stimulation is constant as a function of time, $r(x,t)$ and $e(x,t)$ are the same for all t and can be written as $r(x)$ and $e(x)$. Equation (2) for a recurrent system becomes

$$r(x) = e(x) - \int_{-\infty}^{\infty} r(x') \left[\int_{-\infty}^{t} k(x - x', t - t')dt' \right] dx'. \tag{4}$$

The inner integral is a function only of the distance $x - x'$, indicating the total amount of inhibition being contributed by point x'. This will be called $k(x - x')$. It is equivalent to the coefficient k_{mn} in the usual steady-state equations (1). Equation (4) now becomes:

$$r(x) = e(x) - \int_{-\infty}^{\infty} r(x') k(x - x')dx'. \tag{5}$$

By taking Fourier transforms of both sides and dividing by the transform of the input, one obtains

$$\frac{\widetilde{r(\omega)}}{\widetilde{e(\omega)}} = \frac{1}{1 + \widetilde{k(\omega)}}, \tag{6}$$

where $\widetilde{r(\omega)}$ is the Fourier transform of $r(x)$ as a function of frequency ω and similarly for $\widetilde{e(\omega)}$ and $\widetilde{k(\omega)}$. Therefore $\widetilde{r(\omega)}/\widetilde{e(\omega)}$ is the transfer function of the system. In general, the Fourier transforms $\widetilde{r(\omega)}$ and $\widetilde{e(\omega)}$ are complex numbers with the absolute values representing the amplitude (crest-trough distance) of the response and the angular coordinate in the complex plane representing the phase of the response. However, in this case, $\widetilde{r(\omega)}$ and $\widetilde{e(\omega)}$ have the same phase because k is symmetric, so that the ratio $\widetilde{r(\omega)}/\widetilde{e(\omega)}$ is the real ratio of peak-trough distances.

The nonrecurrent equation (3) can be transformed in the same way to give

$$\frac{\widetilde{r(\omega)}}{\widetilde{e(\omega)}} = 1 - \widetilde{k(\omega)}. \tag{7}$$

Now assume that the total amount of inhibition $\widetilde{k(0)}$ (which equals the integral of $k(x)$ over all x) is less than unity so that the absolute value of $\widetilde{k(\omega)}$ is always less than unity. With this assumption, the condition for amplification can be easily stated: Amplification occurs if and only if $\widetilde{k(\omega)}$ is negative for some ω.

The following analysis of the effects of the inhibitory time course on the responses to stimuli that vary in time, but are uniform in space, bears close formal similarities to the above analysis. Equation (5) is replaced by

$$r(t) = e(t) - \int_{-\infty}^{t} k(t - t')r(t')dt', \tag{8}$$

and equations (6) and (7) follow, as before, where now $\widetilde{k(\omega)}$ is the Fourier transform of the inhibitory time course $k(t)$ rather than of the spatial distribution of inhibition.

The one evident difference from the spatial case is that k no longer is symmetric. In equation (8), only the past history of r, and not its future, influences its present value so that where $\tau < 0$, $k(\tau) = 0$. This means that the point at which the sinusoidal response reaches its crest may differ from that of the stimulus

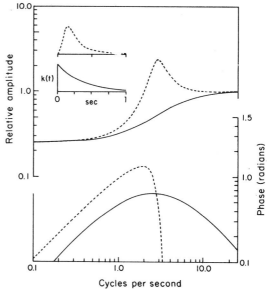

FIG. 3.—The effect of a delay to the maximum inhibition. Normalized transfer functions showing amplitude (*upper graph*) and phase (*lower graph*) for the two inhibitory time courses shown in the inset, an immediate rise to the maximum followed by an exponential decay, and a gradual rise to the maximum followed by a gradual decay. Recurrent network.

by a phase shift. This is reflected in a complex-valued transfer function whose angular coordinate represents the phase shift. Two examples of inhibitory time courses and the resulting transfer functions for a recurrent system are shown in Figure 3. The phase advance at low frequencies, like that shown in the figure, is typical of inhibitory feedback, as inhibition is already shutting off the response by the time the stimulus reaches its maximum.

As is evident from the examples in Figure 3, if $k(t)$ has a maximum away from $t = 0$, then amplification may occur at a frequency about reciprocal to twice the time to the peak of the inhibition. Qualitatively, the reason is the same as for the spatial case above.

A variety of time courses for the inhibitory influences were examined by varying the parameters in the following general expression:

$$
k(t) = \begin{cases} 0 \text{ for } t < \tau_l \\ K\dfrac{1}{n!}\left(\dfrac{t - \tau_l}{\tau_d}\right)^n \exp\left(-\dfrac{t - \tau_l}{\tau_d}\right) \text{ for } t \geq \tau_l \end{cases} \tag{9}
$$

where K is the total or steady-state inhibition, τ_l is the latency before onset of inhibition, τ_d is the relaxation time for final decay, and n indexes the order of onset ($n = 0$ abrupt, $n = 1$ linear, $n = 2$ parabolic, etc.). The time courses in Figure 3 are $n = 0$ and $n = 3$ from this family. The parameters τ_d and n are less easily grasped than the peak time (the time until the maximum inhibition) and spread time (the "standard deviation") of the time course defined by

$$
\tau_s = \left[\overline{(t - \bar{t})^2}\right]^{1/2}, \tag{10}
$$

which also characterize the time course.

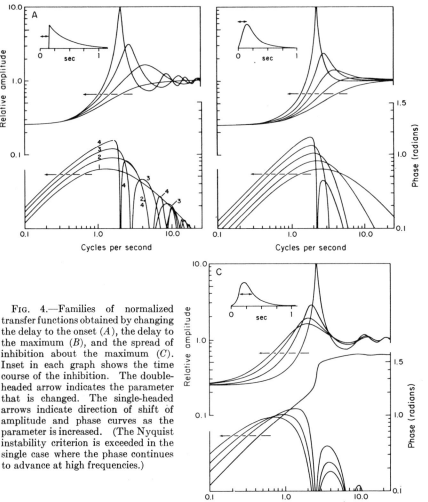

Fig. 4.—Families of normalized transfer functions obtained by changing the delay to the onset (A), the delay to the maximum (B), and the spread of inhibition about the maximum (C). Inset in each graph shows the time course of the inhibition. The double-headed arrow indicates the parameter that is changed. The single-headed arrows indicate direction of shift of amplitude and phase curves as the parameter is increased. (The Nyquist instability criterion is exceeded in the single case where the phase continues to advance at high frequencies.)

The temporal transfer function changes, as expected, with inhibitory latency, peak time, and spread time (Fig. 4). A longer latency (A), or a later peak (B), or a narrower spread (C) gives a stronger amplification maximum, and a longer latency also enhances secondary extrema in the transfer function.

This theory of the response of an inhibitory network to temporal stimuli may be checked experimentally in the eye of *Limulus*. The total inhibitory influence in this case is composed of self-inhibitory (k_s) and lateral inhibitory (k_l) components:

$$k(t) = k_s(t) + k_l(t), \tag{11}$$

$$\widetilde{k(\omega)} = \widetilde{k_s(\omega)} + \widetilde{k_l(\omega)}. \tag{12}$$

Both k_s and k_l may be measured directly[10] and the measured functions may be matched fairly well to ones coming from time courses in the equation (9) family by the following choice of parameters:

For self-inhibition, $K = 3$, $\tau_l = 0$, $\tau_d = 0.5$ sec, $n = 0$.
For lateral inhibition, $\tau_l = 0.1$ sec, $\tau_d = 0.3$ sec, $n = 0$.

The total lateral inhibition, determined by the size of the flickering spot illuminating the eye, is $K = 0$ for a small and $K = 3$ for a large spot. Figure 5A shows the generator-spikes transfer function for small and large spots predicted from equation (6). (The falling-off of the small-spot curve near 10 cps is due to a complication that arises when the driving frequency approaches the mean interspike frequency.[11]) With the large spot (and the resulting lateral inhibition) there is amplification of responses to intermediate frequencies.

In the *Limulus* eye, there is a conversion from light stimulus to generator potential that occurs prior to the inhibitory network. Its transfer function can also be measured directly[10] and is plotted in Figure 5B (for the same mean light intensity as in A). Since the output of the transfer function in B is the input to that in A, multiplying the transfer functions in A and B together gives a predicted transfer function for the complete light-spikes conversion which is plotted in Figure 5C. Also plotted in C is a transfer function for the complete conversion that was measured directly from another preparation under similar conditions.[12] In the phase data (not shown), the agreement between theory and experiment is equally good.

The principles underlying tuning and amplification are general, and similar effects may be expected to occur in any system with negative feedback. For example, Kelly[13] observed a similar amplification in the

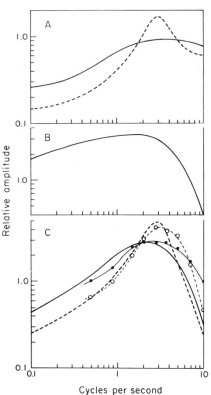

FIG. 5.—Comparison of theoretical and experimental results.

(A) Theoretical generator to spikes transfer function (*solid line*) for no lateral inhibition—that is, a small spot of illumination; and the corresponding transfer function (*dashed line*) for lateral inhibition—that is, a large spot of illumination.

(B) Observed light to generator transfer function.

(C) Theoretical light to spikes transfer functions (A times B) for small spot (*heavy solid line*) and for large spot (*heavy dashed line*). Experimental results for small spot (*filled data points, thin solid line*) and for large spot (*open circle data points, thin dashed line*).

temporal frequency response of the human eye. (Although he attributed the observed effects to ocular tremor, he noted that any other retinal mechanism capable of providing the necessary spatiotemporal interactions would account equally well for the effects.) A similar amplification has also been observed in the transfer function of xerography.[14] It is worth noting, in conclusion, that there is a possibility that reversible variations in the tuning of neural networks in the central nervous system could provide a means for the storage and retrieval of information.

The transfer function shown in Figure 5B is based on an experiment carried out by Jun-ichi Toyoda. We also wish to acknowledge the assistance of F. A. Dodge, Jr., Norman Milkman, and H. K. Hartline.

* This research was supported in part by a research grant (B864) from the National Institute of Neurological Diseases and Blindness, U. S. Public Health Service, and by a research grant (GB-6540X) from the National Science Foundation.

† Present address: Department of Psychology, University of Pennsylvania, Philadelphia.

[1] Hartline, H. K., and F. Ratliff, "Inhibitory interaction of receptor units in the eye of *Limulus*," *J. Gen. Physiol.*, 40, 357–376 (1957).

[2] Hartline, H. K., and F. Ratliff, "Spatial summation of inhibitory influences in the eye of *Limulus*, and the mutual interaction of receptor units," *J. Gen. Physiol.*, 41, 1049–1066 (1958).

[3] Ratliff, F., H. K. Hartline, and W. H. Miller, "Spatial and temporal aspects of retinal inhibitory interaction," *J. Opt. Soc. Am.*, 53, 110–120 (1963).

[4] Lange, David, H. K. Hartline, and F. Ratliff, "The dynamics of lateral inhibition in the compound eye of *Limulus*. II," in *The Functional Organization of the Compound Eye*, ed. C. G. Bernhard (New York: Pergamon Press, 1966), pp. 425–449.

[5] Békésy, G. von, *Sensory Inhibition* (Princeton, N.J.: Princeton University Press, 1967).

[6] Ratliff, F., *Mach Bands: Quantitative Studies on Neural Networks in the Retina* (San Francisco, Calif.: Holden-Day, 1965).

[7] Barlow, R. B., Jr., thesis: "Inhibitory fields in the *Limulus* lateral eye," The Rockefeller University (1967).

[8] Ratliff, F., and H. K. Hartline, "Fields of inhibitory influence of single receptor units in the lateral eye of *Limulus*," *Science*, 126, 1234 (1957).

[9] Ratliff, F., and H. K. Hartline, "The responses of *Limulus* optic nerve fibers to patterns of illumination on the receptor mosaic," *J. Gen. Physiol.*, 42, 1241–1255 (1959).

[10] Toyoda, J., B. W. Knight, and F. A. Dodge, Jr., "A quantitative description of the dynamics of excitation and inhibition in the eye of *Limulus*," manuscript in preparation.

[11] Borsellino, A., R. E. Poppele, and C. A. Terzuolo, "Transfer functions of the slowly adapting stretch receptor organ of crustacea," in *Cold Spring Harbor Symposia on Quantitative Biology*, vol. 30 (1965), pp. 581–586.

[12] Ratliff, F., B. W. Knight, J. Toyoda, and H. K. Hartline, "The enhancement of flicker by lateral inhibition," *Science*, 158, 392–393 (1967).

[13] Kelly, D. H., "Effects of sharp edges in a flickering field," *J. Opt. Soc. Am.*, 49, 730–732 (1959).

[14] Neugebauer, H. E. J., "Development method and modulation transfer function of xerography," *Applied Optics*, 6, 943–945 (1967).

Superposition of excitatory and inhibitory influences in the retina of *Limulus*: effect of delayed inhibition*

FLOYD RATLIFF, B. W. KNIGHT, AND
NORMAN MILKMAN

The Rockefeller University, New York, N.Y.

Reprinted from the PROCEEDINGS OF THE NATIONAL ACADEMY
OF SCIENCES, Vol. 67, no. 3, pp. 1558–1564, November 1970

Abstract. In an optic nerve fiber of the compound eye of the horseshoe crab, *Limulus*, the time course of a train of nerve impulses discharged in response to illumination reflects the interplay of excitatory and inhibitory influences. Responses to sinusoidally modulated excitation and inhibition, as a function of frequency, were measured separately and in combination. A simple linear superposition of the separate frequency responses properly accounts for the composite frequency response for both synchronous and asynchronous modulation of the excitatory and inhibitory influences. In general, the effect on the frequency response of increasing the delay of the inhibitory influence is progressively to shift the maximum amplitude to lower frequencies and gradually to produce pronounced maxima and minima in both the amplitude and phase.

The so-called frequency response of a single ommatidium in the compound eye of *Limulus* expresses the amplitude and phase of variation in the rate of impulse discharge as a function of the frequency of sinusoidal modulation (at a fixed amplitude) of the intensity of incident light. The amplitude curve of the frequency response is unimodal. At low frequency it shows general features of a transducer which applies a "sluggish gain control" to input signals. The amplitude is relatively small at low frequencies, but increases with frequency as the gain control becomes less able to follow the input signal. Since such a gain control still will be reducing the output signal at the moment when the input sinewave reaches its crest, there will usually be a low-frequency phase lead. An eventual high-frequency cut-off and a pronounced phase lag may be anticipated on very general grounds: the time resolution of any real transducer is limited; and the time necessary for internal processing imposes an increasing lag between input cause and output effect as that limit is approached.

The gain control within an ommatidium is partly an adaptation of excitatory processes to the changing light levels[1], and partly self-inhibition[2]. The addition of lateral inhibition by illuminating neighboring ommatidia causes a further decrease in the amplitude of responses to low frequencies and an enhancement, or amplification, at intermediate frequencies.[3] This latter effect is caused by a significant delay to the maxima of the unit inhibitory potentials. At some frequencies, because of this delay, the maxima of inhibition will approach or coincide with the minima of excitation, depressing the rate of discharge there

533

even further, and at the same time minima of inhibition will coincide with maxima of excitation, leaving that rate relatively less affected.[4] The following experiments show the effects of artificially introducing further delays between excitation of one element and inhibition by neighbors. In general, we find that with increasing delays the gain increases at lower frequencies and the frequency response becomes multimodal, as predicted by superposition of independently measured excitatory and inhibitory effects.

Methods and materials. A compound eye of the horseshoe crab, *Limulus*, and about 1 cm of the optic nerve were excised and mounted in a moist chamber. A small strand of the nerve was dissected until a single active fiber from an ommatidium near the center of the eye remained on the cotton wick electrode. The stimulus pattern consisted of a small central spot, confined to that one ommatidium, and a surrounding annulus, each formed by a separate fiber-optics array. After the experiment, the fiber-optics arrays were left in place on the corneal surface of the eye. The soft tissues of the retina were removed and a photograph was taken of the crystalline cones thus exposed on the inner side of the chitinous cornea (Fig. 1). The brightly lit

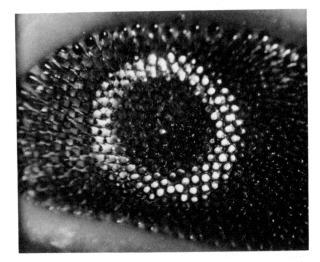

Fig. 1. Pattern of illumination on compound lateral eye of *Limulus* used to obtain results illustrated in Figs. 2–4.

crystalline cones in the photograph are the same as those illuminated during the experiment. The central spot and the surrounding annulus were each illuminated by an independently controlled glow modulator tube. Each tube furnished a light which either could be steady or could be sinusoidally modulated, at some fixed amplitude, about its mean intensity. The frequency of modulation was controlled by a small computer, which also recorded the times at which each light source reached its maximum intensity. The times at which nerve impulses occurred in the isolated nerve fiber were also recorded by the computer, for later processing.

A natural way in which to express the momentary level of activity in a single nerve fiber is in terms of its "instantaneous rate," the reciprocal of the time interval between an impulse and its immediate predecessor. After the experiment this instantaneous rate was calculated by the computer, and expressed as a mean rate plus a modulating sinusoid by a least-squares fitting procedure. The modulating sinusoid was characterized by two parameters: its trough-to-crest *amplitude*, and the *phase* by which its crest differed from the crest of the stimulating light.

In one type of experimental run, the light intensity of the annulus was held constant while that of the central spot was modulated. The impulse data thus collected were processed, as described in the previous paragraph, to determine the amplitude and phase of the response to this flickering light excitation. Interleaved were runs of a second type, in which the central spot was held steady and the surrounding annulus was modulated. This produced a modulation of lateral inhibition upon the central neuron, and hence also produced a modulation of its instantaneous firing rate. In the third type of run, the central spot and the surrounding annulus were both modulated with various delays between the modulation of center and surround. The resulting frequency response was thus a composite of the excitatory modulation and the inhibitory modulation.

Theory and Results. The simplest possible assumption concerning the manner in which the *Limulus* eye treats mixed inputs is that it is a "time-invariant linear system." In essence this assumption asserts that a superposition of individual inputs leads to an output which is the superposition of the corresponding individual outputs. Two nontrivial consequences of this assertion are (*i*) a sinusoidal input leads to a sinusoidal output, whose amplitude and phase may be frequency dependent, and (*ii*) knowledge of output amplitude and phase, at all frequencies and from sinusoidal inputs applied at all input points, completely characterizes the input–output behavior of the system. Recent work[5] suggests that the time-invariant linear assumption should be a good one for the *Limulus* eye under the conditions of this experiment. Thus the separate frequency responses for direct excitation and lateral inhibition shown in Fig. 2 should

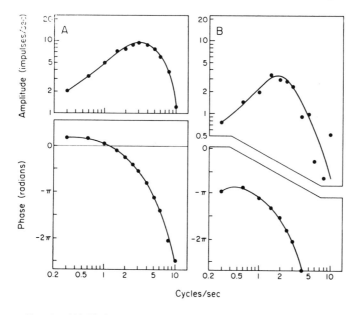

Fig. 2. (*A*) Excitatory frequency response (central spot modulated, annulus steady). (*B*) Inhibitory frequency response (central spot steady, annulus modulated).

enable us to predict the response of the nerve to any combination of light stimuli on the central spot and annulus.

A particularly simple case is that in which the same sinusoidally-modulated light falls on both annulus and central spot. In this case the implications of linear superposition upon both amplitude and phase may be summed up in a single equation using complex numbers. The total response $R_T(f)$ at frequency f is given in terms of the excitatory response $R_E(f)$ and inhibitory response $R_I(f)$ simply by

$$R_T(f) = R_E(f) + R_I(f). \tag{1}$$

Here $R_E(f)$ is the complex number given by

$$R_E(f) = A_E(f) \cdot (\exp i \, \phi_E(f)) \tag{2}$$

where $A_E(f)$ and $\phi_E(f)$ are the excitatory amplitude and phase given in Fig. 2A. $R_I(f)$ is similarly formed from Fig. 2B, and the complex number $R_T(f)$ resulting from Eq. 1 has the amplitude and phase predicted by linear superposition.

A more general case is that in which the sinusoidal waveform stimulating the inhibitory annulus is delayed, by a lag time τ, behind the waveform stimulating the central excitatory spot. This case is of interest for two reasons. First, the time delay may be used to mimic physiological inhibitory delays in other retinas. Second, the addition of an artificial phase shift to the inhibitory

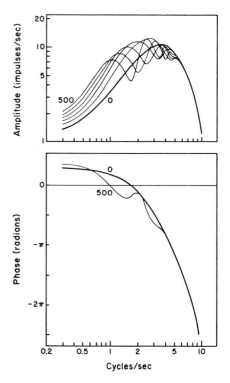

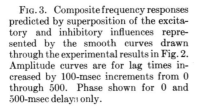

Fig. 3. Composite frequency responses predicted by superposition of the excitatory and inhibitory influences represented by the smooth curves drawn through the experimental results in Fig. 2. Amplitude curves are for lag times increased by 100-msec increments from 0 through 500. Phase shown for 0 and 500-msec delays only.

component of the response may be used to reveal intrinsic phase shift differences between excitation and inhibition.

The frequency-dependent phase lag, introduced by the time lag τ, is equal to the phase lag of the unit-amplitude complex number $\exp(-2\pi i\tau f)$, whence the appropriate generalization of Eq. 1 is

$$R_T(f) = R_E(f) + (\exp(-2\pi i\tau f)) \cdot R_I(f). \tag{3}$$

Equation 1 is recovered for the special case $\tau = 0$. We have fit continuous curves to the data of Fig. 2 by eye, and, using Eq. 2 and 3, have predicted the outcome of the inhibitory-lag experiment using several lag times. The results are shown in Fig. 3.

The introduction of a substantial inhibitory lag time introduces considerable structure into the predicted frequency response curves. An extremum in amplitude is found near any frequency where the excitatory phase differs from the total inhibitory phase (intrinsic plus lag) by a multiple of π radians. Consecutive maxima and minima arise as the inhibitory influence consecutively reinforces and opposes the excitatory influence. The larger the time lag, the smaller the frequency change needed to shift the inhibitory phase from opposition to reinforcement and back.

We tested these theoretical predictions in experiments in which both light sources were modulated. In one type of run the modulations were synchronous.

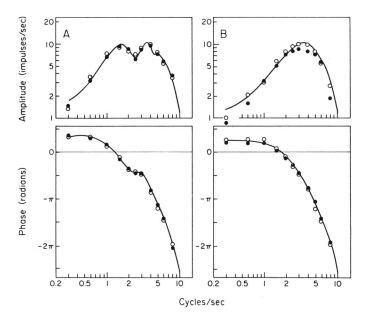

Fig. 4. Comparison of theoretical predictions and experimental observations of composite frequency responses. (*A*) 300-msec delay of sinusoidal modulation of annulus with respect to center. (*B*) 0 delay (synchronous modulation of central spot and annulus).

In the other type, the modulation of the annulus was delayed by 300 msec. The results are shown in Fig. 4. Fig. 4*A* is for the 300 msec delay and Fig. 4*B* for no delay. There are two sets of experimental data: one set (*open dots*), obtained just before the experiment of Fig. 2; the other set (*solid dots*), obtained just after that experiment. The solid lines were predicted from Fig. 2, using Eq. 3.

For detailed comparison with Fig. 3, we show the results of a similar experiment on a different preparation in Fig. 5. The conditions were essentially the same as before, except for a somewhat different configuration of illumination (instead of an annulus, a spot of light adjacent to the test ommatidium) and a greater depth of modulation. Delays of inhibitory modulation with respect to excitation were 0 msec (*open circles*), 100 msec (*open triangles*), 300 msec (*filled circles*), and 400 msec (*filled triangles*). As predicted in Fig. 3, the maximum amplitude shifted progressively to lower frequencies with increasing delays, and pronounced maxima and minima developed. Phase data are shown for 0, 200, and 400 msec only.

Discussion. The frequency response of the *Limulus* retina has many characteristics in common with those of the more complex vertebrate visual system. As Hughes and Maffei[6] and Cleland and Enroth-Cugell[7] have shown in their studies on cat-retinal ganglion cells, the response to sinusoidal stimuli as a function of frequency shows a gradual rise to a maximum followed by a rapid decline. In both the *Limulus* retina and the cat retina, lateral inhibition contributes to the attenuation of responses to low frequencies. In another experiment involving a retinal ganglion cell of a cat, comparable to our experiment on *Limulus*, Maffei, Cervetto, and Fiorentini[8] obtained a result very similar to our Fig. 4*A*. They explain the

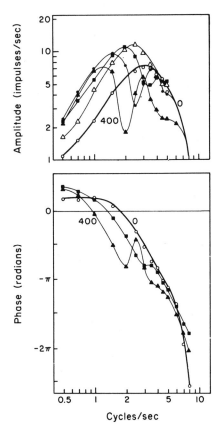

Fig. 5. Composite frequency responses obtained in same type of experiment as in Fig. 4, except for differences in configuration of illumination and depth of modulation.

result in a way equivalent to our Eq. 1. Thus the cat retina furnishes a natural physiological inhibitory time delay which yields a result similar to that which we obtained from the *Limulus* retina by artificially imposing an inhibitory delay externally. For an interpretation of the effects of lateral inhibition on the sensitivity of the human eye to sinusoidal flicker, see Kelly[9] and Fiorentini and Maffei.[10]

Naturally occurring delays, similar to those artificially produced in our experiments, may be of considerable significance in color vision. De Lange[11] found that, for the human subject, sinusoidal red and green stimuli of equal luminance still appear to flicker when 180° out of phase. This flicker cannot be eliminated by merely adjusting the luminance of the two colors; an additional phase shift has to be introduced. Further psychophysical measurements by Walraven and Leebeck[12] and by Kelly[13] strongly suggest that the different color systems introduce different phase shifts. (For a recent study of the temporal characteristics of the color sensitive mechanisms in the human eye, and a brief review of the literature see Green.[14]) A possible mechanism underlying some of the color phenomena described above has recently been discovered by Spekreijse and Norton.[15] They have observed significant natural differences in the phases of intra-retinal S-potentials (goldfish retina) elicited by sinusoidal stimuli of different wavelengths. The importance of delayed lateral inhibition in directionally-sensitive retinal ganglion cells has been pointed out by Barlow and Levick.[16]

We thank F. A. Dodge, Jr. and H. K. Hartline for their assistance.

* This research was supported in part by research grants (EY 00188) from the National Eye Institute, (GM 1789) from the National Institute of General Medical Sciences, and (GB-6540) from the National Science Foundation.

[1] Dodge, F. A., Jr., B. W. Knight, and J. Toyoda, "Voltage noise in *Limulus* visual cells," *Science*, **160**, 88 (1968).

[2] Knight, B. W., J. Toyoda, and F. A. Dodge, Jr., "A quantitative description of the dynamics of excitation and inhibition in the eye of *Limulus*," *J. Gen. Physiol.*, **56**, 421 (1970).

[3] Ratliff, F., B. W. Knight, J. Toyoda, and H. K. Hartline, "Enhancement of flicker by lateral inhibition," *Science*, **158**, 392 (1967).

[4] Ratliff, F., B. W. Knight, and N. Graham, "On tuning and amplification by lateral inhibition," *Proc. Nat. Acad. Sci. USA*, **62**, 733 (1969).

[5] Dodge, F. A., R. M. Shapley, and B. W. Knight, "Linear systems analysis of the *Limulus* retina," *Behav. Sci.*, **15**, 24 (1970).

[6] Hughes, G. W., and L. Maffei, "Retinal ganglion cell response to sinusoidal light stimulation," *J. Neurophysiol.*, **29**, 333 (1966).

[7] Cleland, B., and C. Enroth-Cugell, "Cat retinal ganglion cell responses to changing light intensities: sinusoidal modulation in the time domain," *Acta Physiol. Scand.*, **68**, 365 (1966).

[8] Maffei, L., L. Cervetto, and A. Fiorentini, "Transfer characteristics of excitation and inhibition in cat retinal ganglion cells," *J. Neurophysiol.*, **33**, 276 (1970).

[9] Kelly, D. H., "Flickering patterns and lateral inhibition," *J. Opt. Soc. Amer.*, **59**, 1361 (1969).

[10] Fiorentini, A., and L. Maffei, "Transfer characteristics of excitation and inhibition in the human visual system," *J. Neurophysiol.*, **33**, 285 (1970).

[11] De Lange, H., "Research into the dynamic nature of the human fovea cortex system with intermittent and modulated light. *I*. Attenuation characteristics with white and colored light," *J. Opt. Soc. Amer.*, **48**, 777 (1958); "*II*. Phase shift in brightness and delay in color perception," *J. Opt. Soc. Amer.*, **48**, 784 (1958).

[12] Walraven, P. L., and H. J. Leebeck, "Phase shift of sinusoidally alternating colored stimuli," *J. Opt. Soc. Amer.*, **54**, 78 (1964).

[13] Kelly, D. H., "Visual responses to time-dependent stimuli. *IV*. Effects of chromatic adaptation," *J. Opt. Soc. Amer.*, **52**, 940 (1962).

[14] Green, D. G., "Sinusoidal flicker characteristics of the color-sensitive mechanisms of the eye," *Vision Res.*, **9**, 591 (1969).

[15] Spekreijse, H., and A. L. Norton, "The dynamic characteristics of color coded S-potentials," *J. Gen. Physiol.*, **56**, 1 (1970).

[16] Barlow, H. B., and W. R. Levick, "The mechanism of directionally selective units in the rabbit's retina," *J. Physiol.*, **178**, 477 (1965).

A quantitative description of the dynamics of excitation and inhibition in the eye of *Limulus*

B. W. KNIGHT, JUN-ICHI TOYODA, AND
FREDERICK A. DODGE, JR.

The Rockefeller University, New York, N.Y.

Reprinted from the JOURNAL OF GENERAL PHYSIOLOGY, October 1970
Vol. 56, no. 4, pp. 421–437

ABSTRACT   By means of intracellular microelectrode techniques, we have measured the dynamics of the several processes which translate light stimulation into spike activity in the *Limulus* eye. The transductions from light to voltage and from voltage to spike rate, and the lateral inhibitory transduction from spike rate to voltage, we have characterized by transfer functions. We have checked the appropriateness of treating the eye as a system of linear transducers under our experimental conditions. The response of the eye to a large spot of light undergoing sine flicker has been correctly predicted.

1. INTRODUCTION

The faceted lateral eye of the horseshoe crab, *Limulus polyphemus*, exhibits many functional characteristics in common with the visual systems of more evolved creatures, including man. In this compound eye the relative accessibility of the nerve cells to the techniques of electrophysiology has led to a fairly detailed understanding of the actions of its components, and has made it a particularly attractive model system for the study of sensory neural function. This relatively simple visual organ performs three distinct processing steps upon signals arriving from the outside world. The first step is the translation of light intensity into intracellular voltage. The voltage in turn establishes the rate at which nerve impulses are sent to the brain. Third, the impulse rate is converted back into voltage, to perform the functions of neural inhibition. Here we will present detailed experimental measurements of the time-dependence of the several steps in signal processing which occur in the *Limulus* eye, and will then show how these results lead to a prediction of the time-dependent behavior of the eye as a whole.[1]

The voltage spikes, which travel down the *Limulus* optic nerve fibers toward

---

[1] A recent review article (Dodge, Shapley, and Knight, 1970) discusses this topic briefly.

the brain, originate in the eye near the soma of the neuron (eccentric cell). It was observed by MacNichol (1956) and by Fuortes (1959) that the steady-state spike rate is proportional to the degree of depolarization of the cell. Under conditions of normal functioning this depolarization is the combined effect of several different more peripheral causes. The action of light on the eye is to depolarize the eccentric cell, the result of an increase in membrane conductance that short-circuits the resting polarization of the cell (Tomita, 1956; Fuortes, 1959; Rushton, 1959). The basis of this conductance increase appears to be the superposition of numerous brief, discrete, conductance events which are triggered by absorption of photons (Yeandle, 1958; Fuortes and Yeandle, 1964), and which individually adapt to smaller size in brighter light (Adolph, 1964; Dodge, Knight, and Toyoda, 1968). Opposing the excitatory effect of light is *lateral inhibition* (Hartline, Wagner, and Ratliff, 1956) acting among neighboring eccentric cells. That lateral inhibition depends on the firing of spikes was demonstrated indirectly by quantitative analysis of the inhibitory interaction (Hartline and Ratliff, 1958), and directly by experiments in which inhibition was elicited by antidromic stimulation of the optic nerve (Tomita, 1958). Later, Tomita, Kikuchi, and Tanaka (1960), and Purple (1964; Purple and Dodge, 1965) demonstrated that antidromic inhibition resulted from a hyperpolarizing potential change associated with an increase in membrane conductance; thus lateral inhibition shows the usual features of a classical inhibitory postsynaptic potential. The lateral inhibitory interconnections have been identified anatomically (Hartline, Ratliff, and Miller, 1961), and detailed measurements have been made of the dependence of the inhibitory interaction upon the distance of separation between receptors (Barlow, 1967, 1969). Following the discharge of each spike an eccentric cell also shows a *self-inhibitory* hyperpolarization which is accompanied by a conductance increase, and displays the general features of an inhibitory postsynaptic potential (Stevens, 1964; Purple, 1964; Purple and Dodge, 1965, 1966).

Among the functional characteristics that the eye of *Limulus* and the human eye share are the following: (*a*) great sensitivity to *changes* in light intensity as compared to steady intensity level; (*b*) graded response to a wide range of light intensities (to a factor of about 10^7 in intensities for *Limulus*); (*c*) enhanced response to edges and contours. We note that the presence of self-inhibition should give rise to (*a*) above, the adaptation of the excitatory conductance should give rise to (*a*) and (*b*), and lateral inhibition to (*a*), (*b*), and (*c*). Several models, based on simple assumptions concerning the dynamics of the component processes within the eccentric cell, have yielded reasonable simulated responses to steps of input stimulation (Hartline et al., 1961; Stevens, 1964; Purple, 1964; Purple and Dodge, 1965, 1966; Lange, 1965; Lange, Hartline, and Ratliff, 1966). In this paper we present detailed experimental characterizations of the dynamics of the one excitatory and the two inhibitory processes in the eccentric cell, and from these we predict the dynamics of the entire eye.

Fig. 1, which shows the response of a single fiber to incremental steps in light intensity (Ratliff, Hartline, and Miller, 1963), is a striking illustration of the sensitivity of the *Limulus* eye to changes in intensity. The great relative compression of response to time-independent intensity, shown in Fig. 1, makes the eye's high sensitivity to changes compatible with a wide range of input intensities.

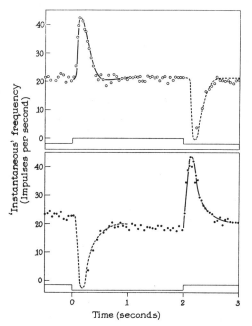

FIGURE 1. Response of the spike rate of an optically isolated eccentric cell to a step in light intensity. In each frame the solid line at "on" is fit to the points, and its reflection gives the dashed line at "off." Lower trace is light intensity. (From Ratliff et al., 1963). Log adapting $I = -0.26$; log I during increment $= 0.0$; log I during decrement $= -0.50$. *Figure reprinted by permission from Journal of the Optical Society of America. 1963. 53:110.*

A less obvious feature of Fig. 1 is crucial to the analysis that will follow. In both frames the response to an intensity decrement is the close mirror image of the response to the corresponding increment. This suggests that we are dealing with a so-called "time-invariant linear" system.

A time-invariant linear system has a property somewhat more general than that shown in Fig. 1. Namely, application of a superposition of individual inputs leads to the corresponding superposition of individual outputs, and the result is independent of the time of application. This is the principle of superposition, which we now assume for simplicity. A consequence of this property may be shown: a sine wave input necessarily leads to a sine wave output at the same frequency but generally with a different amplitude and at a different phase.

Now it is well-known that any physically realizable input can be expressed as a superposition of sine waves, each with its own amplitude and phase. (This is a form of the famous Fourier theorem.) This result, together with the principle of superposition, leads to the following very important conclusion.

Knowledge of the input-output amplitude ratio (amplitude gain) and the input-output phase shift, at all frequencies, completely specifies the input-output dynamics of a time-invariant linear system. This knowledge enables us to predict the system response to any arbitrary input.

2. METHODS

The excised *Limulus* lateral eye was split horizontally with a razor blade to expose the neural tissue behind the individual facets. One half-eye was mounted vertically (with beeswax) to form the fourth side of a three-sided moist chamber, with the exposed tissue facing upward. The chamber was filled with seawater, full enough to just cover the cut. A glass micropipette (3 molar KCl, 10–20 megohms) was lowered into an ommatidium by means of a micromanipulator and under visual control through a dissecting microscope. Electrical recording from the microelectrode was through a unity-gain amplifier with capacitance neutralization and a bridge circuit which permitted direct measurement of pipette and cell resistance and also allowed voltage recording while current was passed into the cell. The eye facets looked horizontally outward from the moist chamber, permitting light stimulation from a single optical fiber, 70 μ in diameter (American Optical Corp.), mounted on another micromanipulator. Earlier multifiber experiments demonstrated that light may be confined to a single facet in this way. The optical fiber was illuminated by a glow-modulator tube (Sylvania R 1131-C). The light intensity was controlled by modulating the repetition rate of 1 msec long light pulses, around a carrier frequency of 400 pulses per sec. Under these operating conditions, no appreciable nonlinear effects arise from the glow-modulator tube. The intensity range was chosen by the use of neutral density filters. Because the effective stimulus intensity was critically dependent on the alignment of the optical fiber to the axis of the ommatidium, we did not calibrate the light by any other method than the response of the eccentric cell. Maximum light intensity typically produced a steady-state firing of 30–40 spikes/sec in an optically isolated ommatidium. Previously reported techniques were used in the experiments in which single nerve fiber recordings were made (Hartline and Graham, 1932), and in those in which the optic nerve was stimulated antidromically (Tomita, 1958; Lange, 1965; Lange et al., 1966). All experiments were done at room temperature (19°–23°C).

In order to limit ourselves to a reasonably uniform population of cells, we accepted only definite eccentric cell recordings (spikes $\geq$ 30 mv). The advent of such an intracellular penetration is accompanied by an unmistakable fusillade of spike activity on the audio-monitor. The isolation of the excitatory process from spike activity was accomplished by the addition of tetrodotoxin to the seawater in the moist chamber.

An automatic timer gated the start of each experimental run and also the span of the light signal. Typically runs were spaced 100 sec apart, with the light on for 17 sec. This timing remained fixed for all runs on any given cell. Sinusoidal modulation was obtained from a function generator (Hewlett-Packard 3300A) whose frequency was set manually for each new run. A phase mark at the crest of each cycle was recorded from a second channel of the function generator.

The occurrence times of nerve spikes and phase marks, and the time course of the intracellular voltage, were recorded by a small computer (CDC 160-A) and stored in a Fortran-compatible format on digital tape. Event times were recorded in terms of the count of a crystal clock which incremented each 200 μsec. Records of the intracellular potential changes were made by feeding the voltage output of a monitoring oscilloscope (Tektronix 502A) to the computer through an analogue-digital converter. The oscilloscope output voltage was sampled every 200 μsec, and was averaged in the computer over 20 msec before storage on tape.

Fig. 2 shows direct graphical transcriptions of the data from individual runs. In the spike records the vertical coordinate is the *"instantaneous frequency"*: the reciprocal of the time interval from the previous spike to the current spike. To a span of each record we have fit, by least squares, a combination of six time functions: a constant, a linear ramp, a cosine and a sine of the input frequency, and a cosine and a sine of twice the input frequency. The constant measures the mean level of the output and the ramp tells the drift of the preparation during a run. Cosine and sine of twice the input frequency measure "harmonic content," which is a check on whether the biological input-output system is responding linearly. The coefficients of cosine and sine at the input frequency are easily converted into amplitude gain and phase—the goal of these experiments. (This gain and phase information vs. frequency we will call the "frequency response" or "transfer function.") In Fig. 2 the least square fits have been superimposed on the raw data. This calculation of fitting coefficients may be regarded as a linear filter applied to the raw data. It proves to be a narrow-pass filter which passes the driving frequency undiminished, and has a bandwidth which is the reciprocal of the time span over which data are taken. This filter has a signal/noise discrimination superior to the familiar computer of average transients: it exploits the fact that a signal of known form lies beneath the noise.

In the experiments reported below, the sinusoidal modulation of the input signal had a peak-to-peak amplitude which was as much as 60% of the mean input signal. (See last frame of Fig. 2.) The second harmonic content of the output rarely exceeded 5% of the amplitude of the output fundamental. The largest harmonic distortions were concurrent with the largest output modulations. We were able, by reducing the input modulation, to spot-check the fact that gain amplitude and phase of the output fundamental were indeed independent of input modulation amplitude under our experimental conditions. This gave us some confidence in treating the *Limulus* eye as a linear system.

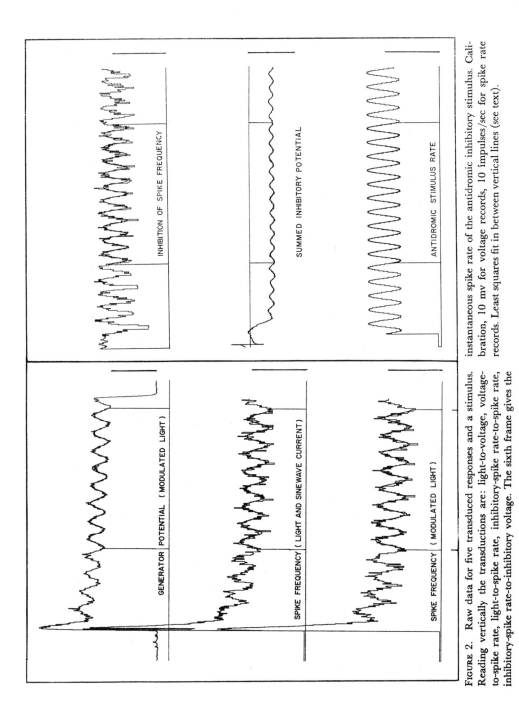

FIGURE 2. Raw data for five transduced responses and a stimulus. Reading vertically the transductions are: light-to-voltage, voltage-to-spike rate, light-to-spike rate, inhibitory-spike rate-to-spike rate, inhibitory-spike rate-to-inhibitory voltage. The sixth frame gives the instantaneous spike rate of the antidromic inhibitory stimulus. Calibration, 10 mv for voltage records, 10 impulses/sec for spike rate records. Least squares fit in between vertical lines (see text).

GENERATOR POTENTIAL (MODULATED LIGHT)

SPIKE FREQUENCY (LIGHT AND SINEWAVE CURRENT)

SPIKE FREQUENCY (MODULATED LIGHT)

INHIBITION OF SPIKE FREQUENCY

SUMMED INHIBITORY POTENTIAL

ANTIDROMIC STIMULUS RATE

In order to display these measurements (Figs. 3–5) we have normalized the amplitude to the value at zero frequency, which was calculated from the modulation depth of the stimulus and the slope of the steady-state stimulus-response relation. This normalization procedure is convenient because it uses only measurements of the incremental response. We can synthesize the empirical frequency response without taking explicit account of such complications as the threshold depolarization for spike firing and the variation of input resistance of the cell with ambient light intensity. Normalization factors for the several experiments are listed in Table I.

TABLE I

NORMALIZATION FACTORS FOR THE EMPIRICAL
FREQUENCY RESPONSE CURVES

Identifier	3/22/66 −0.3 log	4/29/66 −1.3 log	4/29/66 −3.0 log	9/23/66 −1.0 log	9/23/66 −2.6 log
Spike rate parameters (light to spikes)					
Unit amplitude,* sec^{-1}	1.5	1.2	1.2	1.3	1.3
Mean rate, sec^{-1}	17	27	14	35.5	18
Relative stimulus modulation‡	0.19	0.14	0.14	0.23	0.23
Peak-to-peak response at 1 Hz, sec^{-1}	15	10.1	6.2	12.4	8.6
Gains§ at 1 Hz	4.5	2.7	3.1	1.5	2.0
Generator potential parameters					
Unit amplitude,* mv	0.56	0.64	0.64	1.05	1.05
Mean value, mv	14.3	16.1	12.7	21.4	12.7
Relative stimulus modulation‡	0.38	0.28	0.28	0.40	0.40
Peak-to-peak response at 1 Hz, mv	2.05	1.52	1.18	3.64	3.18
Gain§ at 1 Hz	0.38	0.34	0.33	0.42	0.63

* Absolute modulation of response at zero frequency, calculated from slope of steady-state relation and stimulus modulation.
‡ Ratio of peak-to-peak modulation of light intensity to the mean value.
§ Defined as (peak-to-peak response/mean response)/(peak-to-peak stimulus/mean stimulus).

3. RESULTS

Dynamics of the Single Photoreceptor

For convenience, we will refer to any collection of cellular machinery, which modifies the form of a signal, as a "transducer"; the modifying process will be called "transduction." The behavior of the *Limulus* eye arises from three types of neural transducers, which we have isolated experimentally and whose frequency responses we have measured: (a) the transduction of light intensity to intracellular voltage, (b) the transduction from input voltage to spiking rate (this includes self-inhibition), and (c) the lateral inhibitory transduction from spiking rate back into voltage.

In the left frame of Fig. 3 the open circles show the frequency response of the intracellular generator potential, of a single illuminated ommatidium, to sinusoidally flickering light. (See also Pinter, 1966; Dodge et al., 1968.) Nerve spike activity has been abolished by the application of tetrodotoxin.

The frequency response of spike rate, in response to driving voltage, is shown for the same cell by the solid circles in the left frame of Fig. 3. Mean spike rate was maintained by steady light on the receptor, while sinusoidal voltage modulation was achieved by driving a sinusoidal current through the intracellular micropipette.

Both frequency responses show the general features of a transducer which applies a "sluggish gain control" to input signals. The amplitude gain first

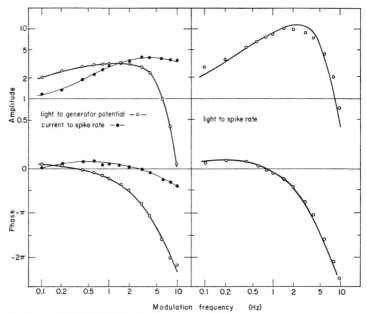

FIGURE 3. Data of 9/23/66 -2.6 log. Left frame, amplitude and phase of frequency response of component transductions, light-to-voltage (open circles) and voltage-to-spike rate (solid circles). Right frame, frequency response of total transduction, light-to-spike rate. Data points from direct measurement, solid curves predicted from left frame.

increases with frequency, as the gain control becomes less able to follow the input signal. Since such a gain control still will be reducing the output signal at the moment when the input sine wave reaches its crest, there will be a low-frequency phase lead. Eventual high-frequency cutoff and phase lag may be anticipated on very general grounds: any real transducer will have a time-resolution limitation; and the time necessary for internal processing will impose a lag between input cause and output effect as that limitation is approached.

Under circumstances of normal operation the sinusoidal output of the light-to-voltage transducer would be the sinusoidal input to the voltage-to-spike rate transducer. Clearly the amplitude gain of the combination should be the product of the amplitude gains of its two components, and the corresponding phase shift should be the algebraic sum of the two component phase shifts. The indicated multiplication and addition have been done, and the results appear as the solid curves in the right frame of Fig. 3. The direct experiment

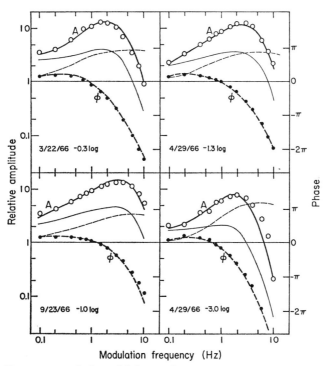

FIGURE 4. Four more predictions of light-to-spike rate frequency response compared with direct measurement (open and closed circles). Thin solid curves, light-to-voltage. Thin dashed curves, voltage-to-spike rate. Heavy curves, light-to-spike rate predicted. Phase data of component transductions are not shown.

has also been done on the same cell: the frequency response of the firing rate to a sinusoidally flickering light has been measured, and is shown by the open circles in the same illustration.

Fig. 4 summarizes the results of four similar experiments. Prediction and measurement are in general agreement in all cases, and show no systematic discrepancies. Thus, by treating the two transducers as time-invariant linear systems, we have correctly predicted their combined effect.

The outcome of a voltage-to-spike rate experiment may be summarized in terms of three parameters: the mean firing rate, the self-inhibitory time constant, and the self-inhibitory strength coefficient. The latter two parameters are evaluated by fitting equation (*d*) (footnote to theoretical section) to the data. The results obtained from 12 *Limulus* eyes are summarized in Table II.

Dynamics of Lateral Inhibition

Under normal operating conditions the frequency response of the lateral inhibitory potential cannot be measured directly. The inhibitory potential is

TABLE II

ESTIMATES OF SELF-INHIBITION PARAMETERS

Identifier	L	Spike rate	Time constant	Self-inhibitory coefficient
		sec^{-1}	sec	
3/16/66	*i*	17	0.75	1.8
3/22/66	−0.3	20	0.70	2.9
4/5/66	*i*	15	0.45	3.5
4/29/66	−3.0	20	0.40	4.0
	−1.3	31	(0.6)*	2.5
9/23/66	−2.6	19	0.50	3.0
	−1.0	34	(0.6)*	2.5
3/30/67	*a*	15	0.50	3.8
4/7/67	*a*	16	0.55	5.0
4/11/67	*a*	19	0.50	4.0
4/14/67	*a*	20	0.80	3.5
4/17/67	*a*	20	0.55	2.5
4/24/67	*a*	19	0.60	3.2
5/2/67	*a*	15	0.45	6.0

L, Background light intensity in terms of logarithm of attenuation of standard source, except:
  i, Modulation superimposed on depolarizing current.
  a, Bright steady light (−0 log) but spike rate diminished by antidromic inhibition.
* Data not fit well by single time constant; estimate given is approximate fit to amplitude at half-maximal value.

written over by the spike activity of the postsynaptic cell. However, an indirect measurement was possible. First, we measured the frequency response of the voltage-to-spike rate transducer as discussed above, using an eye whose optic nerve was prepared for antidromic stimulation of the whole nerve. (The nerve fiber to the impaled cell was severed to prevent antidromic invasion.) Then, with steady light on the recording ommatidium and with no stimulating current passed through the microelectrode, we antidromically stimulated the optic nerve at a rate upon which we imposed a sinusoidal modulation (see last frame of Fig. 2). The resulting modulation in the spike activity of the impaled cell yielded the total transduction from neighbors to test unit: spike rate–to–voltage-to-spike rate. Reversing the earlier procedure, we respectively divided and subtracted these results by the amplitude and phase of the voltage-to-spike rate transduction, to recover the frequency response of the lateral inhibitory synapse. The results for three eyes are shown in Fig. 5.

By altering the intracellular conditions of the impaled eccentric cell, the lateral inhibitory frequency response may be observed directly. The eye was

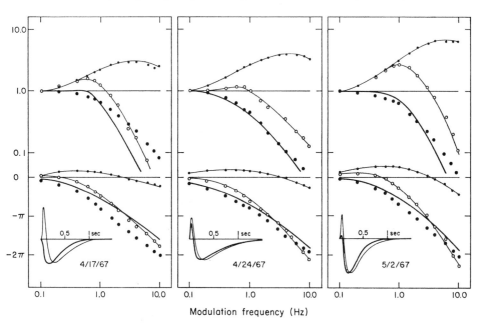

Modulation frequency (Hz)

FIGURE 5. Lateral inhibitory transduction. Small solid circles, voltage-to-spike rate. Open circles, inhibitory-spike rate-to-spike rate. Heavy line, deduced frequency response for inhibitory-spike rate–to–inhibitory-potential transduction in presence of ongoing spike activity in postsynaptic cell. Heavy circles, directly observed inhibitory-spike rate–to–inhibitory-potential in hyperpolarized and quiet cell. Insert, Postsynaptic impulse response predicted by Fourier analysis. Heavy line, active cell. Thin line, hyperpolarized cell.

put in darkness and the cell hyperpolarized to the point at which spike activity ceased. Then the same antidromic stimulation yielded a postsynaptic voltage measurable through the microelectrode. For the three cases of Fig. 5 the directly measured frequency response is shown with solid circles. There is approximate agreement with the indirect measurement, though the departures are systematic.

The insets in Fig. 5 may cast some light on the discrepancy. In the introduction it was mentioned that the frequency response may be used to calculate the response to an arbitrary input. We have used the frequency response

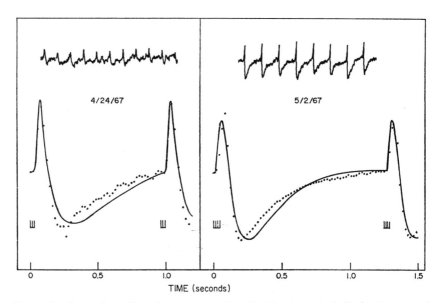

FIGURE 6. Comparison of impulse response predicted by Fourier analysis (line) with averaged transient observed directly (solid circles). Insert shows several cycles of the raw impulse response data. The "impulse" for the left frame consisted of three antidromic whole nerve stimuli spaced at intervals of about 10 msec. In the right frame four such stimuli were used.

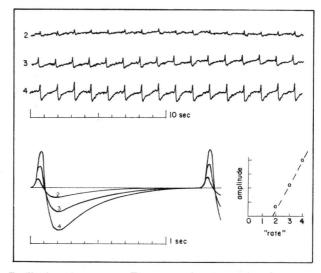

FIGURE 7. Facilitation phenomenon. The averaged postsynaptic voltage response to two, three, and four nerve impulses spaced about 10 msec apart. Beyond threshold the response is linear.

to calculate the response to a brief impulsive input; the result should be the time course of the unit inhibitory postsynaptic potential. In five of the six cases there is a remarkable brief depolarization before the onset of the main inhibitory potential. In all three cells the depolarizing surge is more pronounced when the cell is in the more hyperpolarized condition. This observation is consistent with the notion that the brief depolarization results from an additional postsynaptic permeability change (Kandel and Wachtel, 1968) whose equilibrium potential is positive to the operating voltages within the cell. (By the same token, the hyperpolarizing part of the postsynaptic response is more pronounced when the cell is depolarized. This is not evident in Fig. 5 because the transfer functions have been normalized to unity at zero frequency.)

In the hyperpolarized and quiet cell, the postsynaptic impulse response predicted from frequency information may be compared to that measured directly. The result is shown in Fig. 6. The degree of agreement may be regarded as validation for our treating the lateral inhibitory synapse as a time-invariant linear transducer.

In Fig. 7 are shown the mean postsynaptic voltage responses to two through four closely spaced antidromic impulses. Apparently two stimulating impulses are necessary to facilitate the synapse, which then responds linearly to further increments in input.

4. THEORETICAL

Finally, we use these results to predict the behavior of the entire eye. The time-independent firing rates of the *Limulus* eccentric cells are known to satisfy the Hartline-Ratliff equations (Hartline and Ratliff, 1958):

$$r_m = \epsilon_m - Kr_m - \sum_{n \neq m} k_{mn} r_n , \qquad (1)$$

presented here in a form which includes self-inhibition explicitly. Here r_m is the firing rate of the mth ommatidium, K is its self-inhibitory coefficient, ϵ_m is its excitatory receptor potential expressed in appropriate units, and k_{mn} are the lateral inhibitory coefficients linking it to other ommatidia. Small threshold corrections have been discarded. While the success of these equations is empirical, the three right-hand terms may be interpreted as the three contributions to the intracellular voltage at the site of voltage-to-spike rate transduction. This observation leads to the immediate frequency-dependent generalization of equation 1.

From electrical and control system design it is well-known that a sinusoidally modulated variable may be represented by a complex number fixed in amplitude but advancing in phase at a rate which yields the modulation frequency. The effect of a linear transducer upon that variable is to multiply it by a complex number (the "transfer function") whose amplitude and phase are the amplitude gain and phase of the transducer's frequency response at that frequency. This shorthand scheme is useful because it yields correct results not only for the application of consecutive transductions but also for the addition of several out-of-phase signals. That is exactly what is required to generalize equation 1.

Following this scheme, if I is the modulation in light intensity, then the modulation in receptor potential is given by

$$\epsilon_m = G(f)I \tag{2}$$

where the transfer function $G(f)$ is the complex number whose amplitude and phase are given by the frequency response in Fig. 3 (left frame, open circles), evaluated at the modulation frequency f. The generalization of equation 1 is similarly

$$r_m = \epsilon_m - KT_s(f)r_m - T_l(f) \sum_{n \neq m} k_{mn}r_n . \tag{3}$$

Here T_s and T_l are the self-inhibitory and lateral inhibitory transfer functions so scaled that they are unity when $f = 0$. The amplitude and phase of the lateral inhibitory $T_l(f)$ are given by the spike rate–to–voltage curves of Fig. 5. Fig. 3 (solid circles) determines the form of $T_s(f)$.[2] Now given the ϵ_m

---

[2] Dropping the summation term in (3) easily leads to the determining equation

$$KT_s(f) = \frac{1}{(r/\epsilon)} - 1 \tag{a}$$

where (r/ϵ) is the solid circle frequency response of Fig. 3.

There is a slight approximation in equation (3) because the frequency-dependent transduction effects of the voltage-to-spike rate converter have been ignored. It is easily shown for an exponential inhibitory postsynaptic potential with decrement time τ that

$$T_s = \frac{1}{1 + i\tau\omega} \tag{b}$$

where $\omega = 2\pi f$, whence (a) gives

$$r/\epsilon = \frac{1}{1 + KT_s} = \frac{1}{1 + K\dfrac{1}{1 + i\tau\omega}} \tag{c}$$

which fits the data of Fig. 3 (and similar *Limulus* data) fairly well. (This result is equivalent to the model of Stevens, 1964.) If one assumes that the spikes arise from an integrating voltage-to-frequency converter, an unpleasant perturbation calculation yields the exact transfer function

$$r/\epsilon = \left(\frac{1 - e^{-i\omega/\nu}}{i\omega/\nu}\right) \bigg/ \left(1 + K\left[1 - \frac{(1/\tau\nu)(1 - e^{-i\omega/\nu})}{(e^{1/\tau\nu} - 1)(1 - e^{-(1/\tau+i\omega)/\nu})}\right]\right) \tag{d}$$

where ν is the mean spike rate. Equation (c) is retrieved in the limit $\omega/\nu \to 0$ (Terzuolo, 1969, see pp. 65–69). However, (d) shows a high-frequency amplitude cutoff and phase lag (which (c)

(from equation 2), the equations (3) are in the form of a set of linear simultaneous equations, which at each modulation frequency can be solved for the r_m .

We have tried to use equations 2 and 3 with our data to predict the outcome of another experiment (Ratliff, Knight, Toyoda, and Hartline, 1967), in which first a single ommatidium, and then a circular cluster of 20 ommatidia were stimulated by a flickering light. The firing rate modulation of the central fiber was determined by a single fiber recording. For the calculation we used

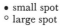

• small spot
∘ large spot

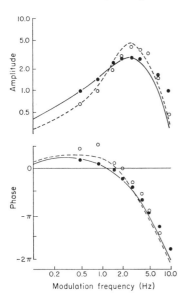

FIGURE 8. Theoretical and observed light-to-spike rate frequency response for a single ommatidium and for the central member of a cluster of 19 interacting ommatidia. Amplitude is given in sec^{-1} peak-to-peak. Mean rate was 25/sec for solid circles and 20/sec for open circles.

the data from two comparable ommatidia: the generator transfer function given in the upper right frame of Fig. 4, and the lateral inhibitory transfer function given in the middle frame of Fig. 5. We used the commonly observed self-inhibitory coefficient value of $K = 3$ and the spatial distribution of lateral inhibition given by Barlow (1969).

A hexagonal array of 19 ommatidia has been assumed. Because there are two axes of symmetry in the Barlow inhibitory distribution, only seven of these ommatidia are mathematically inequivalent. Seven simultaneous equations similar to the set (3) result, and have been solved for a range of frequencies. The frequency response thus obtained for the central ommatidium has been multiplied by the light-to-voltage transfer function. In Fig. 8 this

does not) and in fact fits very well to most of our *Limulus* voltage-to-spike rate transfer function experiments. The predictions which follow utilize the theoretical embellishments which led to (d). However, the difference in result from that of the simpler approximate relation (3) is slight.

theoretical result is compared with the experiment. One remaining parameter, which fixes the scale of the over-all amplitude gain, has been fit by placing the "large spot" theoretical amplitude line through the corresponding data point at 0.5 hz. In the final result, the discrepancies between theory and experiment are small compared to individual variations among ommatidia seen in Figs. 4 and 5.

5. CONCLUSIONS

Over a reasonable range of stimulus illumination, the eye of *Limulus* responds as a linear transducer.

Within the eye three component transductions may be isolated and studied individually. These are the transductions from light to voltage, from voltage-to-spike rate, and the lateral inhibitory transduction from spike rate back to voltage. These are all linear transductions and their individual frequency responses may be measured.

The transductions from light to voltage and from voltage-to-spike rate both have frequency responses whose general form is that of a sluggish gain control.

The lateral inhibitory transduction from spike rate to voltage corresponds to a unit postsynaptic potential which is briefly excitatory before its more pronounced inhibitory phase sets in.

These component frequency responses may be utilized in a time-dependent generalization of the Hartline-Ratliff equations. The over-all dynamic response of an interacting group of ommatidia, to sinusoidal flicker, is predicted properly.

We wish to thank numerous friends who helped us in this project, and in particular Drs. H. K. Hartline, F. Ratliff, and D. Lange.

This work was supported in part by research grants (EY 00188) from the National Eye Institute, (GM 1789), from the National Insitute of General Medical Sciences, and (GB–6540) from the National Science Foundation.

Received for publication 24 April 1970.

REFERENCES

ADOLPH, A. R. 1964. Spontaneous slow potential fluctuations in the *Limulus* photoreceptor. *J. Gen. Physiol.* **48**:297.

BARLOW, R. B., JR. 1967. Inhibitory Fields in the *Limulus* Lateral Eye. Thesis. The Rockefeller University. New York.

BARLOW, R. B., JR. 1969. Inhibitory fields in the *Limulus* lateral eye. *J. Gen. Physiol.* **54**:383.

DODGE, F. A., B. W. KNIGHT, and J. TOYODA. 1968. Voltage noise in Limulus visual cells. *Science* (*Washington*). **160**:88.

DODGE, F. A., R. M. SHAPLEY, and B. W. KNIGHT. 1970. Linear systems analysis of the *Limulus* retina. *Behav. Sci.* **15**:24.

FUORTES, M. G. F. 1959. Initiation of impulses in visual cells of *Limulus*. *J. Physiol.* (*London*). **148**:14.

FUORTES, M. G. F., and S. YEANDLE. 1964. Probability of occurrence of discrete potential waves in the eye of *Limulus*. *J. Gen. Physiol.* **47**:443.

HARTLINE, H. K., and C. H. GRAHAM. 1932. Nerve impulses from single receptors in the eye. *J. Cell. Comp. Physiol.* **1**:277.

HARTLINE, H. K., and F. RATLIFF. 1958. Spatial summation of inhibitory influences in the eye of *Limulus*, and the mutual interaction of receptor units. *J. Gen. Physiol.* **41**:1049.

HARTLINE, H. K., F. RATLIFF, and W. H. MILLER. 1961. Inhibitory interaction in the retina, and its significance in vision. *In* Nervous Inhibition. E. Florey, editor. Pergamon Press, New York. 241.

HARTLINE, H. K., H. G. WAGNER, and F. RATLIFF. 1956. Inhibition in the eye of *Limulus*. *J. Gen. Physiol.* **39**:651.

KANDEL, E. R., and H. WACHTEL. 1968. The functional organization of neural aggregates in *Aplysia*. *In* Physiological and Biochemical Aspects of Nervous Integration. F. D. Carlson, editor. Prentice-Hall, Inc., Englewood Cliffs, N. J. 17.

LANGE, D. 1965. Dynamics of Inhibitory Interaction in the Eye of *Limulus*: Experimental and Theoretical Studies. Thesis. The Rockefeller University. New York.

LANGE, D., H. K. HARTLINE, and F. RATLIFF. 1966 *a*. Inhibitory interaction in the retina: techniques of experimental and theoretical analysis. *Ann. N.Y. Acad. Sci.* **128**:955.

LANGE, D., H. K. HARTLINE, and F. RATLIFF. 1966 *b*. Dynamics of lateral inhibition in the compound eye of *Limulus*. II. *In* The Functional Organization of the Compound Eye. C. G. Bernhard, editor. Pergamon Press, Oxford. 425.

MacNICHOL, E. F., JR. 1956. Visual receptors as biological transducers. *In* Molecular Structure and Functional Activity of Nerve Cells. *Am. Inst. Biol. Sci. Publ. No. 1.* 34–53.

PINTER, R. B. 1966. Sinusoidal and delta function responses of visual cells of the *Limulus* eye. *J. Gen. Physiol.* **49**:565.

PURPLE, R. L. 1964. The Integration of Excitatory and Inhibitory Influences in the Eccentric Cell in the Eye of *Limulus*. Thesis. The Rockefeller University. New York.

PURPLE, R. L., and F. A. DODGE, JR. 1965. Interaction of excitation and inhibition in the eccentric cell in the eye of *Limulus*. *Cold Spring Harbor Symp. Quant. Biol.* **30**:529.

PURPLE, R. L., and F. A. DODGE, JR. 1966. Self inhibition in the eye of *Limulus*. *In* The Functional Organization of the Compound Eye. C. G. Bernhard, editor. Pergamon Press, Oxford. 451.

RATLIFF, F., H. K. HARTLINE, and W. H. MILLER. 1963. Spatial and temporal aspects of retinal inhibitory interaction. *J. Opt. Soc. Amer.* **53**:110.

RATLIFF, F., B. W. KNIGHT, J. TOYODA, and H. K. HARTLINE. 1967. Enhancement of flicker by lateral inhibition. *Science (Washington).* **158**:392.

RUSHTON, W. A. H. 1959. A theoretical treatment of Fuortes' observations upon eccentric cell activity in *Limulus*. *J. Physiol. (London).* **148**:29.

STEVENS, C. F. 1964. A Quantitative Theory of Neural Interactions: Theoretical and Experimental Investigations. Thesis. The Rockefeller University. New York.

TERZUOLO, C. A., editor. 1969. Systems Analysis in Neurophysiology. Proceedings of Conference on Systems Analysis Approach to Neurophysiological Problems. University of Minnesota, Minn.

TOMITA, T. 1956. The nature of action potentials in the lateral eye of the horseshoe crab as revealed by simultaneous intra- and extracellular recording. *Jap. J. Physiol.* **6**:327.

TOMITA, T. 1958. Mechanisms of lateral inhibition in the eye of *Limulus*. *J. Neurophysiol.* **21**:419.

TOMITA, T., R. KIKUCHI, and I. TANAKA. 1960. Excitation and inhibition in lateral eye of horseshoe crab. *In* Electrical Activity of Single Cells. Y. Katsuki, editor. Igaku–shoin, Ltd., Tokyo, 11.

YEANDLE, S. 1958. Electrophysiology of the visual system-discussion. *Am. J. Ophthalmol.* **46**:82.

Fluctuations of the impulse rate in *Limulus* eccentric cells

ROBERT SHAPLEY

The Rockefeller University, New York, N.Y.

Reprinted from the JOURNAL OF GENERAL PHYSIOLOGY
May 1971, Vol. 57, no. 5, pp. 539-556

ABSTRACT   Fluctuations in the discharge of impulses were studied in eccentric cells of the compound eye of the horseshoe crab, *Limulus polyphemus*. A theory is presented which accounts for the variability in the response of the eccentric cell to light. The main idea of this theory is that the source of randomness in the impulse rate is "noise" in the generator potential. Another essential aspect of the theory is that the process which transforms the generator potential "noise" into the impulse rate fluctuations may be treated as a linear filter. These ideas lead directly to Fourier analysis of the fluctuations. Experimental verification of theoretical predictions was obtained by calculation of the variance spectrum of the impulse rate. The variance spectrum of the impulse rate is shown to be the filtered variance spectrum of the generator potential.

INTRODUCTION

Some degree of randomness in the maintained response of a neuron to steady stimulation is characteristic of sensory neurons and neurons of vertebrate and invertebrate central nervous systems. The study of neuronal fluctuations is significant because these fluctuations are widespread, and because they may provide detailed understanding of the function of single neurons (Burns, 1968).

Numerous investigators have studied fluctuations of the maintained response of primary sensory neurons—cells which do not receive convergent input from other neurons (frog muscle spindle [Buller et al., 1953]; *Limulus* visual cells [Ratliff et al., 1968]; cat auditory nerve [Kiang, 1965]; mammalian cutaneous mechanoreceptors [Werner and Mountcastle, 1965]; cat muscle spindle [Stein and Matthews, 1965]; cat chemoreceptors [Biscoe and Taylor, 1962]). The sources of variability in primary sensory cells may not be the same, in detail, as those causing variability in the firing of neurons in the central nervous system. However, because the former are more susceptible to experimental control, they are more suitable for quantitative study than the richly interconnected central neurons.

I have studied the way in which randomness arises in the maintained response to light of eccentric cells in the compound eye of the horseshoe crab.

The axons of the eccentric cells gather to form the optic nerve of the horseshoe crab. As far as we know, these are the only cells in the compound eye which respond to light by firing nerve impulses (Waterman and Wiersma, 1954; Purple, 1964; Behrens and Wulff, 1965). This paper deals with fluctuations due to processes within single eccentric cells. An accompanying paper is concerned with the effect of interactions between eccentric cells.

Ratliff et al. (1968), recording from *Limulus* eccentric cells, found that the variance of the steady-state firing rate in response to electrical stimulation was much smaller than the variance of the response to stimulation by light, and that in the latter case the variance depended on light intensity and light adaptation. These results implied that the randomness in the generator potential, which is probably due to randomness in photon arrival and absorption (Dodge et al., 1968), was responsible for the impulse rate fluctuations. Because the impulse-firing mechanism can be treated as a linear filter for modulated stimuli (Dodge, 1968; Knight et al., 1970), I have used the theory for the linear filtering of stochastic processes to show how fluctuations in impulse rate arise from the generator potential "noise" (Shapley, 1969).

METHODS

The Biological Preparation

This work was done on excised lateral eyes of the horseshoe crab, *Limulus polyphemus*. For intracellular recording, the eye was sliced in half with a razor blade. The slice was parallel to the long axis of the eye and perpendicular to the surface of the eye. The sliced eye formed the fourth wall of a three-sided Plexiglass chamber; it was sealed into place with beeswax. The chamber was filled with artificial seawater. For experiments on generator potentials, the impulse-firing mechanism was poisoned by adding 10^{-6} M tetrodotoxin to the seawater.

Experiments were performed with a micropipette as an intracellular electrode. Micropipettes were filled with 3 molar potassium chloride; they had a resistance of 10–20 megohms measured in seawater. Signals were passed from the micropipette probe to a unity gain negative capacitance bridge amplifier designed by J. P. Hervey. This amplifier has been described by Purple (1964).

In other experiments, nerve fiber recording was done using standard techniques. Bundles of nerve fibers were teased from the *Limulus* optic nerve with glass needles and dissected until a single active fiber was present on the recording electrode. A preamplifier (Tektronix 122) provided a gain of 1000.

Action potentials and/or slow potentials were fed to a Tektronix 502A oscilloscope. The vertical signal output from the oscilloscope was monitored on a loudspeaker. The output of the oscilloscope was also fed into a CDC 160-A digital computer in a manner described below.

Analysis was performed on steady-state responses of eccentric cells which were statistically stationary. This means that statistical parameters of the discharge did not change during the course of one response, or from one experimental run to another.

Stimulus and Stimulus Control

Two sets of stimulus conditions were established. First, different time-varying wave-forms were used to modulate the light intensity illuminating an eccentric cell or the current that was directly driving the cell. Under the second set of stimulus conditions steady stimulation was repeated at constant intervals throughout the experiment. A constant repetition rate was required because statistical measures were obtained by averaging several responses to identical steady stimuli. The responses would be statistically the same only if the cell were in the same adaptation state at the onset of each stimulus presentation.

Stimulus presentation and control were identical to those described by Knight et al. (1970). The stimulus waveform was generated by adding together constant volt-ages with time-varying voltages generated by a waveform generator (Hewlett-Packard 3300A). For stimulation by modulated current the summed voltage was led directly to the bridge stimulus input of the bridge amplifier. For stimulation by modulated light the summed voltage was first fed to a voltage-to-frequency converter with center frequency adjusted to 400 hz. In some experiments a steady light and a sinusoidal current were applied simultaneously to the same cell in order to modulate the activity of the cell around a level of excitation produced by the natural stimulus. For such ex-periments a constant voltage was passed through the voltage-to-frequency converter and the time-varying voltage was led to the bridge amplifier stimulus input and thence to the microelectrode.

The output of the voltage-to-frequency converter triggered a pulse generator (Tektronix 161) which in turn triggered a glow modulator driver. The glow modulator driver, designed by M. Rosetto, provided pulses of constant current, adjustable from 8 to 30 ma, to drive a glow modulator tube (Sylvania R1131C).

The light stimulus was brought to single ommatidia of the compound eye via fiber optics. This method is described by R. Barlow (1969).

A programmed timer was used to control the timing of experimental runs and pro-vide electronic gating and clock signals for on-line computer data acquisition. It was similar to the one described by Milkman and Schoenfeld (1966). The programmed timer provided an input gate signal to alert the computer, and provided the 5 kc clock rate the computer used in the data acquisition program. Seven additional pro-grammable gates were available in the programmed timer to turn stimuli on and off in a prescribed sequence.

Data Processing

The data acquisition program, written for the CDC 160A computer by H. K. Hart-line, Norman Milkman, and David Lange, performed three functions which were particularly important for my experiments. First, the program measured time between pulse events on three separate data channels. Second, it sampled one voltage channel by means of an analogue to digital converter and stored the values of the voltage in memory. These two functions performed on-line took, on the average, a little less than 0.2 msec. Third, at the end of each experimental run the program stored time interval data and voltage data on magnetic tape for later analysis.

The resolution of the measurement of time intervals was 0.2 msec, the length of the clock cycle. This was 1 % accuracy for a firing rate of 50 impulses/sec, one-half % accuracy for 25 impulses/sec.

ANALYTICAL METHODS

Impulse Rate

The primary data for the experiments on impulse firing are intervals between impulses. One way to study the characteristics of neuronal discharge is to convert the list of pulse intervals into a list of instantaneous impulse rate samples. As shown below, in the case of regularly firing neurons, important statistical parameters for the impulse rate are the same as for the impulse intervals. The reason for using the pulse rate, rather than interpulse interval, as a measure of neural activity is that the rate is a more direct measure of the level of excitation of the neuron than the interval.

The algorithm for constructing the impulse rate is illustrated in Fig. 1. For any particular interval between pulses, the reciprocal of the time interval, the impulse rate, is assigned to all the time between the beginning and end of the interval. In effect, in constructing the impulse rate, one is transforming a frequency modulation into an amplitude modulation.

If the instantaneous impulse rate is sampled over equispaced intervals of time, the result is a list of pulse rate samples which can be mathematically manipulated in the same way as periodically sampled continuous functions (one might expect discontinuities in the firing rate at instants when impulses are fired; discontinuities are eliminated by averaging the instantaneous rate before and after an impulse discharge, to obtain a value of the impulse rate for those bins in which an impulse has occurred). If the "sampling" bins are small enough, a negligible amount of information about the statistics of the pulse

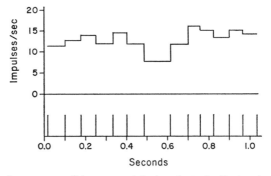

FIGURE 1. Instantaneous firing rate and the impulse train. During the interval between two pulses the impulse rate equals the reciprocal of that interval. The pulse train and impulse rate are plotted on the same time scale.

train will be lost. To be fine enough the sampling interval ought to be less than half the length of the average interspike interval, a limit consistent with the sampling theorem (see Shannon and Weaver, 1949, p. 53, for a discussion of the sampling theorem).

For the purposes of this paper, I have introduced a new unit to replace "impulses per second." This has been done in order to clarify the conception of modulation frequency of the impulse rate, which arises in the Fourier analysis of neuronal firing. The unit is named after E. D. Adrian, who discovered neural pulse frequency coding. 1 adrian equals one impulse/sec. I have used this unit in some of my figures, principally those illustrating spectral analysis of the impulse rate.

SPECTRAL ANALYSIS

Spectral analysis is an analytical tool developed to help understanding of the filtering of signals by linear, time-invariant devices. It has been applied in communication theory to the problem of filtering of stochastic processes (Parzen, 1962; Blackman and Tukey, 1958; Jenkins and Watts, 1968). I used spectral analysis to characterize the fluctuations in the impulse rate and generator potential.

Sinusoidal signals are unchanged in shape, but may be changed in amplitude and shifted in phase, when they are passed through a time-invariant linear filter (Parzen, 1962). Given any time-invariant linear filter, one can characterize it by specifying the response to a unit amplitude sinusoidal signal at each frequency. The function which relates the amplitude and phase of the output to the modulation frequency is called the frequency response.

Also, it is possible to express any continuous, deterministic function of time as a weighted sum of sinusoidal functions of time. The function which relates the relative weighting of each Fourier component to frequency is the Fourier transform of the original function. The operation of a filter on an input function can be expressed as the separate multiplication of each of the Fourier components belonging to the input function by the appropriate value of the frequency response.

For random processes a similar theory can be developed (cf. Bartlett, 1955; Parzen, 1962). A stochastic process is an ensemble of time functions which have some average properties in common but which cannot be determined exactly as a function of time. In an experimental context, this ensemble is composed of the group of noisy records which are measurements of the stochastic process.

One average property of a stochastic process is its autocovariance. The autocovariance is defined as the average product of the deviation of a random variable from its mean, multiplied by the value of the deviation later in time. For the stochastic process $n(t)$ with mean value $\bar{n}$, the autocovariance is defined as $\overline{(n(t) - \bar{n})(n(t + \tau) - \bar{n})}$. The autocovariance is a continuous, deterministic function of time; it depends on the time lag, τ, the lag between the two random variables in the product. The autocovariance is a measure of how rapidly the stochastic process fluctuates around its average value. The value of the autocovariance at zero time lag is the variance of the stochastic process; i.e., $\overline{(n(t) - \bar{n})^2}$.

The autocovariance of a stochastic process can be Fourier analyzed since it is a deterministic function of time. The Fourier transform of the autocovariance is what I call the variance spectrum. This name is appropriate because the value of the variance spectrum at a particular frequency represents the contribution of that frequency to the total variance of the stochastic process. Spectral analysis of stochastic processes was applied first to electrical signals for which variance means power, and so what I call the variance spectrum is more commonly referred to as the power spectrum (Rice, 1944).

The variance (power) spectrum of a stochastic process can also be calculated from direct Fourier analysis of the individual time functions which are members of the ensemble of functions which constitute the stochastic process. The squared amplitudes of the Fourier components must be averaged from many members of the ensemble to obtain the variance spectrum. It is a theorem that the variance spectrum computed in this manner is equal to the variance spectrum calculated from Fourier analysis of the autocovariance (Bartlett, 1955, pp. 159–166).

The function which relates the variance (power) spectrum of a stochastic process put into a linear filter to the spectrum of the output stochastic process is usually called the power transfer function of the filter (using my terminology it ought to be called the variance transfer function). It is the squared absolute value of the frequency response of the filter. The variance spectrum of the output equals the variance spectrum of the input multiplied by the power transfer function.

Spectral Estimation Spectral analysis is often performed on continuous functions of time which have been sampled at equally spaced points in time (Cooley, Lewis, and Welch, 1967). This procedure generates a list of numbers which are the values of the continuous function at the sample times. One can compute the variance spectrum of this list of numbers in the following way. First, one performs a Fourier analysis of the list; this is done by digital computer with subroutines incorporating the fast Fourier transform algorithm (Cooley et al., 1967). The Fourier transform is a list of complex numbers, each number associated with a particular frequency. One calculates the amplitude, or absolute value, of each of these numbers and squares it. The resulting list, of squared amplitudes at a number of evenly spaced points in the frequency domain, is the variance (power) spectrum, of the original list representing the time function.

If the original list is from evenly spaced time samples of a stochastic process, the sample spectrum from one record is not adequate to allow accurate estimation of the spectrum of the stochastic process. One must average several independent spectral estimates from a group of realizations of the stochastic process (cf. Jenkins and Watts, 1968, for details). What this means in a neurophysiological application is that one averages spectral estimates from several experimental runs which have identical stimulus conditions. In order to obtain smooth spectral estimates for stochastic processes I used Welch's method of averaging overlapping sample spectra (Welch, 1967).

The bandwidth of the variance spectrum is set by the frequency of sampling of the continuous signal. The bandwidth is one-half the sampling frequency. In my experiments the sampling frequency was 50 hz, so the bandwidth of the spectrum was 25 hz. The lowest frequency in the spectrum and the frequency resolution are the reciprocal of the record length. The record length was 5.12 sec so that the lowest frequency and frequency resolution were about 0.2 hz. Smoothing reduces the resolution without changing the lowest measurable frequency. The averaged sample spectra were further smoothed to give a frequency resolution of 1 hz. This was accomplished by moving average smoothing of the spectral estimates.

AUTOCORRELATION

The autocorrelation is defined as the autocovariance divided by the variance. Thus the autocorrelation is unity at zero time lag and varies with time lag, typically becoming zero as the time lag becomes large. The autocorrelation can be derived from the variance spectrum and is an equivalent measure of the average temporal pattern of a stochastic process.

The autocorrelation of the impulse rate has a very definite relationship to the serial correlation coefficients of the impulse intervals. The autocorrelation of the impulse rate, $n(t)$, is $\overline{(n(t) - \bar{n})(n(t + \tau) - \bar{n})(n(t) - \bar{n})^2}$.

The impulse rate, n, and pulse interval, s, are related by the equation $n = \dfrac{1}{s}$. In fairly regularly firing nerve cells, where deviations from the mean are not large, for deviations from the mean in pulse rate $\Delta n = n(t) - \bar{n}$ and for deviations in pulse

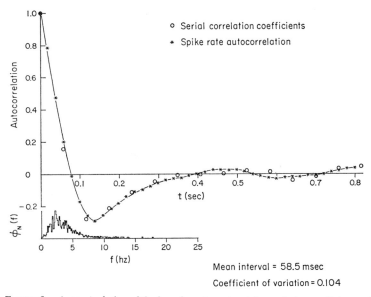

Mean interval = 58.5 msec

Coefficient of variation = 0.104

FIGURE 2.   Autocorrelation of the impulse rate and serial correlation coefficients of pulse intervals. The autocorrelation is plotted as a continuous curve and as asterisks. The serial correlation coefficients are plotted as open circles at times equal to integral multiples of the mean interpulse interval. At the lower left is shown the variance spectrum of the impulse rate, from which the autocorrelation of the impulse rate was calculated by Fourier transformation.

intervals Δs, we can write $\Delta n/\bar{n} = -\Delta s/\bar{s}$. In particular, for the coefficient of varia-
tion, $\sigma_N/\bar{n} = \sigma_s/\bar{s}$. Using the same argument you can show that $r_m = \overline{\Delta S_k \Delta S_{k+m}}/\overline{\Delta S_k^2} = \overline{\Delta n(t)\Delta n(t+\tau)}/\overline{\Delta n(t)^2}$ when $\tau = m\bar{s}$, where $\bar{s}$ is the mean pulse interval, r_m is the mth serial correlation coefficient, and $m = 1, 2, 3 \cdots$. In words, the autocorrelation of the impulse rate equals the interval serial correlation coefficients at time lags which equal an appropriate integral multiple of the mean interval. For example, the auto-correlation of the firing rate at time lag $\tau = 2\bar{s}$ equals the second interval serial cor-relation coefficient.

This is shown for some electronically generated data in Fig. 2.

This means that we can calculate the serial correlation coefficients of the intervals from the variance spectrum of the impulse rate.

RESULTS

Frequency Response of the Current-to-Firing Rate Process

The essential problem of this paper is the relation between noise in the mem-brane potential and variability of the impulse rate. The important mechanism to understand, in connection with this problem, is the process which produces the impulse rate from depolarization. Knight et al. (1970) have shown that this process acts like a linear transducer for small modulated signals; in other words, it can be characterized by its frequency response, $S(f)$. $S(f)$ is defined as the relative modulation (peak to peak divided by the average) of the im-pulse rate divided by the relative modulation of the driving current at the frequency f.

If the fluctuations in the impulse rate are due solely to filtered generator potential fluctuations, and there is no significant extra source of variability in impulse firing, we would predict,

$$\varphi_N(f) = |S(f)|^2 \cdot \varphi_G(f) \tag{1}$$

where $\varphi_G(f)$ is the variance spectrum of the generator potential and $\varphi_N(f)$ is the variance spectrum of the impulse rate. Equation (1) is a consequence of the theory for linear filtering of noise (see Analytical Methods).

Equation (1) is correct if φ_N and φ_G are in the same units. φ_G is expressed in the units of millivolts²/hertz (mv²/hz). φ_N is expressed in the units adrian²/hz; an adrian has been previously defined as 1 impulse/sec. A scale factor with units (adrian/mv)² must be used to convert φ_G from the units of a voltage spectrum to the units of an impulse rate spectrum. This factor was mea-sured as the slope of the steady-state voltage vs. firing rate curve; it lay in the range 1–25 (adrian/mv)² (cf. Fuortes, 1959).

Observations on Filtering of Generator Potential "Noise"

In order to verify this prediction one had to measure, in each eccentric cell, the variance spectrum of the generator potential, $\varphi_G(f)$, the frequency response of the current-to-firing rate process, $S(f)$, and the variance spectrum of the impulse rate, $\varphi_N(f)$.

The shape of a typical $S(f)$ is shown in Fig. 3 (techniques for measurement of $S(f)$ are described in detail in Knight et al., 1970). The logarithms of amplitude and phase are the ordinates and the logarithm of frequency is the abscissa in this graph. The first lobe of the phase shift is a phase lead; at frequencies above 1.5 hz the phase shift changes into a phase lag. The smooth curve

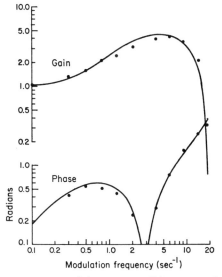

FIGURE 3. Frequency response of the current-to-firing rate mechanism. The amplitude (gain) and phase of the response to a whole range of modulated current stimuli are plotted against frequency of modulation. The points are empirical; the smooth curve is a fit to the points using Knight's (1969) theoretical expression for $S(f)$. The mean impulse rate for this cell was 20 impulses/sec.

drawn through the experimental points is the analytic expression for $S(f)$ derived by Knight (1969) and Knight et al. (1970).[1] The features of the predicted and measured frequency response are a low frequency cutoff, peak in amplitude (gain) at 5 hz, and a high frequency cutoff with a null at the frequency equal to the average impulse rate.

Spectra for both the generator potential, φ_G, and for the impulse rate, φ_N, were both measured in the same cell. Data from such an experiment are shown in Fig. 4. At the upper left is a graph of φ_G, the variance spectrum of the generator potential. Note that in this cell at this light intensity the generator

[1] This analytic expression was fit to the data by the choice of two parameters, the self-inhibitory time constant and self-inhibitory coefficient. The time constant was almost always 0.5 sec while the coefficient, which measured the magnitude of self-inhibition, had values from 2 to 5.

potential spectrum shows little peaking. Below is the predicted impulse rate variance spectrum, φ_N^*. The predicted spectrum is obtained by multiplying each value of the variance spectrum of the generator potential by its appropriate weighting factor—the squared amplitude of $S(f)$ measured in the same cell. The features introduced by filtering are apparent in the figure. The variance spectrum, φ_N^*, is peaked, with a low frequency and high frequency cutoff on either side of the peak.

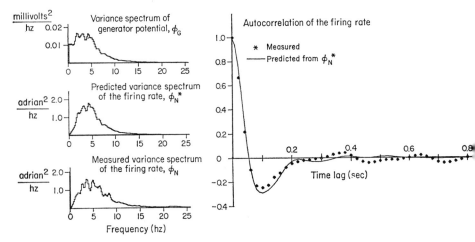

FIGURE 4. Prediction and measurement of the variance spectrum of the impulse rate. Shown in the left column are φ_G and φ_N, the measured generator potential and impulse rate variance spectra. Between them is φ_N^*, the predicted spectrum, obtained by multiplying φ_G by $| S(f) |^2$. The autocorrelations, predicted and measured, are shown at the right. The average rate was 23 impulses/sec.

The measured variance spectrum of the impulse rate, φ_N, is shown at the bottom left of Fig. 4. It appears to have almost exactly the same shape and magnitude as the predicted spectrum, φ_N^*.

We can estimate the degree of agreement of these two spectra, φ_N and φ_N^*, by comparing the differences between them with the amount of error inherent in the calculation of spectral estimates from data. As shown in texts on spectral analysis, if a stochastic process has a Gaussian distribution function, each spectral component is a random variable with a chi-squared distribution. The number of degrees of freedom for this chi-squared distribution is set by the total amount of data and the degree of frequency resolution in the spectrum (see Jenkins and Watts, 1968; Welch, 1967). When this distribution of the spectral components is used, one can calculate a standard error for the variance spectrum. In this experiment 15 estimates were averaged and were smoothed to reduce the standard error by half. This results in an approximate standard error of 10% of the magnitude of the spectral component (the standard error is a constant fraction of the size of the spectral component—the larger the component, the larger the absolute magnitude of the standard error). The predicted and measured variance spectra, φ_N^* and φ_N, agree within 2 SE, over most of the frequency range.

The agreement of the measured variance spectrum of the impulse rate with the predicted spectrum confirms the working hypothesis with which we began. The temporal pattern of variability in the impulse rate originates in the generator potential "noise" and is filtered and therefore shaped by the impulse-firing mechanism.

PREDICTED AND MEASURED AUTOCORRELATION The autocorrelation of the impulse rate for measured data agrees well with the predicted autocorrelation which is calculated from φ_N^*. The two autocorrelation functions, measured and predicted, are shown on the right side of Fig. 4. As shown in the section on Analytical Methods, the autocorrelation of the impulse rate can be calculated from the variance spectrum. It measures in the time domain what the spectrum measures in the frequency domain—the temporal texture of a random process. Since the variance spectra, φ_N and φ_N^*, agree within the inherent error of spectral estimation, it is no accident that the predicted and measured autocorrelation functions also correspond very closely to one another.

It is clear from Fig. 4 that the current-to-firing rate mechanism strongly affects the shape of the variance spectrum. The impulse rate spectrum is far more peaked than the variance spectrum of the generator potential. The filtering of the generator potential also changes the relative amount of variability in the impulse rate; i.e., the size of the coefficient of variation.

The shape of the frequency response, $S(f)$, causes the coefficient of variation of the impulse rate to be greater than the coefficient of variation of the generator potential. Since middle range frequencies are amplified relative to constant or very low frequency stimuli, $S(f)$ is larger than 1 over most of the frequency range where the variance spectrum of the generator potential has large values (cf. Fig. 4). This results in enhancement of the fluctuations relative to the mean—in other words, a higher coefficient of variation for the impulse rate than for the generator potential.

Steady-State Fluctuations and the Frequency Response

Dodge et al. (1968) found that for steady-state fluctuations of the generator potential

$$\varphi_G(f) = \alpha \, | \, G(f) \, |^2 \qquad (2)$$

where $G(f)$ is the frequency response for the transduction, light to generator potential. Also, Knight et al. (1970) showed that $N(f) = S(f) \, G(f)$, where

$N(f)$ is the frequency response of the transduction from light to impulse rate. With the use of these findings and equation 1, we can derive

$$\varphi_N(f) = \beta \mid N(f) \mid^2 \tag{3}$$

The proportionality between variance spectrum and squared frequency response should be carried over to the impulse rate from the generator potential. The results of an experiment which tests this prediction are shown in Fig. 5.

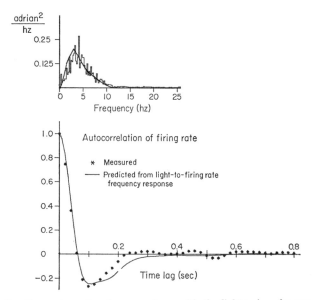

FIGURE 5. Comparison of variance spectrum with the light-to-impulse rate frequency response $N(f)$. This experiment was done with optical stimulation of a single eccentric cell with a small spot of light, steady to measure φ_N and modulated to measure $N(f)$. In the upper graph the jagged curve is φ_N and the smooth curve is $\mid N \mid^2$. $\mid N(f) \mid^2$ is plotted on a vertical scale such that the area under the curve will equal the area under the variance spectrum (the variance). Autocorrelations are shown below.

Probability Densities

Probability density functions for the impulse rate under conditions of steady stimulation by light are well fit by Gaussian functions. This finding is important because the distribution of membrane potential deviations is also Gaussian under the same stimulus conditions.

Fig. 6 shows an impulse rate histogram (estimate of probability density function) and a generator potential histogram for the response to a light whose intensity was 1000 times brighter than the threshold intensity for maintained impulse firing. Both these histograms approximate Gaussian functions; their skewness is close to zero, their kurtosis (fourth moment/ variance squared) is close to three. The interval distribution is positively skewed when the impulse rate has a Gaussian distribution, as one would expect (Shapley, 1970).

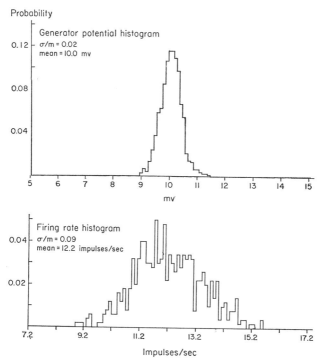

FIGURE 6. Generator potential and impulse rate histograms for the response to steady light. Both responses were recorded from cells stimulated by light intensity 100 to 1000 times brighter than the threshold for maintained discharge. Bin width for the generator potential is 0.1 mv, for the impulse rate 0.1 impulse/sec.

A marked effect occurred in the statistics of a cell stimulated by electric current, which was allowed to dark adapt for over 10 min. The statistics of the impulse rate histogram changed very greatly during dark adaptation, an effect which very convincingly reinforces the view that fluctuations in membrane potential cause the observed variability in impulse firing.

When the cell was light-adapted the membrane potential fluctuations in the dark were very small and symmetrical about the resting potential; under the same conditions the impulse rate histogram was symmetric and approximately Gaussian in shape. The source of the small variability in the firing of a light-adapted, current-driven eccentric cell has not been investigated. I mention the statistical characteristics of the small variability under these experimental conditions to contrast them with the marked changes which occur during dark adaptation.

During dark adaptation, the striking effect which occurs is an increase in the variance of the impulse rate (previously observed by Ratliff et al., 1968), and a marked increase in the skewness of the impulse rate distribution. Under the same conditions of dark adaptation, it is well-known that the membrane potential distribution changes its character, because of the low rate of appearance of large, discrete slow potentials (Yeandle, 1957; Adolph, 1964). These discrete events were occurring at the rate of 2/sec in the eccentric cell whose impulse rate distribution is graphed in Fig. 7. The distribution of the membrane potential in an eccentric cell under the same conditions of dark adapta-

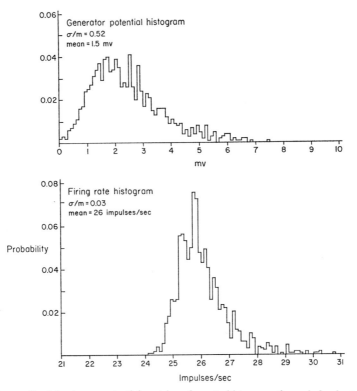

FIGURE 7. Membrane potential and impulse rate histograms for a dark-adapted cell driven by steady current. This figure demonstrates the skewness of the membrane potential and impulse rate in a thoroughly dark-adapted cell. The skewness results from the slow rate of discrete slow potentials which tend to depolarize the cell.

tion is shown in the upper graph of Fig. 7. The skewness of the membrane potential is very obvious. The values of the parameter of skewness, the ratio third moment squared divided by variance cubed, for the histograms of membrane potential and impulse rate, are both about 2.5. This is very significantly different from the value of zero expected for a symmetrical distribution. Both the membrane potential distribution and the impulse rate distribution are positively skewed; the impulse interval distribution is markedly negatively skewed under these conditions.

This large increase in skewness during dark adaptation in the probability density functions of both the membrane potential and impulse rate reinforces even more the idea that random fluctuations in membrane potential underlie the major portion of variability in the impulse rate.

DISCUSSION

The preceding results confirm the hypothesis that membrane potential "noise" causes the variability of the impulse rate. The amount of variability in the response to light, and its temporal pattern, result from the filtering of the generator potential by the current-to-firing rate mechanism.

The current-to-firing rate process is composed of two separate mechanisms—an integration mechanism and self-inhibition (Knight et al., 1970). These two mechanisms account for the shape of $S(f)$, the frequency response for the current-to-firing rate transduction, and therefore they help to shape the variance spectrum of the impulse rate.

The transformation of depolarization into impulse rate is accurately described by an integrate-and-fire model (Knight et al., 1970). In this model, membrane potential (or current through the membrane) is integrated until the integral reaches a threshold and then an impulse is fired and the integral is reset to zero.

There is also a stage of negative feedback or self-inhibition in the *Limulus* eccentric cell (Stevens, 1964; Knight et al., 1970). Purple (1964) showed that each nerve impulse in an eccentric cell triggers a long-lasting hyperpolarization, accompanied by an increase in the conductance of the membrane. The time course of the hyperpolarization is a decaying exponential with a time constant of about half a second.

Self-inhibition is the source of the low frequency cutoff in $S(f)$, and consequently in $\varphi_N(f)$. In other words, self-inhibition causes the negative correlation in the autocorrelation of the impulse rate (see Figs. 4 and 5). Similar persistent negative correlations have been noticed by other investigators working on different neurons; e.g., the work of Geisler and Goldberg (1966) on cells in the superior olivary complex of the cat. As I have already implied, a negative feedback like self-inhibition also has the effect of increasing the coefficient of variation of the impulse rate by inhibiting the DC component of the underlying generator potential more than it inhibits the fluctuations.

While self-inhibition and temporal integration affect the shape of $\varphi_N(f)$, the main determinant of the magnitude and bandwidth of $\varphi_N(f)$ is the generator potential "noise," as characterized by $\varphi_G(f)$ (see Fig. 4).

The generator potential, a depolarization induced by light, appears to be quantized, as if each effectively absorbed photon triggered a unit slow potential fluctuation. The occurrence of the discrete potentials is a random process, presumably reflecting the randomness in the arrival and absorption of photons. The generator potential is therefore the summation of randomly occurring, similarly shaped discrete events. Consequently, at all light intensities, the generator potential has an inherent noisy component (Dodge et al., 1968).

These discrete slow potentials adapt with light intensity, becoming smaller and briefer at higher light intensities (Yeandle, 1957; Adolph, 1964; Dodge et al., 1968). Dodge et al. (1968) showed that the characteristics of the generator potential at all light intensities, its frequency response and variance spectrum, $\varphi_G(f)$, could be accounted for by the summation of the discrete potentials. The effect of intensity on $\varphi_N(f)$ is roughly commensurate with its effect on $\varphi_G(f)$. Thus, diminution of quantal responses at higher light intensities results in a lower coefficient of variation of the impulse rate. An analogous effect should be observed in other neurons; i.e., reduction in the coefficient of variation of the impulse rate whenever there is adaptation in the size of excitatory synaptic potentials. Synaptic "adaptation" might be caused by fatigue, or by presynaptic inhibition. The effect of adaptation on variability of impulse discharge has already been shown by Stein (1967) for a general neuron model and inferred by H. B. Barlow and Levick (1969) from a mathematical model for mammalian retinal ganglion cells.

Finally, my direct measurements of the underlying processes which cause neuronal variability support some of the theoretical speculations of others. In particular, they reinforce the conjectures of Walløe (1968) and Matthews and Stein (1969), that the pattern of the interval serial correlation coefficients should be related to underlying periodicities in the membrane potential.

I am very grateful to Frederick Dodge, Bruce Knight, Floyd Ratliff, and H.K. Hartline for their help and encouragement. This work formed part of a dissertation submitted to The Rockefeller University in fulfillment of the requirements for a Ph.D. degree.

This work was supported by grant B 864 from the National Institute of Neurological Diseases and Blindness, grant GB 654 OX from the National Science Foundation, and by a National Science Foundation Graduate Fellowship.

Received for publication 20 August 1970.

REFERENCES

ADOLPH, A. 1964. Spontaneous slow potential fluctuations in the *Limulus* photoreceptor. *J. Gen. Physiol.* **48**:297.

BARLOW, H. B., and W. R. LEVICK. 1969. Changes in the maintained discharge with adaptation level in the cat retina. *J. Physiol. (London).* **202**:699.

BARLOW, R. 1969. Inhibitory fields in the *Limulus* lateral eye. *J. Gen. Physiol.* **54**:383.

BARTLETT, M. S. 1955. An Introduction to Stochastic Processes. Cambridge University Press, Cambridge.

BEHRENS, M. E., and V. J. WULFF. 1965. Light-initiated responses of retinula and eccentric cells in the *Limulus* lateral eye. *J. Gen. Physiol.* **48**:1081.

BISCOE, T. J., and A. TAYLOR. 1962. Irregularity of discharge of carotid body chemoreceptors. *J. Physiol. (London).* **163**:4P.

BLACKMAN, R. B., and J. W. TUKEY. 1958. The Measurement of Power Spectra. Dover Publications, Inc., New York.

BULLER, A., J. NICHOLLS, and G. STRÖM. 1953. Spontaneous fluctuation in excitability in the muscle spindle of the frog. *J. Physiol. (London).* **122**:409.

BURNS, B. D. 1968. The Uncertain Nervous System. Edward Arnold (Publishers) Ltd., London.

COOLEY, J. W., P. A. W. LEWIS, and P. D. WELCH. 1967. Historical notes on the fast Fourier transform. *IEEE Trans. Audio Electroacoustics.* **AU-15**:76.

DODGE, F. A. 1968. Excitation and inhibition in the eye of *Limulus. In* Optical Data Processing by Organisms and Machines. W. REICHARDT, Academic Press, Inc., New York.

DODGE, F. A., B. W. KNIGHT, and J. TOYODA. 1968. Voltage noise in *Limulus* visual cells. *Science (Washington).* **160**:88.

FUORTES, M. G. F. 1959. Initiation of impulses in visual cells. *J. Physiol. (London).* **148**:14.

GEISLER, C., and J. GOLDBERG. 1966. A stochastic model of the repetitive activity of neurons. *Biophys. J.* **6**:53.

JENKINS, G., and D. WATTS. 1968. Spectral Analysis and Its Applications. Holden-Day, Inc., San Francisco.

KIANG, N. 1965. Discharge Patterns of Single Fibers in the Cat's Auditory Nerve. Massachusetts Institute of Technology Press, Cambridge, Mass.

KNIGHT, B. 1969. Frequency response for sampling integrator and for voltage to frequency converter. *In* Systems Analysis in Neurophysiology (notes from a conference held at Brainerd, Minn. C. Terzuolo, editor).

KNIGHT, B., J. TOYODA, and F. A. DODGE. 1970. A quantitative description of the dynamics of excitation and inhibition in the eye of *Limulus. J. Gen. Physiol.* **56**:421.

MATTHEWS, P. B. C., and R. B. STEIN. 1969. The regularity of primary and secondary muscle spindle afferent discharges. *J. Physiol. (London).* **202**:59.

MILKMAN, N., and R. SCHOENFELD. 1966. A digital programmer for stimuli and computer control in physiological experiments. *Ann. N. Y. Acad. Sci.* **128**:861.

PARZEN, E. 1962. Stochastic Processes. Holden-Day, Inc., San Francisco.

PURPLE, R. 1964. The Integration of Excitatory and Inhibitory Influences in the Eccentric Cell of the Eye of *Limulus*. Ph.D. Thesis. The Rockefeller University, New York.

RATLIFF, F., H. K. HARTLINE, and D. LANGE. 1968. Variability of interspike intervals in optic nerve fibers of *Limulus*: Effect of light and dark adaptation. *Proc. Nat. Acad. Sci. U.S.A.* **60**:392.

RICE, S. O. 1944. Mathematical analysis of random noise. *Bell Teleph. Syst. J.* **23**:282.

SHANNON, C. E., and W. WEAVER. 1949. The Mathematical Theory of Communication. University of Illinois Press, Urbana, Ill.

SHAPLEY, R. 1969. Fluctuations in the response to light of visual neurons in *Limulus. Nature (London).* **221**:437.

SHAPLEY, R. 1970. Variability of Impulse Firing in Eccentric Cells of the *Limulus* Eye. Ph.D. Thesis. The Rockefeller University. New York.

STEIN, R. 1967. Some models of neuronal variability. *Biophys. J.* **7**:37.

STEIN, R., and P. B. C. MATTHEWS. 1965. Differences in variability of discharge frequency between primary and secondary muscle spindle afferent endings of the cat. *Nature (London)*. **208**:1217.

STEVENS, C. 1964. A Quantitative Theory of Neural Interaction: Theoretical and Experimental Investigations. Ph.D. Thesis. The Rockefeller University, New York.

WALLØE, L. 1968. Transfer of Signals through a Second Order Sensory Neuron. Ph.D. Thesis. University of Oslo, Oslo.

WATERMAN, T. H., and C. A. G. WIERSMA. 1954. The functional relation between retinal cells and optic nerve in *Limulus*. *J. Exp. Zool.* **126**:59.

WELCH, P. D. 1967. The use of fast Fourier transform for the estimation of power spectra: A method based on time averaging over short, modified periodograms. *IEEE Trans. Audio Electroacoustics*. **AU-15**:70.

WERNER, G., and V. MOUNTCASTLE. 1965. Neural activity in mechanoreceptive cutaneous afferents: Stimulus response relations, Weber functions, and information transmission. *J. Neurophysiol.* **28**:359.

YEANDLE, S. 1957: Studies on the Slow Potential and the Effects of Cations on the Electrical Responses of the *Limulus* Ommatidium (with an Appendix on the Quantal Nature of the Slow Potential). Ph.D. Thesis. The Johns Hopkins University, Baltimore.

Effects of lateral inhibition on fluctuations of the impulse rate

ROBERT SHAPLEY

The Rockefeller University, New York, N.Y.

Reprinted from the JOURNAL OF GENERAL PHYSIOLOGY, May 1971
Vol. 57, no. 5, pp. 557-575

ABSTRACT   Inhibition from neighboring eccentric cells has an effect on the variability of firing of a given eccentric cell. The reduction in the average impulse rate which is caused by inhibition decreases the variance of the impulse rate. However, this reduction of the average rate increases the coefficient of variation of the impulse rate. Inhibitory synaptic noise should add to the low frequency portion of the variance spectrum of the impulse rate. This occurs because of the slow time course of inhibitory synaptic potentials. As a consequence, inhibition decreases the signal-to-noise ratio for low frequency modulated stimuli.

INTRODUCTION

I have shown in the preceding paper (Shapley, 1971) that, for *Limulus* eccentric cells, stimulated by spots of light which act as purely excitatory stimuli, the variability of neuronal discharge is caused by fluctuations of the generator potential.

As is the case in many other neurons, an eccentric cell can also be influenced by neuronal interaction; illumination of neighboring ommatidia in the *Limulus* eye causes inhibition of the impulse discharge (Ratliff et al., 1963). This lateral inhibition is similar to postsynaptic inhibition in other nervous systems (Purple, 1964; Eccles, 1964). The effects of inhibitory interaction on randomness in the impulse firing of the *Limulus* cells should be similar to the effects of inhibition on other neurons. The effects of inhibition on the variability of neuronal discharge have hardly been studied in other systems.

In this paper, I will present results concerning the effects of lateral inhibition on randomness in impulse firing of eccentric cells. The time course, size, and rate of occurrence of excitatory and inhibitory postsynaptic potentials are important in determining the properties of variability in impulse firing. These factors which influence variability will differ from animal to animal, and from cell to cell within the same animal. For this reason, it is

577

obvious that details of the statistical properties of the activity of *Limulus* visual sensory neurons need not be identical to the characteristics of nerve cells performing different functions in other animals. Nevertheless, there should be general usefulness for the methods of analysis and the qualitative conclusions of this research on the stochastic component of neuronal response resulting from postsynaptic inhibition.

METHODS

These experiments were done mainly on single nerve fiber preparations from the horseshoe crab optic nerve. Techniques for *Limulus* optic nerve fiber recording have been described in the previous paper (Shapley, 1971).

For one part of this investigation, antidromic electrical stimulation of the optic nerve was used to produce lateral inhibition of a single fiber whose activity was monitored. The method used was similar to that described by Tomita (1958) and Lange (1965). The optic nerve was stimulated in air with a bipolar electrode made out of platinum wire. Brief pulses from a pulse generator (Tektronix 161) were passed through an isolation transformer and thence to the stimulating electrodes. Supramaximal electric shocks produced volleys of antidromically conducted nerve impulses in most of the optic nerve fibers. A single fiber was dissected from the nerve at a point closer to the eye than the stimulating electrodes so that it was spared the electrical stimulus.

A typical experiment proceeded as follows. A response of a single unit to a 20 sec light stimulus was recorded. After 2 min the response of the same unit to an identical light stimulus was recorded while the steady antidromic electrical shocks were being produced. The alternating sequence, first control, then inhibited fibers, was repeated 5 to 10 times in order to obtain sufficient data.

In other experiments I measured the effect of naturally evoked lateral inhibition; i.e., lateral inhibition produced by neighboring spots of light. For these experiments the light stimulus on the test receptor was provided by a small single optical wave guide. At a nearby region of the horseshoe crab eye a bundle of light guides was aligned to stimulate a group of receptors. I attempted to place this larger inhibitory spot in order to get the maximum inhibitory effect. The inhibitory light was turned on at the same moment as the test light. Control and inhibitory runs were interleaved, as above.

Measurement of nerve impulse intervals, computation of impulse rate from pulse intervals, calculation of variance spectra—all were performed as previously described (Shapley, 1971). As in the previous paper, eccentric cells were selected for analysis in the event that their responses were statistically stationary. This excluded those cells (a small fraction) whose variability changed with time during an experimental run or from one run to another.

THEORETICAL BACKGROUND

There is a fairly comprehensive mathematical model for the operation of *Limulus* eccentric cells (Knight et al., 1970). A schematic diagram of the model is shown in Fig. 1. The different component processes which determine the response of the cell are labeled in the block diagram. These are: Generator potential, frequency modulation (FM), Self-inhibition, and Lateral inhibition. The first three components and their effects on firing rate variability have been discussed before (Shapley, 1971). In this section I will present the expected effects of lateral inhibition on the stochastic component of neuronal response. Then we can compare the observed results of experiments with these theoretical predictions.

Lateral Inhibition

Lateral inhibition of a given cell's activity is produced by the firing of nerve impulses by neighboring eccentric cells in the *Limulus* compound eye. Knight et al. (1970) have shown that the inhibitory synaptic potential resulting from a single nerve impulse in an inhibitory nerve fiber is biphasic, with a brief

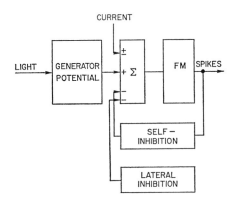

FIGURE 1. Model of an eccentric cell with lateral inhibition. This figure is adapted from Dodge (1968).

depolarizing phase and a prolonged inhibitory hyperpolarization. The time constant for decay of the lateral inhibitory synaptic potential is about one-third of a second, as opposed to about one-half second for decay of a self-inhibitory synaptic potential. The unit lateral inhibitory postsynaptic potential can be considered to be the impulse response of the lateral inhibitory synapse. Toyoda measured both the impulse response and frequency response of the lateral inhibitory synapse (which are related to each other by the Fourier transform). The two functions are shown in Fig. 2. The temporal characteristics of lateral inhibition play an important part in d etermining its effect on neuronal variability, as will be shown in the ensuing discussion.

Variance–Firing Rate Relation

The primary effect of inhibition is to lower the mean firing rate by reducing the average level of membrane depolarization. Such a change in the average rate of firing will affect the variance of the impulse rate. This can be viewed in two ways, in the time domain and in the frequency domain. One can consider that the length of an interval between nerve impulses is an averaging interval; fluctuations of the membrane potential which are rapid enough to be averaged out during the pulse interval will have only a small effect on pulse firing variability—the longer the interval, the more high frequency components will be averaged out. An alternative way of considering the same effect is to view the impulse-firing mechanism as a filter which has a

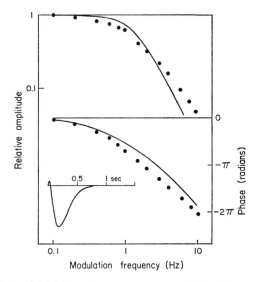

FIGURE 2. Lateral inhibition–frequency response and impulse response. The points were measured by imposing sinusoidal variations in firing of fibers in the optic nerve and measuring the amplitude and phase of the resulting modulation of the lateral inhibitory synaptic potential. The smooth curve is measured similarly, but with the impulse rate of the inhibited cell as the modulated variable. The insert is the impulse response, the Fourier transform of the measured frequency response. This figure is adapted from Dodge (1968).

high frequency cutoff set by the mean firing rate. For instance, as the impulse rate decreases, the bandpass of the filter is narrowed, and, consequently, higher frequency components are filtered out from the impulse rate. Although the latter approach has some limitations, it has proved to be useful for obtaining analytical predictions of the effect of mean impulse rate on the variability of the impulse rate.

The view of an integrate-and-fire mechanism as a linear filter must be applied with caution because of the phenomenon of side bands, or aliasing. These terms refer to the appearance of difference frequency components in the firing rate spectrum when the firing rate is modulated at frequencies which exceed half the mean firing rate. Aliasing does not affect the filter theory of the impulse-firing mechanism, because it is an empirical fact that the side band components do not contribute much variance to impulse rate fluctuations in eccentric cells.

In order to compute the effect of changing the average impulse rate, we must consider the filtering action of the current-to-firing rate mechanism. This involves the contributions of the integrate-and-fire mechanism and self-inhibition. As derived by Knight (1969) and Knight et al. (1970) the frequency response for the current-to-firing rate process is,

$$S(f) = \cfrac{(1 + K_s)(B(f))}{1 + K_s\left[1 - \cfrac{(1/\tau_s f_o)(1 - e^{2\pi i f/f_o})}{(e^{1/\tau_s f_o} - 1)(1 - e^{-(1/\tau_s + 2\pi i f)/f_o})}\right]} \tag{1}$$

$S(f)$ depends on the mean firing rate f_o, and the self-inhibitory coefficient, K_s, and time constant, τ_s. $B(f)$ is the frequency response of an integrate-and-fire device; it depends on f_o.

$$B(f) = \frac{1 - e^{-2\pi i f/f_o}}{2\pi i f/f_o}$$

I have been able to simplify the analytic expression for $S(f)$ by means of an approximation.

If we assume that $\tau_s f_o \gg 1$, which is true over a useful range of the response of eccentric cells, then $e^{1/\tau_s f_o} \approx 1 + 1/\tau_s f_o$, and we can write

$$S(f) \cong \cfrac{(1 + K_s)B(f)}{1 + \cfrac{K_s}{1 + B(-f)2\pi i f\tau_s}}$$

In fact, $S(f))$ can be further approximated to yield

$$S(f) \approx \cfrac{1 + K_s}{1 + \cfrac{K_s}{1 + 2\pi i f\tau_s}} B(f) \tag{2}$$

where the dependence on the mean firing rate is entirely contained in $B(f)$.[1] That equation (2) is a good approximation for $S(f)$ is shown in Fig. 3. $S(f)$ is computed for nominal values of K_s and τ_s, and two values for f_o: 10 adrians (impulses/sec) and 20 adrians. The amplitude and phase of the complex

[1] The approximation, equation (2), turns out to be a refinement of Stevens' original calculation (1964) for the frequency response of a neuron with self-inhibition. It is identical with Stevens' expression except for the important factor $B(f)$.

valued frequency response $S(f)$ are shown. The approximation for $S(f)$ based on equation (2) is plotted as points (+) on the solid curve. The latter is computed from the exact expression, equation (1), which has been shown to fit observed frequency responses. What the approximation ignores is the discrete nature of self-inhibition, the fact that self-inhibitory potentials are phased to the firing of nerve impulses. That it is a good approximation for typical parameter values tells us that the self-inhibitory potentials are long enough so that we can safely ignore the discreteness at moderate firing rates.

The approximate expression for the frequency response is a product of two parts: $B(f)$ which depends on the mean impulse rate, and a function which

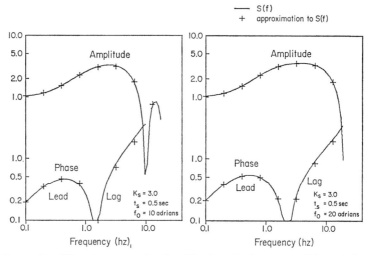

FIGURE 3. $S(f)$ and an approximation. The theoretical current-to-firing rate frequency response is plotted as the smooth curve against frequency. The approximation to $S(f)$ is plotted as crosses at several points on the curve. Values of the parameters are shown in the figure; K_s is the self-inhibitory coefficient, τ_s is the self-inhibitory time constant, f_0 is the mean impulse rate.

does not vary with mean rate. The approximation allows us to predict the effects of changes in mean rate in terms of a single function, $B(f)$.

We can do this by considering the variance spectrum of the impulse rate, $\varphi_N(f)$. As shown previously, the impulse rate variance spectrum is produced by filtering the variance spectrum of the generator potential, $\varphi_G(f)$, through the current-to-firing rate mechanism. This is expressed in the following equation

$$\varphi_N(f) = |S(f)|^2 \cdot \varphi_G(f).$$

Suppose the generator potential variance spectrum remains the same, but the mean impulse rate is changed. Call the original variance spectrum of the impulse rate $\varphi_{N1}(f)$, and the variance spectrum after the rate has been changed $\varphi_{N2}(f)$. Using the approximation of equation (2) and the same notation as for the spectra, $B_1(f)$ for the original impulse rate and $B_2(f)$ for the changed rate, we obtain the following expression

$$\frac{\varphi_{N2}(f)}{\varphi_{N1}(f)} = \frac{|B_2(f)|^2}{|B_1(f)|^2}$$

or

$$\varphi_{N2}(f) = \varphi_{N1}(f) \cdot \frac{|B_2(f)|^2}{|B_1(f)|^2}. \tag{3}$$

The variance can be calculated by integrating the variance spectrum with respect to frequency.

With the use of equation (3) we can calculate the change in variance with average impulse rate, all other variables held fixed. Given $\varphi_N(f)$ at a particular average impulse rate, we can predict the variance (and shape of the variance spectrum) for other mean impulse rates. The curve relating variance with average impulse rate is shown in Fig. 4. The variance increases monotonically with mean firing rate, other things being equal.

In order to check whether this method of calculating the variance–firing rate relation is theoretically correct, I simulated the problem with one of the neuronal analogues which are described in Appendix I. The neuronal analogue is an electronic device which was designed to simulate the mathematical model of the eccentric cell which was diagrammed in Fig. 1. The generator potential variance spectrum, $\varphi_G(f)$, for the neuronal analogue was held fixed while the impulse rate was varied by varying a constant voltage which was added to the noisy simulated generator potential at the summing point of the analogue. The variance and variance spectrum were computed from the impulse rate produced by the analogue. The points marked with an X on Fig. 4 are the values of the variance at different average impulse rates. The analytically calculated curve fits the points fairly well; this indicates that the assumptions used for the calculation are valid.

It is also interesting to consider the effect of varying the average impulse rate on the coefficient of variation of the impulse rate. This relation is also shown in the graph of Fig. 4; it was derived from the variance–firing rate curve. While the variance decreases with decreasing impulse rate, it decreases more slowly than the mean rate; this results in a net increase of the fraction standard deviation/mean, which is the coefficient of variation. Therefore, reductions in average impulse rate decrease the variance of neuronal firing while increasing the coefficient of variation.

Lateral Inhibition As a Noise Source

Besides its effect on the average impulse rate, lateral inhibition should add some extra randomness to the membrane potential of the eccentric cell. During natural stimulation by light, a group of inhibitory cells fire nerve impulses asynchronously and, to some extent, randomly in time. The summed inhibitory synaptic potential should fluctuate because of this effect. The in-

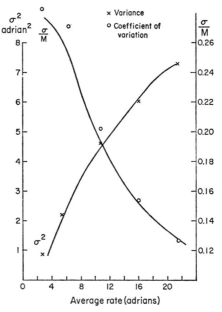

FIGURE 4. Variance (σ^2) and coefficient of variation (σ/m) as functions of mean impulse rate. Variances at different impulse rates of eccentric cell analogue are denoted x. The smooth curve for variance is calculated by filtering the impulse rate variance spectrum at one average rate (16.1 impulses/sec or adrians) by the appropriate filter characteristic for each average impulse rate. The coefficient of variation points (open circles) is calculated from the variance points, and the curve from the variance curve. Note the slope of these curves: positive for the variance, negative for the coefficient of variation.

hibitory synaptic noise is independent of the generator potential, so the variances of the two fluctuating components should add.

The characteristics of the summed inhibitory synaptic potential should depend on two factors: statistical properties of the occurrence of nerve impulses in inhibitory neurons, and the time course of the unit inhibitory synaptic potentials.

The point process which underlies the summed lateral inhibitory potential is a superposition of the impulse trains from each of the nerve fibers which have a synaptic effect. The statistics of this point process, which depends critically on the fact that the individual fibers are almost periodic, have an influence on the variance of the summed synaptic potential. This effect is discussed by Dodge et al. (1970). Summarizing this work we can say that the variance spectrum of the superimposed pulse train will have peaks at the average firing rates of the individual fibers, and at higher harmonics of these average rates. It will therefore differ from a Poisson point process whose variance spectrum is flat.

THE LATERAL INHIBITORY SYNAPSE AS A FILTER   The inhibitory potential, like all summed synaptic potentials, can be viewed as filtered shot noise. The shots are the presynaptic nerve impulses and the filter is the synapse; the unit inhibitory postsynaptic potential is the impulse response of the synaptic filter. The shape of a typical lateral inhibitory postsynaptic potential is shown in Fig. 2; also shown in that figure is the frequency response of the inhibitory synapse. The low pass character of this filter tends to reduce high frequency periodic components in the summed inhibitory potential.

A consequence of the low pass characteristic of the lateral inhibitory synapse is that whatever inhibitory fluctuations there are must be very low frequency fluctuations. So we expect to see additional low frequency components in the impulse rate variance spectrum in an eccentric cell which is influenced by lateral inhibition.

We can get definite predictions for this complicated phenomenon, the effect of inhibitory interaction on neuronal variability, by using the analogue of the eccentric cell (described in Appendix I). Typical neuronal firing in response to purely excitatory stimuli can be simulated. Then a good imitation of naturally occurring lateral inhibition can be produced by feeding a multiple fiber pulse train recorded from a *Limulus* eye into the inhibitory synapse of the analogue.

The results of such an analogue experiment are summarized in the variance spectra of Fig. 5. The control spectrum, characteristic of firing which results from purely excitatory stimuli, shows the low frequency cutoff imposed by self-inhibition and the high frequency cutoff resulting from the integrate-and-fire mechanism. The spectrum of the inhibited impulse rate shows an increase in the size of low frequency components because of added inhibitory "noise" and a lowered high frequency cutoff as a result of the reduction of average impulse rate. If our model is correct, the same kind of change in the pattern of neuronal randomness should be observed in *Limulus* eccentric cells which are inhibited by light-evoked lateral inhibition. Observations on these effects are presented in the next section.

RESULTS

Effect of Reduction in Mean Rate

Inhibition produced by antidromic electrical stimulation reduces the variance of the impulse rate. When the antidromic shock rate is high enough, i.e. greater than 10/sec, the steady-state summed inhibitory potential ought to be practically constant, with very small ripple at the shock rate. Therefore, the change in variance with "antidromic inhibition" should be a measure of the effect on variance of changing the average impulse rate.

The data from such an experiment are displayed in Fig. 6. Two sample records of impulse rate are shown: the lower record is control firing in response to a purely excitatory light stimulus, the upper record is firing in

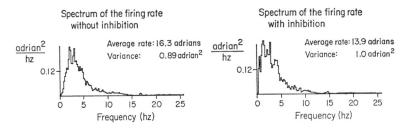

FIGURE 5. Control and inhibited variance spectra, prediction from analogue. The variance spectrum of the inhibited firing has larger low frequency components in the variance, and a more abrupt high frequency cutoff because of the reduction in average rate. These spectra were calculated from data produced by the eccentric cell analogue.

response to the same stimulation by light while the cell is also undergoing steady inhibition elicited by antidromic electric shock of the optic nerve.

The variance of the antidromically inhibited impulse rate is 60% of the variance of the control rate. This drop in variance is associated with a reduction in average impulse rate of 5.2 adrians. The magnitude of the variance reduction predicted by the filter model for the impulse firing mechanism is 59% of the control. The agreement, both qualitatively and quantitatively, of the mathematical model with this experimental result is strong support for the theory.

What seems at first a simpler and more straightforward method for controlling the firing rate, namely DC current injection through a microelectrode, has proved to have more complicated effects than antidromic inhibition. This seems to occur because DC current injected at the cell soma affects the nearby photoreceptor membrane while the inhibitory synaptic potential, which occurs at a point far from the photoreceptor, does not. The inhibitory potential occurs at the point of synaptic contact between eccentric cells, which is close to the impulse firing mechanism and far from the cell soma and photoreceptor membrane (Purple, 1964).

Lateral Inhibition Produced by Light

Lateral inhibition produced by stimulating a neighboring group of receptors with light has a more complex effect than the mere reduction in average impulse rate produced by antidromic inhibition. A record of data

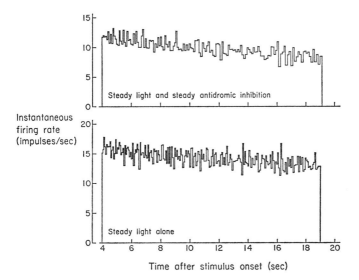

FIGURE 6. Data from an experiment with steady inhibition produced by antidromic electrical stimulation of the optic nerve. The lower record is a response of the cell to excitation by light. The upper record is obtained by using the same excitatory stimulus while shocking the optic nerve at a rate of 20 per sec to produce steady inhibition. The variance of the inhibited firing is reduced compared to the uninhibited firing.

from an experiment which demonstrates this is shown in Fig. 7. The impulse rate of a *Limulus* optic nerve fiber is shown. At time zero a small light illuminated the test receptor. At 4 sec a large spot of light stimulated a neighboring group of receptors and the test cell is inhibited by their activity. Both the pattern and magnitude of the variability in the firing rate were changed by the light-evoked inhibition.

The nature of the effects produced by lateral inhibition can be seen by examination of variance spectra of the impulse rate. Impulse rate spectra for control and inhibited firing are shown in Fig. 8 for two cells which are representative of the many cells on which these measurements were made. The change in the shape of the variance spectra, because of the presence of

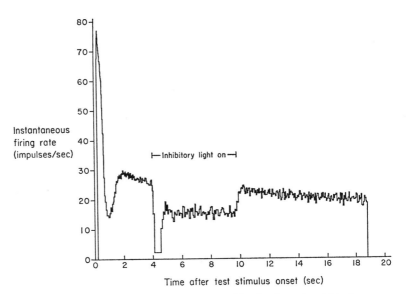

FIGURE 7. Lateral inhibition produced by illumination of neighboring receptors. Shown is the response to excitatory stimulation by light, of 19 sec duration, and superimposed inhibitory flash, of 6 sec duration starting 4 sec after the onset of the excitatory stimulus. In this case the variance is increased by the presence of inhibition.

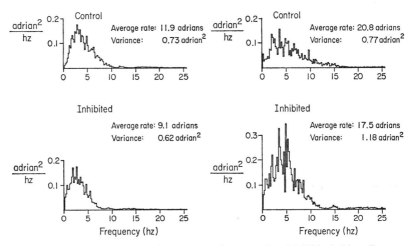

FIGURE 8. Impulse rate variance spectra for control and inhibited firing. Spectra are shown for two different cells. The control spectra are the response of each cell to a purely excitatory stimulus (small steady light). The spectra labeled inhibited are from the response of the cell to the excitatory stimulus presented simultaneously with a stimulus which evoked lateral inhibition (large neighboring spot of light).

lateral inhibition, is very much in agreement with the theoretical predictions advanced in the previous section; to see this, compare Fig. 8 with Fig. 5.

In one of the cases shown, the variance increased during inhibition, in the other it decreased during inhibition. This occurred because the naturally evoked inhibition produced two opposing influences on the variance. Lateral inhibition tends to decrease variance by its reduction of the mean rate, and increase variance by adding an additional noise source to the membrane potential. These two opposing influences can sometimes result in a net increase in variance though more often the balance is on the side of a reduction. Because these effects take place at opposite ends of the variance spectrum, they may be clearly seen in the spectra of Fig. 8.

In both these experiments, reduction of the mean impulse rate by inhibition caused a filtering out of higher frequency components. In opposition to this effect, the noise from inhibition added to low frequency components in the fluctuations of the impulse rate.

Relation between Variance Spectrum and Frequency Response

In the previous paper (Shapley, 1971, equation 3) proportionality was demonstrated between the variance spectrum of the impulse rate, $\varphi_N(f)$, and the squared amplitude of the frequency response for the transduction from light to impulse rate, $N(f)$. In those experiments there was no lateral inhibition because the stimuli were restricted to single ommatidia. Lateral inhibition markedly affects the relation between the frequency response, $N(f)$, and the variance spectrum of steady-state fluctuations.

Fig. 9 shows the results of an experiment designed to measure this effect. The variance spectrum in Fig. 9 is the spectrum of the impulse rate in response to a large spot of steady light intensity. On the same scale, plotted as a smooth curve, is the squared amplitude of the response to sinusoidal modulation of the light at all modulation frequencies. A large spot of light was used in these experiments to provide a substantial amount of lateral inhibition.

In this experiment $\varphi_N(f)$ and $|N(f)|^2$ do not have the same shape, although for experiments in which the stimulus is a small spot of light, $\varphi_N(f)$ is roughly proportional to $|N(f)|^2$. The result of this experiment is consistent with the characteristics of lateral inhibition mentioned in the section on theoretical background. As a component of the response to modulated light, inhibition subtracts from the response to low frequency modulation while enhancing the response to midrange frequencies. As a noise source inhibition adds to the low frequency components of the variance spectrum.

The squared amplitude of the frequency response, $|N(f)|^2$, shows very marked peaking under the conditions of large spot illumination; this is the amplification phenomenon reported and explained by Ratliff et al. (1967, 1969).

Under these conditions the variance spectrum is relatively flat out to the cutoff frequency. This result implies that, in terms of the impulse rate, lateral inhibition reduces the signal-to-noise ratio[2] for low frequency modulated stimuli while maintaining, or even increasing the signal-to-noise ratio for stimuli at the tuning frequency, the peak frequency of the frequency response.

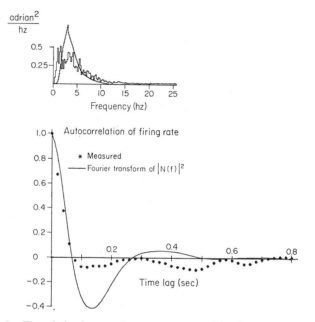

FIGURE 9. The relation between frequency response of the light-to-impulse rate process and the variance spectrum: the effect of lateral inhibition. $| N(f) |^2$ is the smooth curve and $\varphi_N(f)$ is the jagged curve in the upper graph. Below are the respective autocorrelations. Deviations between the spectra are obviously large and significant at low frequencies and at the peak frequency of the frequency response (corresponding to deviations in the autocorrelations at 0.4–0.5 sec, and at 0.15 sec, respectively). The reasons for these discrepancies are commented upon in the text.

DISCUSSION

Lateral inhibition in eccentric cells tends to lower variance of the impulse rate by reduction of average pulse rate; at the same time it tends to increase the variance by adding low frequency fluctuations to the membrane potential

---

[2] I am using the term signal-to-noise ratio in an unconventional way. By signal-to-noise ratio at a given frequency, I mean the ratio $(|N(f)|^2/\varphi_N(f))^{1/2}$. This is the signal-to-noise ratio of the signal plus noise passed through a filter optimally tuned to the frequency f; it is a measure of the optimal performance of which a system is capable. In an uninhibited eccentric cell, typically this ratio is a constant. The usual definition of a signal-to-noise ratio is $| N(f) | /\sigma_N$.

of the neuron. Both these effects are predicted from a phenomenological model of the eccentric cell which has been described above.

The competing effects of lateral inhibition most often result in a net decrease in variance of the impulse rate. The coefficient of variation of the impulse rate, the standard deviation/mean, is invariably increased by the introduction of inhibition.

There are several neuronal models in the literature which contain notions about the sources of neuronal variability similar to the eccentric cell model presented here (Stein, 1967; Gerstein and Mandelbrot, 1964; Geisler and Goldberg, 1966; Calvin and Stevens, 1968). Such models include the assumption that noise in the membrane potential, probably due to randomly arriving synaptic potentials, causes the randomness in neuronal firing. They differ somewhat in degree, but not in kind, from models which involve triggering single nerve impulses off presynaptic pulses arriving on several convergent channels—the pooling models of Bishop et al. (1964) and ten Hoopen (1966). All these models possess a common property, namely that postsynaptic summative inhibition will tend to make the impulse rate relatively more variable, i.e. increase the coefficient of variation, other things being equal. This assertion is proved for one particularly tractable neuronal model, the Gerstein-Mandelbrot model, in Appendix II.

Although the conclusion that relative variability increases with postsynaptic inhibition is implicit in many theories of neuronal mechanisms, it has not been emphasized before. The increased relative variability due to postsynaptic inhibition may be a price the nervous system has to pay for the increased discrimination and tuning, both spatial and temporal, provided by inhibition (Ratliff, 1965; Ratliff et al., 1967, 1969).

However, randomness introduced by inhibition also may serve to mask signals which are not physiologically important. For instance, lateral inhibition in eccentric cells decreases the signal-to-noise ratio (as defined in the section on Results) for low frequency flicker. But it tends to maintain or increase the signal-to-noise ratio at the peak frequency of the frequency response. The *Limulus* eye is sharply tuned to a modulation frequency of 3 hz, while the fluctuations introduced by inhibition are mainly concentrated in the frequency range of zero to 1 hz. So, while variability is designed into the *Limulus* visual system, it still may not degrade the transmission of signals which are important. This may be a design principle in other nervous systems.

APPENDIX I

Analogue Eccentric Cells

The effects on eccentric cells of mixed dynamic excitation and inhibition are complex. In order to simulate these effects, F. A. Dodge has designed electronic analogues of eccentric cells. These machines were used to perform the analogue experiments whose results were shown in Figs. 4 and 5. The analogues conform to the block diagram of Fig. 1.

Each section of the analogue includes a network which imitates, with electrical components, the dynamic behavior of the corresponding part of an eccentric cell. The analogue possesses a summing point which is the output of an operational amplifier. This summing amplifier has as inputs the "generator potential" section, the "current" input, "self-inhibition," and "lateral inhibition."

The output of the summing amplifier drives a voltage-to-frequency converter (FM) which is an integrator circuit in series with a monostable, fast recovery, multivibrator. The output of the multivibrator is the impulse output of the analogue; these pulses are fed back through the "self-inhibition" network to the summing amplifier, or to the "lateral inhibition" network of other analogue eccentric cells.

The generator potential section consists of five stages of low pass RC filtering. The self-inhibition is a single time constant low pass filter; i.e., it produces a decaying exponential for each pulse the analogue fires as a result of stimulation. The lateral inhibition section is somewhat more complicated since it must reproduce a biphasic impulse response. It consists of two different low pass filters in parallel, both feeding yet another filter. The faster of the two parallel stages is inverted before being added to the final filter in order to provide the early positive phase of lateral inhibition. The strengths of self-inhibition and lateral inhibition are set by potentiometers which control how much inhibition each impulse exerts.

The noisy generator potential was simulated with the use of a photomultiplier tube as a white noise generator; the photomultiplier output was fed into the generator potential section.

APPENDIX II

Inhibition and the Gerstein-Mandelbrot Model

WITH THE HELP OF BRUCE KNIGHT

Gerstein and Mandelbrot (1964) proposed that variability in neural impulse firing reflects the random bombardment of excitatory and inhibitory synaptic potentials on the neuron. They assumed that synaptic potentials are very brief, that they are integrated up to a threshold, and that each individual synaptic potential is so small that many are required to sum up to the firing threshold. They derived a probability density function for the impulse intervals, which they wrote:

$$P(t) = Kt^{-3/2} \exp \{-a/t - bt\}$$

K is a normalization constant. The parameter, a, measures the height of the threshold relative to the size of a single synaptic potential, and the parameter, b, measures the difference between the rate of occurrence of excitatory and inhibitory synaptic potentials; i.e., the net rate of drift towards threshold. In order to understand the effects of inhibition, one needs to calculate the coefficient of variation of the Gerstein-Mandelbrot model. This reduces to the problem of calculating the first and second moments of the probability density function.

In order to calculate the moments of $P(t)$ we have to evaluate integrals of the form

$$K \int_0^\infty dt \; t^{n-1/2} \exp\{-a/t - bt\} = \overline{t^{n+1}}$$

where $n = 0$ for the calculation of $\overline{t}$, $n = 1$ for calculation of $\overline{t^2}$.

We simplify the problem by introduction of the parameter, γ, such that $t = \gamma\tau$ and $\gamma = \sqrt{a/b}$. Then, $a/t + bt = a/\gamma\tau + b\gamma\tau = \sqrt{ab} \, (1/\tau + \tau)$. Also, let $z/2 = \sqrt{ab}$. The integrals for the calculation of the moments become

$$K\gamma^{n+1/2} \int_0^\infty d\tau \; \tau^{n-1/2} \exp\left\{-\frac{z}{2}\left(\frac{1}{\tau} + \tau\right)\right\} = \overline{t^{n+1}}.$$

It is possible to show, using the substitution, $\xi = \dfrac{1}{\tau}$, that

$$\int_0^\infty d\tau \; \tau^{n-1/2} \exp\left\{-\frac{z}{2}\left(\frac{1}{\tau} + \tau\right)\right\} = \int_0^\infty d\tau \; \tau^{-n-3/2} \exp\left\{-\frac{z}{2}\left(\frac{1}{\tau} + \tau\right)\right\}$$

or, if we say

$$F_n = K \int_0^\infty d\tau \; \tau^{n-1/2} \exp\left\{-\frac{z}{2}\left(\frac{1}{\tau} + \tau\right)\right\}$$

then $F_n = F_{-n-1}$ and in particular $F_o = F_{-1}$. This implies that $\overline{t} = \gamma = \left(\dfrac{a}{b}\right)^{1/2}$ since calculation of the first moment involves γF_o and calculation of the normalization integral involves F_{-1}.

In order to calculate the second moment, $\overline{t^2}$, we must do a little more. Differentiating with respect to z, we can establish the identity

$$F_{n+1} = -2F_n' - F_{n-1}.$$

It is also possible to show that

$$F_o(z) = \sqrt{2\pi} \; e^{-z}/\sqrt{z}$$

and to calculate from the above identity

$$F_1(z) = \sqrt{\frac{2\pi}{z}} \; e^{-z}\left(1 + \frac{1}{z}\right)$$

this leads finally to the conclusion that

$$\overline{t^2} = \gamma^2\left(1 + \frac{1}{z}\right)$$

where $z = 2 \sqrt{ab}$ or

$$\overline{t^2} = \frac{a}{b} \left(1 + \frac{1}{2 \sqrt{ab}} \right)$$

The variance of the intervals is

$$\sigma^2 = \overline{t^2} - (\bar{t})^2$$
$$= \gamma^2 \left(1 + \frac{1}{z} \right) - \gamma^2$$
$$= \gamma^2 / z$$
$$= \frac{1}{2} \frac{a^{1/2}}{b^{3/2}}$$

and the coefficient of variation is

$$\frac{(\sigma^2)^{1/2}}{\gamma} = \frac{1}{(4ab)^{1/4}}.$$

As Gerstein and Mandelbrot pointed out, when $b = 0$, i.e. when there is no net drift to threshold because inhibition on average balances out excitation, the moments become infinite. A consequence they did not explore is the divergence of the coefficient of variation as net drift approaches zero.

This calculation shows that with a constant, if b is decreased by the introduction of more inhibition, the coefficient of variation will be increased. The quantitative dependence of coefficient of variation on inhibition is not the same for the Gerstein-Mandelbrot model as for the eccentric cell model; the reason is that the Gerstein-Mandelbrot model has identical time constants for excitation and inhibition and the departure from this condition in the *Limulus* cells has significant effects on variability. Nevertheless, it is interesting that postsynaptic inhibition should have the same qualitative effect, an increase of the coefficient of variation, for two such different models of neuronal fluctuations.

I am very grateful to Frederick Dodge, Bruce Knight, Floyd Ratliff, and H. K. Hartline for their help and encouragement. This work formed part of a dissertation submitted to The Rockefeller University in fulfillment of the requirements for a Ph.D. degree.

This work was supported by grant B 864 from the National Institute of Neurological Diseases and Blindness, grant GB 654 OX from the National Science Foundation, and by a National Science Foundation Graduate Fellowship.

Received for publication 20 August 1970.

REFERENCES

BISHOP, P. O., W. R. LEVICK, and W. O. WILLIAMS. 1964. Statistical analysis of the dark discharge in lateral geniculate neurons. *J. Physiol. (London).* **170**:598.

CALVIN, W. H., and C. STEVENS. 1968. Synaptic noise and other sources of randomness in motoneuron interspike intervals. *J. Neurophysiol.* **31**:574.

DODGE, F. A. 1968. Excitation and inhibition in the eye of *Limulus*. *In* Optical Data Processing by Organisms and Machines. W. Reichardt, editor. Academic Press, Inc., New York.

DODGE, F. A., R. M. SHAPLEY, and B. W. KNIGHT. 1970. Linear systems analysis of the *Limulus* retina. *Behav. Sci.* **15**:24.

ECCLES, J. C. 1964. The Physiology of Synapses. Academic Press, Inc., New York.

GEISLER, C., and J. GOLDBERG. 1966. A stochastic model of the repetitive activity of neurons. *Biophys. J.* **6**:53.

GERSTEIN, G. L., and B. MANDELBROT. 1964. Random walk models for the spike activity of a single neuron. *Biophys. J.* **4**:41.

KNIGHT, B. W. 1969. Frequency response for sampling integrator and for voltage to frequency converter. *In* Systems Analysis in Neurophysiology. (notes from the Brainerd, Minn. conference led by C. Terzuolo).

KNIGHT, B., J. TOYODA, and F. A. DODGE. 1970. A quantitative description of the dynamics of excitation and inhibition in the eye of *Limulus*. *J. Gen. Physiol.* **56**:421.

LANGE, G. D. 1965. Dynamics of Inhibitory Interactions in the Eye of *Limulus*. Ph.D. Thesis. The Rockefeller University, New York.

PURPLE, R. 1964. The Integration of Excitatory and Inhibitory Influences in the Eccentric Cell of the Eye of *Limulus*. Ph.D. Thesis. The Rockefeller University, New York.

RATLIFF, F. 1965. Mach Bands: Quantitative Studies on Neural Networks in the Retina. Holden-Day, Inc., San Francisco.

RATLIFF, F., H. K. HARTLINE, and W. H. MILLER. 1963. Spatial and temporal aspects of retinal inhibitory interaction. *J. Opt. Soc. Amer.* **53**:110.

RATLIFF, F., B. KNIGHT, and N. GRAHAM. 1969. On tuning and amplification by lateral inhibition. *Proc. Nat. Acad. Sci. U.S.A.* **62**:733.

RATLIFF, F., B. KNIGHT, J. TOYODA, and H. K. HARTLINE. 1967. Enhancement of flicker by lateral inhibition. *Science. (Washington).* **158**:392.

SHAPLEY, R. 1971. Fluctuations of the impulse rate in *Limulus* eccentric cells. *J. Gen. Physiol.* **57**:539.

STEIN, R. 1967. Some models of neuronal variability. *Biophys. J.* **7**:37.

STEVENS, C. F. 1964. A Quantitative Theory of Neural Interaction. Ph.D. Thesis. The Rockefeller University, New York.

TEN HOOPEN, M. 1966. Multimodal interval distributions. *Kybernetik.* **3**:17.

TOMITA, T. 1958. Mechanism of lateral inhibition in the eye of *Limulus*. *J. Neurophysiol.* **21**:419.

Dynamics of encoding in a population of neurons

B. W. KNIGHT

The Rockefeller University, New York, N.Y.

Reprinted from the JOURNAL OF GENERAL PHYSIOLOGY, June 1972,
Vol. 59, no. 6, pp. 734-766

ABSTRACT   A simple encoder model, which is a reasonable idealization from known electrophysiological properties, yields a population in which the variation of the firing rate with time is a perfect replica of the shape of the input stimulus. A population of noise-free encoders which depart even slightly from the simple model yield a very much degraded copy of the input stimulus. The presence of noise improves the performance of such a population. The firing rate of a population of neurons is related to the firing rate of a single member in a subtle way.

1. INTRODUCTION

In a nervous system it is usual for extremely precise over-all results to arise from the functioning of a collection of components which have very modest precision in their individual construction and behavior. In the human ear, for example, such prodigies as "perfect pitch" are accomplished by a population of neurons which are somewhat haphazard in morphology, and which individually show ragged firing patterns. Apparently it is the collaboration of a large number of units which is responsible for the precision of the over-all result.

In the discussion below, we will examine several models of the process by which a stimulus is encoded to evoke a train of impulses in a single neuron. The behavior of a large population of such neurons will then be explored. The effects that result from variations among members of the population and from irregular behavior of individuals also will be investigated. The most important results will be deduced in section 2, almost without recourse to formal mathematics; the mathematically most difficult results will be presented last. A following paper will compare theoretical results developed here with experiment (Knight, 1972).

This investigation of encoding was undertaken in order to predict quantitatively the inhibitory postsynaptic potential in the visual cell (eccentric cell) of *Limulus*. Here the postsynaptic potential level arises from the pooled effect of nerve impulses arriving from numerous presynaptic neurons. In this well-

597

studied bit of nervous system the dynamics of the various neurological components are known (Knight et al., 1970) well enough to enable us, in principle, to predict the dynamics of the entire eye from stimulus to response. Each small illuminated region of the eye may be conceived as a subpopulation of identical neurons experiencing identical input. In order to determine the effect of this subpopulation upon a particular postsynaptic potential, we must have theoretical tools which enable us to obtain the population response from dynamical laws given initially for individual neurons. The results of this present study yield such tools, and predictions of considerable precision can in fact be made.

The same general problem arises frequently in the consideration of other neural systems. In the visual system of the primate, for example, continuous sensory input apparently is first coded into trains of discrete impulses at the level of the retinal ganglion cells. The next synapse along the major visual pathway, at the lateral geniculate nucleus, apparently is not of the highly convergent type but serves more nearly as a relay station. However, when the geniculate neurons arrive at the visual cortex they give rise to electrophysiological phenomena (Hubel and Wiesel, 1968) which suggest a convergence scheme that bears some close analogies to that of the *Limulus* eccentric cell. Several further layers of population convergence follow, giving rise to neural responses at successive levels of abstraction. Similar statements can be made concerning the secondary visual pathway which conducts impulse trains from the retinal ganglion cells to the superior colliculus.

A similar situation arises in the auditory system. If we conceptually divide the cochlear canal into short sections, we find over the lower half of the frequency range that the mechanical motion of a given section is transcribed into the level of impulse activity in the subpopulation of neurons which arise within it (Brugge et al., 1969), although any given neuron in that subpopulation contributes only a slight fraction of the total activity. The frequency bandwidth for the entire subpopulation greatly exceeds the repetition rate of a single component neuron.

Presumably within the vertebrate central nervous system the remote transmission of information typically is not entrusted to a single neuron, and the multiple channel considerations explored here again will be relevant.

At the motor end of the vertebrate nervous system such considerations again arise. For example, in the spinal stretch reflex circuits of the cat each stretch receptor appears to terminate on all motor neurons of a pool (Mendell and Henneman, 1968).

Three conclusions form the main theme of this paper. The first conclusion is that a particularly simple model for the encoding of a stimulus into nerve impulses yields the result that the variations with time of the firing rate of an entire population can be a perfect time replica of the stimulus. The population firing rate thus has the remarkable property that it may duplicate the stimulus with an indefinitely high degree of fidelity. The second conclusion is that the simple model is essentially unique in this respect, and that more realistic models of encoders are susceptible to spontaneous synchronization, a pathology which makes the temporal variation of the population firing rate a far less useful indicator of the shape of the stimulus. The third conclusion is that this pathology may be thwarted by a population of encoders whose impulse encoding is subject to chance fluctuations. Thus the fact that the encoders are heterogeneous and noisy becomes positively a virtue, which allows the temporal variation of the population firing rate to approach the ideal: a perfect replica of the shape of the stimulus.

In section 2 we will present the "simple integrate-and-fire" model of a neuron. There it will be observed that, in a large population of such neurons, the temporal variation of firing rate of the entire population is a perfect copy of the input stimulus. We will see that this result is still maintained when we introduce individual variations among the members of the population. Finally, we will generalize the model in a way which introduces random fluctuations into the spike train of each individual neuron, and show that the firing rate of the population will still remain a perfect copy of the input stimulus.

In section 3 we investigate the momentary firing rate of a single neuron in the population. If the stimulus is constant, the individual firing rate is proportional to population firing rate. However, if the stimulus is time varying, the single-neuron rate is *not* in fixed proportion to the population rate, nor is it a faithful replica of the input stimulus. It shows two distinct sorts of distortion. The first is nonlinearity in response to large stimulus fluctuations. The second distortion is a phase shift and amplitude attenuation in response to stimulus fluctuations at high frequency. These distortions can be very important when one gathers impulse data from a single nerve fiber, and thereafter tries to deduce the level of impulse activity in an entire population.

In section 4 a determining relationship is discovered between the individual neuron impulse rate and that of a whole population of identical neurons. The result is independent of the impulse encoding model, so long as that model is deterministic (not probabilistic).

Section 5 introduces the "forgetful integrate-and-fire" model for neuron firing. One model feature—infinitely long memory—of the simple integrate-and-fire model, is removed. The introduction of slow decay in memory has slight effect on the single neuron firing rate, but an important new feature appears in the population firing rate: at certain stimulus frequencies, the response of the population is disproportionately large so that the population response is no longer a perfect copy of the stimulus time-course.

Section 6 investigates the response of the forgetful integrate-and-fire model neuron to a periodic stimulus of finite amplitude; emphasis is placed on the phenomenon of "phase locking." Unlike the simple integrate-and-fire case, a population of forgetful neurons will tend to "fall into step," and all fire synchronously at a particular point in the stimulus cycle. The result of section 5, that certain infinitesimal periodic variations in the stimulus lead to disproportionately large responses, was the first hint of this phenomenon.

Section 7 discusses a general theory of the behavior of deterministic encoders in response to periodic stimuli. A ready-made mathematical machinery (created for a different reason) already exists for this problem. A general conclusion emerges: there are two distinct classes of impulse encoders, those which show the tendency to phase lock and those which do not. The class which do not are a slight generalization of the simple integrate-and-fire model, and share the feature of indefinitely extended memory. A population of encoders which do phase lock give the worst possible departure from a perfect copy of the stimulus: their response is in the form of synchronized bursts of impulses, which neither delimit the form of the input stimulus, nor yield more information than does the response of a single encoder. Such encoders also may be brought to the synchronized condition by stimuli which are not periodic.

Section 8 investigates a population of probabilistic (or "stochastic") encoders. A population of such encoders overcomes the phase-locking problem, and in spite of the limitation of finite memory duration, the condition may be approached of a population response rate that gives a perfect representation of the stimulus.

While the following discussion deals with two specific models, these two models do follow from reasonable idealization of the Hodgkin-Huxley equations. In particular, the small-signal frequency response of the impulse encoder in the *Limulus* eccentric cell may be described accurately in terms of a simple integrate-and-fire model (Knight et al., 1970). A slight tendency of this encoder to phase lock to very large signals (see Fig. 5 *b*) suggests that a slightly forgetful integrate-and-fire encoder model would furnish an even more accurate description.

The simple and the forgetful integrate-and-fire models differ in the degree to which a population of such encoders will "fill in" the detailed time profile of a periodic stimulus. (Phase locking is a complete breakdown in this "filling in.") The whole gamut of possibilities in fact arises for different neurons. While at present it is not feasible to record individually from a uniform population of neurons, it is possible to do something equivalent: to record from a single member over repeated stimuli. This has been done, for example, for the retinal ganglion cell (Hughes and Maffei, 1966), in the auditory system (Kiang et al., 1965; Brugge et al., 1969, 1970; Goldberg and Brown, 1969; Rose et al., 1967, 1969; Aitkin et al., 1970), for the innervation of fingertip skin (Mountcastle et al., 1968; Talbot et al., 1967), and for the mammalian muscle spindle (Brown et al., 1967; Matthews and Stein, 1969; Poppele and Bowman, 1970.) (The preceding references are not exhaustive.) The sections that follow should be helpful in the interpretation of these and similar investigations.[1]

2. INTEGRATE-AND-FIRE MODEL

One of the simplest possible impulse encoder models is the following: we imagine a noise-free neuron which contains an internal variable (which we call u) whose value increases at a rate given by the present value of the stimulus [called $s(t)$] which is being encoded. Thus,

$$\frac{du}{dt} = s(t). \qquad (s(t) \geqq 0). \qquad (2.1)$$

When u achieves a criterion level (C), a nerve impulse is fired, u is reset to zero, and the process starts again. In general, larger stimuli will encourage higher firing rates. The Hodgkin-Huxley equations may be made to yield this model in a limiting case.[2]

It is easy to see how a large population of such identical and noiseless encoders will respond to a stimulus. Let us define the "density" $\rho(u)$ by the property that in the population there are a number $\rho(u_1)du$ of encoders for which the value of u falls between u_1 and $u_1 + du$. In Fig. 1 the solid curve indicates how $\rho(u)$ might look at a particular moment. A short time later, those encoders which have not fired will have advanced to larger values of u, and the dashed curve will be obtained. The whole curve marches rigidly to the right. According to equation 2.1, its speed of advance is given by $s(t)$. The rate at which firings occur in the entire population will be the rate at which encoders reach the firing point $u = C$. This will depend jointly on the height of the curve $\rho(u)$ at the point $u = C$, and on the rate of the curve's advance. Thus, the population firing rate r is given by

$$r = s(t)\rho(C). \qquad (2.2)$$

It is an evident property of this model that, if initially the population are not uniformly distributed over u, this condition will persist forever, and even a constant stimulus s will lead to a periodic fluctuation in the population firing

---

[1] Among neurophysiologists the term "phase locking" is frequently used in an unfortunate colloquial way that blurs the distinction between neurons that phase lock and those that do not. Thus, for example, Rose et al. (1967) state very explicitly (footnote 3 of that paper) that they are observing "phase-preference," although the colloquial usage of "locking" appears in their title. Here throughout we use "phase locking" in the strict sense of seeking a fixed phase with respect to the stimulus. In this sense the simple integrate-and-fire model shows phase preference but does not phase lock.

[2] This model was advanced by Partridge (1966). Partridge's comment that "even in a multi-channelled system, considerable distortion could result from the process of pulse rate translation of a dynamic signal" specifically does *not* apply to this model.

rate. The passage of time will not smooth a firing rate which was not smooth initially.

The converse is also true, that if initially the population are uniformly distributed (straight line at ρ_0 in Fig. 1), then they will always remain so. In this case equation 2.2 becomes

$$r = \rho_0 s(t). \tag{2.3}$$

Thus, if the population are uniformly distributed in u, then the population firing rate will be a perfect copy of the stimulus. A more formal derivation of this result will be given near the end of section 4.

The simple preceding discussion deals only with what may be *expected* of an extremely large population of encoders. By choosing a large enough population we may make the fluctuations away from expected behavior arbitrar-

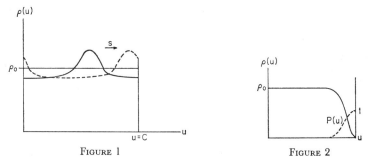

FIGURE 1

FIGURE 2

FIGURE 1. Time-course of the population density function $\rho(u)$.
FIGURE 2. Steady-state population density function, for a stochastic threshold distributed according to the probability function $P(u)$.

ily small. For a finite population questions concerning fluctuations about expected values demand a far more elaborate methodology than we will develop here. Therefore such questions will not be pursued.

So far the discussion has involved a population of neurons which are identical, in the sense that they all have the same firing threshold level C. The generalization to a heterogeneous population, with a distribution of threshold levels, is immediate. Simply divide the population into subpopulations, according to their values of C. The perfect replica argument holds for each subpopulation, and hence for the total.

A word of caution should be added concerning this heterogeneous population model: to achieve the perfect-replica result, each individual subpopulation must be started with a uniform distribution over the internal variable u. This model does not smooth itself.

The simple integrate-and-fire model may be slightly generalized, to include the feature that neurons fire somewhat unpredictably. The generalization might be described as "the integrate-and-fire model with stochastic threshold." Together with equation 2.1, we assume that there is a probability $P(u_1)$ that a particular neuron will fire before its internal variable u reaches the value u_1. The probability $P(u)$ eventually rises to unity, for large enough u. The population density $\rho(u)$ is shown in Fig. 2. The stochastic threshold condition we have postulated may be expressed as

$$\rho(u) = \rho_0(1 - P(u)), \qquad (2.4)$$

which is the content of Fig. 2. According to equation 2.1, individual encoders still advance in u at a speed $s(t)$. In particular, that is their speed of advance at $u = 0$, whence their total rate of appearance at $u = 0$ must be $\rho_0 s(t)$. This must be equal to the population firing rate. Thus equation 2.3 is *still* satisfied, and the population firing rate is again a perfect time replica of the stimulus.

This stochastic model carries one new feature: it tends to randomize the firing times of individual encoders, with respect to one another. Thus, even though the whole population were started synchronously, they would still tend to the time-independent distribution of Fig. 2, and toward the perfect-stimulus-replication behavior.[3]

In sections 5, 6, and 7 we will see that modification of the "simple integrate" law of equation 2.1—even slight modification—will lead to a population of encoders which tend to synchronize among themselves. It is reasonable to suspect that the stochastic feature might offset this tendency. This suggestion will be explored in section 8.

3. INSTANTANEOUS RATE OF A SINGLE UNIT

For a large and homogeneous population of neurons, the "instantaneous rate of a typical single unit" is a well-defined variable at all times, determined by the present state and past history of the entire population. We simply inspect the population for a neuron which currently is firing. The time since its last firing is its instantaneous period, the reciprocal of which is its instantaneous rate.

The single unit rate and the population rate are related in a subtle way. Because it is the single unit rate which usually is observed in the laboratory, and because the single unit rate often is more easily deduced from a theoretical

---

[3] The time of the last firing of a long enough sequence of firings of a given encoder will become uncorrelated with the first firing time. Thus the distribution $\rho(u)$ must become time independent in the limit of long times. It is unreasonable that there should be a second time-independent distribution besides that of equation 2.4. The evolution of the distribution may be reduced to a well-known problem by observing that we are dealing with a so-called "renewal process" in the variable u.

model, we will explore this relationship in this section and the next. The integrate-and-fire model furnishes a start.

Equation 2.1 may be integrated at once, and with the threshold condition, leads immediately to

$$C = \int_{t_n}^{t_{n+1}} dt\, s(t) \tag{3.1}$$

where t_n and t_{n+1} are the times of the nth and $(n + 1)$th impulses, respectively. If the stimulus is constant $(s = s_0)$ then

$$C = (t_{n+1} - t_n)s_0 \tag{3.2}$$

or

$$f_0 = s_0/C \tag{3.3}$$

where f_0 is the instantaneous rate of the single unit. Thus the single unit rate is in fixed linear proportion to the stimulus. This also must be true approximately if s changes by only a very small fraction of its value between two impulses. To find the degree of error we express $s(t)$ as a Taylor series

$$s(t) = s(t_n) + \dot{s}(t_n)(t - t_n) + \cdots \tag{3.4}$$

and equation 3.1 becomes

$$C = \frac{1}{f}s + \frac{1}{2}\frac{1}{f^2}\dot{s} + \cdots \tag{3.5}$$

where f is the single unit rate and the time t_n is implied. Multiplying equation 3.5 by f/C gives

$$f = \frac{1}{C}s + \frac{1}{2}\frac{1}{C\left(\frac{1}{C}s + \frac{1}{2}\frac{1}{Cf}\dot{s} + \cdots\right)}\dot{s} + \cdots \tag{3.6}$$

$$\approx \frac{1}{C}s + \frac{1}{2}\frac{\dot{s}}{s}$$

where the last line assumes $s \gg |\dot{s}/f|$. Now according to equation 3.6, f is no longer a perfect copy of s. It is not even a *linear* copy, in the sense that, for example, doubling the stimulus does not double the rate f. Unlike the population rate, the single unit instantaneous rate is *not* a perfect copy of the stimulus.

Next we investigate the frequency response of the single integrate-and-fire unit's instantaneous rate. Qualitatively, our question is: If the stimulus $s(t)$

fluctuates at a given frequency (the driving frequency), how well does the instantaneous rate $f(t)$ follow? According to equation 3.6 we may at once respond: almost perfectly at very low frequencies; but for driving frequencies which are *not* very low compared to the instantaneous rate, no general answer is known, nor is there known any practical general method for seeking the answer. However, if we confine ourselves to a periodic $s(t)$ which consists of a small fluctuation about a steady mean level then there *is* a general method and an answer in simple terms.

The general method—"linear perturbation theory"—comes in two parts. First, express both the input and output variables as a constant plus a small departure. When these variables are substituted into the mathematical relations which connect them, the strategy will be to ignore all expressions which are small compared to these small departures. An easy example (useful below) will illustrate: instantaneous frequency and instantaneous period [called $T(t)$] are connected by the relation

$$f = 1/T. \tag{3.7}$$

Now let

$$T(t) = T_0 + T_1(t), \quad f(t) = f_0 + f_1(t). \tag{3.8}$$

Note that

$$1/(T_0 + T_1) = 1/T_0 - T_1/T_0^2 + T_1^2/T_0^3 - \cdots. \tag{3.9}$$

If we substitute equation 3.8 into equation 3.7, all that survives is

$$f_1 = -T_1/T_0^2, \tag{3.10}$$

since we knew that $f_0 = 1/T_0$ already, and since T_1^2/T_0^3 and all higher terms are small compared to those in equation 3.10. Note that in equation 3.10 f_1 and T_1 are linearly related. This is a general and important result of the linear perturbation method.

The relation which connects stimulus to period is equation 3.1. In that equation t_{n+1} is the time of the present spike discharge, t_n is the time of the last, and $T = t_{n+1} - t_n$ is the period.

As in equation 3.8, let $s = s_0 + s_1$ and $T = T_0 + T_1$. Now an integral may be interpreted as an area. The relation imposed by equation 3.1 is that the stimulus perturbation s_1 causes a change T_1 in the period just such that the area remains at the unchanged value C. Fig. 3 illustrates this. Equation 3.1 demands *exactly* that the two shaded areas must be equal. This is *almost* properly expressed by the relation

$$\int_{t_{n+1}-T_0}^{t_{n+1}} dt' \, s_1(t') = -s_0 T_1. \tag{3.11}$$

The error is that the integral in equation 3.11 includes the little rectangle with edges $s_1 T_1$ in Fig. 3. But this area is small compared to those in equation 3.11, and its neglect amounts to the linear perturbation approximation.

The time t_{n+1} in equation 3.11 is a perfectly general time, and might as well be called t. When equation 3.11 is solved for T_1 and the result is put into equation 3.10, we obtain

$$f_1(t) = \frac{1}{T_0^2} \int_{t-T_0}^{t} dt' \, \frac{s_1(t')}{s_0},$$
(3.12)

which says that f_1 depends linearly on the recent past history of s_1, and in fact is proportional to the running average of the stimulus perturbation over the last T_0 time units.

The second part of the general method for finding the frequency response

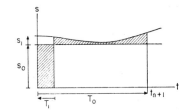

FIGURE 3. Shift T_1 in period due to shift s_1 in stimulus. The two shaded areas must be equal.

to a small fluctuation is to assume an explicit periodic function for $s_1(t)$. We might assume $s_1(t) = s_1(0) \cos \omega t$, for example, where ω is 2π times the driving frequency. Since equation 3.12 is a linear relationship between s_1 and f_1, we are justified in choosing instead

$$s_1(t) = s_1(0)e^{i\omega t}$$
(3.13)

which simplifies formal manipulations (and, in practiced hands, gives a format closer to one's physical intuition). Substituting equation 3.13 in equation 3.12 leads to a very easy integral, and the result is

$$f_1(t) = \frac{s_1(0)e^{i\omega t}}{T_0^2 s_0} \frac{1 - e^{-i\omega T_0}}{i\omega}.$$
(3.14)

Since equation 3.13 reappears in equation 3.14, a bit of rearrangement gives

$$\frac{f_1}{s_1} = \frac{f_0}{s_0} \frac{1 - e^{-i\omega/f_0}}{i\omega/f_0} \equiv \frac{f_0}{s_0} B(\omega/f_0).$$
(3.15)

This expression is the frequency response (or so-called "transfer function") for the transduction from s_1 to f_1. We note first that it is a constant, independent of time, and second that it is independent of the amplitude of s_1. Thirdly, it is a complex number, with an amplitude and a phase. Its amplitude is the ratio of the amplitude of the sinusoidal response f_1 to that of the

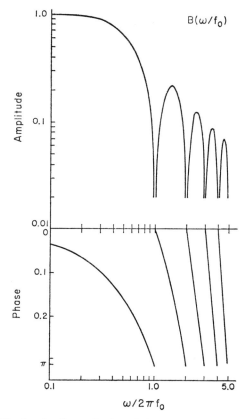

FIGURE 4. The function B, amplitude and phase.

sinusoidal stimulus s_1. Its phase is the phase shift of the crest of the response from the crest of the stimulus. (These facts may be confirmed a bit more laboriously by substituting the cosine form into equation 3.12.) These are all general results of the linear perturbation method. The amplitude and phase of B, over a range of frequencies, are shown in Fig. 4. This sort of frequency response was first recognized in its biological context by Borsellino et al. (1965)[4] and by Partridge (1966). It is also the transfer function of a running averager. Three prominent features deserve comment: (*a*) it shows the perfect time-replica feature at very low frequencies, (*b*) a high-frequency cut-off sets in as the driving frequency $\omega/2\pi$ approaches the unperturbed instantaneous rate f_0, and (*c*) it gives a null at any frequency where the sinusoidal input has a running average of zero, as equation 3.12 would predict.

4. THE RELATION BETWEEN UNIT RATE AND POPULATION RATE

Suppose we have a large population of N neurons, all of which are alike, which do not interact, and which encode their impulse trains, from a common stimulus, according to some law that is deterministic rather than probabilistic. We do *not* assume that the deterministic law is the simple integrate-and-fire model. If the encoding law makes any practical sense, then the time at which a neuron fires for the $(n + 1)$th time will be a monotonic (steadily rising) function of the time it fires for the nth time. Since the neurons are identical, this implies that no neuron can straddle two firings of another neuron with two consecutive firings of its own. That is enough to assure that every neuron in the population fires exactly once between the nth and $(n + 1)$th firings of a given neuron. In symbols,

$$N = \int_{t-T(t)}^{t} dt'\, r(t') \tag{4.1}$$

where $T(t)$ is the instantaneous period of a single unit, as defined in the first paragraph of section 3, N is the total number of neurons in the population, and $r(t)$ is the population rate as in section 2. Equations 4.1 relates the population rate $r(t)$ to a specified single unit period $T(t)$, without making any assumption (except monotonicity) about the encoding law.

Considering the definition of instantaneous period, it is equally true that equation 3.1 may be written

$$C = \int_{t-T(t)}^{t} dt'\, s(t'). \tag{4.2}$$

Now equations 4.1 and 4.2 are identical in form, as N plays the role of C, and r the role of s. The roles of input and output variables have been interchanged, but that is a matter of emphasis, rather than one of mathematics. All the arguments of section 3 apply to equation 4.1. In particular, in the

---

[4] In fact the equipment superimposed such a frequency response upon the biological data. See Poppele and Bowman (1970) for further discussion.

linear perturbation approximation, the frequency response of the population rate to the single unit rate will be

$$\frac{r_1}{f_1} = \frac{r_0}{f_0} \frac{i\omega/f_0}{1 - e^{-i\omega/f_0}}, \qquad (4.3)$$

substantially the inverse of equation 3.15 because input and output have interchanged roles.

The most striking feature of the frequency response equation 4.3 is that it becomes infinite at certain frequencies. The denominator vanishes whenever $\omega/f_0 = 2\pi n$ (where n is any nonzero integer). A "resonance" sets in, leading to a huge amplification whenever the driving frequency gets close enough to a multiple of the single-unit unperturbed rate.[5]

For a population of simple integrate-and-fire neurons, what is the frequency response of the population rate to a small periodic fluctuation in the stimulus? We may combine equations 4.3 and 3.15. Thus

$$\frac{r_1}{s_1} = \left\{\frac{r_1}{f_1}\right\} \left\{\frac{f_1}{s_1}\right\} = \frac{r_0}{s_0}. \qquad (4.4)$$

This is simply a weakened statement of the perfect time-copy property of a population of simple integrate-and-fire encoders. It could have been derived immediately by applying linear perturbation theory to equation 2.3.

The remarkable feature of equation 4.4 is the perfect cancellation of poles and zeros between the two braced terms. The frequency dependence drops out entirely. This will be in striking contrast to the next section, where a different sort of encoder will be investigated.

If the neurons of equation 4.1 should be simple integrate-and-fire encoders, which satisfy equation 4.2, then a solution of equation 4.1 for $r(t)$ is easily found. Let

$$r(t) = \frac{N}{C} s(t). \qquad (4.5)$$

Substitution into equation 4.1 at once yields equation 4.2, which is true by hypothesis. Since $\rho_0 C = N$ (Fig. 1), equation 4.5 is the same as equation 2.3.

Suppose an electronic simple integrate-and-fire circuit is connected to the beam brightener of an oscilloscope. Suppose further that the voltage stimulus,

---

[5] In technical terms, the poles of a frequency response indicate how a system may respond to a vanishingly small stimulus. The poles indicate the "free-running" or undriven behavior of the system. In particular, poles at real ω indicate undamped periodic free responses of the system. In this case the indicated free-running periodic responses are of the sort already mentioned just following equation 2.2. Such periodic free-running responses also may be found in equation 4.1: if T is constant there, r is undetermined to within an additive function which integrates to zero over period T.

a constant voltage plus a sinusoid, also drives the oscilloscope's vertical deflection, and that the horizontal sweep is synchronized to that signal. The experiment should be done at a sweep rate too fast for the eye to follow, and with several cycles of the sinusoid displayed on the scope. If the spike rate is almost identical to the sine frequency, then on the scope face we will see a procession of bright spots voyaging along the sine curve, one to a cycle. The interspot separation will be practically the same when the spots are in the troughs as it is when they are at the crests. But the spots will spend almost all of their time at the crests, and particularly will shun the troughs. The behavior of the single encoder over many cycles shows us what would be the behavior of a population of many encoders over a single cycle.

5. FORGETFUL INTEGRATE-AND-FIRE MODEL

Equation 2.1 is the simplest example of the more general relationship

$$\frac{du}{dt} = F(u, s(t)) \tag{5.1}$$

which might describe the internal dynamics of an encoding neuron. If we interpret u in equation 5.1 as a set of internal variables, and F as a set of functional relationships, the Hodgkin-Huxley equations take this form, with $s(t)$ the input current; the four components of u are the voltage and the three conductance-determining parameters. In designing a neuron encoding model, we should, according to common sense, pick $F(u, s(t))$ in equation 5.1 in such a way that the present value of u depends more strongly on the immediate past history of $s(t)$ than on its more distant past. The Hodgkin-Huxley equations have this property. The simplest example in the form of equation 5.1 with this property is the one-component equation

$$\frac{du}{dt} = -\gamma u + s(t) \tag{5.2}$$

which may be got from the Hodgkin-Huxley equations in a limiting case less drastic than that which yielded equation 2.1. Equation 5.2 carries the feature that the effect of s at time t' upon u at time t will have decremented by a factor of $\exp[-\gamma(t - t')]$.

We complete our encoder model by imposing a firing threshold at the criterion level $u = C$, as before. Equation 5.2 is easily integrated for u, whereupon the threshold condition yields

$$C = \int_{t_n}^{t_{n+1}} dt' e^{-\gamma(t_{n+1} - t')} s(t') \tag{5.3}$$

which should be compared to equation 3.1. Following section 3, if the stimulus is constant ($s = s_0$) integration gives

$$C = +\gamma^{-1}\{1 - \exp[-\gamma(t_{n+1} - t_n)]\}s_0 \qquad (5.4)$$

which may be solved for f_0, giving

$$f_0 = -\gamma/\lg[1 - (\gamma C/s_0)]. \qquad (5.5)$$

We notice that, as we decrease the stimulus s_0, the firing rate f_0 falls to zero at the finite stimulus level $s_0 = \gamma C$. This could be found at once by putting $u = \text{const}$ into equation 5.2, to find the asymptotic value to which u will rise if no threshold is crossed. We see that u rises asymptotically toward the value s_0/γ, which will be below firing threshold if $s_0 < \gamma C$. To compare equation 5.5 to equation 3.3, we expand equation 5.5 about large s_0:

$$f_0 = s_0/C - \gamma/2 + \gamma \cdot 0(\gamma C/s_0). \qquad (5.6)$$

If $s_0 = 2\gamma C$, the first two terms in equation 5.6 differ from the exact result in equation 5.5 by only about 14%. Thus, except very near threshold, the only effect of forgetfulness on the response to a steady stimulus is that the single unit firing rate is offset by a constant amount $-\gamma/2$.

In order to find the single-unit frequency response, it is convenient to express equation 5.3 as

$$C = \int_{t-T(t)}^{t} dt' e^{-\gamma(t-t')}s(t'). \qquad (5.7)$$

The graphical argument of section 3 corresponded to assuming linear perturbations $s = s_0 + s_1(t)$, $T = T_0 + T_1(t)$ in this expression. Substitution into equation 5.7 yields (with $\gamma T_1 \ll 1$)

$$0 = T_1(t)e^{-\gamma T_0}s_0 + \int_{t-T_0}^{t} dt' e^{-\gamma(t-t')}s_1(t') \qquad (5.8)$$

in analogy to equation 3.11; the equation analogous to equation 3.12, which follows, is

$$f_1(t) = \frac{e^{\gamma T_0}}{T_0^2} \int_{t-T_0}^{t} dt' e^{-\gamma(t-t')} \frac{s_1(t')}{s_0}. \qquad (5.9)$$

Notice that f_1 is proportional to a weighted average over past values of s_1, with weights biased in favor of the most recent past.

The second part of the frequency response calculation proceeds much as in section 3, and yields the transfer function

$$\frac{f_1}{s_1} = \frac{f_0}{s_0} e^{\gamma/f_0} \frac{1 - e^{-(i\omega+\gamma)/f_0}}{(i\omega + \gamma)/f_0}, \qquad (5.10)$$

which corresponds to equation 3.15. Equation 5.10 shows two new features. First, if γ is comparable in size to f_0, then even when ω is near zero the perfect copy feature has been lost: f_1/s_1 departs from f_0/s_0 by a factor $(\gamma/f_0)^{-1}(\exp(\gamma/f_0) - 1)$. This reflects the fact that near firing threshold the f_0 vs. s_0 relation in equation 5.5 is nonlinear. Well away from threshold $(\gamma/f_0 \ll 1)$ the frequency response in equation 5.10 looks extremely similar to equation 3.15. However, a second slight discrepancy exists, which will prove important: the frequency response does not quite null at the resonance points $\omega = 2\pi n f_0$, and there equation 5.10 becomes

$$\frac{f_1}{s_1} = \frac{f_0}{s_0} \frac{-i}{2\pi n} \frac{\gamma}{f_0}. \tag{5.11}$$

By hypothesis this is small, but it is not zero.

The frequency response of the population rate to a small periodic fluctuation in stimulus may be found as in equation 4.5:

$$\frac{r_1}{s_1} = \left\{\frac{r_1}{f_1}\right\}\left\{\frac{f_1}{s_1}\right\} = \frac{r_0}{s_0}\left(\frac{i\omega}{i\omega + \gamma}\right)\frac{e^{\gamma/f_0} - e^{-i\omega/f_0}}{1 - e^{-i\omega/f_0}}. \tag{5.12}$$

For small γ this simplifies to

$$\frac{r_1}{s_1} = \frac{r_0}{s_0}\left\{1 + \frac{\gamma/f_0}{1 - e^{-i\omega/f_0}}\right\}. \tag{5.13}$$

The additional term, which is not in equation 4.5, is small under most circumstances, but goes to infinity whenever $\omega/2\pi$ approaches a resonant frequency. If ω is near $2\pi n f_0$ we find

$$\frac{r_1}{s_1} = \frac{r_0}{s_0}\left\{1 - \frac{i\gamma}{\omega - 2\pi n f_0}\right\}. \tag{5.14}$$

Thus the population frequency response of the forgetful integrate-and-fire encoder model, well above threshold, is of the flat perfect time-copy type *except* near the resonant frequencies where it is enormously amplified. The approach of equation 5.14 to equation 4.5, as $\gamma \to 0$, is nonuniform: the peak gets narrower but no less tall. The feature of response climbing to infinity, as the frequency approaches resonance, survives no matter how small a finite value of γ we choose.

We close this section with a comment about the general equation 5.1 with which we started. The degree of forgetfulness it exhibits may be built in by rewriting it as

$$\frac{du}{dt} = F(\gamma u, s(t)) \tag{5.15}$$

where γ is the "forgetfulness parameter" in the sense that if $\gamma = 0$ then equation 5.15 reduces to the simple integrate-and-fire model with input stimulus $F(0, s(t))$. If we assume that γ is small and also that $s(t) = s_0 + s_1(t)$ where s_1 is small, then we may expand F in both small quantities and obtain

$$\frac{du}{dt} = a + bs_1(t) + c\gamma u + \cdots \qquad (5.16)$$

where all the further terms are second or higher order in smallness. This approximate equation closely resembles equation 5.2, and may be put through the same logical procedures to yield essentially the population frequency response equation 5.13. Thus we see that the feature of resonant amplification is not peculiar to the forgetful integrate-and-fire model of equation 5.2, but rather is a common feature intimately associated with the general property of forgetfulness in a deterministic encoder.

6. PHASE LOCKING IN THE FORGETFUL MODEL

For a simple integrate-and-fire encoder, there is no fixed relationship between the phase of a periodic input and the moment at which the encoder fires an impulse. This is so even if the frequency of the periodic stimulus is identical to the firing rate of the encoder.

In equation 3.1 we may add to the stimulus $s(t)$ any other stimulus $s'(t)$ which integrates to zero between the firing times, and the equation will still be satisfied with the firing times unchanged. If all the t_m of equation 3.1 are evenly spaced, and $s(t)$ is periodic over that spacing, then we may let

$$s'(t) = s(t + \tau) - s(t) \qquad (6.1)$$

where τ is arbitrary. The effect of adding equation 6.1 to $s(t)$ is to shift the stimulus pattern by an arbitrary time τ, without shifting the firing times.

For the forgetful integrate-and-fire encoder the situation is altogether different. We may ask under what conditions spike firings will keep in step with a periodic stimulus. Suppose we apply a stimulus which is a constant s_0 plus a sinusoid of fractional amplitude m:

$$s(t) = s_0\{1 + m \operatorname{Re} e^{i(\omega t + \phi)}\}. \qquad (6.2)$$

Since an undetermined phase ϕ has been included in the stimulus, we may start the integral in equation 5.3 at $t_n = 0$ without loosing generality.

$$C = \int_0^T dt' e^{-\gamma(T - t')} s_0\{1 + m \operatorname{Re} e^{i(\omega t' + \phi)}\}. \qquad (6.3)$$

In this equation we intend to see if we can pick the phase ϕ of the driving signal in such a way that the firing period T will be the reciprocal of the driving frequency $\omega/2\pi$. The reason for writing $\cos(\omega t + \phi)$ in that peculiar form in equation 6.2 is that later operations are facilitated and the integral becomes easy:

$$C = e^{-\gamma T} s_0 \left\{ \frac{e^{\gamma T} - 1}{\gamma} + m \operatorname{Re}\left(e^{i\phi} \frac{e^{(\gamma+i\omega)T} - 1}{\gamma + i\omega} \right) \right\}. \tag{6.4}$$

It will be convenient also to write

$$\frac{1}{\gamma + i\omega} = \frac{1}{\sqrt{\gamma^2 + \omega^2}} e^{i\beta} \tag{6.5}$$

where β is the known angle

$$\beta = -\arctan(\omega/\gamma). \tag{6.6}$$

Now we will impose the condition that $s(t)$ is periodic over the firing period T:

$$e^{i\omega T} = 1. \tag{6.7}$$

Under this assumption, can a fixed firing phase ϕ be found such that equation 6.3 or 6.4 is satisfied? Equation 6.4 reduces to

$$C = s_0 \left\{ \frac{1 - e^{-\gamma T}}{\gamma} + \frac{m}{\sqrt{\gamma^2 + \omega^2}} (1 - e^{-\gamma T}) \operatorname{Re} e^{i(\phi+\beta)} \right\}. \tag{6.8}$$

The only unknown in this expression is the phase ϕ, and that appears only in one place. We rearrange equation 6.8 to isolate the unknown, and find

$$\left\{ \frac{C/s_0}{1 - e^{-\gamma T}} - \frac{1}{\gamma} \right\} \frac{\sqrt{\gamma^2 + \omega^2}}{m} = \cos(\phi + \beta). \tag{6.9}$$

Since the cosine is an even function, the extremes of which lie at ± 1, there will be no solution to equation 6.9 for the phase ϕ if the left-hand side is greater than unity in absolute value, but if it is less there will be two solutions.

An easy illustrative example is the case in which the term in braces in equation 6.9 vanishes. According to equation 5.4, that is the case where T is the free-running firing period in the absence of modulation. In this case equation 6.9 is evidently solved by

$$\phi = -\beta \pm \pi/2. \tag{6.10}$$

Since the left-hand side of equation 6.9 need only lie between ± 1, a period somewhat off from the free-running period also will permit a solution of equation 6.9, but a period that is off badly will only solve if the modulation m is made large enough.

If there is only slight memory loss over the firing period ($\gamma T \ll 1$), equation 6.9 becomes

$$\left\{\frac{Cs_0}{T} - 1\right\}\frac{\omega}{\gamma m} = \cos(\phi + \beta). \tag{6.11}$$

The braced term now vanishes if T is the free-running period of the simple integrate-and-fire encoder. We must stick close to that period if equation 6.11 is to have solutions. And, so to speak, twice as close if the encoder becomes only half as forgetful—or we must double the modulation.

In deriving equation 6.11, we have used the implication of equation 6.7 that

$$\omega = 2\pi n/T \tag{6.12}$$

for some integer n. Since ω is a property of the cause, and T a property of the effect, it is of course ω which determines T through equation 6.12, provided equation 6.9 has a solution. The fact that equation 6.9 can be solved for a range of T about the free-running period shows that the firing rate can be "pulled" away from its free-running value by a driving frequency that lies close to a multiple of the free-running firing rate.

What happens if equation 6.9 has no solution? If the modulated part of the stimulus undergoes, for example, two periods of oscillation in a time closely similar to three periods of the free-running encoder, then "frequency pulling" may still occur if the modulation depth is sufficient. More generally, if the sum of k free-running periods falls close to n periods of the driving frequency, a repeating time pattern of k impulses over every n driving cycles may be established. This behavior was noticed and has been treated in detail by Rescigno et al. (1970). The general "n/k" case is very much more difficult in detail[6] than is the "$n/1$" case which led to equation 6.9 above, although very similar conclusions are reached.

If equation 6.9 has any solutions at all, typically it will have two solutions. Both give points in the stimulus cycle at which firings of the encoder will continue in step with the stimulus. These are called "fixed points" because firings continue to occur at them, cycle after cycle. It is not difficult to follow what happens if the encoder is initially fired at a point in the cycle slightly off a solution of equation 6.9 (see Rescigno et al. 1970). The conclusion is that one solution of equation 6.9 yields a stable fixed point, and the other an unstable one. The fixed point on the rising part of the stimulus is stable and

---

[6] Rescigno et al. (1970) is the definitive study of the forgetful model stimulated by a finite sinusoid. The final bit of section 5 in that work must be approached with caution, however. It is unclear whether the final inequality implies necessity or sufficiency, and a result seems to emerge which is in discord with Denjoy's general result (which we meet in section 7 of this paper) concerning "continuity of the turning angle" which claims that "n/k" may take on irrational values.

the one on the falling part is not. An encoder which initially is fired at an arbitrary point in the stimulus cycle will, over a sequence of subsequent firings, choose a sequence of points in the cycle which converge to the stable phase solution of equation 6.9.[7] Thus the stimulus tends to "lock" the firing of the encoder to a fixed phase of the stimulus's own rhythm.

The consequence for a population of forgetful integrate-and-fire encoders is evident and dramatic. The entire population will fall into step with the stimulus, at the stable phase-lock point given by equation 6.9. We saw in the last section that an infinitesimal periodic modulation of the stimulus leads, at the resonant frequencies, to an indefinitely large population response. For a *finite* stimulus modulation the same sort of thing happens not only at the resonant frequencies, but in the whole neighborhoods around those frequencies—the frequency-pulling range—over which equation 6.9 has a solution.

If we view the population of encoders as a transducer the output of which is the population firing rate, this is a very serious matter. The output gives information only on the frequency of the input, plus the fact that the modulation was strong enough for phase locking to occur at that frequency. One or a few encoders could deliver as much information.[8]

7. GENERAL THEORY OF ENCODER PHASE LOCKING[1]

The forgetful integrate-and-fire and the simple integrate-and-fire models show a striking contrast in one feature: in the one model the population of encoders tend to fall into step and fire simultaneously; in the other model they do not. These contrasting behaviors are not specific to the two models we have chosen to analyze in detail. Indeed these two models may be regarded as prototypes of two distinct classes of encoders. This section will show that in fact no further classes exist, so long as we confine ourselves to encoders which are deterministic and depend only on input since the last impulse. Thus the results of the previous sections should be applicable, except for quantitative details, to a wide variety of neural encoders.

Topological methods of a very general nature, discussed in the present section, lead to two conclusions: (a') the most general deterministic impulse encoder which does *not* phase lock to any periodic signal is equivalent to an

---

[7] In the near neighborhood of either the stable fixed point or the adjacent unstable fixed point, the successor to a given impulse steps toward the phase of the stable point and away from the phase of the unstable point. The same must be true over the entire span of phase in between these neighborhoods: the phase of the successor is a continuous function of the phase of the given impulse; the signature of the phase difference can only reverse by passing through zero, which would define another fixed point between the adjacent fixed points. This topological argument illustrates the power of the methods which will be discussed in the next section.

[8] In particular applications phase locking should be advantageous; for example, in the sound direction sense at low frequencies, which depends on the accurate measurement of phase differences between the two ears.

arbitrary continuous transducer followed by a simple integrate-and-fire encoder; and (*b'*) an encoder which *does* phase lock to some specific periodic stimulus will also phase lock to distinct periodic stimuli which are sufficiently similar, and in particular it will phase lock over a finite span of frequencies.

At present the general theory is not in a definitive final form. Two more conclusions strongly suggested but as yet unproven in general are: (*c'*) no forgetful encoder (in the sense of section 5, paragraph 1) can mimic an encoding scheme the last stage of which is an infinite-memory encoder, hence, by conclusion (*a'*) any forgetful encoder must show phase-locking behavior; and (*d'*) any pulse-encoding scheme which shows phase locking in response to some periodic stimulus will also show population synchronization in response to a wide class of reasonable aperiodic stimuli. The tentative conclusions (*c'*) and (*d'*) stand up in explicit cases examined to date. If they hold universally, then they imply that a homogeneous population of deterministic encoders designed on *any* forgetful encoding scheme must eventually fall into a synchronized condition. The remainder of this section outlines the path of reasoning that leads to conclusions (*a'*) and (*b'*).

The general theory of deterministic encoder response to periodic stimuli corresponds to the topological theory of the continuous one-to-one mappings of the circumference of the circle onto itself. In particular the classification of encoders is closely related to the classification of such mappings. Suppose a periodic stimulus $s(t)$ (not necessarily sinusoidal) has a period $T = 2\pi/\omega$. The variable

$$x = t/T \qquad (7.1)$$

ranges from zero to unity over one cycle of the stimulus. We can imagine the ascending values of x as points arrayed around the circumference of a circle. Equation 3.1 or 5.3 is an implicit relation which determines x_{n+1} once x_n has been specified. Both are examples of the general form

$$x_{n+1} = \phi(x_n) \qquad (7.2)$$

where x_{n+1} is some new value which we may place between zero and unity by adopting the obvious cyclic convention. Equation 7.2 expresses a "mapping" in that any point x_n on the circle is mapped uniquely onto a new point x_{n+1}. The position on the circle of the kth successor to x_n will be given by

$$x_{n+k} = \phi(\phi(\cdots\phi(x_n)\cdots)) \equiv \phi^k(x_n). \qquad (7.3)$$

An evident extension of this notation is, for example,

$$x_n = \phi^{-1}(x_{n+1}), \qquad (7.4)$$

and if two mappings are ϕ, ψ, we will sometimes write

$$x' = \chi(x) = \psi(\phi(x)) \quad \text{as} \quad \chi = \psi * \phi. \tag{7.5}$$

The successive application of two one-to-one mappings is a one-to-one mapping; each mapping has an inverse, and there is an identity mapping (do nothing). Technically the mappings form a "group" and their natural classification is in terms of "equivalence classes" in the group theoretic sense.

There is a second way (besides that of equation 7.2) of looking upon the functional relation

$$x' = \psi(x) \tag{7.6}$$

on the circle. It may be looked upon as a reexpression of the same point x in terms of a new coordinate. For example, x might be distance as measured around a circle of unit circumference by an accurate tape measure, and x' that distance as measured by an inaccurate tape measure which is stretched and shrunk over different parts of its range between zero and unity. Then the transformation ψ^{-1} is the correction table to be used with the inaccurate measure.

If x gets changed, as in equation 7.2, by a mapping $\phi(x)$, how does x' get changed? How does the point-to-point mapping, ϕ, look in the primed coordinate system? What is, say, the corresponding $\phi'(x')$? Answer: first change x' to x with the coordinate change ψ^{-1}, then move x to $\phi(x)$ with ϕ, then change the new x back to the new x' with the coordinate change ψ, whence

$$\phi' = \psi * \phi * \psi^{-1}. \tag{7.7}$$

Any two mappings related as ϕ and ϕ' above are said to belong to the same equivalence class. They are, so to speak, the same mapping expressed in terms of alternative coordinates.

To illustrate we look at a particular important class: the "equivalence class of rigid rotations." In equation 7.7 above let ϕ be, in particular,

$$x_X \equiv \phi(x) = x + X \tag{7.8}$$

so that each point x is advanced around the circle rigidly by a constant increment X. Equation 7.7 becomes

$$x'_X = \phi'(x') = \psi(\phi(\psi^{-1}(x'))) = \psi(\psi^{-1}(x') + X) = \psi(x + X) \tag{7.9}$$

which is the generic form of the equivalence class of rigid rotations through the angle X.

There is a remarkable implicit restatement of equation 7.9. Equation 7.8 is trivially rearranged to

$$X = \int_{x}^{x_X} dx. \tag{7.10}$$

In equation 7.6 let $\psi = \sigma^{-1}$. Then we have $dx/dx' = \dot{\sigma}(x')$ where the dot on $\dot{\sigma}$ stands for differentiation. In terms of the x' coordinate equation 7.10 becomes

$$X = \int_{x'}^{x'_x} dx' \dot{\sigma}(x'), \qquad (7.11)$$

the implicit restatement of equation 7.9. But if $\dot{\sigma}$ is regarded as a stimulus this is exactly the equation that determines the phase of the successor impulse x'_x of a simple integrate-and-fire encoder which last fired at x'. The mappings obtained by simple integrate-and-fire encoders, with all possible periodic inputs ($\dot{\sigma}$) and threshold levels (X), are the same as the equivalence classes of the rigid rotations through the various rotation angles X.

There are also equivalence classes distinct from those of the rigid rotations. Equation 5.3, for example, led to equation 6.9, which was solved for the "fixed points" of the mapping; that is, those phase points in the stimulus cycle such that successive impulses appeared at unchanged phase, or in the present language, those points left unmoved by the mapping of equation 7.2. The existence of a fixed point is a co-called "topological property"—it is independent of changes in coordinate system such as equation 7.7. Hence the whole equivalence class will have two fixed points, as surely as any equivalence class of rigid rotations has no fixed points at all (except if X is an integer).

In passing we note that topological considerations demand that if there is a stable fixed point then there must also be an unstable fixed point. If there is a fixed point which the transformation makes other points step *toward* from both sides, somewhere on the circle there must be a fixed point with the opposite property.

Classes also exist which are distinct from rotations and have no fixed points. Consider for example the situation in which equation 5.3 permits phase locking but with two impulses per stimulus cycle. The transformation ϕ has no fixed points, but ϕ^2 has *four* isolated fixed points, as either stable firing position in the cycle will repeat after two firings (see Fig. 5). More generally, an encoding situation which allows a stable time pattern of k spikes to first repeat after n stimulus cycles will yield a mapping whose kth iterate has $2k$ isolated fixed points.

These simple facts will be used in conjunction with a set of deeper results, mostly due to Denjoy (1932; see also Coddington and Levinson, 1955, chapter 17; and Moser, 1968,[9] pp. 41–77), which we cite without proof.

(*a*) Every mapping $\phi(x)$ has associated with it a number (called the "turning angle") defined by

$$\alpha(\phi) = \lim_{n \to \infty} \frac{1}{n} \phi^n(x) \qquad (7.12)$$

which is finite and independent of x. (For purposes of equation 7.12 we do not impose the cyclic convention mentioned at equation 7.2, but alternatively "unroll" the circle along the infinite line.) Given that the limit of equation 7.12 exists, it is easy to see that all members of an equivalence class have the same value of α. It is also instructive to substitute equation 7.8 into equation 7.12 and to calculate directly that the turning angle of a rigid rotation is indeed X.

(*b*) If the mapping ϕ depends continuously on a parameter (in the encoder case the circular driving frequency ω of the stimulus will do) then the turning angle $\alpha(\phi)$ also depends continuously on that parameter.

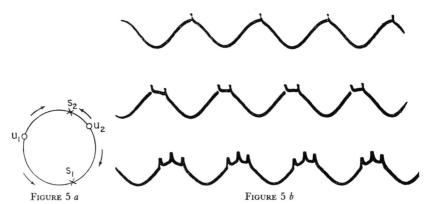

FIGURE 5 *a*   FIGURE 5 *b*

FIGURE 5 *a*. Circle showing two stable fixed points (s_1, s_2) and two unstable fixed points (u_1, u_2) of the mapping ϕ^2.

FIGURE 5 *b*. Phase locking in a sensory neuron (*Limulus* eccentric cell) in response to intracellularly injected current. Top frame: ϕ has one stable fixed point. Middle frame: ϕ^2 has two stable fixed points (as in Fig. 5 *a*). Bottom frame: ϕ^3 has three stable fixed points.

(*c*) The turning angle $\alpha(\phi)$ is either an irrational or a rational number. If α is irrational then ϕ belongs to the equivalence class of rigid rotations with turning angle α.

(*d*) If $\alpha(\phi)$ is rational, say n/k, there are two subcases: either every point x of $\phi^k(x)$ is a fixed point, in which case $\phi(x)$ again belongs to an equivalence class of rigid rotations, or

(*e*) $\phi^k(x)$ has a discrete set of fixed points. In this case a small finite change of a parameter (see [*b*] above) in at least one direction will leave $\alpha(\phi)$ unchanged.[10]

The deep and difficult statement of the lot is (*c*), which asserts that we did not overlook any additional kinds of equivalence classes in our earlier enumeration.

[10] We bar one exceptional case which is unimportant in the application to encoders.

An encoder which never exhibits contingency (*e*) always corresponds to a mapping in the equivalence class of some rotation, and hence to a simple integrate-and-fire encoder receiving some stimulus with the proper period. This substantiates conclusion (*a'*) at the beginning of the section.

The contingency (*e*) is the phase-locking situation, as in Fig. 5, for example. A small enough parameter change simply shifts the positions of the fixed points of ϕ^n, and may be regarded as a coordinate transformation. Hence the equivalence class remains unchanged, and so does the turning angle. The phase-lock condition will likewise persist.[11] Thus any encoder which will phase lock at all will do so over a finite range of frequency (or amplitude, etc.—this is conclusion [*b'*] at the beginning of this section). If we choose a frequency (and amplitude, etc.) at random, we stand a finite chance to draw a phase-locked condition.

We close with a remark concerning tentative conclusions (*c'*) and (*d'*) made at the beginning of this section: suppose two identical encoders, which share the same input signal, fire initially at times that are only slightly separated. Let us follow these encoders through a large number of firings. If the encoders are forgetful in the sense we have used above, then their latest firing times will be more strongly influenced by their very similar recent past histories than by their different initial conditions. Hence we anticipate that their firing times will draw together as their total number of firings increases. We expect them to "fall into step." This heuristic argument explicitly demands the property of forgetfulness, and nowhere asserts that the input signal is periodic.

8. STOCHASTIC ENCODERS

We have seen that one indication of the synchronization phenomenon in a population of deterministic encoders is the resonant amplification of an infinitesimal periodic fluctuation in the stimulus, as shown in equation 5.14. We suggested in sections 1 and 2 that the inclusion of a random process in each encoder should tend to break up this synchronization.[12] In the present section we will verify our suggestion to the extent of showing quantitatively how fluctuations in the firing rate which are nondeterministic, or stochastic, suppress the infinite resonant peaks in the population frequency response.

The frequency response of the population firing rate we will determine in two steps. Following the development for the deterministic case in section 4, first we will derive a relation between the population rate and a complete specification of the firing periods of the individual encoders. The second step

---

[11] We note that $\psi * (\phi^n) * \psi^{-1} = (\psi * \phi * \psi^{-1})^n$ where ψ corresponds to the parameter change. The transformation $\psi * \phi * \psi^{-1}$ has the same turning angle as ϕ does (of course ϕ^n has fixed points and hence turning angle zero). The fact that a ψ may be found to represent the parameter change is called Pliss's theorem and is discussed by Moser.[9]

[12] This idea has been advanced by Stein (1970), and Stein and French (1969).

will be to derive the firing period information from a stochastic model of an individual encoder.

Let us generalize the monotonicity postulate, with which we started section 4, in the following way: we postulate a homogeneous population of stochastic encoders which are such that we *expect* each to fire once between any two consecutive firings of any specified member of the population. The expected total number of firings between two firings of one member is N, the number of encoders in the population. Let $n(T, t)$ be the number of firings between the times $t - T$ and t, and let $Q(T, t)$ be the probability density that an encoder which fires at t also had its last firing at $t - T$. Then our postulate states that

$$N = \int_0^\infty dT Q(T, t) n(T, t). \tag{8.1}$$

Since the number of firings in the span T is related to the population firing rate $r(t)$ by

$$n(T, t) = \int_{t-T}^t dt' r(t'), \tag{8.2}$$

equation 8.1 becomes

$$N = \int_0^\infty dT Q(T, t) \int_{t-T}^t dt' r(t') \tag{8.3}$$

which is the relationship that determines the population firing rate $r(t)$ from the specified encoder period distribution $Q(T, t)$. It is the stochastic analogue of equation 4.1. In the deterministic limit

$$Q(T, t) = \delta(T - T_s(t)), \qquad T_s(t) \text{ a specified function,} \tag{8.4}$$

equation 4.1 is recovered. Or if we assume $r = r_0$ is constant, and $Q = Q_0(T)$, equation 8.3 gives

$$N = r_0 T_0 \tag{8.5}$$

where

$$T_0 = \int_0^\infty dT Q_0(T) T \tag{8.6}$$

is the mean firing period. Equation 8.5 gives the steady rate r_0 in terms of only the first moment T_0 of $Q_0(T)$.

We undertake a perturbation analysis of equation 8.3, and assume

$$r(t) = r_0 + r_1(t), \qquad Q(T, t) = Q_0(T) + Q_1(T, t) \tag{8.7}$$

which gives

$$0 = \int_0^\infty dT Q_0(T) \int_{t-\tau}^t dt' r_1(t') + \int_0^\infty dT Q_1(T, t) \int_{t-\tau}^t dt' r_0 \qquad (8.8)$$

whence

$$\int_0^\infty dT Q_0(T) \int_{t-\tau}^t dt' r_1(t') = -r_0 T_1(t) \qquad (8.9)$$

where the perturbation in mean firing period $T_1(t)$ has a definition analogous to equation 8.6. Again, the perturbation in the population rate depends only on the first moment of the perturbation in the period distribution.

To find the frequency response we assume

$$T_1(t) = T_1(0)e^{i\omega t}, \qquad r_1(t) = r_1(0)e^{i\omega t} \qquad (8.10)$$

and substitution into equation 8.9 gives, with one easy integration,

$$r_1 \int_0^\infty dT Q_0(T) \frac{1 - e^{-i\omega T}}{i\omega} = -r_0 T_1. \qquad (8.11)$$

Since $Q_0(T)$ is a probability density, and integrates to unity, equation 8.11 in turn at once leads to

$$\frac{r_1}{T_1} = -r_0 \frac{i\omega}{1 - \tilde{Q}_0(i\omega)}, \qquad (8.12)$$

where

$$\tilde{Q}_0(i\omega) = \int_0^\infty dT Q_0(T)e^{-i\omega T} \qquad (8.13)$$

is the average value of $\exp(-i\omega T)$ over T, or in probability terminology, the "characteristic function" of Q_0.

Equation 8.12, the frequency response of r_1 to T_1, is the main result of this final theoretical section. As the resonant poles of the deterministic models first arose from the denominator of equation 4.3, we compare the denominator of equation 8.12 to that expression. We notice that a term of the form $\exp(-i\omega T)$ has been replaced by its average over a collection of periods T determined by chance. The difference is very important: although $\exp(-i\omega T)$ has unit length on the complex plane and touches the unit circle, the average of $\exp(-i\omega T)$ over different values of T, its "center of gravity" $\tilde{Q}_0(i\omega)$, must fall *within* the unit circle. Hence the denominator of equation 8.12 cannot vanish. The stochastic feature has taken care of the infinite resonance problem.

Finally, we analyze a specific model which combines the forgetfulness feature of section 5 with the stochastic threshold feature with which we concluded section 2. We assume an internal variable u related to the input stimulus by equation 5.2, and a distribution of firing thresholds C characterized by a probability density $P'(C)$ where P' is the derivative of the probability P that was shown in Fig. 2. As in equation 5.7, the firing threshold C and the period T are related by

$$C = \int_{t-T}^{t} dt' \, e^{-\gamma(t-t')} S(t') \qquad (8.14)$$

and the probability density $Q(T)$ of the random variable T may be found from $P'(C)$ and from equation 8.14 by

$$Q(T) = P'(C(T)) \frac{dC(T)}{dT} \qquad (8.15)$$

according to ordinary probability theory. In equation 8.15 we regard as fixed parameters the time t and the whole past stimulus history $s(t')$ up to that time. To specify our model fully, we may specify either $P'(C)$ or $Q(T)$, as they are related by equation 8.15. For finding the frequency response it is convenient to let $s = s_0$ in equation 8.14 and specify the unperturbed period distribution $Q_0(T_0)$. The reason is that the random variable T_1 is given most conveniently as a function of the random variable T_0. Using $T_0 = 1/f_0$, $T_1 = -T_0^2 f_1$ (equation 3.10), and equation 5.10, we see that

$$T_1 = -\frac{e^{\gamma T_0} - e^{-i\omega T_0}}{i\omega + \gamma} \frac{s_1}{s_0}. \qquad (8.16)$$

The mean value T_1 is thus

$$T_1 = \int_0^\infty dT_0 \, Q_0(T_0) T_1(T_0) = -\frac{\tilde{Q}_0(-\gamma) - \tilde{Q}_0(i\omega)}{i\omega + \gamma} \frac{s_1}{s_0} \qquad (8.17)$$

where $\tilde{Q}_0(-\gamma)$ follows the definition of equation 8.13. Using both equations 8.12 and 8.17, we find that the frequency response of the population rate to the stimulus is

$$\frac{r_1}{s_1} = \frac{r_0}{s_0} \left(\frac{i\omega}{i\omega + \gamma} \right) \frac{\tilde{Q}_0(-\gamma) - \tilde{Q}_0(i\omega)}{1 - \tilde{Q}_0(i\omega)}, \qquad (8.18)$$

which should be compared to the deterministic result of equation 5.12.

A small stochastic effect corresponds to a period distribution $Q_0(T_0)$ which is peaked sharply around the mean period $\bar{T}_0$. We may write

$$e^{-i\omega T_0} = e^{-i\omega \bar{T}_0} e^{-i\omega(T_0 - \bar{T}_0)}$$

$$= e^{-i\omega \bar{T}_0} \left\{ 1 - i\omega(T_0 - \bar{T}_0) - \frac{\omega^2}{2!} (T_0 - \bar{T}_0)^2 + \cdots \right\} \qquad (8.19)$$

and substitution into equation 8.13 yields

$$\tilde{Q}_0(i\omega) \approx e^{-i\omega \bar{T}_0}\left(1 - \frac{\omega^2}{2}\tau^2\right) \qquad (8.20)$$

where

$$\tau = \sqrt{\int_0^\infty dT_0 (T_0 - \bar{T}_0)^2 Q_0(T_0)} \qquad (8.21)$$

measures the distribution's half-width. There is an analogous result for $\tilde{Q}_0(-\gamma)$.

What is the effect of small stochastic fluctuations upon the frequency response near resonance in a population of slightly forgetful encoders? If we assume both γ and τ are small in equation 8.18, we find

$$\frac{r_1}{s_1} = \frac{r_0}{s_0}\left\{1 - \frac{i\gamma}{(\omega - 2\pi n f_0) - i\frac{f_0}{2}(2\pi n f_0 \tau)^2}\right\} \qquad (8.22)$$

by the same approximation that led to equation 5.14. (We have set $f_0 = 1/T_0$.) As we anticipated, the response at resonance is finite, and equation 8.22 converges uniformly to the early perfect time-copy result of equation 4.4 as γ approaches zero. This uniformity is in contrast to the nonuniform convergence found at equation 5.14. The size of the response at resonance is

$$\frac{r_1}{s_1} = \frac{r_0}{s_0}\left\{1 + \frac{2}{(2\pi n)^2}\frac{\gamma/f_0}{(\tau f_0)^2}\right\} \qquad (8.23)$$

and represents a contest between deterministic forgetfulness and irregular firing. We note that the *square* of the small number τf_0 appears in the denominator of equation 8.25, so that in this limit a relatively substantial stochastic spread in firing periods is necessary to control a relatively much smaller degree of forgetfulness, if the perfect time-copy property is to be approximated at resonance. As a rough example consider the case where the internal memory variable u relaxes 10% between typical spikes ($\gamma/f_0 = 0.1$) and the spike periods have a root mean square scatter of 10% about their mean ($\tau f_0 = 0.1$). At the fundamental resonance ($n = 1$), even though the coefficient $2/(2\pi)^2 \approx 0.05$ is small, the resonant response is about 1.5 times the response well away from resonance.

We remark that even though equation 8.22 was derived from a specific model, that result is model independent to within a multiplicative scale factor on γ; the effect of a forgetfulness parameter should first appear through γ to the first power, and the denominator in equation 8.22 followed from equation 8.12 which was model independent.

The half-width τ (equation 8.21) at most may be made equal to the mean T_0, and this happens when $Q_0(T_0)$ is the Poisson distribution

$$Q_0(T_0) = f_0 e^{-f_0 T_0} \tag{8.24}$$

which has the property that successive firing times are completely uncorrelated. In this case it is easy to evaluate the frequency response of equation 8.18 exactly, and the result is

$$\frac{r_1}{s_1} = \frac{r_0}{s_0} \frac{1}{1 - \gamma f_0}, \tag{8.25}$$

which is independent of frequency. In this case the perfect time-copy property is actually achieved for the variation in any stimulus which departs only slightly from its mean.

The frequency response of equation 8.18 also may be calculated exactly for the general "gamma" distribution

$$Q_0(T_0) = \frac{((n+1)f_0)^{n+1}}{n!} T_0^n \, e^{-((n+1)f_0)T_0} \tag{8.26}$$

for which the Poisson and deterministic cases are opposite limits $n = 0$ and $n \to \infty$. We find $n + 1 = (f_0\tau)^{-2}$, and the characteristic function is

$$\tilde{Q}_0(i\omega) = \left(1 + i(f_0\tau)^2 \frac{\omega}{f_0}\right)^{-1/(f_0\tau)^2} \tag{8.27}$$

Fig. 6 gives examples of equation 8.18 which fall between the limiting cases.[13] We see for a very forgetful encoder that an rms stochastic scatter comparable to the forgetfulness coefficient suppresses the resonances very effectively. In the case of $\gamma/f_0 = \tau f_0 = 0.1$, the exact expression of equation 8.27 yields a response ratio of 1.51 between the first resonant peak and zero frequency, as compared to 1.5 calculated from the approximate equation 8.22.

9. CONCLUDING REMARKS

In this investigation we have paid particular attention to the population firing rate of a collection of neurons. Our motivation has been that this rate is essentially what is seen by a postsynaptic neuron. We have confined our consideration to "very large" neuron populations. In a practical sense "very

---

[13] The theoretical results of Fig. 6 may be compared with the hardware analogue results of Stein (1970), and Stein and French (1969).

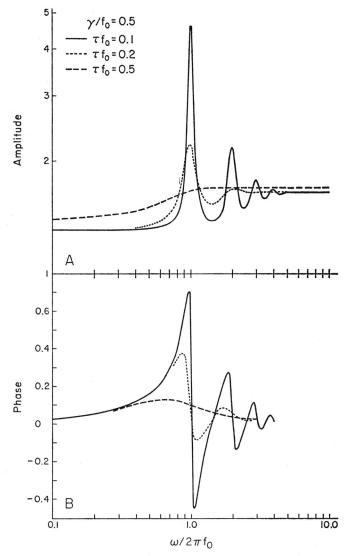

FIGURE 6. Amplitude and phase of population rate frequency response, showing contending effects of forgetfulness and stochastic scatter. Phase is given in radians.

large" means that the population firing rate must exceed the intracellular voltage resolution time of the postsynaptic neuron. The spike encoding schemes we have considered all involve only the stimulus history since the previous spike; this assumption is reasonable for a neuron whose intracellular voltage resolution time is limited by its electrical characteristic time rather than by the decay time of a chemical mediator.

We have reached the following conclusions.

(*a*) A simple encoder model, which is a reasonable idealization of known electrophysiology, yields a population firing rate which is a perfect replica of the input stimulus.

(*b*) A population of noise-free encoders which depart even slightly from the simple encoder model show a tendency to fall into step, and eventually yield a bursting type of population firing which yields a very much degraded copy of the input stimulus.

(*c*) The presence of noise in the encoders counteracts the tendency to synchronize. A slight noise level will retrieve a faithful population response for encoders which depart slightly from the simple model. Large stochastic fluctuations will do the same for a population which departs substantially from the simple model.

In developing these conclusions we have noted that there is a subtle quantitative relation between the firing rate of a single unit and the firing rate of the population from which it is drawn. This relation must be taken into account when the behavior of a population is deduced from observations made on a single cell.

I owe a particular debt to Richard Poppele and Richard Stein, and to Jun-ichi Toyoda who set me on the track of the material in section 2. Others whose thought helped are M. Arbib, E. Bayly, F. A. Dodge, Jr., David Lange, Henry McKean, Jurgen Moser, Richard L. Purple, Morris Schreiber, and Charles F. Stevens.

This research was supported in part by research grants (EY 00188) from the National Eye Institute and (GM1789) from the National Science Foundation.

Received for publication 31 December 1970.

REFERENCES

AITKIN, L. M., D. J. ANDERSON, and J. E. BRUGGE. 1970. Tonotopic organization and discharge characteristics of single neurons in nuclei of the lateral lemniscus of the cat. *J. Neurophysiol.* **32**:421.

BORSELLINO, A., R. E. POPPELE, and C. A. TERZUOLO. 1965. Transfer functions of the slowly adapting stretch receptor organ of Crustacea. *Cold Spring Harbor Symp. Quant. Biol.* **30**:581.

BROWN, M. C., I. ENGBERG, and P. B. C. MATTHEWS. 1967. The relative sensitivity to vibration of muscle receptors of the cat. *J. Physiol. (London).* **192**:773.

BRUGGE, J. F., D. J. ANDERSON, and L. M. AITKIN. 1970. Responses of neurons in the dorsal nucleus of the lateral lemniscus of cat to binaural tonal stimulation. *J. Neurophysiol.* **33**:441.

BRUGGE, J. F., D. J. ANDERSON, J. E. HIND, and J. E. ROSE. 1969. Time structure of discharges in single auditory nerve fibers of the squirrel monkey in response to complex periodic sounds. *J. Neurophysiol.* **32**:386.

CODDINGTON, E. A., and N. LEVINSON. 1955. Theory of ordinary differential equations. McGraw-Hill Book Company, New York.

DENJOY, A. 1932. Sur les courbes definies par les equations differentielles a la surface du tore. *J. Math. Pure Appl.* **11**:333.

GOLDBERG, J. M., and P. B. BROWN. 1969. Response of binaural neurons of dog superior olivary complex to dichotic tonal stimuli: some physiological mechanisms of sound localization. *J. Neurophysiol.* **32**:613.

HUBEL, D. H., and T. N. WIESEL. 1968. Receptive fields and functional architecture of monkey striate cortex. *J. Physiol. (London).* **195**:215.

HUGHES, G. W., and L. MAFFEI. 1966. Retinal ganglion cell response to sinusoidal light stimulation. *J. Neurophysiol.* **39**:333.

KIANG, N. Y.-S., T. WATANABE, E. C. THOMAS, and L. F. CLARK. 1965. Discharge Patterns of Single Fibers in the Cat's Auditory Nerve. The M.I.T. Press, Cambridge, Mass.

KNIGHT, B. W. 1972. The relationship between the firing rate of a single neuron and the level of activity in a population of neurons. Experimental evidence for resonant enhancement in the population response. *J. Gen. Physiol.* **59**:767.

KNIGHT, B. W., J.-I. TOYODA, and F. A. DODGE. 1970. A quantitative description of the dynamics of excitation and inhibition in the eye of *Limulus. J. Gen. Physiol.* **56**:421.

MATTHEWS, P. B. C., and R. B. STEIN. 1969. The sensitivity of muscle spindle afferents to small sinusoidal changes of length. *J. Physiol. (London).* **200**:723.

MENDELL, L. M., and E. HENNEMAN. 1968. Terminals of single Ia fibers: distribution within a pool of 300 homonymous motor neurons. *Science (Washington).* **160**:96.

MOUNTCASTLE, V. B., W. H. TALBOT, H. SAKATA, and J. HYVARINEN. 1968. Cortical neuronal mechanisms in flutter-vibration studied in unanesthetized monkeys. Neuronal periodicity and frequency discrimination. *J. Neurophysiol.* **32**:452.

PARTRIDGE, L. 1966. A possible source of nerve signal distortion arising in pulse rate encoding of signals. *J. Theor. Biol.* **11**:257. (See also Erratum. 1968. *J. Theor. Biol.* **21**:292.)

POPPELE, R. E., and R. J. BOWMAN. 1970. Quantitative description of linear behavior of mammalian muscle spindles. *J. Neurophysiol.* **33**:59.

RESCIGNO, A., R. B. STEIN, R. L. PURPLE, and R. E. POPPELE. 1970. A neuronal model for the discharge patterns produced by cyclic inputs. *Bull. Math. Biophys.* **32**:337.

ROSE, J. E., J. F. BRUGGE, D. J. ANDERSON, and J. E. HIND. 1967. Phase-locked response to low-frequency tones in single auditory nerve fibers of the squirrel monkey. *J. Neurophysiol.* **30**:770.

ROSE, J. E., J. F. BRUGGE, D. J. ANDERSON, and J. E. HIND. 1969. Some possible neural correlates of combination tones. *J. Neurophysiol.* **32**:402.

STEIN, R. B. 1970. The Role of Spike Trains in Transmitting and Distorting Sensory Signals. *In* The Neurosciences. The Rockefeller University Press, New York. 597.

STEIN, R. B., and A. S. FRENCH. 1969. Models for the Transmission of Information by Nerve Cells. *In* Excitatory Synaptic Mechanisms. Oslo University Press, Oslo. 247.

TALBOT, W. H., I. DARIAN-SMITH, H. H. KORNHUBER, and V. B. MOUNTCASTLE. 1967. The sense of flutter-vibration: comparison of the human capacity with response patterns of mechanoreceptive afferents from the monkey hand. *J. Neurophysiol.* **31**:301.

The relationship between the firing rate of a single neuron and the level of activity in a population of neurons

Experimental evidence for resonant enhancement in the population response

B. W. KNIGHT

The Rockefeller University, New York, N.Y.

Reprinted from the JOURNAL OF GENERAL PHYSIOLOGY, June 1972,
Vol. 59, no. 6, pp. 767–778

ABSTRACT A quantitative comparison is made between experiment and the theoretically predicted dynamics of a neuron population. The experiment confirms the theoretical prediction that under appropriate conditions an enlarged resonant response should appear in the activity of the neuron population, near the frequency at which there is minimum modulation in the instantaneous rate of a single neuron. These findings bear on the relationship between the firing rate of a single neuron and the firing rate of a population of neurons.

INTRODUCTION AND RESULTS

The experiment reported here was performed with three objectives. The first was to investigate experimentally the relationship between firing rate of a single neuron and the activity level in a whole population of similar neurons. The second objective was to seek evidence of a "resonant" enhancement in the responsiveness of a neuron population, which was theoretically predicted under specified circumstances, and which might be of some direct physiological interest. The third objective was to attempt a quantitative comparison between data gathered from a real neuron, and several theoretical predictions of a general nature which have been presented in a preceding paper (Knight, 1972). This experiment was done with a single neuron: the response of a homogeneous neuron population to a single cycle of stimulus has been inferred by observing the response pattern of the single neuron again and again over many repeated stimulus cycles.

When one deals with a neuron whose firing is both rapid and regular, it is customary to characterize that neuron's activity by its "instantaneous fre-

631

quency" or "single unit instantaneous firing rate," which is the reciprocal of the interval between impulses. However, if that neuron is firing in response to a periodic input, the period of which is not much longer than the intervals between the impulses with which the neuron responds, then the significance of the single unit instantaneous firing rate becomes less clear. The measure of neural activity which is of direct relevance to physiological effects of that activity not only concerns the time since last firing of a single neuron, but also should be a measure of how many similar neurons are firing at any given phase of the input cycle. If there is convergence upon the next higher order neuron, it will be the momentary level of impulse activity in the entire population which determines the postsynaptic potential in that higher order neuron. In this experiment the single unit rate (measured directly) and the population rate (as inferred from many cycles) in response to a periodic input have been measured simultaneously from a single neuron. Major qualitative differences are found between the two measures of neural activity.

When a neuron fires in response to a periodic input, two important frequencies are involved. One is the frequency of the stimulus input and the other is the "carrier rate" or "center frequency" of the responding neuron, which is the reciprocal of the long-time average of the single unit interpulse interval. The periodic input to the neuron consists of a mean value plus a modulation. In the limit of vanishingly small modulation, the center frequency will be independent of the input modulation frequency, and will depend only on the mean input level and upon the characteristics of the neuron itself. In this limit of small modulation, the response of a homogeneous population of neurons may be analyzed theoretically, in an approximate way that does not require detailed assumptions concerning the underlying machinery of the neurons. A theoretical prediction results: If the input modulation frequency is set close to the center frequency of a single unit, the pooled firing of the neuron population will show an enhanced "resonant" response[1]—a particularly strong modulation in the population's response over the stimulus cycle. This predicted resonant response is specifically a property of the pooled activity of the whole population. The theory predicts that the modulation in the instantaneous rate of a single unit will show the opposite effect: it will drop to a minimum near the point where modulation frequency is equal to center frequency. The experiment bears out these two predictions.

To within experimental error, the frequency responses, of the single unit and population rates, may be measured quantitatively. Theory also predicts what these numbers should be. In its most reduced form, the approximate

---

[1] The word resonance is used in its technical sense here. In technical terms, there exists a real "resonant" frequency (the center frequency) near which there lies a formal complex frequency which makes a denominator vanish in a frequency response expression.

theory compresses all the characteristics of a neuron to two parameters: the "forgetting rate" (γ), and the "coefficient of variation" (c). The forgetting rate γ essentially defines a time scale for discounting old input, in the determination of when the neuron will fire again. The coefficient of variation c is a measure of the fractional random scatter in interpulse interval times. The phenomenon of population resonance is directly related to the process of forgetting: in the limit of no forgetting ($\gamma = 0$) no resonance should appear. In the theory forgetting is included as a simple exponential discounting of old input with the passage of time. The random variability of interpulse intervals (as characterized by the coefficient of variation) has the effect of limiting the height of the resonance, and of increasing its width. In the present experiment the coefficient of variation was measured directly. The choice of forgetting rate was dictated by the data: an attempt was made to obtain a reasonable fit. The comparison of the experiment and the theory is shown in Fig. 1.

Since the experiment yielded frequency responses for both single unit rate and population rate, the data are sufficient to find an empirical transfer function from population rate to single unit rate. The data points in Fig. 2 give this empirical result. Theory also yields an expression, with the interesting feature that it depends only on the coefficient of variation (which was measured) and *not* on the forgetting rate (which was fitted). Thus the theory makes a prediction which contains no free parameters, and is shown by the curves in Fig. 2.

METHODS AND DISCUSSION OF METHODS

A visual neuron, the eccentric cell in the compound lateral eye of the horseshoe crab *Limulus polyphemus*, was chosen for this experiment. The choice was dictated by the sizable body of quantitative information available concerning this neuron (Dodge et al., 1970; Hartline and Ratliff, 1972) and by personal familiarity with the preparation procedures.

The general setup was usual: the excised eye served as the fourth side of a covered moist chamber. Light was led to a single facet of the eye by a narrow (0.4 mm) glass fiber optic bundle, mounted on a micromanipulator. The light came from a glow modulator system. The moist chamber was filled with previously filtered and aerated *Limulus* blood, and a small bundle of nerve fibers, dissected from the optic nerve, was lifted through the air/blood interface and mounted on a cotton wick recording electrode. A single unit was isolated optically, by using the micromanipulator. The signal from the wick electrode went to an AC preamplifier and thence to the amplifier of an oscilloscope. The oscilloscope output drove an audio monitor system and also fed a pulse-height discriminator which interfaced with a small computer (CDC-160A). The glow modulator tube was pulsed at a high frequency

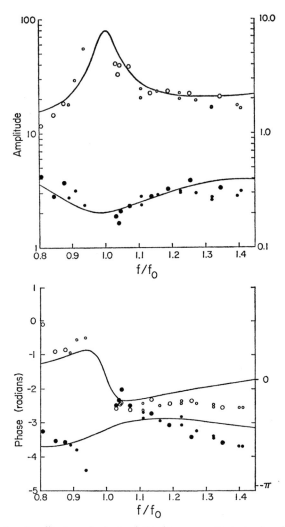

FIGURE 1. Amplitude and phase of the frequency response of a single unit (filled circles) and of the population (open circles). The left-hand ordinate is for the experimental measurements. The solid curves are from the theory, and correspond to the right-hand ordinate. The difference between left-hand and right-hand ordinates reflects the unknown amplitude and phase in the generator potential (see text).

(center frequency, 400/sec). This pulse rate was frequency modulated by a voltage input, which was a constant voltage, plus a sine wave of variable amplitude drawn from a function generator. The function generator also put out a phase mark on another channel at the top of the sine wave, and

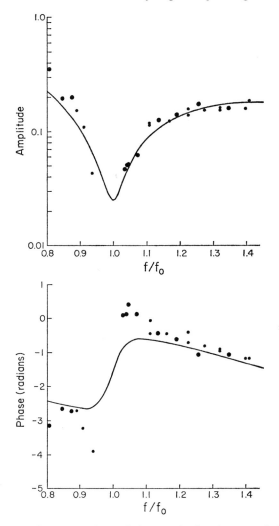

FIGURE 2. Amplitude and phase of the transduction from population response to single unit response. The solid lines are theoretical and the filled circles are from the experiment.

this phase mark was delivered to a second discriminator. To monitor modulation depth, the pulses delivered to the glow modulator tube were also fed to a factor of 16 downcount scaling circuit, the output pulses of which were in turn sent to a third discriminator which interfaced with the computer. At the end of each run, the nerve impulse times were classified according to which consecutive 20 msec time interval in the stimulus cycle they occupied. In this way the computer generated a cycle histogram of the population rate, which it returned through a digital-to-analogue converter, to a second monitoring oscilloscope at the experimental setup. The histogram and the three channels of impulse time information were also stored on magnetic tape by the computer for later processing.

In stimulating the eye it was necessary to abandon the established procedure of light on for about 20 sec and off for about 100 sec per run, which fosters the long-term stability of the preparation but leads to a continuous downward drift in the neuron's center frequency throughout the 20 sec. In this experiment it was necessary to hold the neuron's center frequency at a known level to within a per cent or two during a run, and this demanded that the light be left on continuously. As a result the cell's center frequency gradually declined as the experiment progressed, steadily but slowly, and not appreciably during a 20 sec run. This slow decline proved valuable, and was exploited in performing the experiment: in the theory which this experiment was designed to examine, the sensitive dependence upon frequency is in fact a dependence upon the *ratio* between modulation frequency and center frequency, so it was natural to set a fixed modulation frequency and allow the center frequency to creep past it during the course of the experiment. Proceeding in this way has a particular advantage: the conversion of flickering light to modulated intracellular voltage (generator potential) is frequency dependent, and that frequency dependence is believed to be one of the more stable aspects of this preparation. By working at a single modulation frequency we confine our ignorance of what voltage the impulse encoder sees to a single unknown amplitude and a single unknown phase. The center frequency of the neuron was brought close to 4 impulses/sec by inserting an appropriate neutral density filter in the light path. A fine setting to 4/sec was made by adjusting the duration of the glow modulator pulses. The function generator was set at 3 cps. The neuron's center frequency gradually declined to 2/sec, at which point the experiment was terminated. These firing rates, which are an order of magnitude lower than what is usual for *Limulus* experiments, were chosen for the following reasons. (*a*) The decline in center frequency is gradual at these modest rates. (*b*) The simple theory assumes that irregularities in interpulse interval are uncorrelated, and experiments have shown that eccentric cell impulses become uncorrelated when they are separated by more than about 0.3 sec (Shapley, 1971). (*c*) Since the experiment relies on a stable generator potential, a frequency should be chosen where the generator frequency response is insensitive to parametric changes; the generator amplitude is sensitive to frequency changes above 3 cps (Knight et al., 1970). (*d*) In the usual regime the eccentric cell behaves much like a "simple integrate-and-fire" encoder. That is, it shows only slight memory loss between impulses, as indicated by its lack of any pronounced tendency to phase lock to periodic stimuli. Without memory loss, no resonance should be anticipated. The theory indicates that a lengthened interval would lead to greater memory loss, and a more pronounced resonance; the theoretical resonance height depends on the *ratio* of the forgetting rate to the center frequency. These four considerations set an upper bound on the center frequency and the following one sets a lower bound. (*e*) Near the anticipated resonance, the center frequency must be determined without much more than 1% error, and the computer program is limited to 20 sec of data on any run. Eccentric cell interpulse intervals vary about ±10% (Ratliff et al., 1968); the coefficient of variation of this cell was 0.09. It takes about 60 impulses, or 3/sec, to achieve the necessary error bound.

Because there is substantial random variability in interpulse intervals, the measurement of output modulation faces a serious signal-to-noise problem. For the single unit rate, the problem is at its worst near resonance, where the output modulation drops to small values. It might seem that the problem could be solved by means of a large input modulation. However, the theory (which is a linearized theory) only claims to work in the limit of small modulation. How large a modulation may be used, without causing drastic changes in response, may be estimated from the nonlinear theory without noise, which is given in section 6 of the previous paper (Knight, 1972). The conclusion there is that a result of finite modulation is phase locking, and that this condition is particularly encouraged if (*a*) there is much forgetting between impulses or (*b*) if the modulation frequency is close to center frequency. Of course both are preconditions of this experiment.

These considerations dictated the cycle of operations in the experiment. First, a 20 sec run was taken with no modulation, to determine the center frequency. Then the light modulation was turned up while the sound of the impulse train was monitored on a loudspeaker. Either the unmodulated or the phase-locked response is a monotonous beat on the audio monitor. In between, the beat has a notable nonperiodic texture. When this condition was achieved another run was taken, at the end of which the population cycle histogram was displayed on the monitor oscilloscope. From this display a judgment was made about how to change the modulation. If signal-to-noise was poor the modulation was turned up. If the wave form seen was distorted from sinusoidal, the modulation was turned down. Sometimes no readjustment was necessary. Another run was taken. This pair of modulated runs was followed by an unmodulated run to start the next cycle. The center frequency, which was later related to each modulated run, was the average of the two values obtained before and after.

Subsequently modulation values were extracted from the data by a least-squares fitting procedure described elsewhere (Knight et al., 1970).[2] The modulation in population response was determined in a similar way from the record of the cycle histogram. The frequency responses were calculated in the form (output modulation/mean output)/(input modulation/mean input), which is the form convenient to compare with theory.

The experimental design anticipated discarding the earlier of each pair of modulated runs. This was not always necessary, and conversely sometimes both runs were discarded. The first criterion for discarding came from notes made immediately after each run. The second criterion came from data processing: if harmonic content was excessive, or if the center frequency of the single unit rate was much deviated by the presence of modulation, then that run was rejected. The least-squares procedure also gave a "uniqueness of fit" estimate. The fit to the single unit rate becomes nonunique when phase locking occurs, and some runs were rejected on that basis. Two runs were discarded simply because they were in bad disagreement with all the rest of the data. From a span of 50 modulated runs, 16 runs were discarded and the rest are represented in Figs. 1 and 2. The oversize data points indicate the averages of two consecutive runs in those cases where no modulation readjustment was made. The averaging was done on the fitting coefficients, before reduction to amplitude and phase.

For the theoretical curves of Fig. 1, the value $\gamma/f_0 = 0.75$ (f_0 is center frequency) was chosen because agreement with the experimental points looked reasonable. Higher values give less agreement, but values of γ/f_0 down to 0.5 give agreement comparable to what is shown. In the upper frame of Fig. 1 the theoretical amplitude has been shifted, as shown on the right-hand vertical scale. In the lower frame the phase has been similarly shifted. These two operations adjust for the unknown amplitude and phase in the generator potential modulation. In Fig. 2 there are no adjustable parameters.

THEORETICAL

A detailed theory was developed in the previous paper. In brief outline, here is how the theory may be put into a form to compare with the present experiment. According to the simplest neuron model (integrate-and-fire model) the single unit modulation response is given by the running average of the input modulation:

$$B = \frac{1}{T_0} \int_{-T_0}^{0} dt\, s(t) \tag{1}$$

[2] To determine the modulation in instantaneous frequency, a record was kept of the times at which impulses occurred. To each occurrence time was assigned an instantaneous frequency which was the reciprocal of the time since the previous impulse. An assumed output modulation form was adjusted to give the best possible fit, in the least-squares sense, to the measured instantaneous frequencies at all the impulse occurrence times.

(equation 3.12)[3] where $s(t)$ is the stimulus modulation, B is the response modulation at the moment $t = 0$, and T_0 is the period between impulses in the absence of modulation. If for the stimulus modulation $s(t)$ we substitute the sinusoid exp $(i\omega t)$ the value of which is unity at the moment $t = 0$, we find

$$B = \frac{1}{T_0} \int_{-T_0}^{0} e^{i\omega t}\, dt = \frac{1 - e^{-i\omega T_0}}{i\omega T_0} \tag{2}$$

(equations 3.14 and 3.15). This is the transfer function from the stimulus to the single unit rate. For different reasons it is also *the transfer function from the population rate to the single unit rate* (equation 4.3). If, in the absence of modulation, the interpulse interval T_0 shows random variations, then equation 2 must be replaced by its reasonable generalization

$$B = \frac{1 - \langle e^{-i\omega T_0} \rangle}{i\omega \langle T_0 \rangle} \tag{3}$$

(equation 8.12), which is very nearly the theoretical expression plotted in Fig. 2. If the fluctuations of T_0 from its mean $\bar{T}_0$ are small[4] then we may write

$$\langle e^{-i\omega T_0} \rangle = \langle e^{-i\omega \bar{T}_0} e^{-i\omega (T_0 - \bar{T}_0)} \rangle$$

$$= e^{-i\omega \bar{T}_0} \langle 1 - i\omega (T_0 - \bar{T}_0) + \frac{1}{2!}(-i\omega)^2 (T_0 - \bar{T}_0)^2 + \cdots \rangle \tag{4}$$

(equation 8.19). The means of the first two terms in the pointed brackets are evidently unity and zero, whence

$$\langle e^{-i\omega T_0} \rangle \cong e^{-i\omega \bar{T}_0} \left\{ 1 - \frac{\omega^2}{2} \langle (T_0 - \bar{T}_0)^2 \rangle \right\} \tag{5}$$

(equation 8.20), and equation 3 becomes approximately

$$B = \frac{1 - e^{-i\omega \bar{T}_0} \left\{ 1 - \frac{\omega^2}{2} \langle (T_0 - \bar{T}_0)^2 \rangle \right\}}{i\omega \bar{T}} \tag{6}$$

the amplitude and phase of which are the curves plotted in Fig. 2. The fluctuation term in equation 6 is related to the coefficient of variation c by

$$\langle (T_0 - \bar{T}_0)^2 \rangle = c \bar{T}_0^2 \tag{7}$$

---

[3] Equation numbers with decimal points will refer to corresponding equations in the previous paper (Knight, 1972).
[4] We indicate mean either by pointed brackets or by an overhead bar depending on typographical convenience.

(equation 8.12). The value $c = 0.09$, which persisted throughout the experiment, was used in the calculation. (Fig. 4 of the previous paper [Knight, 1972] shows the analogous result when $c = 0.$)

On rather general theoretical grounds, the behavior of a broad class of real neurons should be typified by the "forgetful integrate-and-fire neuron model." As in equation 2 the single unit frequency response in this model has a numerator containing two terms which represent the present and past limits of an averaging integral. However, in the forgetful model the numerator term representing the present is favored by a weighting factor $\exp(\gamma T_0)$. The full expression is

$$F = \frac{e^{\gamma T_0} - e^{-i\omega T_0}}{(i\omega + \gamma)T_0} \tag{8}$$

(equation 5.10). If the interpulse interval has random scatter, this generalizes to

$$F = \frac{\langle e^{\gamma T_0}\rangle - \langle e^{-i\omega T_0}\rangle}{(i\omega + \gamma)\langle T_0\rangle} \tag{9}$$

(equation 8.17). If again the scatter about the mean is small, this may be approximated by

$$F = \frac{e^{\gamma \bar{T}_0}\left\{1 + \dfrac{\gamma^2}{2}\langle(T_0 - \bar{T}_0)^2\rangle\right\} - e^{-i\omega \bar{T}_0}\left\{1 - \dfrac{\omega^2}{2}\langle(T_0 - \bar{T}_0)^2\rangle\right\}}{(i\omega + \gamma)T_0} \tag{10}$$

in exactly the same way that equation 6 was derived. The value $\gamma T_0 = 0.75$ was substituted into equation 10, which then yielded the theoretical amplitude and phase that are plotted as curves along with the single-unit data in Fig. 1. Finally, the theoretical population response was obtained from

$$P = F/B \tag{11}$$

(equation 8.18), the amplitude and phase of which are plotted along with the population data in Fig. 1. The result should also be compared with Fig. 6 of the previous paper (Knight, 1972) (in that figure the coefficient of variation is given by $\tau f_0 = c$).

In conclusion, here is how B and F are expressed in terms of the modulation frequency f, the center frequency f_0, the forgetting rate γ, and the coefficient of variation c. The expressions are

$$B = \frac{1 - e^{-2\pi i f/f_0}\left(1 - \tfrac{1}{2}(c \cdot 2\pi f/f_0)^2\right)}{2\pi i f/f_0} \tag{12}$$

and

$$F = \frac{e^{\gamma/f_0}\ (1 + \frac{1}{2}(c \cdot \gamma/f_0)^2) - e^{-2\pi i f/f_0}\ (1 - \frac{1}{2}(c \cdot 2\pi f/f_0)^2)}{2\pi i(f/f_0) + (\gamma/f_0)}. \qquad (13)$$

The fact that f and γ appear only in the combinations f/f_0 and γ/f_0 was of course crucial in the design of the experiment.

DISCUSSION

Because of the noise problem inherent in this experiment, there is considerable scatter in the data, and no conclusions should be based on any single point. Nonetheless, there is a substantial similarity between the results of theory and of experiment. In Fig. 1 the most obvious disagreement is in the phase at the upper end of the relative frequency range, where the phase of both single unit and population rates systematically falls behind the predictions of theory. At its greatest this phase lag goes to about a tenth of a cycle (the total height of the phase graph is 6 radians, not quite a full cycle).

The phase lag may be an artifact of the experimental procedure. Between the resonant point at $f/f_0 = 1$ and the last data point on the right, the encoding neuron's time scale, as measured by the center frequency, had become stretched out by some 40%. If the generator potential were likewise "running down" it would introduce the observed phase trend into the data. On the other hand, a real departure of this magnitude from the very simplified theory would be no surprise, and could arise, for example, if the real encoder were to discount past input in a way different from the simple exponential assumed in the model. The fitted value $\gamma/f_0 = 0.75$ corresponds to a characteristic forgetting time of about 0.45 sec, which is quite comparable to the interpulse times in the experiment. Under this circumstance a nonexponential profile for forgetting could yield a substantial departure.

In Fig. 2 the one systematic discrepancy is in the phase near resonance. The abrupt change predicted by theory is exaggerated in the experimental result. This probably is not a breakdown in the theory but rather a result of overmodulation. If the theory were in error we would also expect that the population rate data of Fig. 1 would show a systematic departure of phase near the resonance, since the logical relation among the curves is from the single unit response through the transduction of Fig. 2 (or equation 11) to the population response. This reasoning casts suspicion on the phase data near resonance of the single unit response. There is a second good reason for this suspicion: section 3 of the previous paper (Knight, 1972) indicates that overmodulation will be more severe in the single unit response than in the population response. The severity of the overmodulation problem in the immediate neighborhood of the resonance led to the discarding of all runs that fell within the gap that the figures show there.

Presumably the population resonance does not play a significant role in the normal functioning of the *Limulus* eye. Under normal conditions the eccentric cell center frequency is not far below the flicker-fusion threshold frequency.[5] However, one may speculate how evolution may have exploited the effect in other systems. The population resonance is uniquely suited to the task of frequency discrimination, and one might look for its application in auditory systems, or in the frequency-sensitive electrical sense of certain fish. If the effect were utilized at more than one neuronal level, sharper frequency tuning should be found the farther one went along the sensory pathway.

The data of Fig. 1 show that a population of neurons may carry signals which contain frequencies well beyond the center frequency of any single neuron. These data also show that, as the center frequency is approached or exceeded, the single unit instantaneous frequency if it is used naively becomes an altogether misleading indicator of what the population are doing. Where the population show a maximum response the single unit rate shows a minimum. The results of the experiment were reasonably fit by a simple encoder model: the stochastic and forgetful integrate-and-fire model. This indicates that more detailed knowledge of neuronal impulse encoding may be unnecessary in the further exploration of some aspects of the dynamics of nerve populations.

For their assistance and encouragement I am indebted to H. K. Hartline, to Floyd Ratliff, and to numerous other friends in our laboratory and around The Rockefeller University.

This research was supported in part by Grants EY 188 from the National Eye Institute, GM 1789 from the National Institute of General Medical Sciences, and GB-6540 from the National Science Foundation.

Received for publication 30 December 1971.

REFERENCES

DODGE, F. A., R. M. SHAPLEY, and B. W. KNIGHT. 1970. Linear systems analysis of the *Limulus* retina. *Behav. Sci.* **15**:24.

HARTLINE, H. K., and F. RATLIFF. 1972. Inhibitory interaction in the retina of *Limulus*. *In* Handbook of Sensory Physiology. Springer-Verlag, Berlin. 7(IB).

KNIGHT, B. W. 1972. Dynamics of encoding in a population of neurons. *J. Gen. Physiol.* **59**:734.

KNIGHT, B. W., J.-I. TOYODA, and F. A. DODGE. 1970. A quantitative description of the dynamics of excitation and inhibition in the eye of *Limulus*. *J. Gen. Physiol.* **56**:421.

RATLIFF, F., H. K. HARTLINE, and D. LANGE. 1968. Variability of interspike intervals in optic nerve fibers of *Limulus*: effect of light and dark adaptation. *Proc. Nat. Acad. Sci. U.S.A.* **60**:464.

SHAPLEY, R. M. 1971. Fluctuations of the impulse rate in *Limulus* eccentric cells. *J. Gen. Physiol.* **57**:539.

[5] Unpublished observations of F. A. Dodge, recording from nerve fiber bundles of intact animals in the field, give a center frequency of 6/sec or more. The flicker-fusion frequency is at about 10 cps.

Visual receptors and retinal interaction

H. KEFFER HARTLINE

The Rockefeller University, New York, N.Y.

Reprinted from LES PRIX NOBEL en 1967, The Nobel Foundation, 1968, 1969, pp. 242–269

The neuron is the functional as well as the structural unit of the nervous system. Neurophysiology received an impetus of far-reaching effect in the 1920's, when Adrian and his colleagues developed and exploited methods for recording the activity of single neurons and sensory receptors. Adrian and Bronk were the first to analyze motor function by recording the activity of single fibers dissected from a nerve trunk and Adrian and Zotterman the first to elucidate properties of single sensory receptors (1). These studies laid the foundations for the unitary analysis of nervous function.

My early interest in vision was spurred by another contribution from Adrian's laboratory: his study, with R. Matthews, of the massed discharge of nerve impulses in the eel's optic nerve. (2). I aspired to the obvious extension of this study: application of unitary analysis to the receptors and neurons of the visual system.

Oscillograms of the action potentials in a single nerve fiber are now commonplace. The three shown in Fig. 1 are from an optic nerve fiber whose retinal receptor was stimulated by light, the relative values of which are given at the left of each record. One of the earliest results of unitary analysis was to show that higher intensities are signaled by higher frequencies of discharge of uniform nerve impulses.

In 1931, when C. H. Graham and I sought to apply to an optic nerve the technique developed by Adrian and Bronk for isolating a single fiber, we made a fortunate choice of experimental animal (3). The xiphosuran arachnoid, *Limulus polyphemus,* commonly called "Horseshoe crab", abounds on the eastern coast of North America (4). These "living fossils" have lateral compound eyes that are coarsely faceted and connected to the brain by long optic nerves. The optic nerve in the adults can be frayed into thin bundles which are easy to split until just one active fiber remains. The records in Fig. 1 were obtained from such a preparation.

The sensory structures in the eye of *Limulus* from which the optic nerve fibers arise are clusters of receptor cells, arranged radially around the dendritic process of a bipolar neuron (eccentric cell) (5). Each cluster lies behind its corneal facet and crystalline cone, which give it its own, small visual field (Fig. 2). Each such ommatidium, though not as simple as I once thought, seems to act as a functional receptor unit. Restriction of the stimulating light to one facet elicits discharge in one fiber—the axon of the bipolar neuron whose dendritic process is in intimate contact with the light-sensitive rhabdom that is borne by the encircling retinular cells.

643

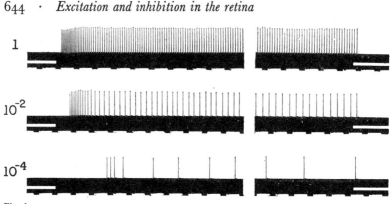

Fig. 1.
Oscillograms of the electrical activity (discharge of nerve impulses) in a single optic nerve, from the lateral eye of *Limulus*, stimulated by illumination of the facet associated with its receptor. Relative values of light intensity given at left. Time marked in 1/5 sec. in trace at bottom of each record; signal marking period of steady illumination blackens out the white band just above time marks. (After Hartline (11)).

Many of the properties of vision that are familiar to us from behavioral experiments on animals, from psychophysical experiments with human subjects, and indeed from our own everyday visual experience find parallels in the responses of the photoreceptor units in the *Limulus* eye. Reciprocity between intensity and duration of short flashes in stimulating single receptors, the spectral sensitivity of individual receptors, the course of light and dark adaption, and threshold uncertainty as related to quantum fluctuations are examples of such parallels. (6).

Two well known and very elementary features of receptor responses appear in the records shown in Fig. 1. The first is that the stimulation intensities cover a wide range; the corresponding steady frequencies of impulse discharge cover only a modest range. Intensity information is considerably compressed in being translated into discharge frequency of the nerve fiber. Our vision, and that of most animals, functions well over an enormous range of ambient light intensity; we may surmise that this capability results in large measure from the inherent properties of the individual receptors.

The second feature to note in Fig. 1 is the high rate of impulse discharge which signals the onset of illumination. After this initial transient the familiar process of sensory adaption sets in to reduce the discharge to a more modest rate. By virtue of this property, a receptor can signal even small changes in intensity while still retaining its ability to function over a wide range of ambient illumination.

This is further illustrated in Fig. 3, which shows the response of a *Limulus* receptor to an increment in light intensity imposed shortly after adaptation to a stronger background light had taken place. This oscillogram was obtained by means of a micropipette electrode thrust into the eccentric cell of the ommatidium (7). It shows both the slow depolarization of the cell—the "generator potential", to use Granit's term (8)—and the train of super-

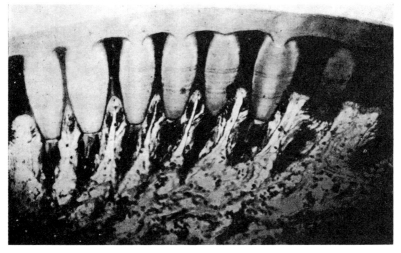

Fig. 2.
Section perpendicular to cornea through a portion (approx. 1 1/2 mm.) of the lateral (compound) eye of *Limulus*, showing 7 ommatidia: the cornea is above; the crystalline cones project downward to the sensory portions of the ommatidia, which have been partially bleached to reveal the retinulae. Fibers of optic nerve and plexus show faintly below. Micrograph by W. H. Miller (cf. (7)).

imposed nerve impulse spikes that are generated in the axon by the local currents from the depolarized cell (9). Both features of the response—the graded depolarization and the frequency of impulse discharge—display exaggerated transients at the onset and cessation of the incremented step in light intensity. The basic mechanism of the receptor is one that emphasizes change.

The response patterns of Figs. 1 and 3 are not faithful representations of

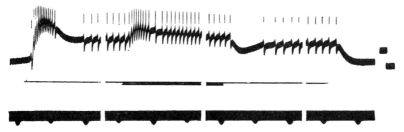

Fig. 3.
Oscillogram of the electrical activity of a receptor unit in the lateral eye of *Limulus*, recorded by a pipette microelectrode in the eccentric cell of an ommatidium, showing "generator potential" and superimposed nerve impulse "spikes". Stimulation by light signalled by black lines above the (1/5 sec.) time marks. Light shone steadily, starting near the beginning of the record; in the middle of the record the light was incremented by approx. 50 %, marked by second black line. Calibration deflection at right = 10 mv. Baseline at beginning of record *ca.* 50 mv. negative with respect to outside cell.

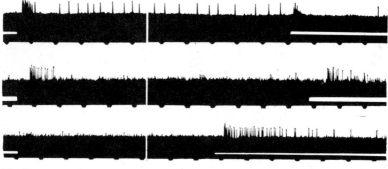

Fig. 4.
Oscillograms of the electrical activity of single optic nerve fibers dissected from the vitreous surface of the retina of a frog's eye. Recording as in Fig. 1. (After Hartline, 1938 (10)).

the light stimuli, which were simple steps of intensity. To some extent, the receptor mechanism distorted the sensory information. This illustrates the broad principle established by the earliest studies of single sensory endings: receptors, by virtue of their inherent properties, operate upon the information they collect from their surroundings to favour certain features of it. The processing of sensory data begins in the receptors.

Successful recording from single fibers in the optic nerve of *Limulus* emboldened me to apply the same methods to the vertebrate eye. The optic nerve of a vertebrate is very different from that of *Limulus;* dissection of bundles of fibers from it seemed a quite hopeless task. Moreover, this was before Granit and his colleagues developed micro-electrodes for retinal recording. But Nature has provided a ready-made dissection of the optic nerve, spreading it in a thin layer over the vitreous surface of the retina. Picking up small bundles from the exposed retina of a frog's eye was easy; splitting one of them until only a single active fiber remained was not too difficult.

The findings were unexpected: different optic nerve fibers responded to light in different ways (Fig. 4). Some fibers gave discharges much like those in *Limulus*, some responded vigorously at onset and again at cessation of illumination or when slight changes in intensity were made, and were otherwise silent. Still other fibers gave no response during illumination, firing a vigorous and prolonged train of impulses only when light was dimmed.

Further study of these responses of single retinal ganglion cells revealed interesting properties. Slight movements of a small spot or shadow elicited responses in some optic nerve fibers if they were within the square millimeter or so of retinal area that is the receptive field of the fiber's ganglion cell (Fig. 5). Convergence of excitatory and inhibitory influences was found to take place within the receptive fields of fibers, and summation of excitation was demonstrated. Receptive fields of fibers were shown to overlap extensively; a given small area of the retina is held in common within the confines of many receptive fields, belonging to fibers of greatly diverse response characteristics (10, 11). Thus there is interaction in the retina, as Granit had

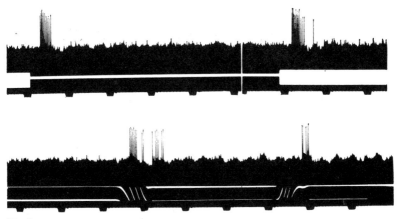

Fig. 5.
Discharge of impulses in a single optic nerve fiber in the frog's retina in response to movements of a spot of light on the retina. Lower record: a small spot (50μ diam.) was moved twice within the fiber's receptive field, about 30 μ each time, as signalled by the white lines crossing the blackened band just above the 1/5 sec. time marks. Upper record: same fiber responded only to light going on and off, when no movement of the spot took place. (Steady light signalled by blackening of band above time marks.) (After Hartline, 1940 (10)).

shown, and as Adrian and Matthews had demonstrated earlier. It is evident that a great deal of elaborate and sophisticated "data processing" takes place in the thin layer of nervous tissue that is the retina.

Since those early observations a wealth of new knowledge has been obtained by workers in many laboratories. From studies of the retinas of mammals as well as cold-blooded vertebrates, from recordings of units, for example, in the ganglionic layers in the eyes of crustaceans and insects, and by the use of various patterns of light, moving and stationary and of various colors, new and surprising properties of retinal neurons have been and are constantly being discovered (12). It is now clear that the retina is even more powerful in the integrative tasks it performs than my early experiments had intimated.

Can we understand how these diverse and complex response patterns, highly specialized for specific tasks, are generated in the retina? Broad Sherringtonian principles can guide us—the interplay of excitatory and inhibitory influences in convergent and divergent pathways, with various spatial distributions, thresholds, time courses (8). But the application of broad principles to specific cases of such complexity is not easy. It is here that comparative physiology can help. The animal world is rich in its variety of visual systems, built in different ways and with different degrees of complexity, although all governed, we are confident, by the same universal, basic principles.

In this, *Limulus* has again proved to be a valuable experimental animal. It, too, has a retina, although a much simpler one than those of the vertebrates

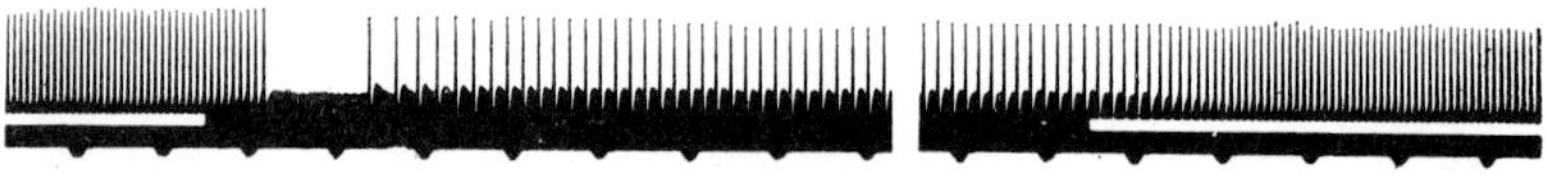

Fig. 6.

Inhibition in the eye of *Limulus*. The train of impulses from a receptor, elicited by steady illumination, was slowed by illumination of a group of 20—30 neighboring receptors in an annular region surrounding it (signalled by blackening of the white band above the 1/5 sec. time marks). (From Hartline et al. (7)).

or higher invertebrates. Interaction in the *Limulus* retina is complex enough to be interesting, yet simple enough to be analyzed with relative ease.

When I first worked with *Limulus,* I thought that the receptor units acted independently of one another. But I soon noticed that extraneous lights in the laboratory, rather than increasing the rate of discharge of impulses from a receptor, often caused a decrease in its activity. Neighboring ommatidia, viewing the extraneous room lights more directly than the receptor on which I was working, could inhibit that receptor quite markedly (13). With my colleagues H. G. Wagner and F. Ratliff, I undertook the investigation of this inhibitory process (14).

An experiment illustrating inhibition in the *Limulus* retina is shown in Fig. 6. Illumination of a small group of ommatida (20—30) in the neighborhood of an arbitrarily chosen, steadily illuminated test receptor caused a substantial slowing of its discharge. After the light on the neighboring receptors was turned off, there was prompt recovery, followed by a small but distinct overshoot—a post inhibitory rebound.

The basic properties of the inhibition in the *Limulus* eye are quickly summarized. The brighter the light on neighboring receptors, the greater is the slowing of the discharge of a receptor being tested. The greater the number of neighboring receptors illuminated, the greater is their effect: there is spatial summation of inhibitory influences. Receptors close to a given receptor inhibit it more strongly, on the average, than do distant ones. Each ommatidium in the eye has its surrounding field of inhibition. The influences are mutual: each receptor, being a neighbor of its neighbors, inhibits and is inhibited by those neighbors. Interaction in the *Limulus* eye, as far as is yet known, is purely inhibitory. Ratliff and I, with many colleagues in our laboratory, have been engaged over the past decade and a half in the analysis of this process (15).

The anatomical basis for the inhibitory influences that are exerted mutually in the *Limulus* eye is a network of nerve fibers—a true retina—lying just behind the layer of ommatidia, and interconnecting them (Fig. 7). It is over this plexus of fiber bundles that run laterally from ommatidium to ommatidium that the inhibitory influences pass: cut these bundles, and the inhibition vanishes. Fibers in these bundles arise as branches of the sensory axons from the ommatidia that traverse the plexus on their way to become the optic nerve; scattered profusely through the plexus are clumps of neuropil, rich in synaptic regions and packed with synaptic vesicles (16).

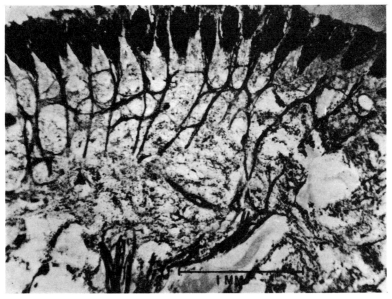

Fig. 7.
Section, perpendicular to the cornea, through part of a lateral eye of an adult *Limulus*. At the top of the figure are shown the heavily pigmented sensory portions of the ommatidia. Bundles of nerve fibers are shown emerging from the ommatidia, with the plexus of interconnecting fibers, and a portion of the optic nerve below. Samuel's silver stain. The chitinous cornea and crystalline cones that appear in Fig. 2 were stripped away prior to fixation. Prepared by W. H. Miller. (From Hartline et al. (14)).

Electrophysiological evidence confirms the synaptic nature of the inhibitory interaction in the *Limulus* retina. Hyperpolarizing potentials are observed by intracellular recording in the eccentric cell of an ommatidium, coincident with inhibition of the receptor (16, 17). Analysis of these and the accompanying conductance changes indicates that these are inhibitory postsynaptic potentials like those met with elsewhere in nervous systems (18, 19).

Before proceeding to a detailed consideration of inhibitory interaction we may ask what roles it might play in vision. One role is enhancement of contrast. Strongly excited receptor elements in brightly lighted regions of the retinal image exert a stronger inhibition on receptors in more dimly lighted regions than the latter exert on the former. Thus the disparity in the actions of the receptors is increased, and contrast enhanced. Since inhibition is stronger between close neighbors than between widely separated ones, steep intensity gradients in the retinal image—edges and contours—will be accentuated by contrast.

"Simultaneous contrast", "border contrast", and the like are well known in visual physiology (20). A century ago Ernst Mach correctly ascribed them to inhibitory interaction in the visual system. Most of us have noted the fluted appearance of uniform steps in intensity, as those in shadows cast by

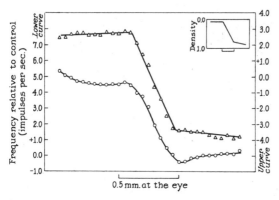

Fig. 8.

Contrast phenomena, analogous to Mach bands, demonstrated by patterns of optic nerve fiber activity in the eye of *Limulus*. The discharge of impulses from a receptor was recorded as the eye was caused to scan slowly a pattern of illumination containing a simple gradient of intensity shown in the inset, upper right. When all the receptors were masked except the one from which activity was being recorded, a faithful representation of the actual physical distribution of light was obtained (upper graph, triangles). With the mask removed, so that all the receptors viewed the pattern, the lower graph (circles) was obtained, with a maximum and a minimum where Mach bands are seen by a human observer viewing the same pattern. (From Ratliff and Hartline (21)).

multiple light sources as, for example, a cluster of candles. The Mach bands flanking a simple gradient are also familiar "illusions" in which contrast is overemphasized by the use of a special pattern of light. Such "distortions" of sensory information ordinarily serve a useful function to accent and "crispen" important features of the visual scene and to sharpen spatial resolution. It is possible to demonstrate analogous distortions of spatial patterns of optic nerve activity in *Limulus,* when its eye views similar patterns of light (Fig. 8). These phenomena are all the result of inhibitory interaction in the visual system.

Inhibitory interaction in the retina is a simple neural mechanism that operates on the sensory data supplied by the receptors, modifying spatial features just as the inherent mechanism of the receptors modifies temporal characteristics. Both of these "data processing" operations are integrative funtions taking place in the earliest phases of the visual process.

Enhancement of contrast is but one consequence of inhibitory interaction. Inhibition plays a pervading and subtle role, in vision as elsewhere in nervous function. To the basic excitation furnished by light, retinal inhibition adds a molding influence, increasing temporal and spatial resolution and supplying a mechanism for increased versatility of response. The opportunity to analyze this process in a retina that is much simpler than those of higher animals should prove helpful in understanding the more complex functions of more complex visual systems.

We begin this analysis (22) with an experiment showing the interaction

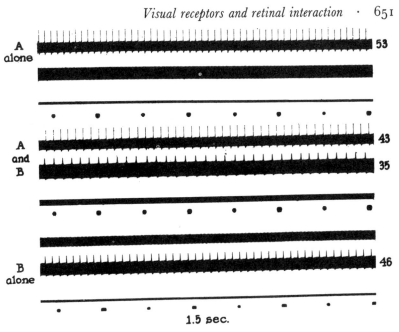

Fig. 9.
Mutual inhibition of receptor units in the eye of *Limulus*. Nerve impulses recorded simultaneously from two optic nerve fibers, showing the discharges when their respective ommatidia were steadily illuminated, separately and together. The numbers on the right give, for the respective cases, the total number of impulses discharged in the period of 1.5 sec. shown. The inhibitory effect on A, 53—43, is to be associated with the concurrent frequency of B, 35; likewise the effect on B, 46—35, is to be associated with the concurrent frequency of A, 43. Time in 1/5 sec. (From Hartline and Ratliff (22)).

of just two ommatidia, Fig. 9. Illuminated together, each of these receptor units discharged impulses at a lower rate than when it was illuminated by itself. For each illuminated alone, its frequency of discharge measures its excitation, e, at the particular intensity being used on it. When both are illuminated together, at the same intensities, we will call their responses r. Analysis shows that the lowering of frequency of each, $e—r$, is to be related quantitatively to the concurrent frequency, r, of the other. It is the output of a receptor unit—its rate of discharge of nerve impulses—that determines how much inhibition it exerts on other units. A receptor that inhibits another receptor affects the very output that in turn inhibits it. Thus the inhibitory interaction is recurrent in its operation, as may be visualized schematically, for just two elements, by Fig. 10. Mathematically, the mutual interaction of two units can be expressed by a pair of simultaneous equations. Measurements of the response of two interacting receptor units, stimulated by various intensities of light in various combinations, permit the construction of two graphs shown in Fig. 11, in which the lowering of frequency of each, $e—r$, is plotted against the concurrent response, r of the other. Evidently the two simultaneous equations that describe the relationship between the re-

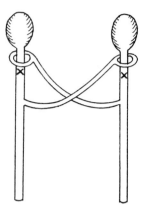

Fig. 10.
Schematic representation of the recurrent nature of mutual inhibition of two receptor units. Excitation of each generates trains of impulses which originate near the point of emergence of the axon from the cell body, marked x. Influences pass back up the recurrent branches of each to exert inhibition on the other at synapses at or near the points of emergence. (From Ratliff et al. (17)).

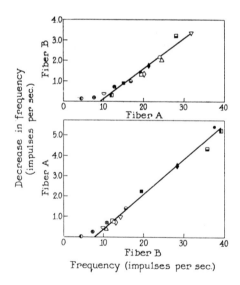

Fig. 11.
Mutual inhibition of two receptor units in the eye of *Limulus*. In each graph, the magnitude of the inhibitory action (decrease in frequency of impulse discharge) exerted on one of the ommatidia is plotted (ordinate) as a function of the concurrent frequency of the other (abscissa), as explained in the legend of Fig. 9. The different pairs of points (identified by the same symbols in the two graphs) were obtained by using various intensities of illumination on the two ommatidia, in various combinations. (From Hartline and Ratliff (22)).

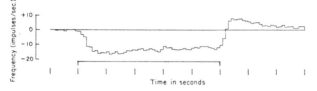

Fig. 12.

Inhibition of a steadily illuminated receptor, elicited artificially by electrical shocks applied to optic nerve fibers from neighboring receptors to generate a train of antidromic volleys of impulses at constant frequency. Frequency of discharge of impulses from the receptor during an experimental run of 9 seconds that included the 5 sec. period of inhibition (signalled by step at bottom) is plotted as ordinate (vs. time as abscissa) after subtracting the frequency of discharge during a "control" run taken over a comparable period, but with no inhibition. The ordinates are given as impulses per second above or below control. Experiment by Lange (32).

sponses of the two interacting receptors are piecewise linear. Considered over the entire range, each relationship is highly non-linear as a result of the fairly abrupt threshold, r^o, below which the steady firing of a receptor exerts no inhibition on its neighbors. Above this threshold, however, a linear relation holds to a fair degree of approximation. The slope of each graph, K, is the inhibitory coefficient measuring the strength of the influence of each element, respectively, on the other.

To describe the interaction of more than two elements, more equations are required. For a group of n interacting receptor units a set of n simultaneous equations, piecewise linear, must be written, and in the equation for each unit inhibitory terms must be introduced and summed to express the inhibition on that particular unit by all of the units that act upon it:

$$r_p = e_p - \sum_{j=1}^{n} K_{p,j}(r_j - r^o_{p,j}) \qquad p = 1,2,...n$$

In this set of equations, r_p is the response of the pth receptor, which if free of inhibition would have discharged impulses at a rate e_p, but which is subjected to the summed inhibitory influences expressed by the linear terms on the right. In each term $K_{p,j}$ is the inhibitory coefficient measuring the action of the jth receptor on the pth; $r^o_{p,j}$ is the associated threshold of that action (23).

In the eye, receptors are deployed spatially, in a mosaic, and the strength of their interaction, as already noted depends on their separation. In general the coefficients K decrease and the thresholds r^o increase with increasing separation of interacting ommatidia in the eye. The spatial distribution of values of the coefficients in the inhibitory field surrounding a small group of receptors has recently been mapped in detail by R. Barlow (24). Such maps will be indispensable in the analysis of the spatial properties of retinal interaction.

The set of simultaneous equations written above provides a succinct and

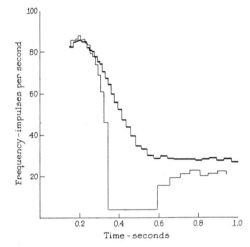

Fig. 13.
"Crispening" of the "on" transient of the discharge of a receptor unit by the inclusion of neighboring receptors in the area illuminated. The upper, heavy curve gives the frequency of discharge of a "test" receptor when it was illuminated alone. The lower curve gives the frequency of discharge of the same receptor when the area of illumination (same intensity as before) was enlarged to include neighboring receptors; the time delay of their inhibitory action on test receptor was long enough that the initial peak of the discharge was unaffected, only the subsequent discharge being reduced to the steady level that reflected the steady state interaction within the entire group. (From Hartline et al., (16)).

useful description of steady state inhibitory interaction in the retina of *Limulus*. Quantitative measurements of the activity of interacting receptors and groups of receptors, in various configurations, are satisfactorily accounted for (17). With measured or postulated inhibitory fields, spatial patterns such as Mach bands are successfully represented (25). Ratliff's recent book treats this subject in detail (20). Von Békésy, using mathematically equivalent formulations to represent inhibitory interaction, has discussed in his recent book (26) the applications to other sensory systems.

Up to this point we have restricted our discussion of inhibitory interaction to the steady state of receptor activity, after all the mutual interactions have come into balance. Whenever, as in the natural world, changes occur in the patterns of light and shade on the retinal mosaic, receptor transients occur, new distributions of excitation are established, and readjustments of the inhibitory interactions are mediated over the retinal network. The interplay of excitation and inhibition is a dynamic process.

Vision itself is a dynamic process. There is little in the world that stands still, at least not as imaged in our retinas, for our eyes are always moving. The visual system is almost exclusively organized to detect change and motion. How can we explain this? How are we to understand, for example, the exquisite sensitivity of some of the frog's retinal fibers to slight movements of the shadow of a fine wire across their receptive fields? Or, what mechan-

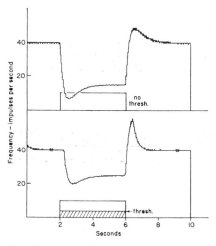

Fig. 14.

Simulations by means of a computer program of the responses of a steadily excited receptor subjected to a period of constant inhibition from neighboring receptors, as in the actual experiment of Fig. 12. The decay constants assigned to the self-inhibitory and lateral-inhibitory influences were respectively 1 sec. and 0.4 sec. For the upper tracing, a threshold of zero was assigned to the lateral inhibition; for the lower tracing, a threshold was introduced that was unrealistically large, considering the strong lateral influence that was assigned. This served to exaggerate, for illustrative purposes, the asymmetries of onset and cessation of inhibition, especially the "post-inhibitory rebound". Cf. (28).

isms can explain the responses that are so highly specific to certain features of the moving pattern, such as curvature of a boundary, size of an object, direction of its motion, etc., as Lettvin and his colleagues, and others, report? (27) Study of visual dynamics in a retina as simple as that of *Limulus* can hardly solve such problems, but it may suggest principles that can be applied toward their solution (28).

If responses are recorded from representative receptors in two interacting groups in a *Limulus* eye, and one group subjected to a small increment in intensity, the other, steadily illuminated, will be disturbed only by the inhibitory influences exerted by the first (29).

Experiments of this kind furnish good examples of dynamic responses that might be encountered in nature. However, they are not suited to quantitative analysis, because the time courses of photoreceptor discharges are difficult to control and those features that are contributed solely by the dynamic properties of the inhibitory interaction are hard to distinguish. Fortunately, lateral inhibition of a receptor unit can be produced artificially by electrical stimulation of the optic nerve fibers from the receptors' neighbors, as Tomita first showed (30). This affords an exact control of temporal factors that is not possible when the neighbors are excited naturally by light.

By this method, sinusoidally modulated inhibition can be exerted on a receptor, and if the influences are above all thresholds, linear systems-analysis

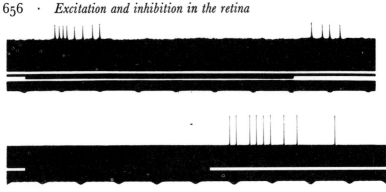

Fig. 15.
Response of a receptor in the eye of *Limulus* imitating the "on—off" and "off" discharges of vertebrate optic nerve fibers. Obtained by the use of special patterns of stimulation under special conditions of adaptation that suppressed the steady discharge but retained the transients at "on" and "off", the latter the consequence of post-inhibitory rebound. Steady illumination of receptor signalled by blackening of white band above 1/5 sec. time marks. (Record by Ratliff and Mueller, cf. (38)).

can be applied (31). Alternatively, abrupt stepwise increments of inhibition can be generated artificially to excite transients of inhibitory systems. Since the latencies and transients of the photic mechanism are thereby avoided, the dynamics of the inhibition itself are revealed (Fig. 12). Inhibition is then seen to set in after an appreciable delay of its own, and often, though not always, with a transient undershoot at the beginning. After the cessation of inhibition, no matter how it is produced, the post-inhibitory rebound we have already noted always occurs; it is a true "off" response (33).

The delayed onset of lateral inhibition has a simple consequence, which appears when a large area of the receptor mosaic is suddenly illuminated (Fig. 13). The first part of the strong "on" transient of each receptor escapes the action of lateral inhibition from its neighbors. After the delay, however, mutual inhibition quickly sets in, sometimes suppressing the discharge for a fraction of a second, before the steady discharge is established, often with minor oscillations, as the receptor adapts and as mutual interactions come into balance (16). This "crispening" of the "on" response is an augmentation of the sensory adaptation that is an inherent property of each individual receptor.

Related to this is the emphasis a short delay in the development of lateral inhibition can give to light fluctuations of a certain frequency occurring over a large retinal area in which there is strong mutual interaction. When the frequency of the fluctuation is such that a minimum of excitation occurs just as the delayed inhibition from the previous maximum comes to its full value, the net fluctuation of the response may actually be amplified, compared to what it would have been had the area been small, with no large numbers of receptors to supply mutual inhibition. The eye of *Limulus* shows such an amplification of response, at about 3 cycles per sec., to a sinusoidally modulated light shining on a large area (34).

Before we can understand fully the dynamics of inhibitory interaction, we must consider a new feature of the inhibitory process in the *Limulus* eye: the inhibition of a receptor unit by its own discharge. This was first analyzed by Stevens (35) and has recently been studied by Purple and Dodge (36). They present evidence that this "self-inhibition" may be a synaptic process like lateral inhibition: following each impulse discharged by an ommatidium, a hyperpolarizing potential appears. Whatever the mechanism underlying it, self-inhibition forms a substantial component of the adaptation process in the *Limulus* receptor, and by tending to oppose any change in the discharge rate of a receptor unit, has a strong influence on the dynamics of receptor action and interaction.

The rise of inhibition, as successive impulses contribute their additive effects, and its decay, resulting presumably from removal or inactivation of inhibitory transmitter, determine the form of the transients exhibited by the interacting system as it adjusts to changing influences. When lateral inhibition is suddenly applied and builds up on a receptor unit, so that its discharge rate drops, its self-inhibition subsides to a new equilibrium, opposing the full effects of the lateral influence. Lateral inhibition has an inherently shorter time constant than self-inhibition, hence the transient in the discharge of a receptor usually is an undershoot when lateral inhibition increases, and a post-inhibitory rebound when it decreases. Non-linearities introduced by the thresholds of lateral inhibition increase the delay in the onset of the inhibition, diminish the undershoot and augment the rebound. Fig. 14 illustrates the two cases, linear and non-linear, by means of a computer simulation, like one devised by Lange (37).

For all of the modifications introduced by inhibitory interaction, patterns of optic nerve activity in *Limulus* remain not too grossly distorted representations of the patterns of light and shade on the receptor mosaic. Although significant integration of sensory data is prominent, the effects are mild, compared to what takes place in more complex retinas. Even in *Limulus,* however, the potentiality for more extreme modifications of optic patterns can be demonstrated. Ratliff and Conrad Mueller (38), by careful adjustments of patterns of light, were able to elicit, from a perfectly normal receptor in *Limulus,* "on-off" and pure "off" responses, shown in Fig. 15. Here, by a contrived interplay of excitation (by light on the receptor) and inhibition (by light on its neighbors), taking advantage of time delays and post-inhibitory rebounds, response patterns simulating some of those observed in the vertebrate retina were "synthesized". What Ratliff and Mueller contrived more or less artificially resembles the dynamic interplay we believe takes place naturally as a result of the complex neural organization in more highly developed retinas and higher visual centers.

The unitary analysis of visual function has yielded substantial knowledge about receptor properties, and about dynamic integrative mechanisms in the retina. In the eye of *Limulus,* the relative simplicity of retinal interaction facilitates its analysis. In more highly organized retinas, a vastly richer integration takes place. Many workers, in many laboratories, are engaged in the study of the diverse and highly specialized responses generated by visual neurons as neural information is processed for transmission to still higher centers. I am confident that the familiar neurophysiological concepts that were needed in the analysis of the simple interaction in the *Limulus* retina will prove useful in elucidating these very complex and very interesting features of visual physiology.

REFERENCES

(1) Adrian, E. D. and D. W. Bronk, *J. Physiol., 66,* 81 (1928); Adrian, E. D. and Y. Zotterman, *J. Physiol., 61,* 151 (1926).

(2) Adrian, E. D. and R. Matthews, *J. Physiol., 63,* 378 (1927); *64,* 279 (1927); *65,* 273 (1928).

(3) Hartline, H. K. and C. H. Graham, *J. Cell. Comp. Physiol., 1,* 277 (1932).

(4) Shuster, C. N.: Xiphosura, in *Encyclopedia of Science and Technology,* McGraw-Hill Book Co., Inc., New York, *14,* 563 (1960); Milne, L. and M. Milne, *The Crab That Crawled Out of the Past,* Atheneum, New York (1965) (popular).

(5) Miller, W. H.: Morphology of the ommatidium of the compound eye of *Limulus, J. Biophys. Biochem. Cyt., 3,* 421 (1957).

(6) Hartline, H. K., *J. Cell. Comp. Physiol., 5,* 229 (1934); Graham, C. H. and H. K. Hartline, *J. Gen. Physiol., 18,* 917 (1935); Hartline, H. K. and P. R. McDonald, *J. Cell. Comp. Physiol., 30,* 225 (1947); Hartline, H. K., Milne, L. J. and I. H. Wagman, *Fed. Proc., 6,* 124 (1947) (Abstr.); see also: Pirenne, M. H.: *Vision and the Eye,* Science Paperback, Associated Book Publishers, Ltd., London, chapter 9. 1967. For short review of earlier papers see (11).

(7) Hartline, H. K., Wagner, H. G. and E. F. MacNichol, Jr., *Cold Spring Harbor Symposia on Quantitative Biology, 17,* 125 (1952).

(8) Granit, R.: *Sensory Mechanisms of the Retina,* Oxford University Press, London (1947); —, *Receptors and sensory perception, Silliman Lectures,* Yale University Press, New Haven, *XII* (1955).

(9) Some of the important recent papers on the generator potential in *Limulus* are: MacNichol, Jr., E. F. in *Molecular Structure and Functional Activity of Nerve Cells,* Publication No. 1 of American Institute of Biological Sciences, 34 (1956); Fuortes, M. G. F., *J. Physiol., 148,* 14 (1959); Rushton, W. A. H., *J. Physiol., 148,* 29 (1959); Purple (18); Fuortes, M. G. F. and A. L. Hodgkin, *J. Physiol. 172,* 239 (1964); Dodge, F. A., Jr., Knight, B. W. and J. Toyoda, *Science* (1968) (in press). Broader coverage of receptor potentials in sense organs may be found in *Cold Spring Harbor Symposia on Quantitative Biology, 30* (1965).

(10) Hartline, H. K., *Am. J. Physiol., 121,* 400 (1938); *130,* 690 (1940); *130,* 700 (1940).

(11) Hartline, H. K.: The neural mechanisms of vision, *The Harvey Lectures,* Series *XXXVII,* 39 (1941—1942).

(12) Examples from this extensive and rapidly growing field: Kuffler, S. W., *J. Neurophysiol., 16,* 37 (1953); Barlow, H. B., *J. Physiol., 119,* 69 (1953); Wagner, H. G., MacNichol, Jr., E. F. and M. L. Wolbarsht, *J. Gen. Physiol., 43,* 45 (1960); Baumgartner, G., *Neurophysiologie und Psychophysik des visuellen Systems,* R. Jung and H. Kornhuber, editors, Springer Verlag, Berlin, 45 (1961); Horridge, G. A., Scholes, J. H., Shaw, S. and J. P. Tunstall, in *The Physiology of the Insect Nervous System,* Treherne, J. E. and J. W. L. Beament, editors, Academic Press (1965); Wiersma, C. A. G. and Y. Yamaguchi, *J. Comp. Neurology, 128,* 333 (1966). See also: (27); see Granit (8) for review of his contributions, and references.

(13) Hartline, H. K., *Fed. Proc., 8,* No. 1, 69 (1949) (Abstr.).

(14) Hartline, H. K., Wagner, H. G. and F. Ratliff, *J. Gen. Physiol., 39,* 651 (1956).

(15) Reviews of this work, in detail, may be found in: Hartline et al. (16) and Ratliff (20).

(16) Hartline, H. K., Ratliff, F. and W. H. Miller, in *Nervous Inhibition,* E. Florey editor, Pergamon Press, New York, 241 (1961).

(17) Ratliff, F., Hartline, H. K. and W. H. Miller, *J. Opt. Soc. Amer., 53,* 110 (1963).

(18) Purple, R. L., *Thesis,* The Rockefeller Institute (1964).

(19) Purple, R. L. and F. A. Dodge, *Cold Spring Harbor Symposia on Quantitative Biology, 30,* 529 (1965).

(20) Ratliff, F.: *Mach Bands: Quantitative Studies on Neural Networks in the Retina,* Holden-Day, Inc., San Francisco, (1965).

(21) Ratliff, F. and H. K. Hartline, *J. Gen. Physiol., 42,* 1241 (1959).

(22) Hartline, H. K. and F. Ratliff, *J. Gen. Physiol., 40,* 357 (1957).

(23) Hartline, H. K. and F. Ratliff, *J. Gen. Physiol., 41,* 1049 (1958). See also: Hartline et al. (16) for restrictions on the equations.

(24) Barlow, R. B., *Thesis,* The Rockefeller University (1967).

(25) Reichardt, W. and G. MacGinitie, *Kybernetik, 1,* 155 (1962); Kirschfeld, K. and W. Reichardt, *Kybernetik, 2,* 43 (1964).

(26) Békésy, G. von: *Sensory Inhibition,* Princeton University Press, Princeton, N. J. (1967).

(27) Lettvin, J. Y., Maturana, H. R., McCulloch, W. S. and W. H. Pitts, *Proc. Inst. Radio Eng., 47,* 1940 (1959); Maturana, H. R., Lettvin, J. Y., McCulloch, W. S. and W. H. Pitts, Anatomy and physiology of vision in the frog *(Rana pipiens), J. Gen. Physiol., 43,* 129 (1960); Grüsser-Cornehls, U., Grüsser, O.-J. and T. H. Bullock, *Science, 141,* 820 (1963); Barlow, H. B., Hill, R. M. and W. R. Levick, *J. Physiol., 173,* 377 (1964); Barlow, H. B. and W. R. Levick, *J. Physiol., 178,* 477 (1965). For discussion of these and related papers see Ratliff (20), chapter 4.

(28) Recent papers on the dynamics of the inhibitory interaction in *Limulus* are: Ratliff, F., Hartline, H. K. and David Lange, in *The Functional Organization of the Compound Eye,* C. G. Bernhard, editor, Pergamon Press, Oxford, 399 (1966); Lange, David, Hartline, H. K. and F. Ratliff, *ibid.,* 425 (1966); Hartline et al. (16); Ratliff, et al. (17) and references in (37).

(29) Ratliff, F., in *Sensory Communication,* W. A. Rosenblith, editor, M. I. T. Press and John Wiley & Sons, New York, 183 (1961).

(30) Tomita, T.: Mechanism of lateral inhibition in the eye of *Limulus, J. Neurophysiol., 21,* 419 (1958).

(31) Dodge, F. A., Jr., Knight, B. W. and J. Toyoda, (in preparation).

(32) Lange, David, *Thesis,* The Rockefeller University (1965).

(33) See discussion by Granit (8) for relation of "off" responses to post-inhibitory rebound.

(34) Ratliff, F., Knight, B. W., Toyoda, J. and H. K. Hartline, *Science, 158,* 392 (1967).

(35) Stevens, C. F., *Thesis,* The Rockefeller Institute (1964).

(36) Purple, R. L. and F. A. Dodge, Jr., in *The Functional Organization of the Compound Eye,* C. G. Bernhard, editor, Pergamon Press, Oxford, 451—464 (1966).

(37) Lange (32); Lange, David, Hartline, H. K. and F. Ratliff, *Ann. N. Y. Ac. Sci., 128,* 955 (1966).

(38) Ratliff, F. and C. G. Mueller, *Science, 126,* 840 (1957).

Subject Index

Name Index